Acta Neurochirurgica Supplement 120

Series Editor
H.-J. Steiger

For further volumes:
http://www.springer.com/series/4

Javier Fandino • Serge Marbacher
Ali-Reza Fathi • Carl Muroi • Emanuela Keller
Editors

Neurovascular Events After Subarachnoid Hemorrhage

Towards Experimental and Clinical Standardisation

Springer

Editors
Javier Fandino
Department of Neurosurgery
Kantonsspital Aarau
Aarau
Switzerland

Serge Marbacher
Department of Neurosurgery
Kantonsspital Aarau
Aarau
Switzerland

Ali-Reza Fathi
Department of Neurosurgery
Kantonsspital Aarau
Aarau
Switzerland

Carl Muroi
Department of Neurosurgery
Kantonsspital Aarau
Aarau
Switzerland

Emanuela Keller
Department of Neurosurgery
Neurointensive Care Unit
University Hospital Zurich
Zurich
Switzerland

ISBN 978-3-319-04980-9 ISBN 978-3-319-04981-6 (eBook)
DOI 10.1007/978-3-319-04981-6
Springer Cham Heidelberg New York Dordrecht London

Library of Congress Control Number: 2014951213

Printed on acid-free paper

Springer is part of Springer Science+Business Media (www.springer.com)

Preface

Forty-two years after the first International Conference on Cerebral Vasospasm (ICCV) was held in Jackson, Mississippi, USA, a new horizon of translational research and interdisciplinary interests motivated our community to change the name of this traditional meeting. It was in fact during the last ICCV in Cincinnati, OH, USA, in 2011, that a new name arose to embrace all disciplines and events related to subarachnoid hemorrhage. After celebrating venues on all five continents, we had the privilege to hold the newly baptized *12th Conference on Neurovascular Events After Subarachnoid Hemorrhage* (former ICCV) in Lucerne, Switzerland. During a magical week, from July 10 to 12, 2013, surrounded by the beautiful Lake of Lucerne and the Swiss Alps, more than 300 participants had the opportunity to meet and exchange experiences and visions, which will led us *Toward Experimental and Clinical Standardization* in this field. This book contains the proceedings of the Conference. We were motivated by the superb quality of 102 submitted abstracts, most of them included in this book. The collection of papers were divided into topical chapters: Aneurysm Formation, Early Brain Injury and Neuroprotection, Macro- and Microcirculatory Disturbances, Pathophysiology of DIND, Imaging and Endovascular Management, Techniques and Surgical Innovations, Neurocritical Care, and Clinical Trials. For the first time the Conference included a session on Animals Models which allowed the participants to have an overview of all experimental techniques routinely used worldwide. This summary will contribute to the standardization of laboratory techniques and will enable the application of data into clinical trials in a more reliable fashion. We want to acknowledge the authors of the chapters of this book and would like to express our deepest gratitude to all of those who made the meeting in Lucerne possible, especially Mrs. Anna Scrowther and Mrs. Antonella Ricci. Finally, we are indebted to our institution, the Kantonsspital Aarau, and its CEO, Mr. Hans Leuenberger, for the support and encouragement throughout the organization of the conference. This book will contribute to a better understanding of cerebrovascular events related to subarachnoid hemorrhage.

Aarau, Switzerland — Javier Fandino

Acknowledgment

This volume has been made possible thanks to a generous educational grant from the Kantonsspital Aarau Education and Research Fund.

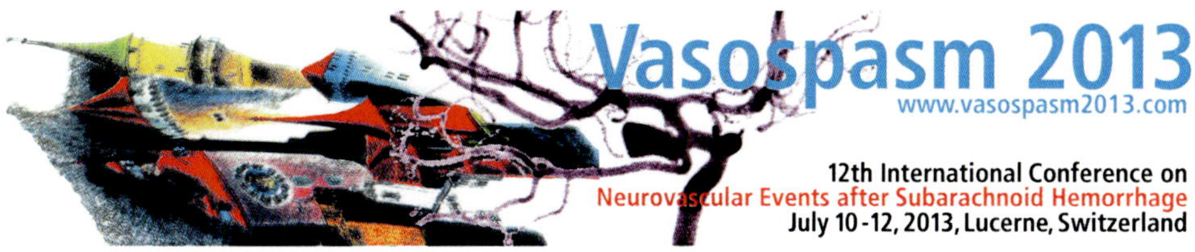

Contents

Vasospasm: My First 25 Years—What Worked? What Didn't? What Next?

R. Loch Macdonald

Abstract Angiographic vasospasm as a complication of aneurysmal and other types of subarachnoid hemorrhage (SAH) was identified about 62 years ago. It is now hypothesized that angiographic vasospasm contributes to delayed cerebral ischemia (DCI) by multiple pathways, including reduced blood flow from angiographic vasospasm as well as microcirculatory constriction, microthrombosis, cortical spreading ischemia, and delayed effects of early brain injury. It is likely that other factors, such as systemic complications, effects of the subarachnoid blood, brain collateral and anastomotic blood flow, and the genetic and epigenetic makeup of the patient, contribute to the individual's response to SAH. Treatment of aneurysmal SAH and DCI includes neurocritical care management, early aneurysm repair, prophylactic administration of nimodipine, and rescue therapies (induced hypertension and balloon or pharmacologic angioplasty) if the patient develops DCI. Well-designed clinical trials of tirilazad, clasozentan, antiplatelet drugs, and magnesium have been conducted using more than a 1,000 patients each. Some of these drugs have almost purely vascular effects; other drugs are theoretically neuroprotective as well, but they share in common the ability to reduce angiographic vasospasm and, in many cases, DCI, but have no effect on clinical outcome. Experimental research in SAH continues to identify new targets for therapy. Challenges for the future will be to identify the most promising drugs to advance from preclinical studies and to understand why clinical trials have so frequently failed to show drug benefit on clinical outcome. Similar issues with treatment of ischemic stroke are being addressed by suggestions for improving the quality of experimental studies, collaborative preclinical trials, and multinational, multicenter clinical studies that can rapidly include many patients and be large enough to account for numerous factors that conspire to disrupt clinical trials.

Keywords Subarachnoid hemorrhage • Vasospasm • Brain injury

R.L. Macdonald, MD, PhD
Division of Neurosurgery, St. Michael's Hospital, 30 Bond St., Toronto, ON M5B 1W8, Canada

Labatt Family Center of Excellence in Brain Injury and Trauma Research, Keenan Research Center of the Li Ka Shing Knowledge Institute of St. Michael's Hospital, Toronto, ON, Canada

Department of Surgery, Institute of Medical Science, University of Toronto, Toronto, ON, Canada
e-mail: macdonaldlo@smh.ca

History

There have been at least 12 meetings focused on angiographic vasospasm and now on additional causes of neurological injury after subarachnoid hemorrhage (SAH) (Table 1). The first meeting was arranged by Robert R. Smith and James T. Robertson in Jackson, MS, in 1972. Echlin [18] wrote there was an earlier meeting in Bari, Italy, in 1970, chaired by Umberto Izzo, medical director of the Ospedali di Acquaviva, and Vincente Lombardi, also from the Ospedali di Acquaviva. The focus of these meetings has expanded as knowledge about the pathophysiology of brain injury after SAH has been gained. The honored guests and many participants at these meetings were or are leaders who have generated the knowledge that has led to improvement in outcomes of patients with SAH. I thank the organizing committee for recognizing me as an honored guest. I do not feel that I necessarily deserve it yet; I believe this honor would fit someone who made a definitive advance in terms of pharmacologic or other treatment for SAH, but few have met this high bar.

J. Fandino et al. (eds.), *Neurovascular Events After Subarachnoid Hemorrhage*, Acta Neurochirurgica Supplement, Vol. 120,
DOI 10.1007/978-3-319-04981-6_1, © Springer International Publishing Switzerland 2015

Table 1 Meetings on angiographic vasospasm, delayed cerebral ischemia, and early brain injury

Meeting title	Location, organizer(s)	Honored guest(s)	Topics	Resulting book
Subarachnoid Hemorrhage and Cerebrovascular Spasm. The First International Workshop	Jackson, Mississippi, USA, 1972, Robert R. Smith, 18 attendees	Dedicated to Francis A. Echlin	Mainly focused on acute effects of blood, prostaglandins on large cerebral arteries	Smith, R.R., Robertson, J.T., eds. Subarachnoid Hemorrhage and Cerebrovascular Spasm. The First 'International' Workshop. Springfield: Charles C. Thomas Publisher, 1975.
2nd International Workshop on Cerebral Arterial Spasm	Amsterdam, The Netherlands, 1979, A.J.M. van der Werf, 200 participants	C. Miller Fisher	More understanding of vascular contraction, animal models focused on in vitro and large animal in vivo, time course of angiographic vasospasm and effect on cerebral blood flow recognized, dependence on subarachnoid clot and its removal suggested; treatments suggested were antiplatelet agents, nitroprusside, hydrocortisone, induced hypertension	Wilkins, R.H., ed. Cerebral Arterial Spasm. Proceedings of the Second International Workshop. Amsterdam, Netherlands, Baltimore: Williams & Wilkins, 1980.
3rd International Symposium on Cerebral Vasospasm	Charlottesville, Virginia, USA, 1987, Neal Kassell, 197 contributors	Keiji Sano (Honored guest), Charles G. Drake, (Honorary president)	Transcranial Doppler, role of the endothelium, brain microvessels examined, free radicals, prostaglandins, platelets; treatments included clot removal (fibrinolysis), intracisternal irrigation, papaverine and nimodipine, as well as systemic nimodipine, nicardipine, balloon angioplasty	Wilkins, R.H., ed. Cerebral Vasospasm. Proceedings of the III International Symposium in Charlottesville. New York, Raven Press, 1988.
4th International Conference on Cerebral Vasospasm	Tokyo, Japan, 1990, Keiji Sano, K. Takakura, Tomio Sasaki	Bryce K.A. Weir	Transcranial Doppler, smooth muscle contraction and biology, hemoglobin, perivascular nerves, inflammation, endothelium and endothelin; treatments included cisternal irrigation and fibrinolysis, hemodynamic therapy, steroids, immunosuppression, balloon angioplasty, nimodipine, nicardipine, fasudil	Sano, K., Takakura, K., Kassell, N.F., Sasaki, T., eds. Cerebral Vasospasm. Proceedings of the International Conference on Cerebral Vasospasm, Tokyo, 1990: University of Tokyo Press.
5th International Conference on Cerebral Vasospasm	Edmonton and Jasper, Alberta, Canada, 1993, Bryce Weir	Neal Kassell	Cerebral hemodynamics, other causes of delayed ischemia, smooth muscle contraction and biology, hemoglobin, free radicals, nitric oxide, endothelins, structural changes; treatments similar to last meeting, but in addition tirilazad, FUT-175	Findlay, J.M., ed. Cerebral Vasospasm. Proceedings of the V International Conference on Cerebral Vasospasm, Edmonton, Amsterdam: Elsevier Publishing Company, 1993
6th International Conference on Cerebral Vasospasm	Sydney, Australia, 1997, Nicholas Dorsch	Robert R. Smith	Experimental pathophysiology and treatments, mostly the same targets as above, in addition iron chelators, biomarker studies; new treatments included ebselen and flunarazine	Dorsch NWC (ed): Cerebral Vasospasm VI. Proceedings of the VIth International Conference on Cerebral Vasospasm. Oslington, Leichhardt, Australia, 1999
7th International Conference on Cerebral Vasospasm	Interlaken, Switzerland, 2000, Rolf Seiler, 75 participants	Helge Nornes	Vascular biology, nitric oxide, endothelins, gene therapy, magnetic resonance imaging, microdialysis; treatments included cisternal drugs, intraarterial pharmacologic or balloon angioplasty, nicardipine pellets	R.W. Seiler, H.-J. Steiger (eds): Cerebral vasospasm. Acta Neurochirurgica, Supplement 77, Springer, Wien New York, 2001

8th International Conference on Cerebral Vasospasm	Chicago, Illinois, USA, 2003, R. Loch Macdonald, 90 participants	Shigeharu Suzuki, Tomio Ohta	Vascular biology, inflammation, computed tomographic perfusion, biomarkers; treatments included magnesium, phosphodiesterase inhibitors, lumbar drainage, cisternal drugs	Macdonald RL (ed): Cerebral Vasospasm. Advances in Research and Treatment. New York, Thieme Medical Publishers, 2005
9th International Conference on Cerebral Vasospasm	Istanbul, Turkey, 2006, Talat Kiris, 75–100 participants	None	Much discussion of vascular biology, electrophysiology, noninvasive monitoring; treatments included clazosentan, magnesium, fasudil, statins, cilostazol	Kiris T, Zhang JH (eds): Cerebral Vasospasm. New Strategies in Research and Treatment. Springer-Verlag, Wien, Acta Neurochir Suppl, 2008
10th International Conference on Cerebral Vasospasm	Chongqing, China, 2009, Hua Feng, 90 participants	Nicholas Dorsch (Honored guest), Ryszard Pluta (distinguished keynote speaker)	Early brain injury, apoptosis, microvascular changes, cortical spreading depolarization, systemic effects of subarachnoid hemorrhage; treatments included statins, phosphodiesterase inhibitors, osteopontin, minocycline, many others discussed above	Feng H, Mao Y, Zhang JH (eds): Early Brain Injury or Cerebral Vasospasm. Volume 1: Pathophysiology. Acta Neurochir Suppl 110/1, Springer, New York, 2011 Feng H, Mao Y, Zhang JH (eds): Early Brain Injury or Cerebral Vasospasm. Volume 2: Clinical Management. Acta Neurochir Suppl 110/2, Springer, New York, 2011
11th International Conference on Neurovascular Events after Subarachnoid Hemorrhage	Cincinatti, Ohio, USA, 2011, Mario Zuccarello, Joseph F. Clark	Frank H. Mayfield	Clinical trials discussed (clazosentan, nicardipine pellets, magnesium, sodium nitrite), neuromonitoring, neurocritical care, spreading depolarizations, early brain injury, microcirculation	Zuccarello M, Clark JF, Pyne-Geithman G, Andaluz N, Hartings JA, Adeoye OM (eds): Cerebral Vasospasm: Neurovascular Events After Subarachnoid Hemorrhage. Acta Neurochir Suppl 115, Springer, New York, 2013
12th International Conference on Neurovascular Events after Subarachnoid Hemorrhage	Lucerne, Switzerland, 2013, Javier Fandino, 300 participants	R. Loch Macdonald	Early brain injury, neuroprotection, macrocirculation and microcirculation, inflammation, spreading depolarization, animal models, nitric oxide, neurocritical care; new treatments (nimodipine microparticles, albumin)	Fandino J, Marbacher S, Fathi AR, Muroi C, Keller E (eds): Neurovascular Events After Subarachnoid Hemorrhage - Towards Experimental and Clinical Standardisation. Acta Neurochir Suppl. Springer, Wien, 2014

What Worked: Etiology and Pathogenesis

The response to SAH includes an acute increase in intracranial pressure to varying degrees, as well as deposition of blood into the subarachnoid space or other brain compartments [38] (Fig. 1). Figure 1 summarizes some of the current pathways and processes leading to poor outcomes after SAH; these are discussed below and were demonstrated statistically in one study [57]. There can be transient global (and possibly focal) cerebral ischemia, and the pathogenesis of early brain injury probably includes some combination of effects of ischemia and the subarachnoid blood [46]. Animal models demonstrate that the etiology of angiographic vasospasm is a subarachnoid blood clot, and that removal of the clot, even in humans, lessens angiographic vasospasm [33]. The effect of clot removal on early brain injury has not been studied; the relative contributions of ischemia and subarachnoid blood to early brain injury are unknown.

Angiographic vasospasm correlates strongly with delayed cerebral infarction, although the correlation is imperfect, and it is theorized that multiple other processes contribute to whether a patient develops delayed cerebral ischemia (DCI) after SAH [6, 7]. Cortical spreading ischemia is one such process and has been documented in animal models and humans with SAH [16]. Associative evidence that it contributes to DCI is that nimodipine, an effective treatment to improve outcome after SAH, reduced cortical spreading ischemia in animals [17]. Microthrombi also have been demonstrated in the brain after experimental and clinical SAH [48]. It is a reasonable hypothesis that they contribute to brain injury, and nimodipine also could abrogate this process through its fibrinolytic activity [59]. On the other hand, clinical trials of antiplatelet drugs, which should reduce microthrombosis, have not documented marked improvements in outcome [15].

The relationship between microthrombi and microcirculatory constriction after SAH is not fully worked out yet.

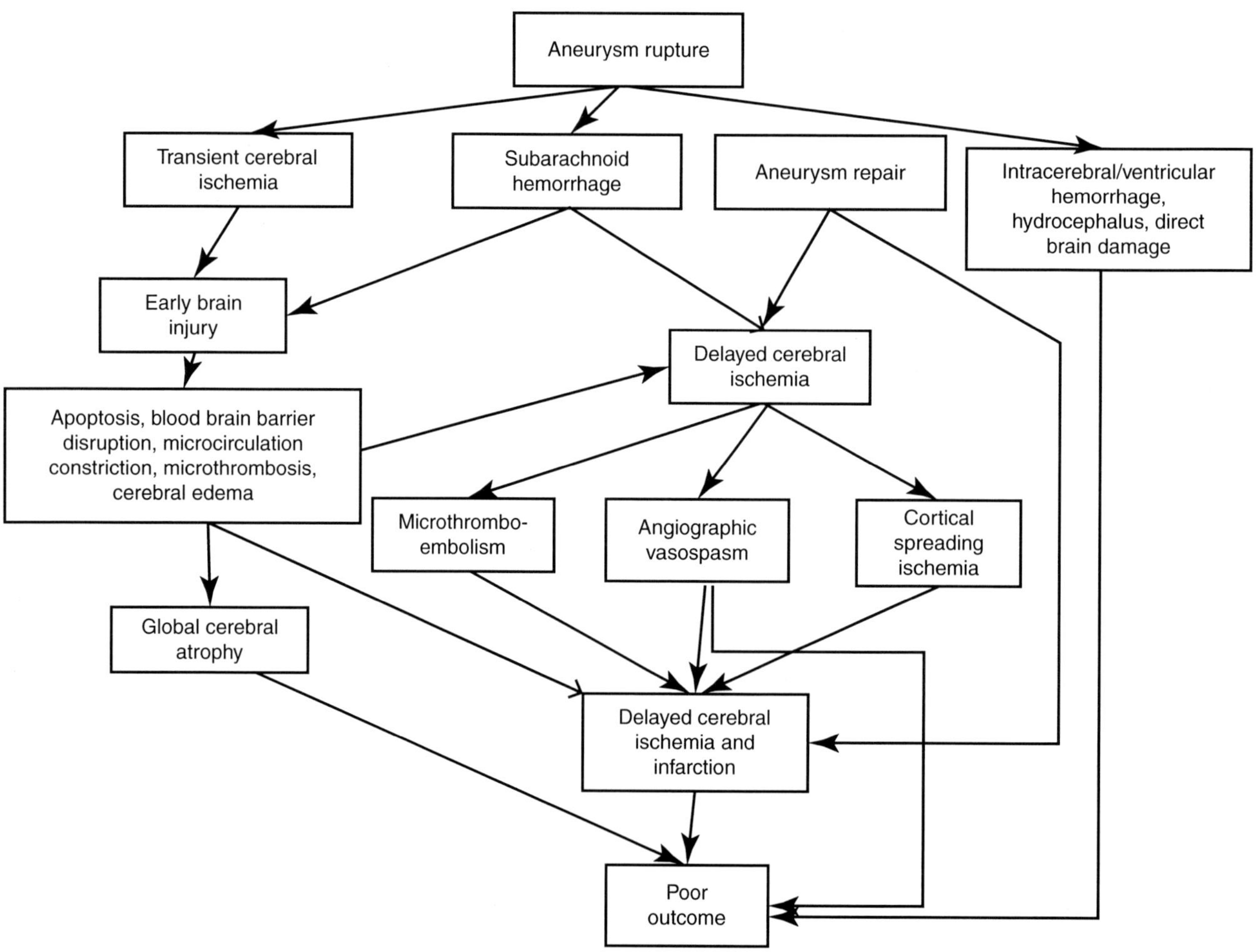

Fig. 1 Some aspects of the pathophysiology of SAH

Studies in animals show that subarachnoid blood alone causes pial arteriolar constriction, thrombosis, and blood brain barrier disruption [12]. These effects occur acutely, but also have been documented days after experimental SAH as well as acutely in penetrating blood vessels [22]. The extent to which these events occur in humans is not well studied [54].

Some evidence links early brain injury with DCI. Worse admission neurological grade, which means worse early brain injury, increases the risk of DCI [40]. Loss of consciousness at the time of SAH, which also should reflect an acute brain injury, also may increase the risk of DCI [9].

The pathogenesis of early brain injury after experimental SAH includes neuronal and endothelial cell apoptosis [23]. Humans dying 0–33 days after SAH exhibited neuronal apoptosis in the dentate gyrus [43]. About half of patients with SAH and no focal cerebral lesions were found to have cerebral atrophy on computed tomography (CT) scans weeks after SAH [50]. It is of note that many of these patients had good clinical grades and did not develop DCI, leading to the hypothesis that early brain injury diffusely injures the brain. To the extent that initial clinical grade reflects early brain injury, population-based studies suggest that the initial effect of the SAH contributes significantly to poor outcome [3].

The impact of the aneurysm repair procedure on clinical outcome has been investigated decades ago, although a lot has changed since then, prompting renewed interest [21, 53]. In one randomized clinical trial, 43 % of patients undergoing neurosurgical clipping of ruptured aneurysms experienced neurological deterioration immediately after surgery [41]. Deterioration was associated with poor outcome. The contribution of DCI to poor outcome is underestimated if only mortality is considered, because most patients can be saved with aggressive interventions including decompressive craniectomy. This comes with a high cost, both financial and in terms of morbidity. Rescue therapy costs approximately US $40,000 and DCI at least doubles the risk of poor outcome [4, 13].

What Worked: Diagnosis

Understanding the time course of angiographic vasospasm and DCI was fundamentally important [62]. It led to the differentiation of DCI from perioperative complications, and to the concept, which is now widely applied, that the aneurysm could be repaired early after rupture without more risk than if performed days later. I described previously the history of the discovery of the other fundamental finding that subarachnoid clot on CT scan is the best predictor of angiographic vasospasm and DCI [37]. Studies showing no relationship fail to account for clot clearance over time, lack of correlation between transcranial Doppler ultrasound and angiographic vasospasm, and numerous other factors.

Consensus has been obtained on definitions for angiographic vasospasm, DCI, and delayed cerebral infarction (Table 2) [60]. The authors wrote that angiographic vasospasm might be an appropriate surrogate outcome measure for proof-of-principle studies. Phase 2 and 3 clinical trials were recommended to use delayed cerebral infarction and a clinical outcome measure. There are limitations to this approach, however (vide infra). The definition and diagnosis of DCI was believed to be subjective and to probably have high interobserver variability.

A group of specialists who manage patients with SAH was convened in 2010 [10]. The GRADE system was used to assess evidence for different diagnostic tools for DCI [26]. While catheter angiography remains the gold standard for diagnosis of angiographic vasospasm, its limitations are that it does not assess brain perfusion or metabolism very well or at all, and it is invasive and complicated and time consuming to obtain. The current trend is to use CT angiography and perfusion to diagnose angiographic vasospasm and DCI [61]. Complications from contrast administration are uncommon but reported. Risk of developing cancer from radiation also has to be considered. Smith-Bindman and colleagues estimated that for every 8,100 CT scans in women of median age 40 years, one radiation-induced cancer would develop [47].

Table 2 Results of an international consensus on definitions of angiographic vasospasm and DCI [60]

Term	Definition	Comments
Angiographic vasospasm	Describes a radiologic test showing artery narrowing	This is the recommended term for artery narrowing on computed tomographic, magnetic resonance, or catheter angiography
Delayed cerebral ischemia	Focal neurologic deficit or decrease of at least 2 points in Glasgow coma scale, lasting longer than 1 h, with no identifiable cause, such as the aneurysm repair procedure, rebleeding, infections, seizures, hyponatremia, or hydrocephalus	The threshold for diagnosis and the duration of deficit are empirically derived and not based on scientific evidence. Detection in comatose or sedated patients can be difficult
Delayed cerebral infarction	Cerebral infarction on computed tomography scan, magnetic resonance imaging, or autopsy, present after the time of DCI within 6 weeks of SAH and not 24–48 h after aneurysm repair procedure	Does not include encephalomalacia from intracerebral hemorrhage or ventricular drains. Presumably includes only lesions consistent with arterial territories

For men, the corresponding number was 11,080 CT scans. Transcranial Doppler ultrasound is still used, although its limitations are recognized.

What Worked: Treatment

Guidelines for management of SAH from the American Heart Association list nimodipine (class 1, level of evidence A), maintenance of euvolemia (class 1, level of evidence B), endovascular coiling (class 1, level of evidence B), and, if the patient develops DCI, then induction of hypertension (class 1, level of evidence B) as recommended at the highest class of evidence [5]. Nimodipine and endovascular aneurysm repair appear to have contributed to improved outcome after SAH; indeed, mortality has declined 0.9 % per year from about 50 to 35 % over the past two decades [36]. But, have other changes in management contributed? The American Heart Association Guidelines also recommend not using prophylactic hemodynamic manipulations; administering fludrocortisone acetate and hypertonic saline to treat hyponatremia; controlling the blood pressure before aneurysm repair; neurologic, transcranial Doppler, and hemodynamic monitoring; treatment of hydrocephalus; prophylactic anticonvulsants; rescue therapy with balloon or pharmacologic angioplasty; and avoidance of hypoglycemia, fever, hypovolemia and hypervolemia at class 2–3, level of evidence B [5]. European guidelines are similar but they do not address all of the same factors [49]. The main difference in the European guidelines is induced hypertension for treatment of DCI was considered to have no evidence for its use [49]. A potentially important factor that is not mentioned in the American Heart Association guidelines is timing of ruptured aneurysm repair, perhaps because it is considered standard of care to repair the aneurysm immediately [5]. European guidelines suggest repair as soon as possible, independent of grading [49]. The evidence is not based on large randomized trials. Despite this, early aneurysm repair has been associated with reduction in mortality caused by rebleeding, resulting in other factors, such as the effects of the SAH and medical complications, contributing increasingly to mortality [32]. Combining the better medical management of patients with SAH and procedures that can reduce mortality, such as decompressive craniectomy, led to a shift to a greater portion of mortality being caused by the SAH itself and by medical complications. As noted above, however, morbidity from DCI remains high.

Of the treatments for SAH that have been subjected to metaanalysis, two, fasudil and intrathecal fibrinolysis, are not widely used despite evidence to suggest they improve outcome [33, 35].

Some Noteable Failures

Treatments for DCI that have undergone metaanalysis include corticosteroids, antiplatelet drugs, calcium channel antagonists, hemodynamic therapy, statins, tirilazad, intrathecal fibrinolytics, fasudil, endothelin receptor antagonists, and magnesium [8, 14, 15, 20, 24, 25, 28, 33, 35, 56]. Antiplatelet drugs, tirilazad, endothelin receptor antagonists, and magnesium have been studied in randomized trials totaling at least 1,385; 3,821; 2,024; and 2,401 patients, respectively [38]. There are limitations to the metaanalyses including the quality of the data in some studies and combining different drugs and doses together. It is notable, however, that tirilazad, endothelin receptor antagonists (principally clazosentan), and magnesium reduced DCI, but had no effect on clinical outcome. Why the drugs did not improve outcome has been discussed (Table 3) [38]. Statins and corticosteroids have probably not been adequately studied, but sample sizes seem adequate for tirilazad, clazosentan, and magnesium. The modified Rankin scale may or may not be very sensitive, but it did detect a difference in outcome between clipping and coiling in the International Subarachnoid Aneurysm Trial [42]. The issue of rescue therapy warrants discussion.

Table 3 Some possible reasons for failure of drugs to improve outcome in clinical trials of SAH

1. The drug is truly ineffective
2. The dose, timing, and duration of administration, route of administration, etc. were wrong
3. The sample size was too small
4. The outcome measure was insensitive or did not detect a clinically meaningful improvement in outcome
5. The drug benefit was offset by drug adverse effects
6. Rescue therapy was as effective in the placebo group as the drug was in the treatment group, leading to no overall difference in outcome
7. Practice misalignment led to application of the drug to patients who could not benefit from the drug or who were at increased risk of adverse effects
8. The wrong patient subgroup was studied
9. The drug was not manufactured properly, randomization codes were wrong, etc.

If rescue therapy is effective, then unless the drug treatment being tested is very effective, increased use of rescue therapy in the placebo groups will reduce the difference in clinical outcome between the groups. On one hand, it seems impossible to withhold rescue therapy but, on the other hand, European guidelines do not strongly support use of induced hypertension, and there is even an ongoing randomized trial comparing induced hypertension to no induced hypertension (NCT01613235, www.clinicaltrials.gov).

What Next?

There are many examples of great successes in treatment of diseases such as acquired immunodeficiency syndrome and breast cancer. Another example of success is cystic fibrosis, from which median survival has increased from 6 months in 1959 to 27 years in 2007 [2]. This is an orphan disease, as is SAH. It has the advantage for study of having a known molecular target. In addition and in common with some other successfully treated conditions, there is a very well-organized and -funded patient advocacy group that generates $10 million a year in the United States for research. The Cystic Fibrosis Foundation provides many research tools and candidate preclinical drugs to researchers for free. Can those of us studying SAH learn something from them?

When examining causes for the unsuccessful clinical trials, the question arises regarding which of the numerous preclinical treatments to advance into clinical trials. At this meeting alone, papers and posters describe 19 experimental treatments for SAH that have not been studied or have had only limited study in humans (inhaled nitric oxide, minocycline, pitavastatin, melatonin, deferoxamine, valproic acid, intrathecal magnesium, cilostazol, eicosapentanoic acid, ADAMTS13, rhinacanthin, curcumin, ecdysterone, baivalein, molsidomine, exercise, cystatin C, imatinib, and Ro 25-6981). Guidelines have been proposed for the conduct of experimental studies and there is evidence that studies that do not follow these guidelines overestimate the benefit of the treatment [31, 34]. I support adherence to the guidelines. They reflect good scientific design; however, bear in mind that the studies of nimodipine, which is the only US Food and Drug Administration-approved treatment for SAH, would probably not qualify for study in humans and the animal studies often showed it did not affect its suspected mechanism of action, angiographic vasospasm [19]. There is also the implication that animal models exist or can be created that are externally valid or, in other words, that efficacy in the animal model would translate to humans if the guidelines were followed [55]. Whether this is true in SAH remains to be seen. Adhering to at least some of the guideline recommendations is going to be necessary because granting agencies are requiring this to some extent. The recommendations for multiple studies in multiple laboratories will require increased cooperation between investigators and centers. Dirnagl et al. noted that this already occurs in some fields such as physics (and astronomy), where some obvious barriers such as authorship, student independence, intellectual property, collaboration of funding bodies between countries, communications, governance, and monitoring have been overcome [11].

Moving to clinical trials, there is the question of the outcome measure (Table 3). The modified Rankin scale has been used in a SAH clinical trial with a positive result, but whether adding cognitive assessments would disclose differences in outcome in the group of patients classified as good outcome patients, generally modified Rankin score 0–2 in other SAH studies, is an open question [45]. There is little agreement about what cognitive tests to use to assess outcome after SAH, and the number of studies is almost the same as the number of tests used [1]. National and international cooperation might be recommended here. Another reason for this is the observation that, among models of prognostic factors for outcome after SAH, one study of 3,567 patients found that a detailed logistic regression explained only 36 % of the variance in outcome [44]. What is the cause of the rest of the variation? Why do some patients with angiographic vasospasm not develop DCI? Why does one grade 4 patient recover and the other die? In addition to the probable multifactorial pathogenesis, there are physiologic differences in anatomy and blood flow and genetic and epigenetic variations that affect individual responses to SAH, but this personalized approach to medicine is only beginning to be studied in SAH [30, 58]. Ultimately, treatments might need to be adjusted depending on the genetic makeup of the patient, as in other diseases where personalized medicine has already been applied. Some of these discoveries required large, multinational collaborative efforts [29, 63]. Practice misalignment also may result from differing patient responses [52]. Some clinical trials in SAH focus on the treatment, with varying degrees of patient subgroup selection, taking a pragmatic approach [51]. Another option is to focus on very specific hypotheses and more on the individual characteristics of the patient and pathology, which is the explanatory trial (Fig. 2). There is no correct answer, although success was seen in a narrowly focused neuroprotection trial in humans [27]. Finally, it is of note that 34 years ago, clinical use of steroids was described at the second vasospasm meeting. Their use is still being investigated in SAH in small, single-center studies. Why don't we know the answer to whether they are efficacious in SAH or not, three decades later? Would it be beneficial to cooperate nationally and internationally to pool clinical, genetic, radiologic, and such data, develop common definitions and data elements, both retrospectively and then on a prospective basis? The SAH international trialists repository seeks to do this [39].

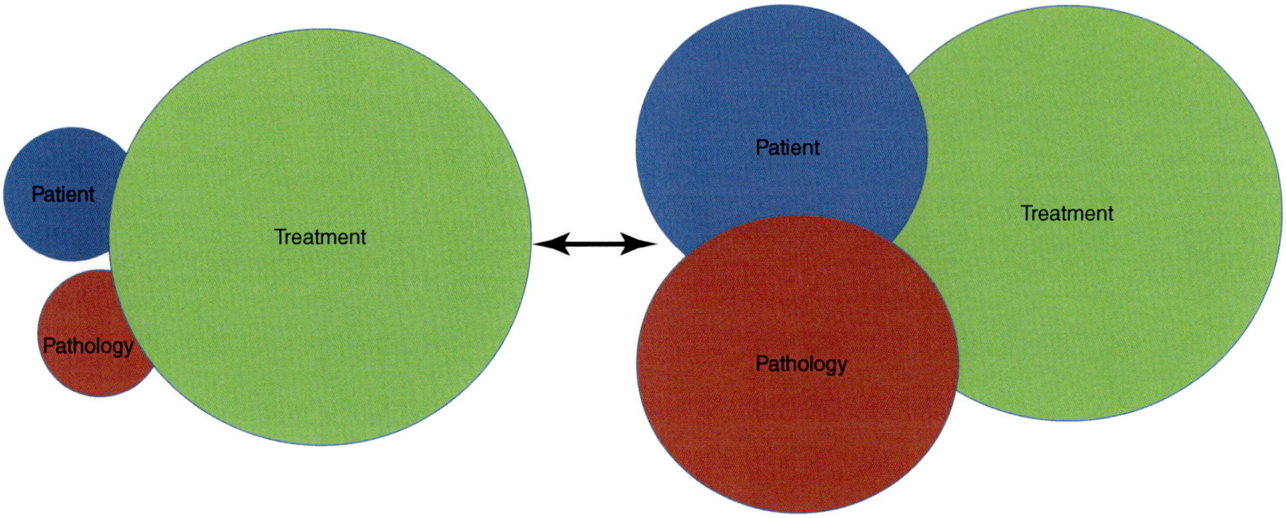

Fig. 2 Simplistic view of pragmatic versus explanatory clinical trials, presented in detail by Thorpe et al. [51]. Clinical trials may be pragmatic and focus on administering a single treatment to unselected patients with little attention to patient- or pathology-related factors or they may be explanatory and test a very specific hypothesis in a well-defined patient subgroup

Summary

The pathophysiology of DCI is probably complex and multifactorial. Progress has been made in improving outcome but there is still no cure for DCI. Many promising preclinical treatments were described at this meeting and others are in early stage clinical trials. To reduce the chances of failure of translation, it has been recommended that the quality of preclinical studies be improved, and that treatments be studied in collaboration between multiple laboratories. Similarly, on the clinical side, many centers already work together, but it may be beneficial for investigators to work cooperatively to develop common definitions and outcome measures, and to redefine these as new data become available. Funding agencies are increasingly interested in this approach and it may be beneficial from the position of a relatively uncommon disease such as SAH for garnering philanthropic and other sources of support.

Conclusion

Outcome from aneurysmal SAH has improved in the past decades, in association with introduction of nimodipine pharmacologic prophylaxis, early aneurysm repair and endovascular coiling. Advances in treatment of angiographic vasospasm and DCI also have likely contributed, but they are less well based on randomized clinical trials. Further reductions in morbidity and mortality will require cooperative efforts of centers around the world to bring new therapies identified in preclinical studies into the clinic.

Acknowledgements RLM receives grant support from the Physicians Services Incorporated Foundation, Brain Aneurysm Foundation, Canadian Stroke Network, Canadian Institutes of Health Research, and Heart and Stroke Foundation of Ontario.

Conflict of Interest Statement RLM is Chief Scientific Officer of Edge Therapeutics.

References

1. Al-Khindi T, Macdonald RL, Schweizer TA (2010) Cognitive and functional outcome after aneurysmal subarachnoid hemorrhage. Stroke 41:e519–e536
2. Barr HL, Britton J, Smyth AR, Fogarty AW (2011) Association between socioeconomic status, sex, and age at death from cystic fibrosis in England and Wales (1959 to 2008): cross sectional study. BMJ 343:d4662
3. Broderick JP, Brott TG, Duldner JE, Tomsick T, Leach A (1994) Initial and recurrent bleeding are the major causes of death following subarachnoid hemorrhage. Stroke 25:1342–1347
4. Chou CH, Reed SD, Allsbrook JS, Steele JL, Schulman KA, Alexander MJ (2010) Costs of vasospasm in patients with aneurysmal subarachnoid hemorrhage. Neurosurgery 67:345–352
5. Connolly ES Jr, Rabinstein AA, Carhuapoma JR, Derdeyn CP, Dion J, Higashida RT, Hoh BL, Kirkness CJ, Naidech AM, Ogilvy CS, Patel AB, Thompson BG, Vespa P (2012) Guidelines for the management of aneurysmal subarachnoid hemorrhage: a guideline for healthcare professionals from the American Heart Association/American Stroke Association. Stroke 43:1711–1737
6. Crowley RW, Medel R, Dumont AS, Ilodigwe D, Kassell NF, Mayer SA, Ruefenacht D, Schmiedek P, Weidauer S, Pasqualin A, Macdonald RL (2011) Angiographic vasospasm is strongly correlated with cerebral infarction after subarachnoid hemorrhage. Stroke 42:919–923
7. Dankbaar JW, Rijsdijk M, van der Schaaf IC, Velthuis BK, Wermer MJ, Rinkel GJ (2009) Relationship between vasospasm, cerebral perfusion, and delayed cerebral ischemia after aneurysmal subarachnoid hemorrhage. Neuroradiology 51:813–819

8. Dankbaar JW, Slooter AJ, Rinkel GJ, van der Schaaf IC (2010) Effect of different components of triple-H therapy on cerebral perfusion in patients with aneurysmal subarachnoid haemorrhage: a systematic review. Crit Care 14:R23
9. de Rooij NK, Rinkel GJ, Dankbaar JW, Frijns CJ (2013) Delayed cerebral ischemia after subarachnoid hemorrhage: a systematic review of clinical, laboratory, and radiological predictors. Stroke 44:43–54
10. Diringer MN, Bleck TP, Claude HJ III, Menon D, Shutter L, Vespa P, Bruder N, Connolly ES Jr, Citerio G, Gress D, Hanggi D, Hoh BL, Lanzino G, Le RP, Rabinstein A, Schmutzhard E, Stocchetti N, Suarez JI, Treggiari M, Tseng MY, Vergouwen MD, Wolf S, Zipfel G (2011) Critical care management of patients following aneurysmal subarachnoid hemorrhage: recommendations from the Neurocritical Care Society's Multidisciplinary Consensus Conference. Neurocrit Care 15:211–240
11. Dirnagl U, Hakim A, Macleod M, Fisher M, Howells D, Alan SM, Steinberg G, Planas A, Boltze J, Savitz S, Iadecola C, Meairs S (2013) A concerted appeal for international cooperation in preclinical stroke research. Stroke 44:1754–1760
12. Doczi T, Joo F, Adam G, Bozoky B, Szerdahelyi P (1986) Blood-brain barrier damage during the acute stage of subarachnoid hemorrhage, as exemplified by a new animal model. Neurosurgery 18:733–739
13. Dorhout Mees SM, Kerr RS, Rinkel GJ, Algra A, Molyneux AJ (2012) Occurrence and impact of delayed cerebral ischemia after coiling and after clipping in the International Subarachnoid Aneurysm Trial (ISAT). J Neurol 259:679–683
14. Dorhout Mees SM, Rinkel GJ, Feigin VL, Algra A, van den Bergh WM, Vermeulen M, van Gijn J (2007) Calcium antagonists for aneurysmal subarachnoid haemorrhage. Cochrane Database Syst Rev 3:CD000277
15. Dorhout Mees SM, van den Bergh WM, Algra A, Rinkel GJ (2007) Antiplatelet therapy for aneurysmal subarachnoid haemorrhage. Cochrane Database Syst Rev 4:CD006184
16. Dreier JP (2011) The role of spreading depression, spreading depolarization and spreading ischemia in neurological disease. Nat Med 17:439–447
17. Dreier JP, Windmuller O, Petzold G, Lindauer U, Einhaupl KM, Dirnagl U (2002) Ischemia triggered by red blood cell products in the subarachnoid space is inhibited by nimodipine administration or moderate volume expansion/hemodilution in rats. Neurosurgery 51:1457–1465
18. Echlin FA (1980) Some historical remarks. In: Wilkins RH (ed) Cerebral arterial spasm. Williams and Wilkins, Baltimore, pp 1–6
19. Espinosa F, Weir B, Overton T, Castor W, Grace M, Boisvert D (1984) A randomized placebo-controlled double-blind trial of nimodipine after SAH in monkeys. Part 1: clinical and radiological findings. J Neurosurg 60:1167–1175
20. Feigin V, Anderson N, Rinkel G, Algra A, van Gijn J, Bennett DA (2005) Corticosteroids for aneurysmal subarachnoid haemorrhage and primary intracerebral haemorrhage. Cochrane Database Syst Rev 3:CD004583
21. Findlay JM, Deagle GM (1998) Causes of morbidity and mortality following intracranial aneurysm rupture. Can J Neurol Sci 25:209–215
22. Friedrich B, Muller F, Feiler S, Scholler K, Plesnila N (2012) Experimental subarachnoid hemorrhage causes early and long-lasting microarterial constriction and microthrombosis: an in-vivo microscopy study. J Cereb Blood Flow Metab 32:447–455
23. Fujii M, Yan J, Rolland WB, Soejima Y, Caner B, Zhang JH (2013) Early brain injury, an evolving frontier in subarachnoid hemorrhage research. Transl Stroke Res 4:432–446
24. Golan E, Vasquez DN, Ferguson ND, Adhikari NK, Scales DC (2013) Prophylactic magnesium for improving neurologic outcome after aneurysmal subarachnoid hemorrhage: systematic review and meta-analysis. J Crit Care 28:173–181
25. Guo J, Shi Z, Yang K, Tian JH, Jiang L (2012) Endothelin receptor antagonists for subarachnoid hemorrhage. Cochrane Database Syst Rev 9:CD008354
26. Guyatt GH, Oxman AD, Vist GE, Kunz R, Falck-Ytter Y, Alonso-Coello P, Schunemann HJ (2008) GRADE: an emerging consensus on rating quality of evidence and strength of recommendations. BMJ 336:924–926
27. Hill MD, Martin RH, Mikulis D, Wong JH, Silver FL, terBrugge KG, Milot G, Clark WM, Macdonald RL, Kelly ME, Boulton M, Fleetwood I, McDougall C, Gunnarsson T, Chow M, Lum C, Dodd R, Poublanc J, Krings T, Demchuk AM, Goyal M, Anderson R, Bishop J, Garman D, Tymianski M (2012) Safety and efficacy of NA-1 in patients with iatrogenic stroke after endovascular aneurysm repair (ENACT): a phase 2, randomised, double-blind, placebo-controlled trial. Lancet Neurol 11:942–950
28. Jang YG, Ilodigwe D, Macdonald RL (2009) Metaanalysis of tirilazad mesylate in patients with aneurysmal subarachnoid hemorrhage. Neurocrit Care 10:141–147
29. Jones DT, Jager N, Kool M, Zichner T, Hutter B, Sultan M, Cho YJ, Pugh TJ, Hovestadt V, Stutz AM, Rausch T, Warnatz HJ, Ryzhova M, Bender S, Sturm D, Pleier S, Cin H, Pfaff E, Sieber L, Wittmann A, Remke M, Witt H, Hutter S, Tzaridis T, Weischenfeldt J, Raeder B, Avci M, Amstislavskiy V, Zapatka M, Weber UD, Wang Q, Lasitschka B, Bartholomae CC, Schmidt M, von Kalle C, Ast V, Lawerenz C, Eils J, Kabbe R, Benes V, van Sluis P, Koster J, Volckmann R, Shih D, Betts MJ, Russell RB, Coco S, Tonini GP, Schuller U, Hans V, Graf N, Kim YJ, Monoranu C, Roggendorf W, Unterberg A, Herold-Mende C, Milde T, Kulozik AE, von Deimling A, Witt O, Maass E, Rossler J, Ebinger M, Schuhmann MU, Fruhwald MC, Hasselblatt M, Jabado N, Rutkowski S, von Bueren AO, Williamson D, Clifford SC, McCabe MG, Collins VP, Wolf S, Wiemann S, Lehrach H, Brors B, Scheurlen W, Felsberg J, Reifenberger G, Northcott PA, Taylor MD, Meyerson M, Pomeroy SL, Yaspo ML, Korbel JO, Korshunov A, Eils R, Pfister SM, Lichter P (2012) Dissecting the genomic complexity underlying medulloblastoma. Nature 488:100–105
30. Khurana VG, Sohni YR, Mangrum WI, McClelland RL, O'Kane DJ, Meyer FB, Meissner I (2004) Endothelial nitric oxide synthase gene polymorphisms predict susceptibility to aneurysmal subarachnoid hemorrhage and cerebral vasospasm. J Cereb Blood Flow Metab 24:291–297
31. Kilkenny C, Browne WJ, Cuthill IC, Emerson M, Altman DG (2010) Improving bioscience research reporting: the ARRIVE guidelines for reporting animal research. PLoS Biol 8:e1000412
32. Komotar RJ, Schmidt JM, Starke RM, Claassen J, Wartenberg KE, Lee K, Badjatia N, Connolly ES Jr, Mayer SA (2009) Resuscitation and critical care of poor-grade subarachnoid hemorrhage. Neurosurgery 64:397–410
33. Kramer AH, Fletcher JJ (2011) Locally-administered intrathecal thrombolytics following aneurysmal subarachnoid hemorrhage: a systematic review and meta-analysis. Neurocrit Care 14: 489–499
34. Lapchak PA, Zhang JH, Noble-Haeusslein LJ (2013) RIGOR guidelines: escalating STAIR and STEPS for effective translational research. Transl Stroke Res 4:279–285
35. Liu GJ, Wang ZJ, Wang YF, Xu LL, Wang XL, Liu Y, Luo GJ, He GH, Zeng YJ (2012) Systematic assessment and meta-analysis of the efficacy and safety of fasudil in the treatment of cerebral vasospasm in patients with subarachnoid hemorrhage. Eur J Clin Pharmacol 68:131–139
36. Lovelock CE, Rinkel GJ, Rothwell PM (2010) Time trends in outcome of subarachnoid hemorrhage: population-based study and systematic review. Neurology 74:1494–1501
37. Macdonald RL (2013) History and definition of delayed cerebral ischemia. Acta Neurochir Suppl 115:3–7
38. Macdonald RL (2014) Delayed neurological deterioration after subarachnoid haemorrhage. Nat Rev Neurol 10:44–58

39. Macdonald RL, Cusimano MD, Etminan N, Hanggi D, Hasan D, Ilodigwe D, Jaja B, Lantigua H, Le RP, Lo B, Louffat-Olivares A, Mayer S, Molyneux A, Quinn A, Schweizer TA, Schenk T, Spears J, Todd M, Torner J, Vergouwen MD, Wong GK (2013) Subarachnoid Hemorrhage International Trialists Data Repository (SAHIT). World Neurosurg 79:418–422
40. Macdonald RL, Rosengart A, Huo D, Karrison T (2003) Factors associated with the development of vasospasm after planned surgical treatment of aneurysmal subarachnoid hemorrhage. J Neurosurg 99:644–652
41. Mahaney KB, Todd MM, Bayman EO, Torner JC (2012) Acute postoperative neurological deterioration associated with surgery for ruptured intracranial aneurysm: incidence, predictors, and outcomes. J Neurosurg 116:1267–1278
42. Molyneux A, Kerr R, Stratton I, Sandercock P, Clarke M, Shrimpton J, Holman R (2002) International Subarachnoid Aneurysm Trial (ISAT) of neurosurgical clipping versus endovascular coiling in 2143 patients with ruptured intracranial aneurysms: a randomised trial. Lancet 360:1267–1274
43. Nau R, Haase S, Bunkowski S, Bruck W (2002) Neuronal apoptosis in the dentate gyrus in humans with subarachnoid hemorrhage and cerebral hypoxia. Brain Pathol 12:329–336
44. Rosengart AJ, Schultheiss KE, Tolentino J, Macdonald RL (2007) Prognostic factors for outcome in patients with aneurysmal subarachnoid hemorrhage. Stroke 38:2315–2321
45. Scott RB, Eccles F, Molyneux AJ, Kerr RS, Rothwell PM, Carpenter K (2010) Improved cognitive outcomes with endovascular coiling of ruptured intracranial aneurysms: neuropsychological outcomes from the International Subarachnoid Aneurysm Trial (ISAT). Stroke 41:1743–1747
46. Sehba FA, Hou J, Pluta RM, Zhang JH (2012) The importance of early brain injury after subarachnoid hemorrhage. Prog Neurobiol 97:14–37
47. Smith-Bindman R, Lipson J, Marcus R, Kim KP, Mahesh M, Gould R, de Berrington GA, Miglioretti DL (2009) Radiation dose associated with common computed tomography examinations and the associated lifetime attributable risk of cancer. Arch Intern Med 169:2078–2086
48. Stein SC, Browne KD, Chen XH, Smith DH, Graham DI (2006) Thromboembolism and delayed cerebral ischemia after subarachnoid hemorrhage: an autopsy study. Neurosurgery 59:781–787
49. Steiner T, Juvela S, Unterberg A, Jung C, Forsting M, Rinkel G (2013) European stroke organization guidelines for the management of intracranial aneurysms and subarachnoid haemorrhage. Cerebrovasc Dis 35:93–112
50. Tam AK, Ilodigwe D, Li Z, Schweizer TA, Macdonald RL (2013) Global cerebral atrophy after subarachnoid hemorrhage: a possible marker of acute brain injury and assessment of its impact on outcome. Acta Neurochir Suppl 115:17–21
51. Thorpe KE, Zwarenstein M, Oxman AD, Treweek S, Furberg CD, Altman DG, Tunis S, Bergel E, Harvey I, Magid DJ, Chalkidou K (2009) A pragmatic-explanatory continuum indicator summary (PRECIS): a tool to help trial designers. CMAJ 180:E47–E57
52. Tobin MJ (2008) Counterpoint: evidence-based medicine lacks a sound scientific base. Chest 133:1071–1074
53. Tucker WS (1987) The relationship between timing of surgery and operative complications in aneurysmal subarachnoid hemorrhage. Can J Neurol Sci 14:84–87
54. Uhl E, Lehmberg J, Steiger HJ, Messmer K (2003) Intraoperative detection of early microvasospasm in patients with subarachnoid hemorrhage by using orthogonal polarization spectral imaging. Neurosurgery 52:1307–1315
55. van der Worp HB, Howells DW, Sena ES, Porritt MJ, Rewell S, O'Collins V, Macleod MR (2010) Can animal models of disease reliably inform human studies? PLoS Med 7:e1000245
56. Vergouwen MD, de Haan RJ, Vermeulen M, Roos YB (2010) Effect of statin treatment on vasospasm, delayed cerebral ischemia, and functional outcome in patients with aneurysmal subarachnoid hemorrhage: a systematic review and meta-analysis update. Stroke 41:e47–e52
57. Vergouwen MD, Etminan N, Ilodigwe D, Macdonald RL (2011) Lower incidence of cerebral infarction correlates with improved functional outcome after aneurysmal subarachnoid hemorrhage. J Cereb Blood Flow Metab 31:1545–1553
58. Vergouwen MD, Frijns CJ, Roos YB, Rinkel GJ, Baas F, Vermeulen M (2004) Plasminogen activator inhibitor-1 4G allele in the 4G/5G promoter polymorphism increases the occurrence of cerebral ischemia after aneurysmal subarachnoid hemorrhage. Stroke 35:1280–1283
59. Vergouwen MD, Vermeulen M, de Haan RJ, Levi M, Roos YB (2007) Dihydropyridine calcium antagonists increase fibrinolytic activity: a systematic review. J Cereb Blood Flow Metab 27:1293–1308
60. Vergouwen MD, Vermeulen M, van Gijn J, Rinkel GJ, Wijdicks EF, Muizelaar JP, Mendelow AD, Juvela S, Yonas H, terBrugge KG, Macdonald RL, Diringer MN, Broderick JP, Dreier JP, Roos YB (2010) Definition of delayed cerebral ischemia after aneurysmal subarachnoid hemorrhage as an outcome event in clinical trials and observational studies: proposal of a multidisciplinary research group. Stroke 41:2391–2395
61. Washington CW, Zipfel GJ (2011) Detection and monitoring of vasospasm and delayed cerebral ischemia: a review and assessment of the literature. Neurocrit Care 15:312–317
62. Weir B, Grace M, Hansen J, Rothberg C (1978) Time course of vasospasm in man. J Neurosurg 48:173–178
63. Yasuno K, Bilguvar K, Bijlenga P, Low SK, Krischek B, Auburger G, Simon M, Krex D, Arlier Z, Nayak N, Ruigrok YM, Niemela M, Tajima A, von Und Zu FM, Doczi T, Wirjatijasa F, Hata A, Blasco J, Oszvald A, Kasuya H, Zilani G, Schoch B, Singh P, Stuer C, Risselada R, Beck J, Sola T, Ricciardi F, Aromaa A, Illig T, Schreiber S, van Duijn CM, van den Berg LH, Perret C, Proust C, Roder C, Ozturk AK, Gaal E, Berg D, Geisen C, Friedrich CM, Summers P, Frangi AF, State MW, Wichmann HE, Breteler MM, Wijmenga C, Mane S, Peltonen L, Elio V, Sturkenboom MC, Lawford P, Byrne J, Macho J, Sandalcioglu EI, Meyer B, Raabe A, Steinmetz H, Rufenacht D, Jaaskelainen JE, Hernesniemi J, Rinkel GJ, Zembutsu H, Inoue I, Palotie A, Cambien F, Nakamura Y, Lifton RP, Gunel M (2010) Genome-wide association study of intracranial aneurysm identifies three new risk loci. Nat Genet 42:420–425

Aneurysm Formation

Molecular Basis for Intracranial Aneurysm Formation

Miyuki Fukuda and Tomohiro Aoki

Abstract Intracranial aneurysm (IA) is a socially important disease both because it has a high prevalence and because of the severity of resultant subarachnoid hemorrhages after IA rupture. The major concern of current IA treatment is the lack medical therapies that are less invasive than surgical procedures for many patients. The current situation is mostly caused by a lack of knowledge regarding the regulating mechanisms of IA formation. Hemodynamic stress, especially high wall shear stress, loaded on arterial bifurcation sites is recognized as a trigger of IA formation from studies performed in the field of fluid dynamics. On the other hand, many studies using human specimens have also revealed the presence of active inflammatory responses, such as the infiltration of macrophages, in the pathogenesis of IA. Because of these findings, recent experimental studies, mainly using animal models of IA, have revealed some of the molecular mechanisms linking hemodynamic stress and long-lasting inflammation in IA walls. Currently, we propose that IA is a chronic inflammatory disease regulated by a positive feedback loop consisting of the cyclooxygenase (COX)-2 – prostaglandin (PG) E_2 – prostaglandin E receptor 2 (EP2) – nuclear factor (NF)-κB signaling pathway triggered under hemodynamic stress and macrophage infiltration via NF-κB-mediated monocyte chemoattractant protein (MCP)-1 induction. These findings indicate future directions for the development of therapeutic drugs for IAs.

Keywords Intracranial aneurysm • Subarachnoid hemorrhage • Inflammation • Nuclear factor (NF)-κB • Macrophage • Prostaglandin • Cyclooxygenase-2 (COX-2) • EP2 • Monocyte chemoattractant protein-1 (MCP-1) • Statin

Findings from Studies Performed with Human Intracranial Aneurysms

Recent studies in the field of fluid dynamics demonstrated the close interactions of hemodynamics with intracranial aneurysm (IAs) [10]. For example, among various parameters of hemodynamics, high wall shear stress loaded on the arterial bifurcation sites, where IAs are formed, is associated with IA formation and growth [10]. High wall shear stress can, therefore, be recognized as a trigger of IA formation.

On the other hand, in the field of histopathological analyses, gene linkage analyses and comprehensive gene expression analyses have revealed that active inflammatory responses, such as macrophage infiltration and the expression of various cytokines, are present in human IAs [8]. For example, Shi et al. [11] analyzed gene expression profiles in human IA lesions using a microarray technique and revealed that inflammation-related biological pathways, inflammatory response and apoptosis, were associated with IA development. Consistent with this, they also confirmed the upregulation of proinflammatory genes in human IA walls, including interleukin (IL)-1β, tumor necrosis factor (TNF)-α, vascular cell adhesion molecule (VCAM)-1, C-X-C chemokine receptor type 4 (CXCR4), and chemokine ligand (CCL) 5 [11].

M. Fukuda
Department of Neurosurgery, Kyoto University Graduate School of Medicine, Kyoto Japan

Department of Pharmacology, Kyoto University Graduate School of Medicine, Kyoto Japan

Core Research for Evolutional Science and Technology (CREST), Kyoto University Graduate School of Medicine, Kyoto Japan

T. Aoki (✉)
Department of Pharmacology, Kyoto University Graduate School of Medicine, Kyoto Japan

Core Research for Evolutional Science and Technology (CREST), Kyoto University Graduate School of Medicine, Kyoto Japan

Innovation Center for Immunoregulation Technologies and Drugs (AK Project), Kyoto University Graduate School of Medicine, Konoe-cho Yoshida, Sakyo-ku, Kyoto city, Kyoto 606-8501, Japan
e-mail: tomoaoki@kuhp.kyoto-u.ac.jp

J. Fandino et al. (eds.), *Neurovascular Events After Subarachnoid Hemorrhage*, Acta Neurochirurgica Supplement, Vol. 120,
DOI 10.1007/978-3-319-04981-6_2,

However, studies using human IA specimens have considerable limitations, such as the heterogeneity of individual genetic backgrounds and the difficulty of pathological analyses at each period of IA formation from the same patient, in elucidating the mechanisms underlying IA formation and development. We, therefore, have developed experimental models of IA to overcome this situation.

Molecular Mechanisms Regulating IA Formation Through Linking Hemodynamic Stress and Long-Lasting Inflammation

We established experimental models of IAs by increasing the hemodynamics at the bifurcation sites of cerebral arteries through the ligation of the carotid artery and salt overloading [5]. Because experimental IA and human IA share histological similarities characterized by the degeneration of the arterial wall, the disruption of internal elastic lamina, and the infiltration of inflammatory cells, these animal models are suitable for analyses of the pathogenesis of IAs. Indeed, results from recent experimental studies using these models remarkably accelerated our understanding of the mechanisms regulating IA formation and development.

Through the studies using animal models, we identified nuclear factor (NF)-κB as a critical transcription factor for IA formation [1, 8]. NF-κB leads the induction of various proinflammatory genes, such as monocyte chemoattractant protein (MCP)-1, a factor that recruits macrophages in IA walls [7, 8]. Macrophages recruited in cerebral arterial walls by NF-κB-mediated MCP-1 induction produce a large amount of cytokines and proteinases and exacerbate the inflammation associated with IA formation and growth [7, 8]. However, how high wall shear stress induces NF-κB-mediated inflammation and how the inflammation becomes chronic remain to be elucidated.

We recently demonstrated that the positive feedback loop consisting of the cyclooxygenase (COX)-2 – prostaglandin (PG) E_2 – prostaglandin E receptor 2 (EP2) – NF-κB signaling pathway is formed under high wall shear stress and induces a long-lasting (chronic) inflammation in IA walls [6, 7]. As previously discussed, at the sites of IA formation, which are mostly at arterial bifurcations, high wall shear stress is loaded and recognized as a trigger of IA formation [7]. An in vitro study, using a primary culture of endothelial cells from human carotid arteries, demonstrated the induction of COX-2, a prostaglandin-producing enzyme, and its receptor, EP2, under high wall shear stress. Both COX-2 and EP2 expression were also consistently upregulated in experimentally induced IAs during IA formation and their expression was well colocalized in endothelial cells where wall shear stress was loaded. Here, because either the administration of Celecoxib (a selective COX-2 inhibitor) or EP2 deficiency significantly suppressed both IA formation and inflammatory responses in IA walls, such as NF-κB activation and macrophage infiltration, the shear stress-activated prostaglandin pathway was identified as a mediator of NF-κB-induced inflammation during IA formation. Indeed, in endothelial cells, treatment with PGE_2 or a selective EP2 agonist activated NF-κB and its target, MCP-1. Importantly, COX-2 inhibition suppressed EP2 expression, and vice versa. Thus, once hemodynamic stress induces COX-2 expression in endothelial cells at the bifurcation sites of cerebral arteries, the positive feedback loop consisting of COX-2 – PGE_2 – EP2 – NF-κB was formed, resulting in the amplification and the chronicity of inflammation (Fig. 1).

Future Prospects for the Development of Therapeutic Drugs for IA

The recent experimental results indicate that NF-κB is a potential therapeutic target for IA treatment [4]. The significant suppression of IA formation and growth in animals with NF-κB deficiency or treated with a NF-κB inhibitor, decoy oligonucleotides, further supports this notion [1].

Statins (3-hydroxy-3 methylglutaryl coenzyme A reductase inhibitors) were originally developed as therapeutic drugs for lipid metabolic abnormality. In addition, statins are well recognized as having powerful anti-inflammatory and especially anti-NF-κB effects; known as the pleiotropic effect of statins. Encouraged by this pleiotropic effect of statins, we administered Pitavastatin, one of the statins, to our rat model of IA and demonstrated that Pitavastatin treatment effectively prevented the growth of IAs in rats [3]. Pitavastatin treatment remarkably suppressed the inflammatory responses in IA walls, characterized by NF-κB activation and subsequent induction of the expression of NF-κB-regulating genes, such as MCP-1, VCAM-1, and IL-1β [3]. Furthermore, Pitavastatin treatment effectively inhibited the degenerative change of IA walls, suggesting a preventive effect of Pitavastatin against the rupture of IAs [3]. Other kinds of statins, Simvastatin and Pravastatin, also successfully prevented IA growth through inhibition of inflammation in IA walls, suggesting that statins are potential therapeutic drugs for IAs [2, 9].

Because of these findings from experimental animals, we examined the preventive effect of statins for the rupture of human IAs in a case-controlled clinical study in Japan. As a result, we clarified the inverse relationship between the usage of statins and the occurrence of aneurysmal subarachnoid hemorrhage in the Japanese population. Statins were administered in 9.4 % of cases with ruptured IAs and 26.0 % of cases with unruptured IAs. The usage of statins, therefore, significantly prevented the rupture of preexisting IAs with a relative odds ratio of 0.3 [12].

These studies suggest the potential of statins as therapeutic drugs to prevent the growth and rupture of IAs.

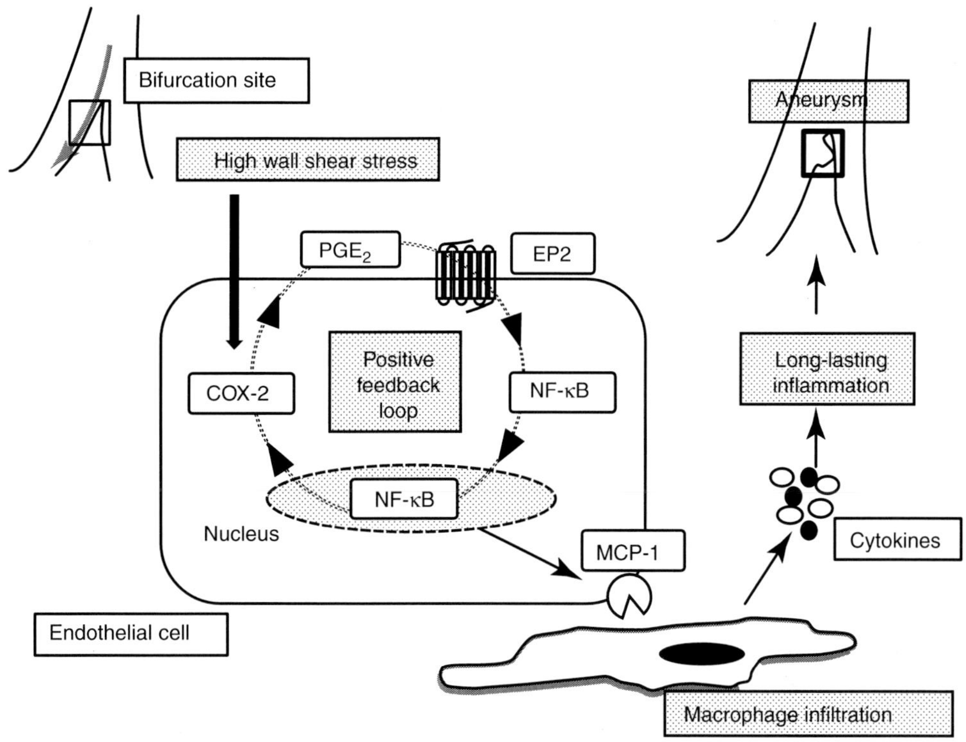

Fig. 1 Schema demonstrating our hypothesis for the potential mechanisms underlying the chronicity of inflammation contributing to intracranial aneurysm formation. Note the positive feedback loop consisting of PGE_2 – NF-κB signaling under hemodynamic stress and macrophage infiltration via NF-κB-mediated MCP-1 induction

Conclusion

Recent experimental studies using an animal model of IA have revealed the crucial role of long-lasting inflammation in its pathogenesis. In this process, prostaglandin-mediated NF-κB activation plays the role to trigger and amplify the inflammatory responses in IA lesion suggesting the potential of NF-κB as a therapeutic target for IA treatment. Indeed, recent case-control study has demonstrated the suppressive effect of statins on rupture of IAs in human cases through their potent anti-NF-κB effect. In near future, a medical treatment of IA is supposed to be established.

Acknowledgment The authors are grateful to all of the researchers, collaborators, technical assistants, and secretaries contributing to our studies cited in the present manuscript. We also express our sincere gratitude to the grants supporting our research.

Conflict of Interest Statement We declare that we have no conflict of interest.

References

1. Aoki T, Kataoka H, Shimamura M, Nakagami H, Wakayama K, Moriwaki T, Ishibashi R, Nozaki K, Morishita R, Hashimoto N (2007) NF-κB is a key mediator of cerebral aneurysm formation. Circulation 116:2830–2840
2. Aoki T, Kataoka H, Ishibashi R, Nozaki K, Hashimoto N (2008) Simvastatin suppresses the progression of experimentally induced cerebral aneurysms in rats. Stroke 39:1276–1285
3. Aoki T, Kataoka H, Ishibashi R, Nakagami H, Nozaki K, Morishita R, Hashimoto N (2009) Pitavastatin suppresses formation and progression of cerebral aneurysms through inhibition of the nuclear factor kappaB pathway. Neurosurgery 64:357–365
4. Aoki T, Nishimura M (2010) Targeting chronic inflammation in cerebral aneurysms focusing on NFκB as a putative target of medical therapy. Expert Opin Ther Targets 14:265–273
5. Aoki T, Nishimura M (2011) The development and the use of experimental animal models to study the underlying mechanisms of CA formation. J Biomed Biotechnol. doi:10.1155/2011/535921
6. Aoki T, Nishimura M, Matsuoka T, Yamamoto K, Furuyashiki T, Kataoka H, Kitaoka S, Ishibashi R, Ishibazawa A, Miyamoto S, Morishita R, Ando J, Hashimoto N, Nozaki K, Narumiya S (2011) PGE_2-EP2 signaling in endothelium is activated by haemodynamic stress and induces cerebral aneurysm through an amplifying loop via NF-κB. Br J Pharmacol 163:1237–1249
7. Aoki T, Narumiya S (2012) Prostaglandins and chronic inflammation. Trends Pharmacol Sci 33:304–311
8. Kataoka H, Aoki T (2010) Molecular basis for the development of intracranial aneurysm. Expert Rev Neurother 10:173–187
9. Kimura N, Shimizu H, Eldawoody H, Nakayama T, Saito A, Tominaga T, Takahashi A (2010) Effect of olmesartan and pravastatin on experimental cerebral aneurysms in rats. Brain Res 1322: 144–152
10. Meng H, Tutino VM, Xiang J, Siddiqui A (2013) High WSS or low WSS? Complex interactions of hemodynamics with intracranial aneurysm initiation, growth, and rupture: toward a unifying hypothesis. Am J Neuroradiol. doi:10.3174/ajnr.A3558
11. Shi C, Awad IA, Jafari N, Lin S, Du P, Hage ZA, Shenkar R, Getch CC, Bredel M, Batjer HH, Bendok BR (2009) Genomics of human intracranial aneurysm wall. Stroke 40:1252–1261
12. Yoshimura Y, Murakami Y, Saitoh M, Yokoi T, Aoki T, Miura K, Ueshima H, Nozaki K, SSS Research Group (2013) Statin use and risk of cerebral aneurysm rupture: a hospital-based case-control study in Japan. J Stroke Cerebrovasc Dis. doi:10.1016/j.jstrokecerebrovasdis.2013.04.022

Aneurysm Wall Thickness Measurements of Experimental Aneurysms: In Vivo High-Field MR Imaging Versus Direct Microscopy

Camillo Sherif, Günther Kleinpeter, Michel Loyoddin, Georg Mach, Roberto Plasenzotti, Thomas Haider, Erwin Herbich, and Martin Krssak

Abstract *Background:* Thin cerebral aneurysm wall thickness (AWT) is connected to high aneurysm rupture risk. MR imaging of AWT leads to overestimations. The aim of the present study was to quantify MR inaccuracy by comparison with accurate light microscopic measurements.

Methods: In 13 experimental microsurgical bifurcation aneurysms in rabbits, 3 Tesla (3 T)-MR imaging using contrast-enhanced T1 Flash sequences (resolution: $0.4 \times 0.4 \times 1.5$ mm^3) was performed. The aneurysms were retrieved immediately after MR acquisition, cut longitudinally, and calibrated photographs were obtained. AWT (dome, neck) and parent vessel thickness (PVT) were measured on the MR images and microscopic photographs by independent investigators. All parameters were statistically compared (Wilcoxon test, Spearman correlation).

Results: AWT and PVT could be imaged and measured in all aneurysms with good quality. Comparison with the "real" light microscopic measurements showed a progressive tendency of MR AWT overestimation with smaller AWT: AWT at the dome (0.24 ± 0.06 mm vs. MR 0.30 ± 0.08 mm; $p = 0.0078$; $R = 0.6125$), AWT at the neck (0.25 ± 0.07 mm vs. MR 0.29 ± 0.07 mm; $p = 0.0469$; $R = 0.7451$), and PVT (0.46 ± 0.06 mm vs. MR 0.48 ± 0.06 mm; $p = 0.5$; $R = 0.8568$).

Conclusion: In this experimental setting, 3 T-MR imaging of cerebral AWT showed unacceptable inaccuracies only below the image resolution threshold. Theoretically, AWT for clinical usage could be classified in ranges, defined by the maximum image resolution.

Keywords Aneurysm • Wall thickness • High-field MR • Risk

Introduction

The risk assessment and treatment indications of unruptured aneurysms remain controversial and additional predictive parameters are clinically needed. A potential parameter could be aneurysm wall thickness (AWT). Although we know that thin aneurysm walls are correlated with higher rupture risks [3], few studies have focused on MR image-based

C. Sherif, MD (✉)
Department of Neurosurgery, Krankenanstalt Rudolfstiftung, Juchgasse 25, A-1030 Wien, Vienna, Austria

Department of Neurosurgery, Cerebrovascular Research Group, Krankenanstalt Rudolfstiftung, Vienna, Austria

Department of Neurosurgery, Ludwig Boltzmann Cluster for Cardiovascular Research, Vienna, Austria
e-mail: camillo.sherif@cerebrovascular.at

G. Kleinpeter, MD
Department of Neurosurgery, Krankenanstalt Rudolfstiftung, Juchgasse 25, A-1030 Wien, Vienna, Austria

Cerebrovascular Research Group, Krankenanstalt Rudolfstiftung, Vienna, Austria

M. Loyoddin, MD
Department of Neurosurgery, Krankenanstalt Rudolfstiftung, Juchgasse 25, A-1030 Wien, Vienna, Austria

G. Mach
Cerebrovascular Research Group, Krankenanstalt Rudolfstiftung, Vienna, Austria

Institute for Electrotechniques, University of Technology, Vienna, Austria

R. Plasenzotti • E. Herbich
Department of Biomedical Research, Medical University of Vienna, Vienna, Austria

T. Haider
Cerebrovascular Research Group, Krankenanstalt Rudolfstiftung, Vienna, Austria

M. Krssak
MR Center of Excellence, Medical University of Vienna, Vienna, Austria

J. Fandino et al. (eds.), *Neurovascular Events After Subarachnoid Hemorrhage*, Acta Neurochirurgica Supplement, Vol. 120, DOI 10.1007/978-3-319-04981-6_3,

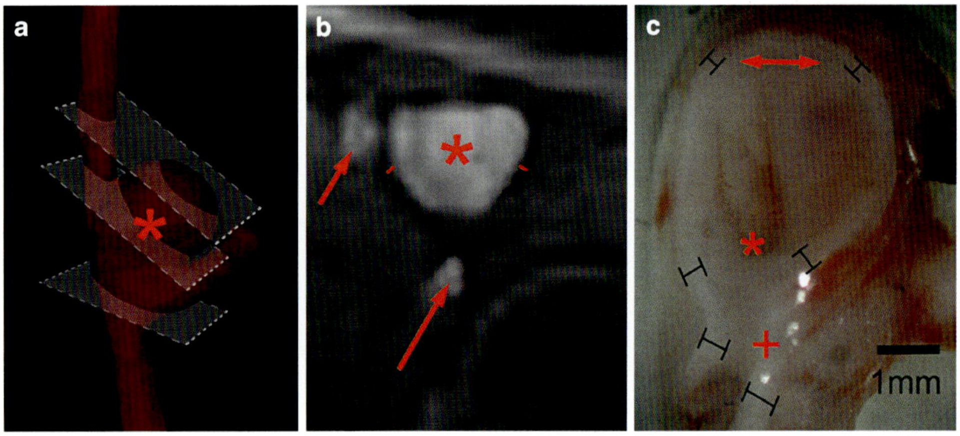

Fig. 1 (**a**) Three-dimensional reconstruction of the MR images. The *asterisk* shows the aneurysm sac. The *planes* define the points of measurements. (**b**) MR image showing the aneurysm sac (*asterisk*) and the parent vessels (*arrows*). The points of measurements are marked by *red small lines*. (**c**) Histologic image of the longitudinally cut aneurysm: the corresponding points of measurements were defined by their exact distance to the neck plane as seen on the MR image in (a). All measurement points were defined and mutually rechecked by two independent blinded researchers: AWT at the dome (*arrow*), AWT at the neck (*asterisk*), and PVT (*cross*)

human cerebral AWT measurements [1, 6]. Despite promising results, there have been theoretical and methodological shortcomings, showing a tendency toward AWT overestimation [10]. Because of ethical limitations using human subjects, no published studies have yet assessed the relative accuracy of MR-based AWT with "real" in vivo measurement. However, this comparison would better determine the clinical relevance of the MR methodological inaccuracies. Thus, the purpose of this investigation was to evaluate and quantify the inaccuracy of MR-based AWT evaluations by comparison with histologic measurements of "fresh" aneurysm walls in experimental aneurysms.

Materials and Methods

In 13 New Zealand White rabbits, saccular bifurcation aneurysms formed by a venous pouch of the external jugular vein were created using well-established techniques [5, 7, 8]. Four weeks after aneurysm creation, the rabbits were anesthetized, and MR images were obtained with well-established algorithms for 3 Tesla (3 T) high-resolution, three-dimensional MR imaging in rabbits (Medspec, Bruker Biospin, Ettlingen, Germany) [9]. A single dose (0.03 mmol/kg) of vascular contrast agent (Vasovist; Schering, Germany) was administered by intravenous bolus before image acquisition. MR images were acquired using 3D FLASH (Fast Low Angle Shot) T1-weighted sequences, with an image resolution of $0.41 \times 0.4 \times 1.5$ mm^3. The aneurysms were retrieved immediately after MR image acquisition. Within a few minutes, digitized color micrographs were taken at 3× and 10× magnification.

For each parameter (AWT at the neck; AWT at the dome; PVT), two measurement points were defined on both MR and histologic images (see Fig. 1). To guarantee valid and precise correspondence, the measurement points were determined and mutually rechecked by two blinded investigators. Then the points were measured on MR and histologic images. For each parameter, both measurement points were used to calculate a mean value. Mean values were then rounded to the nearest 0.1 mm. All measurements were performed using the software CoilControl 3D® (NVtec Ltd., Vienna, Austria). The MR versus histometric parameters were compared with the nonparametric 2-tailed Wilcoxon paired signed-rank test. Agreements between MR image and microscopic measurements were assessed using a Spearman rank correlation (r).

Results

There was a clear tendency toward overestimating AWT in MR images with decreasing wall thickness. Statistically significant differences were seen between MR and light microscopic images at the aneurysm dome and at the neck, but not for measurements of PVT. The mean microscopic AWT measurement at the dome was 0.24 ± 0.06 mm vs. 0.30 ± 0.068 mm for MR imaging ($p = 0.0078$). The mean microscopic AWT measurement at the neck reached 0.25 ± 0.07 mm vs. 0.29 ± 0.07 mm for MR imaging ($p = 0.0469$). The mean microscopic PVT measurement was 0.46 ± 0.06 mm vs. 0.47 ± 0.06 mm for MR imaging ($p = 0.5$). Spearman correlation showed better agreement with increasing wall thickness: AWT at dome $R = 0.6125$, AWT at the neck $R = 0.7451$, PVT $R = 0.8568$.

Discussion

Clinical Background

We face an increasing number of incidentally found aneurysms. However, parameters for personalized risk assessment are rare. In addition to the description of epidemiological and aneurysm geometry features, the first clinical attempts of individualized risk assessment were performed using fluid dynamic simulations [4]. However, in the literature, highly contradicting findings are found, such as high versus low shear stress theories as potential causes for aneurysm rupture [2].

Aneurysm wall thickness (AWT) might serve as another clinical parameter because a histologic examination by Frösen et al. [3] showed that decreasing AWT seems to be closely correlated with increased aneurysm rupture risk. However, few authors have focused on human cerebral AWT measurements. Boussel et al. [1] introduced an indirect method of AWT evaluation by measuring the inner and outer aneurysm volumes in an effort to describe the dangerous progression of fusiform basilar aneurysmal disease. Park et al. [6] assessed the wall of saccular cerebral aneurysms in 14 patients using a 2D double-inversion recovery black-blood sequence (BBDI) at 1.5 T, reporting a resolution of $0.48 \times 0.58 \times 3$ mm^3. Although promising, these studies were not without criticism because of perceived methodological shortcomings. Steinmann et al. [10] stated that black-blood imaging is not acceptable for clinical AWT measurements because of its potential for overestimation. They encouraged further ex vivo and in vivo imaging studies to demonstrate the true capabilities and limitations of MR imaging for resolving the wall thickness and morphology of unruptured cerebral aneurysms.

Aneurysm Wall Thickness Measurements

Because of the known limitations of black-blood imaging, we used contrast-enhanced 3D FLASH T1-weighted sequences. 3D sequences were used to minimize partial volume effects. We also found a clear tendency of measurements made from 3-T MR images to overestimate AWT. This overestimation was closely connected to measurement values below the image resolution threshold. Above the image resolution threshold, reasonable values were obtained. Therefore, clinical utility of MR estimates of AWT may be reasonable if measurement ranges defined by the maximum MR resolution are used. In the current study, this would mean a classification of 0–0.4, 0.41–0.8, 0.81–1.2 mm, etc. Additionally, a combination of AWT measurements with shear stress simulations could lead to a better understanding of the interactions between flow-related physical forces and aneurysm wall reactions.

Limitations

The results of our study, particularly with respect to applicability in human subjects, may be limited. Additionally, the act of sectioning the aneurysm may lead to aneurysm wall deformations. Another possible source of bias would be failure of proper correspondence of the MR image and light microscopy measurement points.

Conclusions

In this experimental setting, measurements made from 3-T MR images of cerebral AWT showed considerable inaccuracies below the image resolution threshold. For clinical application, AWT should be classified in ranges, defined by the maximum image resolution. Further experimental and human studies, especially combining AWT with aneurysmal flow and shear stress simulations, are needed to better define the clinical role of AWT as a risk factor for aneurysm rupture.

Funding This study was funded by the Medical Scientific Fund of the Major of the City of Vienna.

Conflict of Interest Statement Sherif and Mach are shareholders of NVTec. Ltd., Vienna, Austria.

References

1. Boussel L, Wintermark M, Martin A, Dispensa B, VanTijen R, Leach J, Rayz V, Acevedo-Bolton G, Lawton M, Higashida R, Smith W, Young W, Saloner D (2008) Monitoring serial change in the lumen and outer wall of vertebrobasilar aneurysms. AJNR 29:259–264
2. Cebral J, Mut F, Weir J, Putman C (2011) Quantitative characterization of the hemodynamic environment in ruptured and unruptured brain aneurysms. AJNR 32:145–151
3. Frösen J, Piippo A, Paetau A, Kangasniemi M, Niemelä M, Hernesniemi J, Jääskeläinen J (2004) Remodeling of saccular cerebral artery aneurysm wall is associated with rupture: histological analysis of 24 unruptured and 42 ruptured cases. Stroke 35: 2287–2293
4. Lall R, Eddleman C, Bendok B, Batjer H (2009) Unruptured intracranial aneurysms and the assessment of rupture risk based on anatomical and morphologic factors: sifting through the sands of data. Neurosurg Focus 26(E2):1–5
5. Marbacher S, Erhardt S, Ai Schläppi J, Coluccia D, Remonda L, Fandino J, Sherif C (2011) Complex bi-lobular, bi-saccular, and broad-necked microsurgical aneurysms formation in the rabbit

bifurcation model for the study of upcoming endovascular techniques. AJNR 32:772–777
6. Park J, Lee C, Sim K, Huh J, Park J (2009) Imaging of the walls of saccular cerebral aneurysms with double inversion recovery black-blood sequence. J Magn Reson Imaging 30:1179–1183
7. Sherif C, Fandino J, Erhardt S, Di Ieva A, Killer M, Kleinpeter G, Marbacher S (2011) Microsurgical arterial-bifurcation aneurysms in the rabbit model: technical aspects. J Vis Exp 51:2718. doi:10.3791/2718
8. Sherif C, Marbacher S, Erhardt S, Fandino J (2011) Improved microsurgical creation of venous-pouch arterial-bifurcation aneurysms in rabbits. AJNR 32:165–169
9. Sherif C, Marbacher S, Fandino J (2009) High-resolution three-dimensional 3 T magnetic resonance angiography for the evaluation of experimental aneurysms in the rabbit. Neurol Res 31:869–872
10. Steinman D, Antiga L, Wasserman B (2010) Overestimation of cerebral aneurysm wall thickness by black blood MRI? J Magn Reson Imaging 31:766

Early Brain Injury and Neuroprotection

Early Events After Aneurysmal Subarachnoid Hemorrhage

Fatima A. Sehba and Victor Friedrich

Abstract The first 72 h after aneurysmal subarachnoid hemorrhage (SAH) is a critical period for the patient. Most of the deaths in the SAH patient population occur during this time, and a number of key events activate and trigger mechanisms that not only contribute to early brain injury but evolve over time and participate in the delayed complications. This review highlights the contribution of key events to the early brain injury and to overall outcome after SAH.

Keywords Aneurysmal subarachnoid hemorrhage • Early events • Chemical brain injury • Cerebral ischemia • Cerebral hyperemia • Intracranial hypertension

Introduction

Aneurysmal subarachnoid hemorrhage (SAH) accounts for 5 % of all stroke cases. SAH victims are in the prime of their lives, with a mean age of approximately 55 years of age [1]. Epidemiological and population-based studies show that the first 72 h are most crucial for survival and outcome (Fig. 1). During this period, patient mortality is substantial (45 %) and patient status relates well with the overall outcome. The overall consensus is that early treatment is essential to reduce injury and extend survival in this patient population.

Two phases of injury after SAH are recognized: the early phase, which begins at aneurysmal rupture and extends through the first 3 days, and the delayed phase, which appears 3–14 days later and is characterized by delayed vasospasm and delayed neurological deficits. Studies show that early injury is the product of the events that occur at or immediately after SAH. These *key* events can broadly be categorized as: blood release, acute reactive hyperemia, and transient global ischemia (Fig. 2). Each of these event triggers mechanisms that are specific to it or are shared among the events to create early brain injury (Fig. 3). These mechanisms may evolve with time and contribute to delayed phase complications. Here, we briefly review key events after SAH and the mechanisms that they activate.

F.A. Sehba, PhD (✉)
Departments of Neurosurgery and Neurosciences,
Mount Sinai School of Medicine,
1 Gustave L. Levy Place, New York, NY 10029, USA
e-mail: fatima.sehba@mssm.edu

V. Friedrich, PhD
Department of Neuroscience, Mount Sinai School of Medicine,
1. Gustave L. Levy Place, New York, NY 10029, USA

Subarachnoid Blood

The volume of subarachnoid blood correlates with the patient's status at admission and with neurological deficits and clinical outcome [2]. Blood can damage the brain by inducing mechanical and chemical trauma (Fig. 3a).

Mechanical Trauma

Mechanical trauma occurs as blood that is released under high pressure stretches the subarachnoid space, compresses the surrounding arteries, and elevates the intracranial pressure. Cerebral vasculature is very sensitive to changes in local environment and vessels constrict as they come in contact with blood. A short-lived constriction of large cerebral arteries is frequently observed in the first minutes after experimental SAH [3]. Blood, in addition, obstructs the passage of cerebrospinal fluid (CSF) and hence increases the risk of acute hydrocephalus, which is observed in as many as 50 % of SAH patients and is associated with poor outcome [4].

J. Fandino et al. (eds.), *Neurovascular Events After Subarachnoid Hemorrhage*, Acta Neurochirurgica Supplement, Vol. 120,
DOI 10.1007/978-3-319-04981-6_4, © Springer International Publishing Switzerland 2015

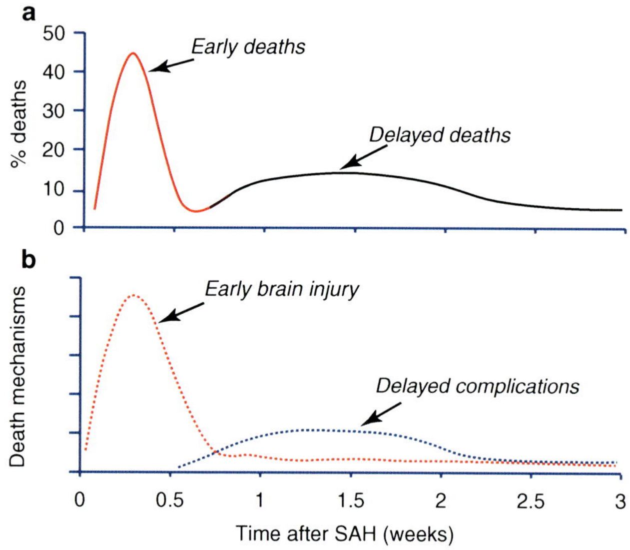

Fig. 1 Post SAH patient mortality and underlying mechanisms: mortality in SAH patients is greatest in the early phase (**a**). Although early mortality results from early activating mechanisms, delayed mortality is the product of both the early and the delayed developing complications (**b**). See text for explanation

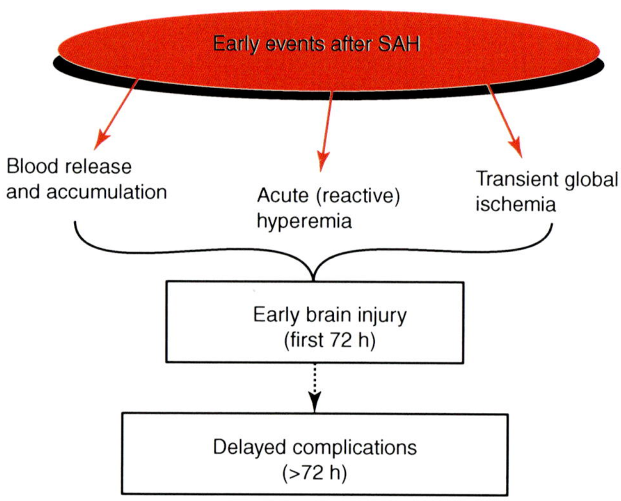

Fig. 2 The early events after SAH: broadly, early events after SAH can be divided as: release of blood, acute reactive hyperemia representing the Cushing response, and transient global ischemia. Each of these events triggers mechanisms that contribute to early brain injury and evolve with time to participate in delayed complications after SAH

Chemical Trauma

Chemical trauma is created by the products of subarachnoid blood lysis. Blood lysis begins within minutes after SAH and results in the appearance of oxyhemoglobin and xanthochromia in the CSF. Hence, xanthochromia is often used for clinical SAH diagnosis when CT scan results are negative [5]. At least three major products of clot lysis are implicated in SAH pathology: oxyhemoglobin, iron, and the recently discovered bilirubin oxidation products (BOXes).

Oxyhemoglobin

Oxyhemoglobin levels peak in the CSF at 24 h after SAH and decrease thereafter (from animal and patient cerebral microdialysis studies). Oxyhemoglobin is a potent spasmogen and is implicated in early arterial constriction and in delayed vasospasm after SAH [2, 6]. Studies that report that in vivo (subarachnoid space) and in vitro (basilar artery) exposure to oxyhemoglobin creates ultrastructural alterations in vascular morphology similar to those documented early after SAH support this implication [7]. These alterations include the appearance of cell craters, blebs, and vacuoles in endothelial cells and detachment of endothelium from the basement membrane [8]. Oxyhemoglobin is also cytotoxic to endothelial cells and astrocytes [9, 10]. The mechanisms underlying oxyhemoglobin-induced constriction include scavenging and creating a deficiency of nitric oxide (endothelial and neuronal) [11], suppression of voltage-dependent potassium currents [12], and an increase in endothelin (ET)-1 production [13].

Heme Metabolism Products

Heme is metabolized by heme oxygenase (HO)-1 into iron, biliverdin, and carbon monoxide [14].

Iron

Approximately 70 % (1,800 mg) of the body's iron is bound to hemoglobin in the form of heme; each hemoglobin molecule has four heme groups. As a result, a substantial amount of iron is released into the subarachnoid space after lysis of subarachnoid blood. HO-1 (see above) is upregulated and the expression of ferritin, an iron-binding protein, increases 1–3 days after SAH [15, 16]. The ferritin level in the CSF is considered a good diagnostic measure for SAH patients who present late to the clinic [17]. After SAH, ferritin expression increases in microglia, neurons, and cells in the adventitia of the arterial wall [15, 16, 18]. Lee et al. used an iron chelator, deferoxamine, to establish a role of iron in oxidative injury after SAH [18]. In this experiment, deferoxamine administered 3–6 h after SAH reduced cerebral iron deposits, HO-1 and ferritin expression, oxidative stress and neuronal apoptosis, and extended animal survival [18].

Bilirubin Oxidation Products (BOXes)

BOXes, as the name indicates, are formed upon oxidative degradation of bilirubin [19]. Bilirubin is formed by the action of biliverdin reductase on biliverdin (a product of heme metabolism; see above). BOXes are potent vasoconstrictors and are present in significantly higher concentration in the CSF of SAH patients who develop vasospasm than in the CSF of the patients who do not [20]. Hence, BOXes are being studied for their possible contribution to the pathogenesis of delayed vasospasm. A role of BOXes in early brain injury is anticipated but remains to be elucidated.

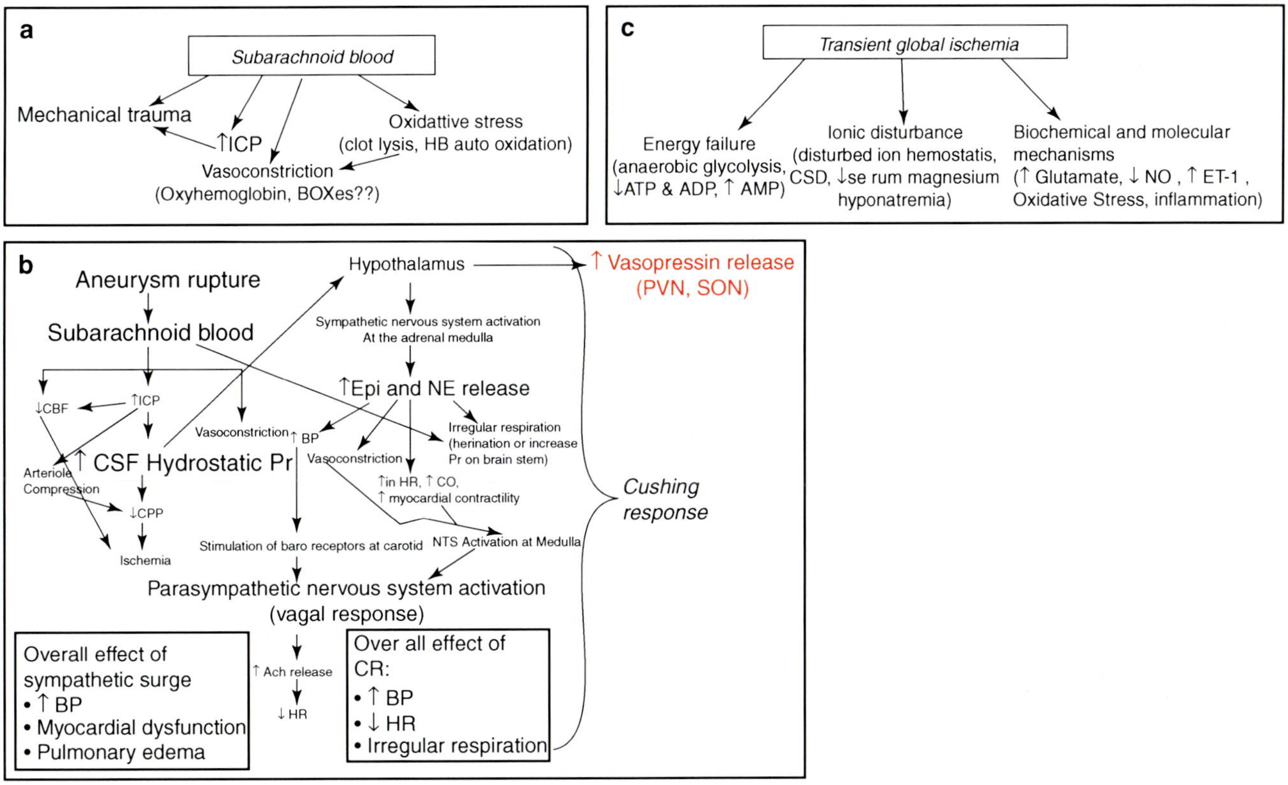

Fig. 3 Mechanisms of early brain injury after SAH: (**a**) outlines the mechanism by which subarachnoid blood participates in early brain injury after SAH; (**b**) outlines the triggers of the Cushing response (CR) after SAH, mechanisms that the CR activates, and the complications that follow; and (**c**) outlines the main mechanism by which transient global ischemia contributes to early brain injury after SAH

Acute Reactive Hyperemia; Cushing Response (CR)

The Cushing response (CR) is a compensatory hypothalamus-mediated response to a rise in intracranial pressure (ICP). The severity of the CR at SAH depends on the magnitude of rise in ICP, which in turn depends upon the volume of subarachnoid blood. The CR acts to maintain the difference between blood pressure (BP) and ICP to oppose drops in cerebral blood flow (cerebral perfusion pressure (CPP) = BP − ICP); however, it is not always successful [21]. In SAH patients, the CR is mostly observed as a sympathetic surge with increased serum epinephrine (EP) and/or norepinephrine (NE) levels. Two major complications, myocardial dysfunction and pulmonary edema, are associated with sympathetic surge [22] (Fig. 3b). These complications develop early after SAH and are often associated with poor patient outcome.

Cardiac Complications

In most SAH patients, cardiac complications appear immediately or develop within a few hours after aneurysmal rupture [22]. These complications include electrocardiographic (ECG) abnormalities, cardiac arrhythmias, and myocardial damage. ECG abnormalities develop within the first 48 h after SAH and reappear at rebleed [23–25]. Prominent ECG abnormalities include P wave abnormalities, prolonged QT interval, ST segment, and T-wave and are associated with poor neurologic grade on admission [26]. Cardiac arrhythmias can occur as the first symptom of acute SAH and are life threatening in 5–10 % of cases [27]. Major rhythmic abnormalities include sinus tachycardia, sinus bradycardia, and premature atrial and ventricular beats [25]. Myocardial injury is found in approximately 30–60 % of SAH patients and is associated with higher mortality [28–30]. Serum creatine kinase (CK)-MB and troponin-1 concentrations that are associated with myocardial injury are frequently increased within 24–48 h in SAH patients [28–30]. In addition, contraction band necrosis, myocardial fragmentation, and focal myocytolysis in the myocardium is found in autopsy of patients who died early after SAH [29–32]. In animals, increased serum CK-MB and cardiac troponin-1 are found as early as 10 min [33], and myocardial damage at 3 h, after SAH [32].

Pulmonary Complications

Pulmonary edema, also called neurogenic pulmonary edema, occurs in 10 % of all SAH cases and is a predominant complication in poor grade (Hunt and Hess grade III–V) patients [34]. Pulmonary edema usually develops within hours after SAH; however, a delayed form that appears 3–5 days after SAH is also reported [35]. In animals, leakage of lung capillaries occurs 8 min after injection of blood into the cisterna magna [36]. The nature of mechanisms underlying SAH-related pulmonary edema are cardiogenic (myocardial dysfunction leading to a raised hydrostatic pressure and fluid retention), noncardiogenic (such as acute lung injury or acute respiratory distress syndrome), and neurogenic (pressure of blood on respiratory centers at SAH) [34, 35].

Transient Global Ischemia (TGI)

Ischemia after SAH affects the entire brain and appears early. Mechanisms triggered by SAH-induced transient global ischemia (TGI) can be broadly classified as energy failure, ionic disturbances, and biochemical and molecular mechanisms (Fig. 3c). A brief description of these mechanisms is given below; for a review that is more detailed, an interested reader is referred to recent reviews [37, 38].

Energy Failure

Energy failure after SAH is mostly observed as changes in cerebral energy metabolism as detected in cerebral microdialysis studies. In addition, depletion of high-energy phosphate stores (fall in ATP and ADP and rise in AMP) in the cerebral cortex is noted as early as 6 h after experimental SAH [39, 40]. Cerebral microdialysis studies in animals have established that energy metabolism is disturbed within minutes after SAH, causing depletion of pyruvate and glucose and rises in lactate and in the lactate-to-pyruvate ratio [41, 42]. Similar findings are made in clinical SAH. Sarrafzadeh and colleagues noted that the lactate-to-pyruvate ratio remains significantly high for the first 8 days after SAH in patients with acute ischemic neurological deficits [42].

Ionic Changes

Energy is required to fuel ATPases to maintain ionic homeostasis across cell membranes. After SAH, as brain energy stores deplete, rapid alterations in ionic distributions across the membranes of brain cells and of cerebral vascular cells occur. In metabolically active neurons and astrocytes, as Na^+K^+-ATPases cease to work, intracellular Na^+ rises and, on reaching a critical point, reverses the operation of the Na^+–Ca^{2+} exchange carrier, creating increases in intracellular Ca^{2+} and extracellular K^+. Changes in neuronal ionic content promotes the cortical spreading depolarization and disturbed neurovascular coupling that contributes to the acute pathophysiology of SAH and the later-occurring delayed ischemic neurological deficits (DINDs) [43]. In cerebral endothelial and smooth muscle cells, a pathological rise in intracellular calcium promotes constriction [44, 45]. Other pathological consequences of rises in intracellular calcium include the release of neurotransmitters such as glutamate and activation of enzymes, including ones that are detrimental to cells, such as inducible nitric oxide (NO) synthase (iNOS) and caspases [46, 47].

Biochemical and Molecular Mechanisms

Although the list of biochemical and molecular mechanisms that activate early and contribute to SAH pathology is long, the key mechanisms are as follows:

Extracellular Glutamate

Animal cerebral microdialysis studies show that interstitial glutamate concentration increases after SAH, reaches a peak at 40 min, and is associated with early pathology [48, 49]. Clinically, microdialysis studies have found that, during the first 8 days after SAH, the cerebral glutamate concentration correlates with early and delayed status of SAH patients; the concentration is greatest in the patients who develop acute ischemic neurological deficits, and is elevated (although not as much) in patients who develop delayed ischemic neuronal deficits [42].

Nitric Oxide (NO)

Cerebral NO levels are altered after SAH. Cerebral NO levels decrease in animals minutes after SAH and increase at 24 h [11, 50]. Sehba et al. found that an NO donor administered early after SAH recovers the cerebral blood flow (CBF) reduction and prevents ischemic glutamate release in animals after SAH [49]. In the clinic, the initial increase in cerebral NO has not been studied, but an increase in NO level in the CSF at 24 h after SAH has been established [51, 52]. Patients with low NO levels in the CSF at 0–12 days after SAH are more prone to develop delayed vasospasm [51, 52].

Endothelin (ET)-1

An increase in CSF ET-1 is observed within minutes in animals and within 24 h in patients after SAH [53]. Because ET-1 is a potent spasmogen that produces long-lasting constriction, the potential of receptor antagonists in preventing the pathogenesis of delayed vasospasm after SAH was evaluated. These clinical trials successfully reduced/inhibited development of the delayed vasospasm but did not improve patient's outcomes [54, 55].

Inflammation

The status of acute mediators of inflammation, cells of the immune system (such as neutrophils and platelets), pro-inflammatory cytokines (interleukin (IL)-1β, IL-6, tumor necrosis factor (TNF)-α, and others), and adhesion molecules (intercellular adhesion molecule (ICAM)-1, P and S-selectins, and others), is studied after SAH. Animal studies establish overt vascular neutrophil accumulation, serum cytokine concentration, and expression of adhesion molecules within the hours after SAH and their associations with early brain injury [37]. In patients, similar increases in serum and CSF cytokines and in soluble forms of adhesion molecules (within 1–3 days from ictus) are established and associated with hyperthermia, vascular spasm, and unfavorable outcome [56–58].

Oxidative Stress

Oxidative stress after SAH is observed as the presence of lipid peroxidation products, decreased activities of enzymatic and non-enzymatic antioxidant systems, and generation of reactive oxidative species. In experimental animals, oxidative stress is present within the first 24 h [59] and, in patients, within the first 72 h after SAH [60]. In patients, an increase in lipid peroxidation products during the early phase of SAH is associated with the pathogenesis of delayed vasospasm and with poor outcome [61, 62].

Conclusion

In conclusion, a number of key events are activated within the first 72 h after SAH and trigger mechanisms that contribute to early brain injury and are also associated with delayed vasospasm and overall outcomes of patients. A better understanding of early mechanisms and their timely prevention may provide a superior strategy to improve clinical outcome in this patient population.

Conflict of Interest Statement We declare that we have no conflict of interest.

References

1. Le Roux PD, Winn HR (1998) Management of the ruptured aneurysm. Neurosurg Clin N Am 9:525–540
2. Macdonald RL, Weir BK (1991) A review of hemoglobin and the pathogenesis of cerebral vasospasm. Stroke 22:971–982
3. Simeone FA, Ryan KG, Cotter JR (1968) Prolonged experimental cerebral vasospasm. J Neurosurg 29:357–366
4. Dupont S, Rabinstein AA (2013) Extent of acute hydrocephalus after subarachnoid hemorrhage as a risk factor for poor functional outcome. Neurol Res 35:107–110
5. Vermeulen M, van Gijn J (1990) The diagnosis of subarachnoid haemorrhage. J Neurol Neurosurg Psychiatry 53:365–372
6. Ishiguro M, Murakami K, Link T, Zvarova K, Tranmer BI, Morielli AD, Wellman GC (2008) Acute and chronic effects of oxyhemoglobin on voltage-dependent ion channels in cerebral arteries. Acta Neurochir Suppl 104:99–102
7. Sehba FA, Friedrich V (2013) Cerebral microvasculature is an early target of subarachnoid hemorrhage. Acta Neurochir Suppl 115:199–205
8. Kajikawa H, Ohta T, Yoshikawa Y, Funatsu N, Yamamoto M, Someda K (1979) Cerebral vasospasm and hemoglobins – clinical and experimental studies. Neurol Med Chir (Tokyo) 19:61–71
9. Meguro T, Chen B, Lancon J, Zhang JH (2001) Oxyhemoglobin induces caspase-mediated cell death in cerebral endothelial cells. J Neurochem 77:1128–1135
10. Rollins S, Perkins E, Mandybur G, Zhang JH (2002) Oxyhemoglobin produces necrosis, not apoptosis, in astrocytes. Brain Res 945:41–49
11. Sehba FA, Schwartz AY, Chereshnev I, Bederson JB (2000) Acute decrease in cerebral nitric oxide levels after subarachnoid hemorrhage. J Cereb Blood Flow Metab 20:604–611
12. Ishiguro M, Morielli AD, Zvarova K, Tranmer BI, Penar PL, Wellman GC (2006) Oxyhemoglobin-induced suppression of voltage-dependent K+ channels in cerebral arteries by enhanced tyrosine kinase activity. Circ Res 99:1252–1260
13. Ohlstein EH, Storer BL (1992) Oxyhemoglobin stimulation of endothelin production in cultured endothelial cells. J Neurosurg 77:274–278
14. Maines MD (1997) The heme oxygenase system: a regulator of second messenger gases. Annu Rev Pharmacol Toxicol 37: 517–554
15. Ozawa H, Nishida A, Mito T, Takashima S (1994) Immunohistochemical study of ferritin-positive cells in the cerebellar cortex with subarachnoidal hemorrhage in neonates. Brain Res 651:345–348
16. Ono S, Zhang ZD, Marton LS, Yamini B, Windmeyer E, Johns L, Kowalczuk A, Lin G, Macdonald RL (2000) Heme oxygenase-1 and ferritin are increased in cerebral arteries after subarachnoid hemorrhage in monkeys. J Cereb Blood Flow Metab 20:1066–1076
17. Petzold A, Worthington V, Appleby I, Kerr ME, Kitchen N, Smith M (2011) Cerebrospinal fluid ferritin level, a sensitive diagnostic test in late-presenting subarachnoid hemorrhage. J Stroke Cerebrovasc Dis 20:489–493
18. Lee JY, Keep RF, He Y, Sagher O, Hua Y, Xi G (2010) Hemoglobin and iron handling in brain after subarachnoid hemorrhage and the effect of deferoxamine on early brain injury. J Cereb Blood Flow Metab 30:1793–1803
19. Kranc KR, Pyne GJ, Tao L, Claridge TD, Harris DA, Cadoux-Hudson TA, Turnbull JJ, Schofield CJ, Clark JF (2000) Oxidative degradation of bilirubin produces vasoactive compounds. Eur J Biochem 267:7094–7101
20. Pyne-Geithman GJ, Morgan CJ, Wagner K, Dulaney EM, Carrozzella J, Kanter DS, Zuccarello M, Clark JF (2005) Bilirubin production and oxidation in CSF of patients with cerebral vasospasm after subarachnoid hemorrhage. J Cereb Blood Flow Metab 25:1070–1077
21. Brinker T, Seifert V, Dietz H (1992) Cerebral blood flow and intracranial pressure during experimental subarachnoid haemorrhage. Acta Neurochir 115:47–52
22. Lee VH, Oh JK, Mulvagh SL, Wijdicks EF (2006) Mechanisms in neurogenic stress cardiomyopathy after aneurysmal subarachnoid hemorrhage. Neurocrit Care 5:243–249
23. Brouwers PJ, Wijdicks EF, Hasan D, Vermeulen M, Wever EF, Frericks H, van Gijn J (1989) Serial electrocardiographic recording in aneurysmal subarachnoid hemorrhage. Stroke 20:1162–1167
24. Eisalo A, Perasalo J, Halonen PI (1972) Electrocardiographic abnormalities and some laboratory findings in patients with subarachnoid haemorrhage. Br Heart J 34:217–226

25. Frontera JA, Parra A, Shimbo D, Fernandez A, Schmidt JM, Peter P, Claassen J, Wartenberg KE, Rincon F, Badjatia N, Naidech A, Connolly ES, Mayer SA (2008) Cardiac arrhythmias after subarachnoid hemorrhage: risk factors and impact on outcome. Cerebrovasc Dis 26:71–78
26. Sakr YL, Lim N, Amaral AC, Ghosn I, Carvalho FB, Renard M, Vincent JL (2004) Relation of ECG changes to neurological outcome in patients with aneurysmal subarachnoid hemorrhage. Int J Cardiol 96:369–373
27. van der Kleij FG, Henselmans JM, van de Loosdrecht AA (1999) Cardiac arrhythmia as initial presentation of aneurysmal subarachnoid hemorrhage. Neth J Med 55:242–246
28. Norris JW, Hachinski VC, Myers MG, Callow J, Wong T, Moore RW (1979) Serum cardiac enzymes in stroke. Stroke 10:548–553
29. Fabinyi G, Hunt D, McKinley L (1977) Myocardial creatine kinase isoenzyme in serum after subarachnoid haemorrhage. J Neurol Neurosurg Psychiatry 40:818–820
30. Zhu BL, Ishikawa T, Michiue T, Li DR, Zhao D, Bessho Y, Kamikodai Y, Tsuda K, Okazaki S, Maeda H (2007) Postmortem cardiac troponin I and creatine kinase MB levels in the blood and pericardial fluid as markers of myocardial damage in medicolegal autopsy. Leg Med (Tokyo) 9:241–250
31. Kolin A, Norris JW (1984) Myocardial damage from acute cerebral lesions. Stroke 15:990–993
32. Sato K, Masuda T, Izumi T (1999) Subarachnoid hemorrhage and myocardial damage clinical and experimental studies. Jpn Heart J 40:683–701
33. Masuda T, Sato K, Yamamoto S, Matsuyama N, Shimohama T, Matsunaga A, Obuchi S, Shiba Y, Shimizu S, Izumi T (2002) Sympathetic nervous activity and myocardial damage immediately after subarachnoid hemorrhage in a unique animal model. Stroke 33:1671–1676
34. Muroi C, Keller M, Pangalu A, Fortunati M, Yonekawa Y, Keller E (2008) Neurogenic pulmonary edema in patients with subarachnoid hemorrhage. J Neurosurg Anesthesiol 20:188–192
35. McLaughlin N, Bojanowski MW, Girard F, Denault A (2005) Pulmonary edema and cardiac dysfunction following subarachnoid hemorrhage. Can J Neurol Sci 32:178–185
36. Walder B, Brundler MA, Totsch M, Elia N, Morel DR (2002) Influence of the type and rate of subarachnoid fluid infusion on lethal neurogenic pulmonary edema in rats. J Neurosurg Anesthesiol 14:194–203
37. Sehba FA, Pluta RM, Zhang JH (2011) Metamorphosis of subarachnoid hemorrhage research: from delayed vasospasm to early brain injury. Mol Neurobiol 43:27–40
38. Sehba FA, Hou J, Pluta RM, Zhang JH (2012) The importance of early brain injury after subarachnoid hemorrhage. Prog Neurobiol 97:14–37
39. Fein JM (1976) Brain energetics and circulatory control after subarachnoid hemorrhage. J Neurosurg 45:498–507
40. Fein JM (1978) Brain energetics and cerebral death. Ann N Y Acad Sci 315:97–104
41. Gewirtz RJ, Dhillon HS, Goes SE, DeAtley SM, Scheff SW (1999) Lactate and free fatty acids after subarachnoid hemorrhage. Brain Res 840:84–91
42. Sarrafzadeh AS, Sakowitz OW, Kiening KL, Benndorf G, Lanksch WR, Unterberg AW (2002) Bedside microdialysis: a tool to monitor cerebral metabolism in subarachnoid hemorrhage patients? Crit Care Med 30:1062–1070
43. Dreier JP, Drenckhahn C, Woitzik J, Major S, Offenhauser N, Weber-Carstens S, Wolf S, Strong AJ, Vajkoczy P, Hartings JA (2013) Spreading ischemia after aneurysmal subarachnoid hemorrhage. Acta Neurochir Suppl 115:125–129
44. Kohno K, Sakaki S, Ohue S, Kumon Y, Matsuoka K (1991) Intracellular calcium levels in canine basilar artery smooth muscle following experimental subarachnoid hemorrhage: an electron microscopic cytochemical study. Acta Neuropathol 81:664–669
45. Wang J, Ohta S, Sakaki S, Araki N, Matsuda S, Sakanaka M (1994) Changes in Ca(++)-ATPase activity in smooth-muscle cell membranes of the canine basilar artery with experimental subarachnoid hemorrhage. J Neurosurg 80:269–275
46. Hubschmann OR (1987) The role of calcium in parenchymal cell injury in subarachnoid haemorrhage. Neurol Res 9:265–269
47. Sakaki S, Ohue S, Kohno K, Takeda S (1989) Impairment of vascular reactivity and changes in intracellular calcium and calmodulin levels of smooth muscle cells in canine basilar arteries after subarachnoid hemorrhage. Neurosurgery 25:753–761
48. Bederson JB, Levy AL, Ding WH, Kahn R, DiPerna CA, Jenkins AL 3rd, Vallabhajosyula P (1998) Acute vasoconstriction after subarachnoid hemorrhage. Neurosurgery 42:352–360
49. Sehba FA, Ding WH, Chereshnev I, Bederson JB (1999) Effects of S-nitrosoglutathione on acute vasoconstriction and glutamate release after subarachnoid hemorrhage. Stroke 30:1955–1961
50. Yatsushige H, Calvert JW, Cahill J, Zhang JH (2006) Limited role of inducible nitric oxide synthase in blood-brain barrier function after experimental subarachnoid hemorrhage. J Neurotrauma 23:1874–1882
51. Durmaz R, Ozkara E, Kanbak G, Arslan O, Dokumacioğlu A, Kartkaya K, Atasoy M (2008) Nitric oxide level and adenosine deaminase activity in cerebrospinal fluid of patients with subarachnoid hemorrhage. Turk Neurosurg 18:157–164
52. Jung CS, Oldfield EH, Harvey-White J, Espey MG, Zimmermann M, Seifert V, Pluta RM (2007) Association of an endogenous inhibitor of nitric oxide synthase with cerebral vasospasm in patients with aneurysmal subarachnoid hemorrhage. J Neurosurg 107:945–950
53. Wang X, Zhu C, Zhang G, Lu Y (1995) Changes of endothelin during cerebral vasospasm after experimental subarachnoid hemorrhage. Chin Med J (Engl) 108:586–590
54. Kramer A, Fletcher J (2009) Do endothelin-receptor antagonists prevent delayed neurological deficits and poor outcomes after aneurysmal subarachnoid hemorrhage?: a meta-analysis. Stroke 40:3403–3406
55. Etminan N, Vergouwen MD, Ilodigwe D, Macdonald RL (2011) Effect of pharmaceutical treatment on vasospasm, delayed cerebral ischemia, and clinical outcome in patients with aneurysmal subarachnoid hemorrhage: a systematic review and meta-analysis. J Cereb Blood Flow Metab 31:1443–1451
56. Mathiesen T, Edner G, Ulfarsson E, Andersson B (1997) Cerebrospinal fluid interleukin-1 receptor antagonist and tumor necrosis factor-alpha following subarachnoid hemorrhage. J Neurosurg 87:215–220
57. Dumont AS, Dumont RJ, Chow MM, Lin CL, Calisaneller T, Ley KF, Kassell NF, Lee KS (2003) Cerebral vasospasm after subarachnoid hemorrhage: putative role of inflammation. Neurosurgery 53:123–133; discussion 133–135
58. Kaynar MY, Tanriverdi T, Kafadar AM, Kacira T, Uzun H, Aydin S, Gumustas K, Dirican A, Kuday C (2004) Detection of soluble intercellular adhesion molecule-1 and vascular cell adhesion molecule-1 in both cerebrospinal fluid and serum of patients after aneurysmal subarachnoid hemorrhage. J Neurosurg 101:1030–1036
59. Gaetani P, Marzatico F, Rodriguez Y, Baena R, Pacchiarini L, Vigano T, Grignani G, Crivellari MT, Benzi G (1990) Arachidonic acid metabolism and pathophysiologic aspects of subarachnoid hemorrhage in rats. Stroke 21:328–332
60. Lin CL, Hsu YT, Lin TK, Morrow JD, Hsu JC, Hsu YH, Hsieh TC, Tsay PK, Yen HC (2006) Increased levels of F2-isoprostanes following aneurysmal subarachnoid hemorrhage in humans. Free Radic Biol Med 40:1466–1473
61. Kamezaki T, Yanaka K, Nagase S, Fujita K, Kato N, Nose T (2002) Increased levels of lipid peroxides as predictive of symptomatic vasospasm and poor outcome after aneurysmal subarachnoid hemorrhage. J Neurosurg 97:1302–1305
62. Hsieh YP, Lin CL, Shiue AL, Yin H, Morrow JD, Hsu JC, Hsieh TC, Wei HJ, Yen HC (2009) Correlation of F4-neuroprostanes levels in cerebrospinal fluid with outcome of aneurysmal subarachnoid hemorrhage in humans. Free Radic Biol Med 47:814–824

Mouse Genetic Background Is Associated with Variation in Secondary Complications After Subarachnoid Hemorrhage

Josephine A. D'Abbondanza, Elliot Lass, Jinglu Ai, and R. Loch Macdonald

Abstract Spontaneous subarachnoid hemorrhage (SAH) is a form of hemorrhagic stroke that accounts for approximately 7 % of all strokes worldwide and is associated with mortality in approximately 35 % of cases and morbidity in many of the survivors. Studies have suggested that genetic variations may affect the pathophysiology of SAH. The goal of this study was to investigate the effect of mouse genetic background on brain injury and large artery vasospasm after SAH. SAH was induced in seven inbred strains of mice, and the degree of large artery vasospasm and brain injury was assessed. After 48 h, SAH mice showed a significant reduction in middle cerebral artery diameter and increased neuronal injury in the cerebral cortex compared with sham-operated controls. Mouse strains also demonstrated variable degrees of vasospasm and brain injury. This data suggests that different genetic factors influence how much brain injury and vasospasm occur after SAH. Future investigations may provide insight into the causes of these differences between strains and into which genetic contributors may be responsible for vasospasm and brain injury after SAH.

Keywords Subarachnoid hemorrhage • Mice • Vasospasm • Brain injury

J.A. D'Abbondanza, MSc • R.L. Macdonald, MD, PhD (✉)
Division of Neurosurgery, St. Michael's Hospital,
30 Bond St., Toronto, ON M5B 1W8, Canada

Labatt Family Centre of Excellence in Brain Injury and Trauma Research, Keenan Research Centre of the Li Ka Shing Knowledge Institute of St. Michael's Hospital, Toronto, ON, Canada

Department of Surgery, Institute of Medical Science, University of Toronto, Toronto, ON, Canada
e-mail: macdonaldlo@smh.ca

E. Lass, BSc • J. Ai, MD, PhD
Division of Neurosurgery, St. Michael's Hospital,
30 Bond St., Toronto, ON M5B 1W8, Canada

Labatt Family Centre of Excellence in Brain Injury and Trauma Research, Keenan Research Centre of the Li Ka Shing Knowledge Institute of St. Michael's Hospital, Toronto, ON, Canada

Introduction

Subarachnoid hemorrhage (SAH) is a form of hemorrhagic stroke that can occur traumatically or spontaneously. The most common cause of spontaneous SAH is a ruptured intracranial aneurysm. SAH is associated with significant morbidity and mortality and, even with appropriate treatment, patients often experience secondary complications, such as angiographic vasospasm (aVSP) and delayed cerebral ischemia (DCI). Mouse models have been used extensively to study the pathophysiological changes that occur after SAH. Although these models are fairly successful at mimicking some of the secondary complications of SAH, there is still limited knowledge regarding how genetic variation may impact outcome after aneurysm rupture.

Previous studies of SAH in mice used predominately the C57BL/6J strain [3, 9] as well as transgenic mice with a mixed genetic background [12, 15]. Inherent genetic differences in susceptibility to stroke may mask the effects of gene mutations with the use of different background strains [5]. Although backcrossing over 12 generations is suggested to eliminate genetic heterogeneities, this may not be sufficient if the genes contributing to stroke sensitivity are located close to the mutated genes of interest [5]. The genetic background of mice has also been shown to influence spatial learning [18], excitotoxic cell death [14], the inflammatory response [16], neurogenesis [16], and brain and vascular anatomy [1, 4, 7, 10, 11, 17, 20].

In a model of hindlimb ischemia, BALB/c mice had worse flow (poor collaterals), worse recovery, less angiogenesis, and lower tumor necrosis factor (TNF)-α expression compared with C57BL/6 mice [2]. In addition, BALB/c mice had an almost complete absence of collaterals in the pial circulation and suffered greater ischemic damage of the cortex after middle cerebral artery occlusion (MCAO) compared with C57BL/6J mice [2]. This suggests that interstrain variability may be influenced by differences in collateral density. Research on ischemic stroke demonstrated that

DOI 10.1007/978-3-319-04981-6_5,

there are differences in infarct volume depending on the mouse strain used [6]. Keum and Marchuk induced cerebral infarction by permanent MCAO in 16 inbred mouse strains and performed genome-wide linkage analysis for infarct volume as a quantitative trait. They found a significant locus on mouse chromosome 7 that was responsible for the majority of the infarct volume variants, as well as loci on chromosomes 1 and 8 that accounted for a lesser degree of the difference.

There has been much research focused on identifying biomarkers and substances that make individuals susceptible to SAH; however, to our knowledge, no studies have been conducted on factors that may determine variation in a patient's injury sensitivity after SAH or that are aimed at finding genes that may alter susceptibility to brain injury and aVSP after SAH. Although a locus for sensitivity to cerebral infarction was found in a model of ischemic stroke [6], no similar studies have been conducted in experimental SAH. Studies of SAH in genetically manipulated mice represent an artificial state that may not accurately mirror the effect of the genetic variation if it occurred naturally. Therefore, to identify genes that may contribute to differences in the response to an injury, it may be useful to observe changes in a natural state. This study aims to identify how genetic background in inbred mouse strains results in variation in aVSP and brain injury after experimental SAH.

Methods

Animals and SAH Model

All experimental protocols were approved by the Animal Care Committee at St. Michael's Hospital, Toronto, Canada and were conducted in accordance with the regulations of the Canadian Counsel on Animal Care. We used 72 male mice weighing 20–25 g from seven inbred strains: C57BL6/J, DBA/2J, FVB/NJ, A/J, 129S/SvImJ, KK/HIJ, and BALB/c (Jackson Laboratories, Bar Harbor, ME, USA). Animals were anesthetized with spontaneous inhalation of isofluorane (5 % induction; 2–3 % maintenance) with an oxygen flow rate of 1 L/min. Body temperature was maintained at 37.0±0.5 °C with a homeothermic heating pad and rectal temperature probe (Harvard apparatus, Holliston, MA, USA).

The SAH model was performed according to a previously published protocol [13]. Briefly, the head was fixed in a stereotactic frame equipped with a mouse adaptor (Harvard apparatus) and stereotactic manipulators to hold a laser Doppler flow probe (BLT21, Transonics Systems, New York, NY, USA) and a 27-gauge spinal needle (BD Biosciences, San Jose, CA, USA). An incision was made in the midline of the anterior scalp to expose the skull and a burr hole was drilled 4.5 mm anterior to the bregma and lateral to the midline using a 0.9-mm STARRETT drill (TRANSCAT, New York, NY, USA) angled ventrally at 40°.

For the SAH group ($n=5$ per strain), nonautologous blood (80 µl) was withdrawn from a donor mouse of the same strain. Donor mice were anesthetized with an intraperitoneal injection of ketamine (120 mg/kg) and xylazine (30 mg/kg). The spinal needle was advanced at a 40° angle through the burr hole until the base of the skull was contacted (~5 mm) and withdrawn (~0.5–1 mm) to position the needle in the prechiasmatic cistern. Sixty microliters of the nonautologous blood was manually injected through the spinal needle over 10 s. The sham-operated group ($n=5$/strain) underwent the same procedure as the SAH group but the spinal needle was inserted without blood injection. Animals were sacrificed 48 h after SAH or sham surgery. They were anesthetized with an intraperitoneal injection of ketamine (120 mg/kg) and xylazine (30 mg/kg). Mice were perfused through the left cardiac ventricle with 0.9 % NaCl (1 ml), followed by 4 % paraformaldehyde in phosphate-buffered saline (5 ml). Brain sections were processed, embedded in paraffin, and cut into 5-µm-thick sections using a microtome (Leica, Wetzlar, Germany).

Hematoxylin and Eosin Staining

Brain sections were deparaffinized in xylene and rehydrated with decreasing concentrations of ethanol solutions. Slides were stained with hematoxylin and eosin, and coverslipped with a xylene-based mounting medium (Permount, Sigma-Aldrich, St. Louis, MO, USA). Samples were viewed using a light microscope (Olympus, Center Valley, PA, USA) and images were taken using constant parameters.

Fluoro-Jade B Staining

Fluoro-jade B (Histo-Chem, Jefferson, AR, USA) staining was performed according to a previously published protocol [13]. After deparaffinization and rehydration, the slides were incubated in 0.06 % potassium permanganate (VWR International, Strasbourg, France) for 15 min. Slides were then rinsed in deionized water and immersed in 0.001 % fluoro-jade B in 0.1 % acetic acid for 30 min. Slides were washed and dried at 60±1 °C for 15 min. Xylene was used to clear the slides and they were coverslipped with a nonaqueous, low fluorescence, styrene-based mounting medium

(Sigma-Aldrich). Slides were viewed under a light microscope with a fluorescent module (Olympus) and images were taken using constant parameters.

Data Quantification and Statistical Analysis

Images of the middle cerebral artery (MCA) were taken at 200× magnification and the lumen area and thickness of the MCA wall were quantified using Image J (NIH, Bethesda, MD, USA). After calibration, the MCA lumen area was outlined and measured with the free-hand tool. Artery wall thickness was measured at four equally spaced points around the circumference and averaged. To determine fluoro-jade B staining, we took images at 200× magnification of the entire cerebral cortex, hippocampus, and the basal ganglia, thalamus, and midbrain. Two blinded observers counted the number of degenerated neurons in these regions and measured the degree of MCA VSP; these values were averaged. Quantification was performed on all sham control and SAH samples.

All statistical analyses were performed using SigmaStat 3.1 (Systat Software Inc., San Jose, CA, USA). Data are presented as means ± standard error of the mean (SEM). Student's *t*-test was performed when two groups were compared and ANOVA was used when assessing significance across multiple groups. If the ANOVA was significant, pairwise comparisons were performed using Fisher LSD.

Results

Mortality

Mortality was 3 % (2 of 72 mice). Both deaths occurred in the SAH group immediately after blood injection in one KK/HIJ and one DBA/2J mouse. These mice did not survive to tissue collection (48 h) and were not included in analyses. No mortality was observed in sham-operated animals.

MCA Vasospasm

At 48 h, sham controls had no evidence of MCA contraction and the artery had a normal histological appearance. SAH mice had a large reduction in the lumen of the MCA and an increase in artery wall thickness with a corrugated appearance. The MCA lumen/wall thickness ratio was considerably smaller in SAH mice compared with their sham counterparts; this was statistically significant across all strains except DBA/2J and KK/HIJ (Student's *t*-test, $P<0.05$; Fig. 1). The MCA lumen/wall thickness ratio in sham mice was variable across strains but did not differ significantly. The level of vasoconstriction observed after SAH was similar across strains and was not statistically significant (ANOVA, $P>0.05$; Fig. 1). 129S1/SvImJ mice had the least MCA vasoconstriction, whereas FVB/NJ mice had the most.

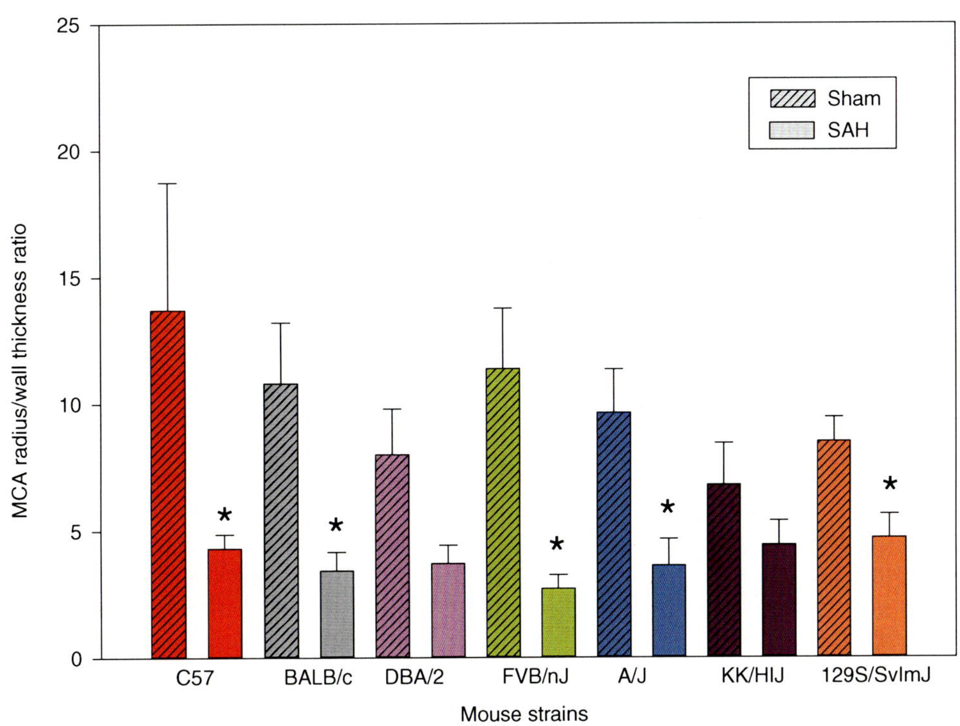

Fig. 1 MCA vasospasm in seven inbred mouse strains after sham and SAH surgery. Data expressed as mean MCA radius/wall thickness ratio ± SEM, * $P<0.05$, $n=5$ control and 5 SAH/strain

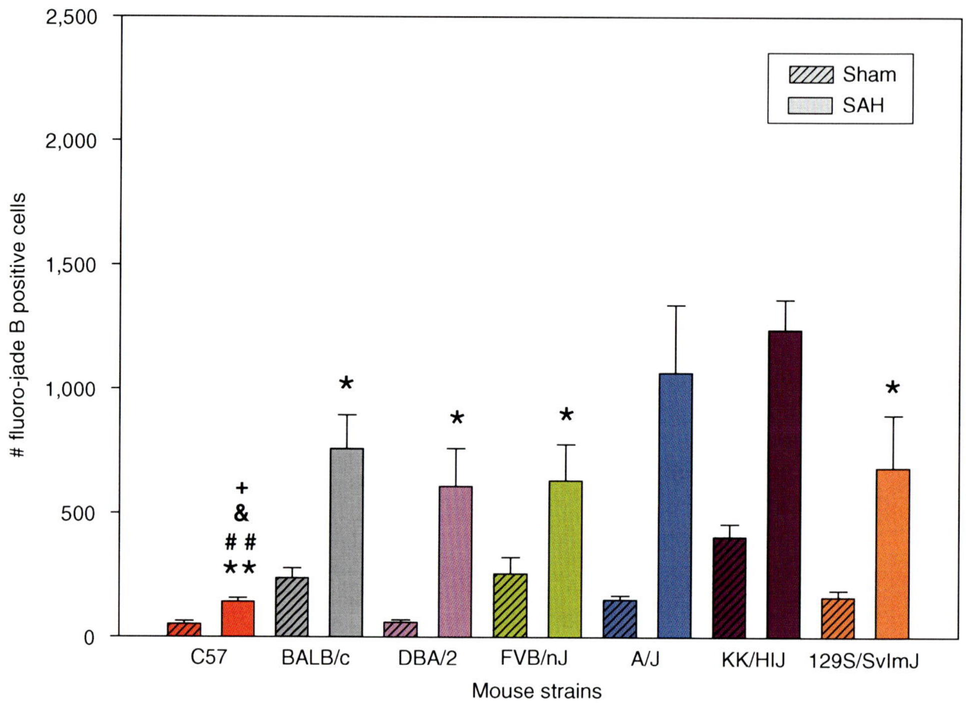

Fig. 2 Total number of fluoro-jade B-positive cells in coronal sections of seven inbred mouse strains after sham or SAH surgery. Data expressed as mean ± SEM, * $P<0.05$ compared with KK/HIJ, ** $P<0.001$ compared with KK/HIJ, ## $P<0.05$ compared with A/J, and $P<0.05$ compared with BALB/c, + $P<0.05$ compared with 129S1/SvImJ, ANOVA (Fisher LSD), $n=5$ control and 5 SAH/strain

Neuronal Degeneration

All SAH animals exhibited fluoro-jade B-positive cells in molecular layers 1 and 2 of the cerebral cortex and in the hippocampus and dentate gyrus. Sham animals had few to no fluoro-jade B-positive cells present. All SAH animals differed significantly from sham controls (Student's t-test, $P<0.05$). KK/HIJ mice had the greatest number of damaged neurons, whereas C57BL/6J mice had the least amount of brain damage (Fig. 2). Across strains, the difference in brain damage differed significantly between KK/HIJ and BALB/c, DBA/2J, FVB/NJ, and 129S1/SvImJ mice (ANOVA, Fisher LSD, $P<0.05$) and C57BL/6J mice ($P<0.001$). C57BL/6J mice also differed from A/J ($P<0.001$), BALB/c, and 129S1/SvImJ mice ($P<0.05$, Fig. 2).

Discussion

Previous work in ischemic stroke has demonstrated that inherent genetic differences in mice can contribute to differences in cerebral infarction [6]. Other studies have also identified differences across mouse strains in performance during the Morris water maze [17], neurogenesis [16], and natural brain and vascular anatomy [1, 4, 7, 10, 11, 17, 20]. Here we show that genetic background in seven inbred mouse strains can contribute to variation in the severity of aVSP and neuronal injury after experimental SAH.

In the current experiments, aVSP and brain injury were assessed in C57BL/6J, BALB/c, DBA/2J, FVB/NJ, A/J, KK/HIJ, and 129S1/SvImJ mouse strains. Forty-eight hours after SAH, strains showed differences in the severity of MCA VSP. All strains differed significantly from sham controls, except DBA/2J and KK/HIJ mouse strains (Student's t-test, $P<0.05$). 129S1/SvImJ mice had the least aVSP (largest MCA radius/wall thickness ratio), whereas FVB/NJ mice had the greatest aVSP (smallest MCA radius/wall thickness ratio); however, these differences were not statistically significant (Fig. 1). Differences across strains were also observed in terms of the total number of fluoro-jade B-positive neurons. All mice differed significantly from sham controls, with KK/HIJ and C57BL/6J mice showing the most and least neuronal degeneration, respectively (ANOVA, Fisher LSD, $P<0.05$; Fig. 2).

These underlying strain characteristics have important implications for the conduct of studies using mouse models. These findings suggest that because differences in VSP and brain injury have at least some genetic basis, experimental findings between different mouse strains should be compared with caution. Also, although transgenic technology is useful for the study of specific gene function, these mice are often a hybrid of multiple strains. Therefore, the amalgamation of traits may alter the reported levels of aVSP or neuronal injury, rather than what may be seen in the strain's natural state. It is suggested that backcrossing over 12 generations can eliminate genetic heterogeneities; however, this may not be sufficient if genes responsible for stroke sensitivity are located close to the mutated genes of interest [5]. Therefore, avoiding interstrain crosses may give the truest representation of results.

Across numerous mouse studies, the C57BL/6J strain tends to be more successful at enduring injury compared with other strains [6, 8, 11, 17]. This has implications for future experimental models. The C57BL/6J strain is most common in SAH studies, so the degree of brain injury and aVSP detected may be less than if other strains were used. Identifying the most appropriate strain to model human SAH is important for translational studies. It is possible that a strain exhibiting more brain injury may be a better representation of clinical SAH because approximately 10–15 % of patients with spontaneous aneurysmal SAH die before reaching the hospital [19]. More importantly, identifying the genetic basis for the variation in aVSP and brain injury between strains may lead to insight into the pathogenesis of these complications and potentially even to treatments for SAH.

Conclusion

Mouse genetic background can influence the degree of brain injury and aVSP after experimental SAH. FVB/NJ and 129S1/SvImJ mice had the most and least severe aVSP, while KK/HIJ and C57BL/6J had the most and least neuronal damage, respectively. These findings are important for animal modeling of disease, and suggest that the mouse strain used may alter the results of SAH studies. Identifying the appropriate strain to model human SAH is essential for translation from bench-to-bedside. Future investigations into the genetic factors that modify brain injury and aVSP across mouse strains may strengthen our understanding of secondary complications after clinical SAH.

Acknowledgments RLM receives grant support from the Physicians Services Incorporated Foundation, Brain Aneurysm Foundation, Canadian Stroke Network, Canadian Institutes of Health Research, and the Heart and Stroke Foundation of Ontario.

Conflict of Interest Statement RLM is Chief Scientific Officer of Edge Therapeutics. The remaining authors declare no conflict of interest.

References

1. Barone FC, Knudsen DJ, Nelson AH, Feuerstein GZ, Willette RN (1993) Mouse strain differences in susceptibility to cerebral ischemia are related to cerebral vascular anatomy. J Cereb Blood Flow Metab 13:683–692
2. Chalothorn D, Clayton JA, Zhang H, Pomp D, Faber JE (2007) Collateral density, remodeling, and VEGF-A expression differ widely between mouse strains. Physiol Genomics 30:179–191
3. Feiler S, Friedrich B, Scholler K, Thal SC, Plesnila N (2010) Standardized induction of subarachnoid hemorrhage in mice by intracranial pressure monitoring. J Neurosci Methods 190:164–170
4. Fujii M, Hara H, Meng W, Vonsattel JP, Huang Z, Moskowitz MA (1997) Strain-related differences in susceptibility to transient forebrain ischemia in SV-129 and C57black/6 mice. Stroke 28:1805–1810; discussion 1811
5. Gerlai R (1996) Gene-targeting studies of mammalian behavior: is it the mutation or the background genotype? Trends Neurosci 19:177–181
6. Keum S, Marchuk DA (2009) A locus mapping to mouse chromosome 7 determines infarct volume in a mouse model of ischemic stroke. Circ Cardiovasc Genet 2:591–598
7. Kitagawa K, Matsumoto M, Yang G, Mabuchi T, Yagita Y, Hori M, Yanagihara T (1998) Cerebral ischemia after bilateral carotid artery occlusion and intraluminal suture occlusion in mice: evaluation of the patency of the posterior communicating artery. J Cereb Blood Flow Metab 18:570–579
8. Lambertsen KL, Gregersen R, Finsen B (2002) Microglial-macrophage synthesis of tumor necrosis factor after focal cerebral ischemia in mice is strain dependent. J Cereb Blood Flow Metab 22:785–797
9. Lin CL, Calisaneller T, Ukita N, Dumont AS, Kassell NF, Lee KS (2003) A murine model of subarachnoid hemorrhage-induced cerebral vasospasm. J Neurosci Methods 123:89–97
10. Maeda K, Hata R, Hossmann KA (1999) Regional metabolic disturbances and cerebrovascular anatomy after permanent middle cerebral artery occlusion in C57black/6 and SV129 mice. Neurobiol Dis 6:101–108
11. Majid A, He YY, Gidday JM, Kaplan SS, Gonzales ER, Park TS, Fenstermacher JD, Wei L, Choi DW, Hsu CY (2000) Differences in vulnerability to permanent focal cerebral ischemia among 3 common mouse strains. Stroke 31:2707–2714
12. Sabri M, Ai J, Lakovic K, Macdonald RL (2013) Mechanisms of microthrombosis and microcirculatory constriction after experimental subarachnoid hemorrhage. Acta Neurochir Suppl 115:185–192
13. Sabri M, Jeon H, Ai J, Tariq A, Shang X, Chen G, Macdonald RL (2009) Anterior circulation mouse model of subarachnoid hemorrhage. Brain Res 1295:179–185
14. Schauwecker PE, Steward O (1997) Genetic determinants of susceptibility to excitotoxic cell death: implications for gene targeting approaches. Proc Natl Acad Sci U S A 94:4103–4108
15. Sehba FA, Flores R, Muller A, Friedrich V, Chen JF, Britz GW, Winn HR, Bederson JB (2010) Adenosine A(2A) receptors in early ischemic vascular injury after subarachnoid hemorrhage. Laboratory investigation. J Neurosurg 113:826–834
16. Steward O, Schauwecker PE, Guth L, Zhang Z, Fujiki M, Inman D, Wrathall J, Kempermann G, Gage FH, Saatman KE, Raghupathi R, McIntosh T (1999) Genetic approaches to neurotrauma research: opportunities and potential pitfalls of murine models. Exp Neurol 157:19–42
17. Sugimori H, Yao H, Ooboshi H, Ibayashi S, Iida M (2004) Krypton laser-induced photothrombotic distal middle cerebral artery occlusion without craniectomy in mice. Brain Res Brain Res Protoc 13:189–196
18. Upchurch M, Wehner JM (1988) DBA/2Ibg mice are incapable of cholinergically-based learning in the Morris water task. Pharmacol Biochem Behav 29:325–329
19. van Gijn J, Kerr RS, Rinkel GJ (2007) Subarachnoid haemorrhage. Lancet 369:306–318
20. Yang G, Kitagawa K, Matsushita K, Mabuchi T, Yagita Y, Yanagihara T, Matsumoto M (1997) C57BL/6 strain is most susceptible to cerebral ischemia following bilateral common carotid occlusion among seven mouse strains: selective neuronal death in the murine transient forebrain ischemia. Brain Res 752:209–218

The Value of Perfusion Computed Tomography (PCT) Imaging After Aneurysmal Subarachnoid Hemorrhage: A Review of the Current Data

Kerim Beseoglu, Nima Etminan, and Daniel Hänggi

Abstract *Background and Purpose*: The estimation of the extent of early brain injury (EBI) and sensitive detection of delayed cerebral ischemia (DCI) remains a major challenge in the context of aneurysmal subarachnoid hemorrhage (aSAH). Cerebral perfusion computed tomography (PCT) imaging is increasingly used as an additional diagnostic tool to monitor early brain injury as well as delayed cerebral ischemia after aSAH. Here, we review the current literature as well as the resulting implications and illustrate our institutional experience with PCT imaging in this context.

Methods: The current literature on PCT imaging for SAH was identified based on a search of the PubMed database. Patient cohorts were dichotomized according to the time of PCT after ictus into early PCT (<72 h after ictus) and subsequent PCT (>72 h after ictus). The specific aspects and findings of PCT at different times are compared and discussed.

Results: Sixteen relevant publications were identified, nine of which focused on early PCT and seven on subsequent PCT diagnostics after aSAH. Early PCT provided relevant details on the extent of EBI and identified patients at risk for developing DCI, whereas subsequent PCT imaging facilitated the monitoring and detection of DCI.

Conclusions: The present review demonstrates that PCT imaging is able to detect EBI as well as DCI in patients experiencing aSAH. As a consequence, this technique should be routinely implemented in monitoring strategies for this patient population.

K. Beseoglu, MD (✉) • N. Etminan, MD • D. Hänggi, MD
Department of Neurosurgery, Medical Faculty,
Heinrich-Heine-University, Moorenstrasse 5,
Düsseldorf 40225, Germany
e-mail: beseoglu@med.uni-duesseldorf.de

Keywords Perfusion-CT • SAH • Functional outcome • Early brain injury • Delayed cerebral ischemia

Introduction

The extent of primary or early brain injury (EBI) and the incidence of delayed cerebral ischemia (DCI) are predominant determinants for neurological outcome in patients after aneurysmal subarachnoid hemorrhage (aSAH) [5, 20]. Several noninvasive and invasive modalities have been used to monitor patients for EBI as well as DCI [3]. Within the last years, different clinical studies reported the use of perfusion computed tomography (PCT) in patients suffering from aSAH and, in general, suggest that PCT imaging in this context may provide data that is more comprehensive on macrocirculatory and microcirculatory impairment, as opposed to angiographic imaging of large proximal cerebral vessels [21]. The goal of the present article is to provide an overview of currently available data for PCT monitoring after aSAH.

Methods

A Medline search was conducted for articles published through July 2013 with the key words "subarachnoid hemorrhage" combined with (1) perfusion CT, (2) delayed cerebral ischemia, (3) vasospasm and/or (3) early brain injury, limited to publications in English and excluding animal studies. Case reports, reviews, and comments were not included in the present review. Subsequently, the resulting publications were dichotomized according to the time of PCT after initial aSAH into (a) early PCT, defined as PCT within 72 h after ictus, and (b) subsequent or follow-up PCT, defined as after 3 days but within the first 14 days.

DOI 10.1007/978-3-319-04981-6_6,

Results

A total of 16 studies were identified that evaluated the role of PCT after aSAH, nine in the early phase and seven with subsequent analysis (Table 1).

Summary of Early PCT Data

In the first 72 h after aSAH, the majority of patients demonstrated changes in cerebral blood flow (CBF) and cerebral blood volume (CBV), which suggests an impaired autoregulation [11]. This reduction of CBF may persist over the initial phase after hemorrhage, independent from intracranial pressure and/or cerebral perfusion pressure. Additionally, a strong correlation between impaired global perfusion and clinical presentation at admission was demonstrated using Xenon-enhanced CT imaging [15]. In line with the aforementioned decrease in CBF, a prolongation of mean transit time (MTT) was reported. Early MTT prolongation significantly correlated with early mortality and occurrence of angiographic vasospasm [9]. These findings were confirmed by data reporting an association of prolonged early MTT in the thalami with poor outcome [17]. Moreover, a global MTT prolongation in the first hours after aSAH was reported as an independent predictor for poor outcome [16].

Table 1 Tabular overview of recent relevant publications focusing on PCT after aSAH sorted by scanning time after ictus. The size of the patient cohort and the key finding of the respective publication are given

Time of PCT	Publication	Patient cohort	Time of scan	Key finding
Early PCT	Tateyama et al. [16]	21 patients	<3 h	Global MTT prolongation is an independent predictor of outcome
	Tsuang et al. [17]	38 patients	<6 h	Early bilateral prolonged MTT at the thalami is associated with poor outcome
	Etminan et al. [4]	79 patients	<12 h	Subarachnoid clot volume and early MTT prolongation have an amplified risk for DCI and poor outcome
	Schubert et al. [15]	17 patients	<12 h	The first 12 h after aSAH are characterized by reduction of CBF independent of ICP or CPP
	Honda et al. [6]	94 patients	24–72 h	Higher CBF and lower MTT was found in patients with favorable outcome
	Nabavi et al. [11]	15 patients	<48 h	The majority of patients showed changes in CBF and CBV with time suggestive of disturbed autoregulation
	Van der Schaaf et al. [19]	45 patients	<72 h	The development of DCI is related to brain perfusion assessed by PCT shortly after aSAH
	Sanelli et al. [13]	75 patients	<72 h	CBF reduction and MTT prolongation can be demonstrated early in aSAH patients who later develop vasospasm
	Van Asch et al. [18]	138 patients	<72 h	Acute hydrocephalus after aSAH reduces CBF in the deep grey matter and periventricular white matter
Follow-up PCT	Sanelli et al. [14]	97 patients	Day 6–8	CBF and MTT at days 6–8 have the highest diagnostic accuracy for DCI
	Pham et al. [12]	38 patients	>3 days, <14 days	Time to peak in PCT is a sensitive and early predictor of secondary cerebral infarction
	Dankbaar et al. [2]	42 patients	<3 days to 14 days	CBF and MTT values worsening precedes DCI
	Wintermark et al. [22]	27 patients	<3 days to 14 days	MTT represents the most sensitive parameter to detect vasospasm
	Kunze et al. [8]	53 patients	>3 days, <14 days	Repeatedly obtained PCT is a valuable tool to detect DCI
	Aralasmak et al. [1]	55 patients	Day 3 to day 15	PCT indicates high likelihood of perfusion abnormality in case of macrovascular vasospasm
	Moftakhar et al. [10]	14 patients	Day 1–15	High agreement between DSA and PCT for detection of DCI

MTT mean transit time, *DCI* delayed cerebral ischemia, *aSAH* aneurismal subarachnoid hemorrhage, *CBF* cerebral blood flow, *ICP* intracranial pressure, *CPP* cerebral perfusion pressure, *CBV* cerebral blood volume, *DSA* digital subtraction angiography

Additionally, we recently reported that the risk for new cerebral infarction and poor outcome is higher in patients with concomitant large subarachnoid clot volumes and ultra-early MTT prolongation, as opposed to sole MTT prolongation. Using a risk model based on these two variables, we defined three different risk groups for outcome prediction [4]. Changes in early cerebral perfusion, as detected by PCT, can be related to the risk for DCI because patients developing DCI show significantly more asymmetry in perfusion between the hemispheres in semiquantitative data sets [19]. An early reduction of CBF and prolongation of MTT within the first 72 h after aSAH was related to the incidence of subsequent DCI [13]. This was also supported by our own data [4]. Correspondingly, patients with favorable outcomes had increased CBF and lower MTT values. Thus, discriminant analysis of these parameters can predict patient outcome with fair probability [6]. Interestingly, early PCT can also show the effect of acute hydrocephalus on the CBF in the periventricular white matter and deep grey matter [18].

Summary of Subsequent PCT Data

For the period after the first 3 days after SAH ictus, a routine PCT screening is warranted, because perfusion changes may precede occurrence of DCI at several days [12]. A worsening of absolute and relative CBF and MTT values before the actual onset of clinical DCI has been demonstrated, with MTT being the most sensitive parameter for the diagnosis of angiographic vasospasm [22]. Here, increasing asymmetry between the hemispheres was found to be an important indicator for DCI [2]. In addition to MTT prolongation, time to peak (TTP) has been also reported as a sensitive and early predictor of DCI [12]. Standardized PCT screening from the immediate time after aSAH to day 14 or, if necessary, extended over 14 days is recommended [8]. A high agreement between digital subtraction angiography (DSA) and PCT for detection of DCI has been demonstrated; however, the highest diagnostic accuracy for DCI has been demonstrated for PCT at day 6–8 [10, 14]. At this time, positive and negative predictive values for detecting impeding DCI are comparable to DSA [7]. In case of angiographic vessel narrowing exceeding 50 %, PCT demonstrates a high likelihood of perfusion abnormality in the corresponding vascular territory [1].

Conclusion

The present review illustrates that PCT imaging is able to provide additional insight into the extent of EBI as well as the detection of DCI in patients suffering from aSAH. Thus, this technique should be routinely implemented in monitoring strategies for this patient population.

Conflict of Interest Statement We declare that we have no conflict of interest.

References

1. Aralasmak A, Akyuz M, Ozkaynak C, Sindel T, Tuncer R (2009) CT angiography and perfusion imaging in patients with subarachnoid hemorrhage: correlation of vasospasm to perfusion abnormality. Neuroradiology 51(2):85–93
2. Dankbaar JW, de Rooij NK, Smit EJ, Velthuis BK, Frijns CJ, Rinkel GJ, van der Schaaf IC (2011) Changes in cerebral perfusion around the time of delayed cerebral ischemia in subarachnoid hemorrhage patients. Cerebrovasc Dis 32(2):133–140
3. Diringer MN, Bleck TP, Claude Hemphill J 3rd, Menon D, Shutter L, Vespa P, Bruder N, Connolly ES Jr, Citerio G, Gress D, Hanggi D, Hoh BL, Lanzino G, Le Roux P, Rabinstein A, Schmutzhard E, Stocchetti N, Suarez JI, Treggiari M, Tseng MY, Vergouwen MD, Wolf S, Zipfel G (2011) Critical care management of patients following aneurysmal subarachnoid hemorrhage: recommendations from the Neurocritical Care Society's Multidisciplinary Consensus Conference. Neurocrit Care 15(2):211–240
4. Etminan N, Beseoglu K, Heiroth HJ, Turowski B, Steiger HJ, Hanggi D (2013) Early perfusion computerized tomography imaging as a radiographic surrogate for delayed cerebral ischemia and functional outcome after subarachnoid hemorrhage. Stroke 44(5):1260–1266
5. Fergusen S, Macdonald RL (2007) Predictors of cerebral infarction in patients with aneurysmal subarachnoid hemorrhage. Neurosurgery 60(4):658–667; discussion 667
6. Honda M, Sase S, Yokota K, Ichibayashi R, Yoshihara K, Sakata Y, Masuda H, Uekusa H, Seiki Y, Kishi T (2012) Early cerebral circulatory disturbance in patients suffering subarachnoid hemorrhage prior to the delayed cerebral vasospasm stage: xenon computed tomography and perfusion computed tomography study. Neurol Med Chir (Tokyo) 52(7):488–494
7. Killeen RP, Mushlin AI, Johnson CE, Comunale JP, Tsiouris AJ, Delaney H, Dunning A, Sanelli PC (2011) Comparison of CT perfusion and digital subtraction angiography in the evaluation of delayed cerebral ischemia. Acad Radiol 18(9):1094–1100
8. Kunze E, Pham M, Raslan F, Stetter C, Lee JY, Solymosi L, Ernestus RI, Vince GH, Westermaier T (2012) Value of perfusion CT, transcranial Doppler sonography, and neurological examination to detect delayed vasospasm after aneurysmal subarachnoid hemorrhage. Radiol Res Pract 2012:231206
9. Laslo AM, Eastwood JD, Pakkiri P, Chen F, Lee TY (2008) CT perfusion-derived mean transit time predicts early mortality and delayed vasospasm after experimental subarachnoid hemorrhage. AJNR Am J Neuroradiol 29(1):79–85
10. Moftakhar R, Rowley HA, Turk A, Niemann DB, Kienitz BA, Van Gomple J, Baskaya MK (2006) Utility of computed tomography perfusion in detection of cerebral vasospasm in patients with subarachnoid hemorrhage. Neurosurg Focus 21(3):E6
11. Nabavi DG, LeBlanc LM, Baxter B, Lee DH, Fox AJ, Lownie SP, Ferguson GG, Craen RA, Gelb AW, Lee TY (2001) Monitoring cerebral perfusion after subarachnoid hemorrhage using CT. Neuroradiology 43(1):7–16
12. Pham M, Johnson A, Bartsch AJ, Lindner C, Mullges W, Roosen K, Solymosi L, Bendszus M (2007) CT perfusion predicts secondary cerebral infarction after aneurysmal subarachnoid hemorrhage. Neurology 69(8):762–765

13. Sanelli PC, Jou A, Gold R, Reichman M, Greenberg E, John M, Cayci Z, Ugorec I, Rosengart A (2011) Using CT perfusion during the early baseline period in aneurysmal subarachnoid hemorrhage to assess for development of vasospasm. Neuroradiology 53(6): 425–434
14. Sanelli PC, Ugorec I, Johnson CE, Tan J, Segal AZ, Fink M, Heier LA, Tsiouris AJ, Comunale JP, John M, Stieg PE, Zimmerman RD, Mushlin AI (2011) Using quantitative CT perfusion for evaluation of delayed cerebral ischemia following aneurysmal subarachnoid hemorrhage. AJNR Am J Neuroradiol 32(11):2047–2053
15. Schubert GA, Seiz M, Hegewald AA, Manville J, Thome C (2009) Acute hypoperfusion immediately after subarachnoid hemorrhage: a xenon contrast-enhanced CT study. J Neurotrauma 26(12): 2225–2231
16. Tateyama K, Kobayashi S, Murai Y, Teramoto A (2013) Assessment of cerebral circulation in the acute phase of subarachnoid hemorrhage using perfusion computed tomography. J Nippon Med Sch 80(2):110–118
17. Tsuang FY, Chen JY, Lee CW, Li CH, Lee JE, Lai DM, Hu FC, Tu YK, Hsieh ST, Wang KC (2012) Risk profile of patients with poor-grade aneurysmal subarachnoid hemorrhage using early perfusion computed tomography. World Neurosurg 78(5):455–461
18. van Asch CJ, van der Schaaf IC, Rinkel GJ (2010) Acute hydrocephalus and cerebral perfusion after aneurysmal subarachnoid hemorrhage. AJNR Am J Neuroradiol 31(1):67–70
19. van der Schaaf I, Wermer MJ, van der Graaf Y, Hoff RG, Rinkel GJ, Velthuis BK (2006) CT after subarachnoid hemorrhage: relation of cerebral perfusion to delayed cerebral ischemia. Neurology 66(10):1533–1538
20. Vergouwen MD (2011) Vasospasm versus delayed cerebral ischemia as an outcome event in clinical trials and observational studies. Neurocrit Care 15(2):308–311
21. Washington CW, Zipfel GJ (2011) Detection and monitoring of vasospasm and delayed cerebral ischemia: a review and assessment of the literature. Neurocrit Care 15(2):312–317
22. Wintermark M, Ko NU, Smith WS, Liu S, Higashida RT, Dillon WP (2006) Vasospasm after subarachnoid hemorrhage: utility of perfusion CT and CT angiography on diagnosis and management. AJNR Am J Neuroradiol 27(1):26–34

Neurovascular Events After Subarachnoid Hemorrhage: Focusing on Subcellular Organelles

Sheng Chen, Haijian Wu, Jiping Tang, Jianmin Zhang, and John H. Zhang

Abstract Subarachnoid hemorrhage (SAH) is a devastating condition with high morbidity and mortality rates due to the lack of effective therapy. Early brain injury (EBI) and cerebral vasospasm (CVS) are the two most important pathophysiological mechanisms for brain injury and poor outcomes for patients with SAH. CVS has traditionally been considered the sole cause of delayed ischemic neurological deficits after SAH. However, the failure of antivasospastic therapy in patients with SAH supported changing the research target from CVS to other mechanisms. Currently, more attention has been focused on global brain injury within 3 days after ictus, designated as EBI. The dysfunction of subcellular organelles, such as endoplasmic reticulum stress, mitochondrial failure, and autophagy–lysosomal system activation, has developed during EBI and delayed brain injury after SAH. To our knowledge, there is a lack of review articles addressing the direction of organelle dysfunction after SAH. In this review, we discuss the roles of organelle dysfunction in the pathogenesis of SAH and present the opportunity to develop novel therapeutic strategies of SAH via modulating the functions of organelles.

Keywords Organelles • Subarachnoid Hemorrhage • Early Brain Injury • Cerebral Vasospasm • Therapy

S. Chen, MD
Department of Neurosurgery, Second Affiliated Hospital, School of Medicine, Zhejiang University, Hangzhou, Zhejiang, China

Department of Physiology and Pharmacology, Loma Linda University, 11041 Campus St, Loma Linda, CA 92354, USA

H. Wu, BS • J. Zhang, MD
Department of Neurosurgery, Second Affiliated Hospital, School of Medicine, Zhejiang University, Hangzhou, Zhejiang, China

J. Tang, MD • J.H. Zhang, MD, PhD (✉)
Department of Physiology and Pharmacology, Loma Linda University, 11041 Campus St, Loma Linda, CA 92354, USA
e-mail: johnzhang3910@yahoo.com

Introduction

Subarachnoid hemorrhage (SAH), which only accounts for 5 % of stroke, is often a devastating condition because of significant morbidity and mortality [58, 73]. Among SAH, 85 % are caused by intracranial ruptured aneurysms, termed spontaneous aneurysmal SAH [63]. Although much progress has been made with the surgical clip and endovascular coil for intracranial ruptured aneurysms over the last decade, long-term outcomes for patients with SAH are still unsatisfactory [9, 49]. Further elucidation of the pathogenesis is helpful for developing novel therapeutic interventions for SAH.

To date, early brain injury (EBI) and cerebral vasospasm (CVS) are the two most important determinants for poor outcome in patients with SAH [43, 55]. CVS, which occurs between 3 and 14 days after SAH [11], is traditionally considered the sole cause of delayed ischemic neurological deficits (DINDs) [23, 51]. Endothelin (ET)-1, a potent vasoconstrictor, plays a key role in CVS after SAH [53]. However, randomized, double-blind, placebo-controlled trials demonstrated that the ET-1 receptor antagonist, clazosentan, which can significantly ameliorate angiographic vasospasm, failed to improve functional outcomes in patients with SAH [35, 36]. Furthermore, CVS was a common imaging finding in approximately 70 % of patients with SAH, but only one-third of those patients went on to suffer from DINDs [1]. Those findings suggest that SAH-induced DINDs may be a result of multiple factors. The importance of EBI (which occurs within the first 72 h after SAH) has recently been emphasized because of its potentially critical role in the pathophysiology of SAH [5]. Inflammation, oxidative stress, excitotoxicity, and impaired ionic homeostasis (but not mechanical force) have all been proposed as having a role in EBI and other types of stroke [56, 60]. To date, studies of the alteration of organelles after SAH have included endoplasmic reticulum

The authors Sheng Chen and Haijian Wu contributed equally to this work.

DOI 10.1007/978-3-319-04981-6_7,

(ER) stress, mitochondrial dysfunction, and activation of the autophagy–lysosomal system. Neurobehavioral deficits were dependent on the disturbance of organelles in several kinds of cerebral cells. A new review focusing on disturbance or alteration of organelle function is helpful in understanding the pathophysiology of SAH [16]. Targeting organelles may provide a novel therapeutic potential for SAH treatment.

Appropriate animal models are imperative in understanding the pathogenesis of and treatment strategies for SAH [61]. This review summarizes preclinical evidence of the functional alteration of subcellular organelles in the pathogenesis of SAH. This is followed by a discussion of future research directions in developing new therapeutic strategies of SAH via modulating the organelles.

The Functional Alteration of Organelles Within the Progression of SAH

The main subcellular organelles in central nervous system (CNS) cells are the nucleus, ER, mitochondria, lysosomes, ribosomes, and Golgi body. Experimental studies have demonstrated that some subcellular organelles, including the ER, mitochondria, and autophagy–lysosomal system, have altered functions after SAH and are implicated in the pathophysiology of SAH. In the following sections, we describe the underlying roles of these organelles in SAH (Fig. 1).

Nucleus: Transcription Factor Activation

The Nuclear Factor-Erythroid 2-Related Factor 2 (Nrf2)-Antioxidant Response Element (ARE) Signaling

The nuclear factor-erythroid 2-related factor 2 (Nrf2)–antioxidant response element (ARE) pathway was the key regulator in maintaining cellular homeostasis via antioxidant defense, making it a therapeutic candidate for SAH [3]. Nrf2 is a cap 'n' collar (CNC) transcription factor, which possesses a basic region leucine zipper structure [76]. In the latent state, Nrf2 is sequestered by Kelch-like erythroid cell-derived protein with CNC homology-associated protein 1 (Keap1)-dependent ubiquitination–proteasomal degradation in the cytoplasm. Modifying critical cysteine thiols of Keap1 and Nrf2 by some oxidants promotes Nrf2 dissociation from the Keap1/Nrf2 complex and translocation into nuclei. Subsequently, Nrf2 binds to ARE in the promoter of cytoprotective genes leading to upregulated expression of relevant proteins, such as heme oxygenase-1, NAD(P)H:quinone oxidoreductase 1, and glutathione-*S*-transferase [34, 64].

Evidence from experimental SAH research indicates a protective role of the Nrf2/ARE pathway in EBI and CVS after SAH. Nrf2/ARE signaling was activated during the EBI period after SAH [66, 74]. Post-SAH treatment with melatonin and recombinant human erythropoietin reduced brain edema and improved neurobehavioral outcome via activating the Nrf2/ARE pathway and modulating oxidative stress after SAH, making these drugs promising for treatment. In addition, an elevated level of Nrf2 was detected in endothelial and smooth muscle cells in the basilar arterial walls [65]. The activation of Nrf2 increased in the arterial wall, parallel to the development of basilar artery vasospasm, in a double-injection SAH rabbit model. Because of the elevated expression of Nrf2, the Nrf2/ARE pathway was hypothesized to prevent CVS after SAH [78]. In an in vitro SAH model, sulforaphane, an agonist of the Nrf2–ARE pathway, can inhibit oxyhemoglobin (OxyHb)-induced inflammatory cytokine, such as interleukin (IL)-1β, IL-6, and tumor necrosis factor (TNF)-α, release in vascular smooth muscle cells [77]. Oxyhemoglobin-induced inflammation was aggravated in astrocytes from Nrf2-knockout mice via nuclear factor (NF)-κB signaling [45]. Thus, the Nrf2/ARE pathway may exert anti-inflammatory and antioxidative effects that contribute to alleviation of EBI and CVS after SAH. However, additional in vivo experiments using Nrf2 agonists or antagonists are required to further investigate the role of Nrf2 on SAH-induced brain injury.

NF-κB Signaling

NF-κB signaling is involved in various CNS disorders because it regulates immune and inflammatory responses including infection, brain trauma, neurodegenerative diseases, and stroke [48, 54]. In mammalian cells, the NF-κB family of transcription factors consists of five members, Rel A (p65), c-Rel, Rel B, p50, and p52. Under inactive conditions, NF-κB is sequestered in the cytoplasm by binding with IκB family members. The IκB kinase (IKK) enzyme complex can phosphorylate IκB proteins to release active NF-κB, leading to translocation of NF-κB into the nucleus. Subsequently, NF-κB dimmers (p50–p65) are free to bind to the promoters of genes of inflammatory mediators and increase the release of those mediators [42]. An in vitro study demonstrated that the phosphorylation of IκB diminishes its association with NF-κB, leading to NF-κB translocation into the nucleus, where NF-κB binds to the promoter of nitric oxide synthase (NOS)-2 in endothelial cells [8].

NF-κB signaling in SAH has been explored and some trials are ongoing trials. Toll-like receptor (TLR)-4 is an important upstream receptor of NF-κB. At the acute stage of SAH, TLR4/NF-κB signaling is significantly activated, suggesting that this pathway may regulate the inflammatory response in experimental SAH [33]. Post-SAH administration of progesterone attenuated EBI via suppressing the activation of

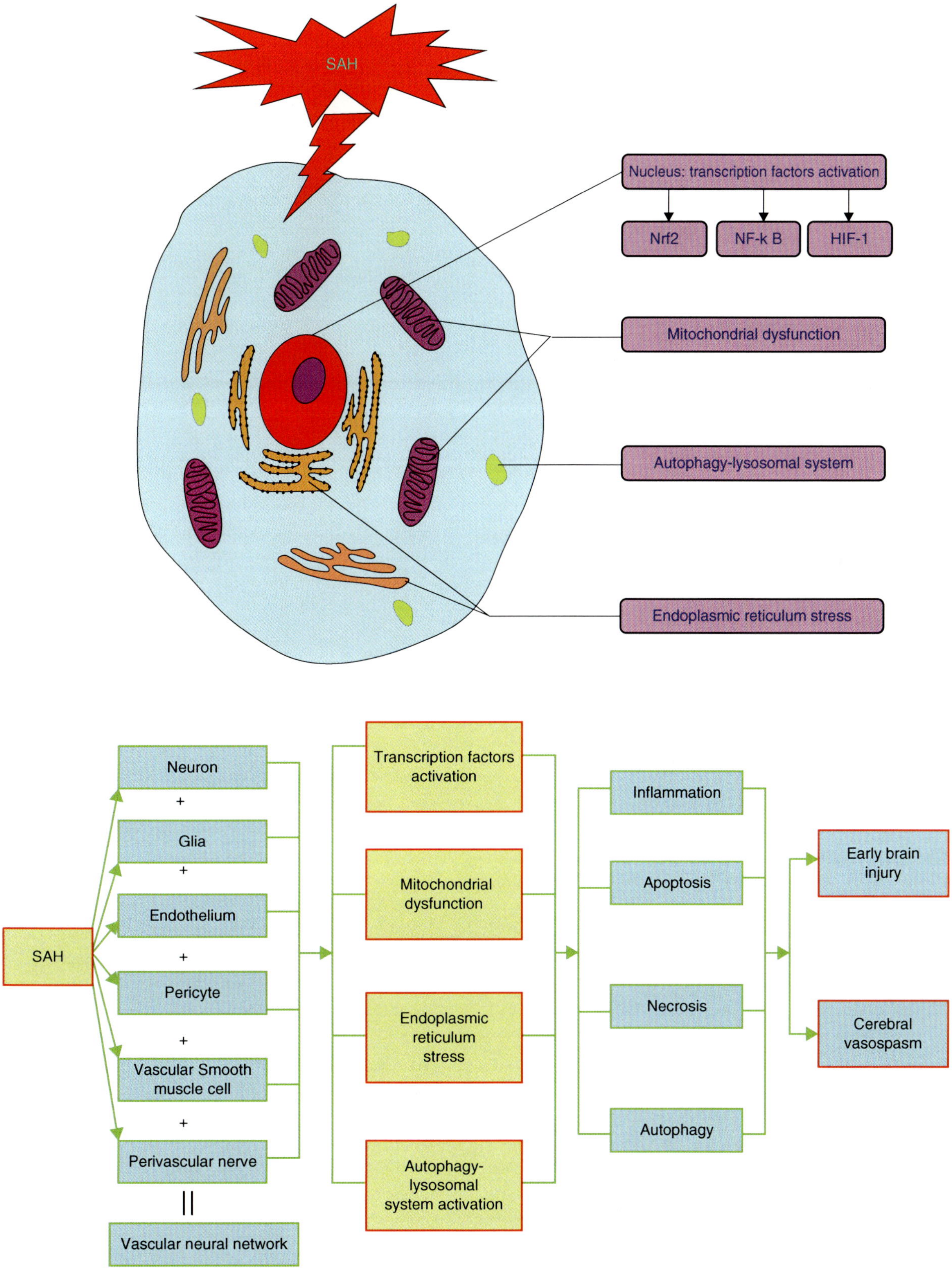

Fig. 1 The functional disturbance of organelles in the pathogenesis of SAH. The components of the vascular neural network of the brain, including neurons, glia, endothelium, pericytes, vascular smooth muscle cells, and perivascular nerves, all suffer from SAH-induced injuries. The dysfunctions/functional alterations of the organelles that take place are in the transcription factors (e.g., Nrf2, NF-κB, and HIF-1), mitochondrial dysfunction, endoplasmic reticulum stress, and the autophagy–lysosomal system. These pathophysiologic cascades play a critical role in inflammation, apoptosis, necrosis, and autophagy in brain parenchyma after SAH

TLR4/NF-κB signaling in the cortex after SAH [68]. p65, a nuclear NF-κB subunit, was overexpressed in the basilar artery, which indicated that the NF-κB-mediated inflammatory response may also facilitate the development of CVS after SAH. Intracisternal administration of pyrrolidine dithiocarbamate, an inhibitor of NF-kB, reduced the levels of TNF-α, IL-1β, intercellular adhesion molecule (ICAM)-1, and vascular cell adhesion molecule (VCAM)-1 and alleviated CVS in a rat model of SAH [79]. In addition, Nle4, DPhe7-α-MSH (NDP-MSH) and trehalose exerted protective effects on CVS via inhibiting NF-κB signaling in the basilar artery [13, 15]. Similarly, 6-mercaptopurine increased the level of IκB, downregulating NF-κB activity. Thus, 6-mercaptopurine was capable of hindering the production of inflammatory cytokines (e.g., IL-1β, IL-6, and TNF-α) after SAH. The anti-inflammatory effect of 6-mercaptopurine contributed to its antivasospastic property in SAH animals [7]. Furthermore, because of the association of p65 with the estrogen receptor, 17β-estradiol blocked the binding of p65 to the gene target inducible NOS (iNOS). Therefore, this hormone drug reduced iNOS and showed a neuroprotective effect on CVS [57]. The activation of NF-κB was biphasic in a single injection rabbit SAH model. The peaks of NF-κB activity occurred around day 3 and day 10 after SAH. The first peak plays a prominent role in neuronal injury, but the exact role of the second peak requires additional investigation [72].

In conclusion, these data indicated an essential role of the NF-κB pathway in the pathogenesis of EBI and CVS after SAH.

Hypoxia-Inducible Factor (HIF)-1

HIF-1 is a critical regulator of cellular adaptation to hypoxic stress and is a heterodimeric DNA-binding complex composed of one α- and one β-subunit [30, 37]. Cytoplasmic HIF-1α is continuously degraded via ubiquitination in normoxic conditions. However, in hypoxia, the proteasomal degradation of HIF-1α is inhibited, leading to HIF-1α accumulation. Nondegraded HIF-1α recruits HIF-1β to form the functional HIF complex, which enters the nucleus. HIF-1 binds in the location of hypoxia response elements to induce the transcription activation of these genes (e.g., erythropoietin, vascular endothelial growth factor (VEGF), and heme oxygenase (HO)-1) [2].

During the EBI, the expression of HIF-1α, VEGF, and BNIP3 were increased in the hippocampus and cortex [44]. Hyperbaric oxygen reduced the expression of HIF-1α and its target genes (including VEGF and BNIP3), which resulted in fewer apoptotic cells [12]. A recent study demonstrated that HIF-1α may exert a deleterious effect in EBI by upregulating its downstream proteins BNIP3 and VEGF, resulting in cell apoptosis, blood brain barrier (BBB) disruption, and brain edema [69]. However, 3-(5′-hydroxymethyl-2′-furyl)-1-benzylinda-zole (YC-1), a HIF-1α inhibitor, increased cell apoptosis in the hippocampus and increased cognitive function damage in SAH rats, suggesting that HIF-1α might exert beneficial effects in SAH [10].

In the brainstem, an upregulated HIF-1α protein level, but not mRNA level, was detected in the acute (10 min) and chronic (7 days) phases of SAH. The difference in levels between protein and mRNA is not yet clear. Deferoxamine promoted the expression and activity of HIF-1α, which ameliorated basilar artery vasospasm [20]. Additionally, isoflurane significantly attenuated vasospasm by increasing endothelial HIF-1 and iNOS in SAH mice [38]. Conversely, HIF-1α was suggested as an important contributor in the development of CVS in other studies. 2-Methoxyestradiol might reduce CVS and improve neurological deficient via inhibiting HIF-1α/VEGF and HIF-1α/BNIP3 apoptotic pathways after SAH [70].

To date, both beneficial and detrimental effects of HIF-1α have been found in SAH. Therefore, the exact mechanism of HIF-1α in the pathogenesis of SAH is not yet fully elucidated.

Mitochondrial Dysfunction

Mitochondria, the double-membrane organelle, are the primary energy-generating systems in most eukaryotic cells. Mitochondria play a vital role in cellular bioenergetics, function, and survival [29]. Mitochondrial dysfunction leads to a serial of detrimental consequences, including collapse of the mitochondrial inner transmembrane potential, disruption of mitochondrial biogenesis, overproduction of reactive oxygen species, outflow of matrix calcium, and release of apoptogenic proteins [6, 25]. Mitochondrial disturbance, as a starting mechanism, results in apoptosis and necrosis.

Mitochondrial dysfunction in neuronal cells of the cortex has been described in EBI. SB203580, a p38-specific inhibitor, might prevent mitochondrial depolarization, increase ATP content and decrease cytochrome *c* release. SB203580 administration attenuated mitochondrial impairment-induced neuronal apoptosis [21]. However, the molecular mechanism of SB203580 in the amelioration of mitochondrial dysfunction is not yet fully elucidated. Tea polyphenols inhibited mitochondrial membrane potential polarization, leading to increased ATP content, and blocked cytochrome *c* release in the cerebral cortex [41]. Taken together, mitochondrial dysfunction likely plays an important role in the pathogenesis of SAH, especially in apoptosis.

Autophagy–Lysosomal System

The lysosome, an acidic organelle, is the terminal proteolytic compartment in cells. It can degrade macromolecules from endocytosis, phagocytosis, and autophagy [32, 52]. Autophagy, a lysosomal degradation pathway, is involved in protein degradation and clearing, defective organelle turnover, and cellular remodeling [39]. Some sequential processes of autophagy are phagophores, autophagosomes, the fusing of autophagosomes with lysosomes, degradation, and recycling/reuse of degradative products [40, 62]. Microtubule-associated protein light chain-3 (LC-3) is an autophagosome biomarker. Beclin-1 is a Bcl-2-interacting protein required for autophagy [26].

Increasing attention has been paid to the diverse role of autophagy in CNS disorders. Appropriate autophagic activity can facilitate the clearance of the dysfunctional/aging macromolecules and organelles, thus it can promote neuronal survival, whereas excessive autophagy induces cell death and is detrimental [59].

The activation of autophagy in neurons was detected in the EBI period after SAH [28]. The autophagy activity in cortical neurons peaked at 24 h and recovered at 48 h after SAH. Rapamycin, an autophagy activator, ameliorated cortical neuronal apoptosis, brain edema, and BBB breakdown by increasing autophagy-related signaling (LC-3 and beclin-1) 24 h after SAH. Conversely, 3-methyladenine, an autophagy inhibitor, decreased the level of autophagy-related proteins and worsened neurological deficits [67]. Furthermore, simvastatin suppressed apoptosis and attenuated EBI via enhancing autophagy [75]. The activation of autophagy prevented activation of SAH-induced neuronal caspase-dependent and -independent pathways to inhibit apoptosis [22]. However, the mutual link between autophagy and apoptosis after SAH is still unclear and needs to be further investigated.

The role of autophagy in the pathogenesis of cerebral CVS after SAH also has been investigated. Cystatin C increased LC-3 in the artery wall 48 h after SAH, which attenuated SAH-induced CVS [31].

Taken together, these data indicate that autophagy may be a potential effective target for preventing EBI and CVS after SAH, but that more investigation focusing on the precise mechanism is required.

ER Stress

The ER is a cellular organelle with a network of tubular membranes and is responsible for calcium storage and signaling as well as for protein folding and processing [46]. Once the ER is impaired by some pathophysiological insult, unfolded proteins accumulate in the lumen of the ER [24]. To cope with lethal conditions, the ER has a variety of stress responses, including unfolded protein response, ER overload response, and ER-associated degradation. Those responses can block the new synthesis of unfolded proteins, but can also promote the degradation of unfolded or misfolded proteins, which is important for restoring normal ER function. At the same time, ER stress can also cause a disturbance in ER function and eventually lead to apoptosis of the affected cells [47].

ER dysfunction is involved in the pathogenesis of CNS disorders, including SAH [46, 50]. The p53-upregulated modulator of apoptosis (PUMA) promotes apoptosis of endothelial cell and results in BBB disruption after SAH. PUMA siRNA suppressed the expression of ER-related proteins in microvascular endothelial cells of the hippocampus [71]. Further studies are likely to yield the exact mechanisms behind PUMA, ER stress, and apoptosis. C/EBP homologous protein (CHOP) overexpression was recently found to possibly play an important role in the ER stress-induced apoptotic cascades after SAH. CHOP silencing by small interfering RNA is capable of inhibiting apoptosis, reducing BBB disruption, and improving neurological function after SAH [17].

ER stress plays a critical role in the development of CVS as well. CHOP was elevated in the basilar artery after SAH. CHOP knockout by its siRNA could reduce bim and cleaved caspase-3 while increasing bcl-2 in vascular tissues; therefore, suppressing endothelial apoptosis and ameliorating CVS after SAH [18]. Overall, ER stress may be an important response in EBI and CVS after SAH.

Future Directions and Conclusion

The incomplete knowledge of the mechanisms of SAH and loose translational research hinder the development of targeted therapies for this devastating disease [27]. Currently, the significance of functional disturbance of organelles in the pathophysiology of SAH is emerging. Further identification of the precise roles of each organelle in SAH pathogenesis will help to elucidate the exact molecular mechanisms and create hope in discovering effective treatments for this devastating form of stroke. Electron microscopy or other imaging technologies will be useful in observing the phenotypic transformation of organelles after SAH. Organelle-specific manipulations may be effective for SAH therapy. Furthermore, because organelles are a collection of interrelated components, multitarget therapeutic strategies that focus on multiple organelles is likely to be more efficient for SAH treatment. Moreover, considering the significance of EBI on the outcome of SAH, more efforts on EBI are required to develop a novel treatment paradigm [14, 51]. Finally, sex differences in the organelles need to be emphasized in experimental studies [4, 19].

In conclusion, the functional disturbance of organelles contributes to the pathogenesis of EBI and CVS after SAH by transcription factor entry into the nucleus, ER stress, mitochondrial dysfunction, and autophagy–lysosomal system activation. The crosstalk among these organelles and their exact roles in SAH remain unclear. Further exploration to address these issues will broaden our knowledge of the pathogenesis of SAH and facilitate the development of novel therapeutic strategies for SAH.

Acknowledgement This study was supported by a National Institutes of Health grant (NS053407) to JH Zhang and by a National Natural Science Foundation of China grant (No.81171096) to JM Zhang.

Conflict of Interest Statement We declare that we have no conflict of interest.

References

1. Alaraj A, Charbel FT, Amin-Hanjani S (2009) Peri-operative measures for treatment and prevention of cerebral vasospasm following subarachnoid hemorrhage. Neurol Res 31:651–659
2. Bain JM, Moore L, Ren Z, Simonishvili S, Levison SW (2013) Vascular endothelial growth factors A and C are induced in the SVZ following neonatal hypoxia-ischemia and exert different effects on neonatal glial progenitors. Transl Stroke Res 4:158–170
3. Baird L, Dinkova-Kostova AT (2011) The cytoprotective role of the Keap1-Nrf2 pathway. Arch Toxicol 85:241–272
4. Bramlett HM (2013) Importance of sex in the pathophysiology and treatment of acute CNS repair. Transl Stroke Res 4:379–380
5. Caner B, Hou J, Altay O, Fuj M 2nd, Zhang JH (2012) Transition of research focus from vasospasm to early brain injury after subarachnoid hemorrhage. J Neurochem 123(Suppl 2):12–21
6. Chan DC (2006) Mitochondria: dynamic organelles in disease, aging, and development. Cell 125:1241–1252
7. Chang CZ, Wu SC, Lin CL, Hwang SL, Kwan AL (2012) Purine anti-metabolite attenuates nuclear factor kappaB and related pro-inflammatory cytokines in experimental vasospasm. Acta Neurochir (Wien) 154:1877–1885
8. Chen LC, Hsu C, Chiueh CC, Lee WS (2012) Ferrous citrate up-regulates the NOS2 through nuclear translocation of NFkappaB induced by free radicals generation in mouse cerebral endothelial cells. PLoS One 7:e46239
9. Coppadoro A, Citerio G (2011) Subarachnoid hemorrhage: an update for the intensivist. Minerva Anestesiol 77:74–84
10. Dong Y, Li Y, Feng D, Wang J, Wen H, Liu D, Zhao D, Liu H, Gao G, Yin Z, Qin H (2013) Protective effect of HIF-1alpha against hippocampal apoptosis and cognitive dysfunction in an experimental rat model of subarachnoid hemorrhage. Brain Res 1517:114–121
11. Dorsch NW, King MT (1994) A review of cerebral vasospasm in aneurysmal subarachnoid haemorrhage part I: incidence and effects. J Clin Neurosci 1:19–26
12. Dzietko M, Derugin N, Wendland MF, Vexler ZS, Ferriero DM (2013) Delayed VEGF treatment enhances angiogenesis and recovery after neonatal focal rodent stroke. Transl Stroke Res 4:189–200
13. Echigo R, Shimohata N, Karatsu K, Yano F, Kayasuga-Kariya Y, Fujisawa A, Ohto T, Kita Y, Nakamura M, Suzuki S, Mochizuki M, Shimizu T, Chung UI, Sasaki N (2012) Trehalose treatment suppresses inflammation, oxidative stress, and vasospasm induced by experimental subarachnoid hemorrhage. J Transl Med 10:80
14. Fujii M, Yan J, Rolland WB, Soejima Y, Caner B, Zhang JH (2013) Early brain injury, an evolving frontier in subarachnoid hemorrhage research. Transl Stroke Res 4:432–446
15. Gatti S, Lonati C, Acerbi F, Sordi A, Leonardi P, Carlin A, Gaini SM, Catania A (2012) Protective action of NDP-MSH in experimental subarachnoid hemorrhage. Exp Neurol 234:230–238
16. Gump W, Laskowitz DT (2008) Management of post-subarachnoid hemorrhage vasospasm. Curr Atheroscler Rep 10:354–360
17. He Z, Ostrowski RP, Sun X, Ma Q, Huang B, Zhan Y, Zhang JH (2012) CHOP silencing reduces acute brain injury in the rat model of subarachnoid hemorrhage. Stroke 43:484–490
18. He Z, Ostrowski RP, Sun X, Ma Q, Tang J, Zhang JH (2012) Targeting C/EBP homologous protein with siRNA attenuates cerebral vasospasm after experimental subarachnoid hemorrhage. Exp Neurol 238:218–224
19. Herson PS, Palmateer J, Hurn PD (2013) Biological sex and mechanisms of ischemic brain injury. Transl Stroke Res 4:413–419
20. Hishikawa T, Ono S, Ogawa T, Tokunaga K, Sugiu K, Date I (2008) Effects of deferoxamine-activated hypoxia-inducible factor-1 on the brainstem after subarachnoid hemorrhage in rats. Neurosurgery 62:232–240; discussion 240–231
21. Huang L, Wan J, Chen Y, Wang Z, Hui L, Li Y, Xu D, Zhou W (2013) Inhibitory effects of p38 inhibitor against mitochondrial dysfunction in the early brain injury after subarachnoid hemorrhage in mice. Brain Res 1517:133–140
22. Jing CH, Wang L, Liu PP, Wu C, Ruan D, Chen G (2012) Autophagy activation is associated with neuroprotection against apoptosis via a mitochondrial pathway in a rat model of subarachnoid hemorrhage. Neuroscience 213:144–153
23. Kassell NF, Sasaki T, Colohan AR, Nazar G (1985) Cerebral vasospasm following aneurysmal subarachnoid hemorrhage. Stroke 16:562–572
24. Kaufman RJ (1999) Stress signaling from the lumen of the endoplasmic reticulum: coordination of gene transcriptional and translational controls. Genes Dev 13:1211–1233
25. Kroemer G, Dallaporta B, Resche-Rigon M (1998) The mitochondrial death/life regulator in apoptosis and necrosis. Annu Rev Physiol 60:619–642
26. Kumari S, Anderson L, Farmer S, Mehta SL, Li PA (2012) Hyperglycemia alters mitochondrial fission and fusion proteins in mice subjected to cerebral ischemia and reperfusion. Transl Stroke Res 3:296–304
27. Lapchak PA, Zhang JH, Noble-Haeusslein LJ (2013) RIGOR guidelines: escalating STAIR and STEPS for effective translational research. Transl Stroke Res 4:279–285
28. Lee JY, He Y, Sagher O, Keep R, Hua Y, Xi G (2009) Activated autophagy pathway in experimental subarachnoid hemorrhage. Brain Res 1287:126–135
29. Lin MT, Beal MF (2006) Mitochondrial dysfunction and oxidative stress in neurodegenerative diseases. Nature 443:787–795
30. Lisy K, Peet DJ (2008) Turn me on: regulating HIF transcriptional activity. Cell Death Differ 15:642–649
31. Liu Y, Cai H, Wang Z, Li J, Wang K, Yu Z, Chen G (2013) Induction of autophagy by cystatin C: a potential mechanism for prevention of cerebral vasospasm after experimental subarachnoid hemorrhage. Eur J Med Res 18:21
32. Luzio JP, Pryor PR, Bright NA (2007) Lysosomes: fusion and function. Nat Rev Mol Cell Biol 8:622–632
33. Ma CX, Yin WN, Cai BW, Wu J, Wang JY, He M, Sun H, Ding JL, You C (2009) Toll-like receptor 4/nuclear factor-kappa B signaling detected in brain after early subarachnoid hemorrhage. Chin Med J (Engl) 122:1575–1581
34. Ma Q (2013) Role of nrf2 in oxidative stress and toxicity. Annu Rev Pharmacol Toxicol 53:401–426
35. Macdonald RL, Higashida RT, Keller E, Mayer SA, Molyneux A, Raabe A, Vajkoczy P, Wanke I, Bach D, Frey A, Marr A, Roux S,

Kassell N (2011) Clazosentan, an endothelin receptor antagonist, in patients with aneurysmal subarachnoid haemorrhage undergoing surgical clipping: a randomised, double-blind, placebo-controlled phase 3 trial (CONSCIOUS-2). Lancet Neurol 10:618–625

36. Macdonald RL, Kassell NF, Mayer S, Ruefenacht D, Schmiedek P, Weidauer S, Frey A, Roux S, Pasqualin A (2008) Clazosentan to overcome neurological ischemia and infarction occurring after subarachnoid hemorrhage (CONSCIOUS-1): randomized, double-blind, placebo-controlled phase 2 dose-finding trial. Stroke 39:3015–3021
37. Majmundar AJ, Wong WJ, Simon MC (2010) Hypoxia-inducible factors and the response to hypoxic stress. Mol Cell 40:294–309
38. Milner E, Harries MD, Vellimana AK, Gidday JM, Han BH, Zipfel GJ (2013) Post-conditioning with isoflurane reduces SAH-induced vasospasm and microthrombosis via hypoxia-inducible factor 1 and nitric oxide synthase. Neurosurgery 60(Suppl 1):181
39. Mizushima N (2005) The pleiotropic role of autophagy: from protein metabolism to bactericide. Cell Death Differ 12(Suppl 2):1535–1541
40. Mizushima N (2007) Autophagy: process and function. Genes Dev 21:2861–2873
41. Mo H, Chen Y, Huang L, Zhang H, Li J, Zhou W (2013) Neuroprotective effect of tea polyphenols on oxyhemoglobin induced subarachnoid hemorrhage in mice. Oxid Med Cell Longev 2013:743938
42. Napetschnig J, Wu H (2013) Molecular basis of NF-kappaB signaling. Annu Rev Biophys 42:443–468
43. Naraoka M, Munakata A, Matsuda N, Shimamura N, Ohkuma H (2013) Suppression of the Rho/Rho-kinase pathway and prevention of cerebral vasospasm by combination treatment with statin and fasudil after subarachnoid hemorrhage in rabbit. Transl Stroke Res 4:368–374
44. Ostrowski RP, Colohan AR, Zhang JH (2005) Mechanisms of hyperbaric oxygen-induced neuroprotection in a rat model of subarachnoid hemorrhage. J Cereb Blood Flow Metab 25:554–571
45. Pan H, Wang H, Zhu L, Mao L, Qiao L, Su X (2011) Depletion of Nrf2 enhances inflammation induced by oxyhemoglobin in cultured mice astrocytes. Neurochem Res 36:2434–2441
46. Paschen W (2003) Endoplasmic reticulum: a primary target in various acute disorders and degenerative diseases of the brain. Cell Calcium 34:365–383
47. Paschen W, Mengesdorf T (2005) Cellular abnormalities linked to endoplasmic reticulum dysfunction in cerebrovascular disease–therapeutic potential. Pharmacol Ther 108:362–375
48. Pasparakis M (2009) Regulation of tissue homeostasis by NF-kappaB signalling: implications for inflammatory diseases. Nat Rev Immunol 9:778–788
49. Rinkel GJ, Algra A (2011) Long-term outcomes of patients with aneurysmal subarachnoid haemorrhage. Lancet Neurol 10:349–356
50. Roussel BD, Kruppa AJ, Miranda E, Crowther DC, Lomas DA, Marciniak SJ (2013) Endoplasmic reticulum dysfunction in neurological disease. Lancet Neurol 12:105–118
51. Rowland MJ, Hadjipavlou G, Kelly M, Westbrook J, Pattinson KT (2012) Delayed cerebral ischaemia after subarachnoid haemorrhage: looking beyond vasospasm. Br J Anaesth 109:315–329
52. Saftig P, Klumperman J (2009) Lysosome biogenesis and lysosomal membrane proteins: trafficking meets function. Nat Rev Mol Cell Biol 10:623–635
53. Saggu R (2013) Characterisation of Endothelin-1-Induced intra-striatal lesions within the juvenile and adult rat brain using MRI and 31P MRS. Transl Stroke Res 4:351–367
54. Sarkar FH, Li Y, Wang Z, Kong D (2008) NF-kappaB signaling pathway and its therapeutic implications in human diseases. Int Rev Immunol 27:293–319
55. Sehba FA, Hou J, Pluta RM, Zhang JH (2012) The importance of early brain injury after subarachnoid hemorrhage. Prog Neurobiol 97:14–37
56. Sehba FA, Pluta RM, Zhang JH (2011) Metamorphosis of subarachnoid hemorrhage research: from delayed vasospasm to early brain injury. Mol Neurobiol 43:27–40
57. Shih HC, Lin CL, Lee TY, Lee WS, Hsu C (2006) 17beta-Estradiol inhibits subarachnoid hemorrhage-induced inducible nitric oxide synthase gene expression by interfering with the nuclear factor kappa B transactivation. Stroke 37:3025–3031
58. Simard JM, Tosun C, Ivanova S, Kurland DB, Hong C, Radecki L, Gisriel C, Mehta R, Schreibman D, Gerzanich V (2012) Heparin reduces neuroinflammation and transsynaptic neuronal apoptosis in a model of subarachnoid hemorrhage. Transl Stroke Res 3:155–165
59. Smith CM, Chen Y, Sullivan ML, Kochanek PM, Clark RS (2011) Autophagy in acute brain injury: feast, famine, or folly? Neurobiol Dis 43:52–59
60. Switzer JA, Sikora A, Ergul A, Waller JL, Hess DC, Fagan SC (2012) Minocycline prevents IL-6 increase after acute ischemic stroke. Transl Stroke Res 3:363–368
61. Tajiri N, Dailey T, Metcalf C, Mosley YI, Lau T, Staples M, van Loveren H, Kim SU, Yamashima T, Yasuhara T, Date I, Kaneko Y, Borlongan CV (2013) In vivo animal stroke models: a rationale for rodent and non-human primate models. Transl Stroke Res 4:308–321
62. Uchiyama Y, Shibata M, Koike M, Yoshimura K, Sasaki M (2008) Autophagy-physiology and pathophysiology. Histochem Cell Biol 129:407–420
63. van Gijn J, Kerr RS, Rinkel GJ (2007) Subarachnoid haemorrhage. Lancet 369:306–318
64. Vomhof-Dekrey EE, Picklo MJ Sr (2012) The Nrf2-antioxidant response element pathway: a target for regulating energy metabolism. J Nutr Biochem 23:1201–1206
65. Wang Z, Chen G, Zhu WW, Zhou D (2010) Activation of nuclear factor-erythroid 2-related factor 2 (Nrf2) in the basilar artery after subarachnoid hemorrhage in rats. Ann Clin Lab Sci 40:233–239
66. Wang Z, Ma C, Meng CJ, Zhu GQ, Sun XB, Huo L, Zhang J, Liu HX, He WC, Shen XM, Shu Z, Chen G (2012) Melatonin activates the Nrf2-ARE pathway when it protects against early brain injury in a subarachnoid hemorrhage model. J Pineal Res 53:129–137
67. Wang Z, Shi XY, Yin J, Zuo G, Zhang J, Chen G (2012) Role of autophagy in early brain injury after experimental subarachnoid hemorrhage. J Mol Neurosci 46:192–202
68. Wang Z, Zuo G, Shi XY, Zhang J, Fang Q, Chen G (2011) Progesterone administration modulates cortical TLR4/NF-kappaB signaling pathway after subarachnoid hemorrhage in male rats. Mediators Inflamm 2011:848309
69. Wu C, Hu Q, Chen J, Yan F, Li J, Wang L, Mo H, Gu C, Zhang P, Chen G (2013) Inhibiting HIF-1alpha by 2ME2 ameliorates early brain injury after experimental subarachnoid hemorrhage in rats. Biochem Biophys Res Commun 437:469–474
70. Yan J, Chen C, Lei J, Yang L, Wang K, Liu J, Zhou C (2006) 2-Methoxyestradiol reduces cerebral vasospasm after 48 hours of experimental subarachnoid hemorrhage in rats. Exp Neurol 202:348–356
71. Yan J, Li L, Khatibi NH, Yang L, Wang K, Zhang W, Martin RD, Han J, Zhang J, Zhou C (2011) Blood-brain barrier disruption following subarchnoid hemorrhage may be facilitated through PUMA induction of endothelial cell apoptosis from the endoplasmic reticulum. Exp Neurol 230:240–247
72. You WC, Li W, Zhuang Z, Tang Y, Lu HC, Ji XJ, Shen W, Shi JX, Zhou ML (2012) Biphasic activation of nuclear factor-kappa B in experimental models of subarachnoid hemorrhage in vivo and in vitro. Mediators Inflamm 2012:786242

73. Zacharia BE, Hickman ZL, Grobelny BT, DeRosa P, Kotchetkov I, Ducruet AF, Connolly ES Jr (2010) Epidemiology of aneurysmal subarachnoid hemorrhage. Neurosurg Clin N Am 21:221–233
74. Zhang J, Zhu Y, Zhou D, Wang Z, Chen G (2010) Recombinant human erythropoietin (rhEPO) alleviates early brain injury following subarachnoid hemorrhage in rats: possible involvement of Nrf2-ARE pathway. Cytokine 52:252–257
75. Zhao H, Ji Z, Tang D, Yan C, Zhao W, Gao C (2013) Role of autophagy in early brain injury after subarachnoid hemorrhage in rats. Mol Biol Rep 40:819–827
76. Zhao X, Aronowski J (2013) Nrf2 to pre-condition the brain against injury caused by products of hemolysis after ICH. Transl Stroke Res 4:71–75
77. Zhao XD, Zhou YT, Lu XJ (2013) Sulforaphane enhances the activity of the Nrf2-ARE pathway and attenuates inflammation in OxyHb-induced rat vascular smooth muscle cells. Inflamm Res 62:857–863
78. Zhao XD, Zhou YT, Zhang X, Wang XL, Qi W, Zhuang Z, Su XF, Shi JX (2010) Expression of NF-E2-related factor 2 (Nrf2) in the basilar artery after experimental subarachnoid hemorrhage in rabbits: a preliminary study. Brain Res 1358:221–227
79. Zhou ML, Shi JX, Hang CH, Cheng HL, Qi XP, Mao L, Chen KF, Yin HX (2007) Potential contribution of nuclear factor-kappaB to cerebral vasospasm after experimental subarachnoid hemorrhage in rabbits. J Cereb Blood Flow Metab 27:1583–1592

Effects of Diltiazem on Sympathetic Activity in Patients with Aneurysmal Subarachnoid Hemorrhage

Takeshi Ogura, Ririko Takeda, Hidetoshi Ooigawa, Hiroyuki Nakajima, and Hiroki Kurita

Abstract This study evaluated the effect of diltiazem, a calcium antagonist, on sympathetic activity in patients with aneurysmal subarachnoid hemorrhage (SAH) during the hyperacute stage. Of patients with aneurysmal SAH who underwent aneurysm repair between August 2008 and June 2011, 119 consecutive patients were enrolled in this prospective study. On admission, patients were assigned to an antihypertensive treatment receiving continuous infusion of diltiazem (67 patients) or nicardipine (52 patients). Plasma levels of adrenaline (AD), noradrenaline (NA), and dopamine (DP) were repeatedly measured using high-performance liquid chromatography (HPLC). There were no significant differences in patient characteristics or aneurysm topography between the two groups. In all patients, acute surge of catecholamines was observed with mutual correlation. However, patients receiving diltiazem exhibited a significantly lower plasma concentration of DP than those receiving nicardipine, 3 and 6 h after admission. A similar trend was observed for NA, but the difference was not significant at 6 h. Conversely, the concentration of AD was similar between the two groups. Diltiazem may suppress sympathetic activity in the hyperacute stage of aneurysmal SAH. Further studies are needed to verify the beneficial effect of diltiazem in patients with SAH.

Keywords Catecholamine surge • Diltiazem • Subarachnoid hemorrhage • Cerebral vasospasm

T. Ogura • R. Takeda • H. Ooigawa • H. Nakajima
H. Kurita, MD, PhD (✉)
Department of Cerebrovascular Surgery,
International Medical Center, Saitama Medical University,
1397-1 Yamane, Hidaka, Saitama 350-1298, Japan
e-mail: hkurita@saitama-med.ac.jp

Introduction

Subarachnoid hemorrhage (SAH) is a serious condition associated with a high rate of mortality and morbidity. The plasma concentration of catecholamines often increases rapidly and excessively after the onset of SAH, causing harmful sympathetic reactions, including ECG abnormalities and pulmonary edema [2, 3, 10, 12, 15, 16, 18, 20]. These systemic insults can affect patient outcomes, and direct or indirect effects of catecholamines on cerebral vessels have been proposed as a predictor of poor prognosis [4, 5, 17].

Among Ca^{2+} channel blockers, diltiazem and nicardipine are widely used in Japan for the control of blood pressure during the hyperacute phase of SAH. Diltiazem is known to inhibit catecholamine release in the sympathetic nervous system in coma conditions [9, 13, 14, 20]. The aim of this study is to evaluate the effect of diltiazem on sympathetic activity in patients with hyperacute SAH.

Patients and Methods

Of patients with aneurysmal SAH who underwent aneurysm repair between August 2008 and June 2011, 119 consecutive patients were enrolled in this prospective study (38 men and 81 women; age range, 31–97 years; mean, 62 years). Baseline demographics (age and sex), physiological parameters (blood pressure, heart rate), and neurological grading (Hunt & Kosnic grade) were recorded on admission. Diagnosis of SAH was made by CT scan, and the amount of subarachnoid blood was categorized according to the Fisher scale.

All patients underwent strict blood pressure control (<140 mmHg) using continuous venous infusion of diltiazem (5–15 μg/ml/min) or nicardipine (0.5–6 μg/ml/min) immediately after admission. Principally, the antihypertensives were selected randomly, but the patient's condition, including heart rate and ECG abnormalities, were considered in some cases. All patients were sedated with continuous intravenous infusion of propofol before aneurysm treatment. Blood samples were collected at 0, 3, and 6 h after admission and plasma concentrations of dopamine (DP), noradrenaline (NA), and adrenaline (AD) were measured by high-performance liquid chromatography (HPLC) [7]. The limit of detection for plasma catecholamines was 0.02 ng/ml.

The ruptured aneurysms were repaired by surgical clipping (75 patients) or endovascular coiling (44 patients), depending on the aneurysm and hematoma topography. The blood samples were collected before surgery, in consideration of the influence of anesthesia and surgical insults on the sympathetic nervous system.

Data were analyzed using commercially available software (SigmaPlot). The significance of differences between the diltiazem and nicardipine groups at each time point was determined using a two-tailed multiple *t*-test with Bonferroni correction. The corrected significance level p value is $0.05/3=0.017$. The present study was approved by the Committee on Human Research at Saitama International Medical Center, and informed consent was obtained from all patients or family members for the acquisition of blood samples.

Results

The basic characteristics of patients in the two groups are shown in Table 1. There were no significant differences in patient characteristics that might affect serum catecholamine values [18].

Immediately after the onset of SAH, markedly high levels of AD were seen, which then rapidly decreased to the normal range within 6 h. There were no significant differences between the two groups at any time point (Fig. 1a). Patients receiving diltiazem exhibited lower plasma concentrations of NA and DP than those receiving nicardipine at 3 and 6 h. The difference was not significant for NA levels ($p=0.021$, $P=0.368$, respectively) (Fig. 1b), but a significant difference was observed in DP levels at 3 h ($p=0.002$, $p=0.029$, respectively) (Fig. 1c).

Table 1 Characteristics of patients in each treatment group

	Diltiazem	Nicardipine	
Number of patients	67	52	
Male/Female	23/44	15/37	n.s.
Age	59 ± 12	62 ± 12	n.s.
Blood pressure (on admission)			
Systolic	164 ± 30	167 ± 24	n.s.
Diastolic	87 ± 18	87 ± 16	n.s.
Time after onset	4.6 ± 4.6	4.7 ± 5.7	n.s.
Hunt & Kosnic grade	2.8 ± 1.0	2.7 ± 1.0	n.s.
Fisher scale (1+2/3+4)	5/62	4/48	n.s.

Discussion

The present study demonstrated that diltiazem may be more repressive than nicardipine against the acute surge of NA and DP in patients with SAH. NA and DP are mainly derived from sympathetic nerve endings [5] and our findings support the notion that diltiazem exerted inhibitory effects on the sympathetic nervous system. The primary action of Ca^{2+} channel blockers is to inhibit the Ca^{2+} influx through voltage-dependent calcium channels in the plasma membrane that leads to relaxation and vasodilation of vascular smooth muscle [1]. Previous studies have shown that the inhibition of Ca^{2+} channels can decrease catecholamine release by inhibiting neurotransmitter release at adrenergic nerve terminals [6, 11]. Several authors reported that diltiazem might have an inhibitory effect on sympathetic transmission through some extra actions in addition to the inhibition of Ca^{2+} influx into the adrenergic nerve endings [8, 16], although the mechanism remains to be elucidated.

We have demonstrated previously that AD concentrations were markedly high immediately after SAH onset and decreased rapidly, whereas NA and DP concentrations had a significant time delay until their peak occurred compared with AD [17, 19]. The discrepancy of response to diltiazem among catecholamines may arise from the difference in the time course of when diltiazem affects the activated sympathetic nervous system. Further controlled clinical trials are needed to establish the beneficial effect of diltiazem in patients with aneurysmal SAH.

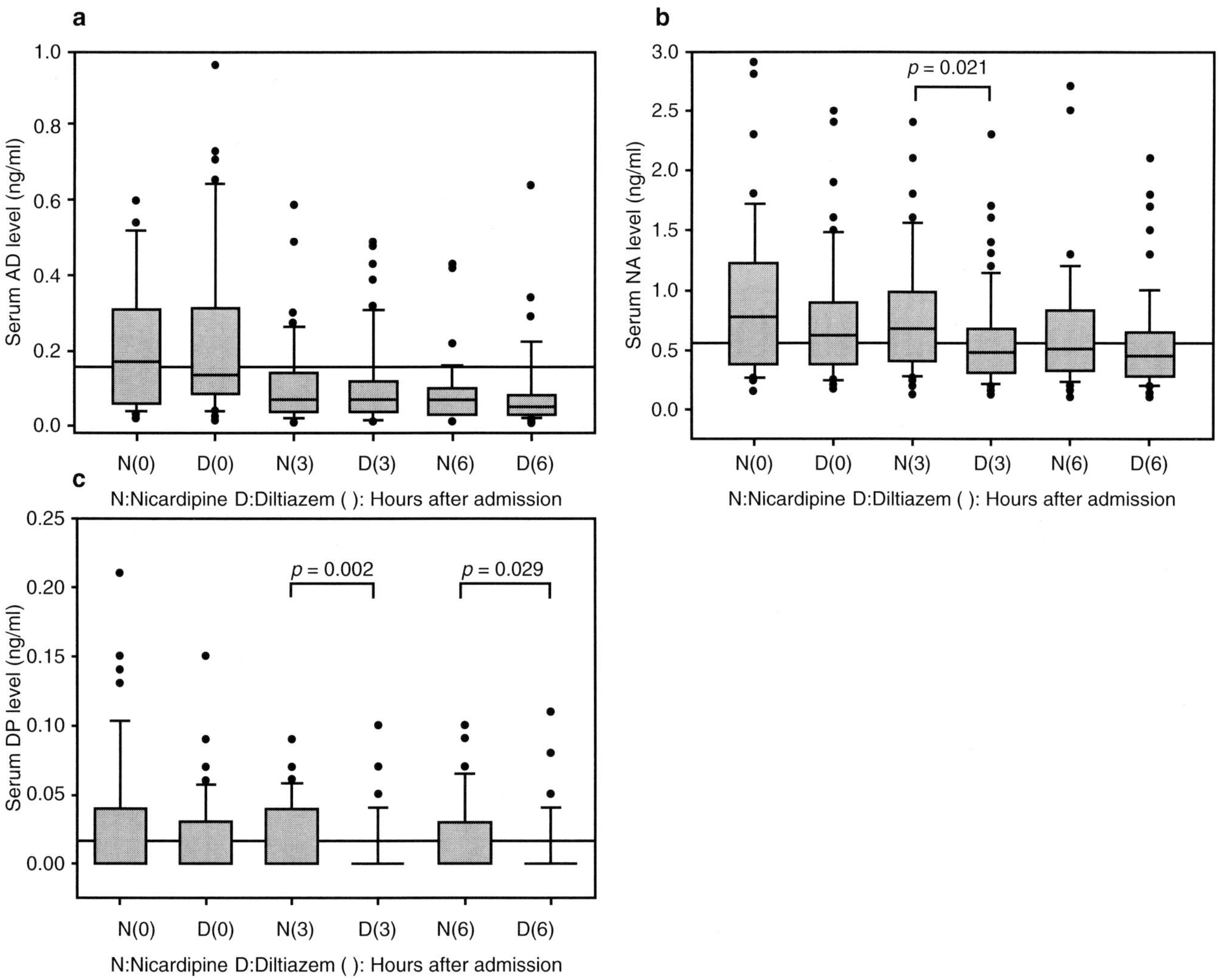

Fig. 1 Time course of the changes in AD (**a**), NA (**b**), and DP (**c**) concentration between the two treated groups. Concentrations below the detection limit (0.02 ng/ml) were assigned a value of zero. The *horizontal line* represents the upper limit of normal

Conclusion

Our preliminary data indicate that diltiazem can suppress sympathetic activity and may contribute favorable outcome to patients with SAH.

Conflict of Interest Statement All authors have no financial affiliations or conflicts of interest to announce.

References

1. Fleckenstein A (1977) Specific pharmacology of calcium in myocardium, cardiac pacemakers and vascular smooth muscle. Annu Rev Pharmacol Toxicol 17:149–166
2. Fukui S, Katoh H, Tsuzuki N, Ishihara S, Otani N, Ooigawa H, Toyooka T, Ohnuki A, Miyazawa T, Nawashiro H, Shima K (2003) Multivariate analysis of risk factors for QT prolongation following subarachnoid hemorrhage. Crit Care 7:7–12
3. Frontera JA, Parra A, Shimbo D, Fernandez A, Schmidt JM, Peter P, Claassen J, Wartenberg KE, Rincon F, Badjatia N, Naidech A, Connolly ES, Mayer SA (2008) Cardiac arrhythmias after subarachnoid hemorrhage: Risk factors and impact on outcome. Cerebrovasc Dis 26:71–78
4. Gao C, Liu X, Shi H, Xu S, Ji Z, Wang C, Wu P, Liu Z, Zhao S (2009) Relationship between sympathetic nervous activity and inflammatory response after subarachnoid hemorrhage in a perforating canine model. Auton Neurosci 147:70–74
5. Goldstein D, Holmes C (2009) Neuronal source of plasma dopamine. Clin Chem 54:1864–1871
6. Grossman E, Messerli FH (2010) Effect of calcium antagonists on plasma norepinephrine levels, heart rate, and blood pressure. Am J Cardiol 80:1453–1458

7. Holmes C, Eisenhofer G, Goldstein DS (1994) Improved assay for plasma dihydroxyphenylacetic acid and other catechols using high-performance liquid chromatography with electro-chemical detection. J Chromatog B Biomed Appl 653:131–138
8. Houlihan LM, Slater EY, Beadle DJ, Lukas RJ, Bermudez I (2000) Effects of Diltiazem on human nicotinic acetylcholine and GABA A receptors. Neuropharmacology 39:2533–2542
9. Isojima K, Takase B, Arakawa K, Shibuya T, Satomura K, Mizuno K, Kurita A, Nakamura H (1991) Effects of Diltiazem on hemodynamics, plasma catecholamine and rennin activity during exercise in hypertension. J Cardiol 21:383–390
10. Isotani E, Sato Y, Kubota Y, Ohno K, Otomo Y (2008) Monitoring of the cardiopulmonary function by Picco plus after subarachnoid hemorrhage. Neurosurg Emerg 13:174–181
11. Kato H, Takata Y (2000) Differential effects of Ca antagonists on the noradrenaline release and contraction evoked by nerve stimulation in the presence of 4-aminopyridine. Br J Pharmacol 90:191–201
12. Khechinashvili G, Asplund K (2000) Electrocardiographic changes in patients with acute stroke: a systematic review. Cerebrovasc Dis 14:67–76
13. Leenen FH, Fourney A (1996) Comparison of the effects of amlodipine and Diltiazem on 24-hour blood pressure, plasma catecholamines, and left ventricular mass. Am J Cardiol 78:203–207
14. Moussouttas M, Huynh TT, Khoury J, Lai EW, Dombrowski K, Pello S, Pacak K (2012) Cerebrospinal fluid catecholamine levels as predictors of outcome in subarachnoid hemorrhage. Cerebrovasc Dis 33:173–181
15. Naredi S, Lambert G, Eden E, Zall M, Runnerstam B, Rydenhag B, Friberg P (2000) Increased sympathetic nervous activity in patients with nontraumatic subarachnoid hemorrhage. Stroke 31:901–906
16. Obata T (2006) Diltiazem, an antagonist of calcium channels, reduces norepinephrine in the rat myocardium. Bioelectrochemistry 69:234–236
17. Ogura T, Satoh A, Ooigawa H, Sugiyama T, Takeda R, Fushihara G, Yoshikawa S, Okada D, Suzuki H, Araki R, Ishihara S, Nishikawa R, Kurita H (2012) Characteristics and prognostic value of acute catecholamine surge in patients with aneurysmal subarachnoid hemorrhage. Neurol Res 34:490–498
18. Saito R, Takahashi T, Noshita N, Narisawa A, Negi K, Takei K, Kaneko U (2010) Takotsubo cardiomyopathy induced by dobutamine infusion during hypertensive therapy for symptomatic vasospasm after subarachnoid hemorrhage. Neurol Med Chir 50: 393–395
19. Satoh A, Nakamura H, Kobayashi S, Miyata A, Matsutani M (2005) Management of severe subarachnoid hemorrhage; significance of assessment of both neurological and systemic insults at acute stage. Acta Neurochir Suppl 94:59–63
20. Shigihara A, Iwama H, Kawamae K (1992) Effects of Diltiazem hydrochloride on patients with ruptured cerebral aneurysm. ICU CCU 16:435–440

Haemoglobin Scavenging After Subarachnoid Haemorrhage

A. Durnford, J. Dunbar, J. Galea, D. Bulters, J.A.R. Nicoll, D. Boche, and I. Galea

Abstract Rapid and effective clearance of cell-free haemoglobin after subarachnoid haemorrhage (SAH) is important to prevent vasospasm and neurotoxicity and improve long-term outcome. Haemoglobin is avidly bound by haptoglobin, and the complex is cleared by CD163 expressed on the membrane surface of macrophages. We studied the kinetics of haemoglobin and haptoglobin in cerebrospinal fluid after SAH. We show that haemoglobin levels rise gradually after SAH. Haptoglobin levels rise acutely with aneurysmal rupture as a result of injection of blood into the subarachnoid space. Although levels decline as haemoglobin scavenging occurs, complete depletion of haptoglobin does not occur and levels start rising again, indicating saturation of CD163 sites available for haptoglobin–haemoglobin clearance. In a preliminary neuropathological study we demonstrate that meningeal CD163 expression is upregulated after SAH, in keeping with a proinflammatory state. However, loss of CD163 occurs in meningeal areas with overlying blood compared with areas without overlying blood. Becauses ADAM17 is the enzyme responsible for shedding membrane-bound CD163, its inhibition may be a potential therapeutic strategy after SAH.

A. Durnford (✉) • J. Dunbar • D. Bulters • D. Boche • I. Galea
Clinical Neurosciences, Clinical and Experimental Sciences, Faculty of Medicine, University of Southampton, Southampton, UK
e-mail: andrew.durnford@uhs.nhs.uk

J. Galea
Department of Neurosurgery, Manchester Academic Health Sciences Centre, Manchester, UK

J.A.R. Nicoll
Clinical Neurosciences, Clinical and Experimental Sciences, Faculty of Medicine, University of Southampton, Southampton, UK

Department of Cellular Pathology, University Hospital Southampton NHS Foundation Trust, Southampton, UK

Keywords Subarachnoid haemorrhage • Vasospasm • Haemoglobin • Haptoglobin • Delayed neurological deficit

Introduction

Spontaneous subarachnoid haemorrhage (SAH) is an acute cerebrovascular event that causes significant morbidity and mortality. The majority of cases result from ruptured intracranial aneurysms. After SAH, evidence suggests that extracellular haemoglobin (Hb) released from erythrocytes within the subarachnoid space is the agent responsible for poor outcomes [9], mediated by effects on cerebral vessels and neurons, leading to ischemia caused by vasospasm and direct neurotoxicity.

Outside the brain, the CD163-haptoglobin axis is responsible for Hb scavenging. Haptoglobin has a very high affinity for Hb. The resulting haptoglobin–Hb complex formation uncovers a neoepitope on haptoglobin that enables recognition of the complex by CD163 expressed on the membrane surface of myeloid cells [8]. This results in receptor-mediated endocytosis of the complex and further intracellular degradation of Hb into bilirubin. ADAM17 enzyme is coexpressed by CD163-expressing myeloid cells and proteolytically cleaves CD163 from the cell membrane surface, resulting in constitutive circulating levels of soluble CD163 [3]. ADAM17 may be upregulated by ischemia [2] and inflammation [7], which results in increased soluble CD163 shedding.

In the brain, CD163 is expressed by perivascular and meningeal macrophages in both rodents and humans [4, 5]; these macrophages are strategically located to scavenge blood products after SAH. We have recently shown saturation of the CD163–haptoglobin system after SAH [6] by examining cerebrospinal fluid (CSF) from patients with SAH and healthy individuals. We demonstrated that CSF haptoglobin coexisted with free uncomplexed Hb, suggesting that

J. Fandino et al. (eds.), *Neurovascular Events After Subarachnoid Hemorrhage*, Acta Neurochirurgica Supplement, Vol. 120,
DOI 10.1007/978-3-319-04981-6_9,

CD163-mediated clearance of haptoglobin–Hb complexes was saturated after SAH. This could be secondary to purely overwhelming CD163 sites available for binding in the central nervous system, proteolytic loss of membrane-bound CD163 mediated by ADAM17, or both. Preliminary evidence suggested that CD163 was indeed being shed because CSF soluble CD163 levels were higher after SAH compared with controls, and most of it was synthesised intrathecally. We could not examine the levels of membrane-bound CD163 available for binding in these patients because this requires availability of tissue for immunohistochemistry or Western blot, and only CSF was available from these patients.

Here we sought additional evidence for saturation of the CD163–haptoglobin system by examining the kinetics of CSF Hb and haptoglobin levels with time. We also examined post-mortem tissue from brains of SAH and control patients to determine the level of membrane-bound CD163.

Materials and Methods

Cerebrospinal fluid (CSF) from patients with SAH ($n=30$) and control individuals ($n=20$) was analysed by derivative spectrophotometry for Hb and enzyme-linked immunosorbent assay for haptoglobin (AssayPro, MO, USA). In patients with SAH, CSF was obtained from external ventricular drains on insertion. However, unlike serial samples taken after drainage, these CSF samples therefore truly reflect the composition of CSF at different time points after SAH. Control individuals were patients with non-inflammatory/non-haemorrhagic conditions undergoing lumbar puncture; their CSF was subsequently found to be normal with respect to protein, glucose, cell count, cytology, albumin CSF/serum quotient and isoelectric focusing for oligoclonal bands. Samples were collected with Research Ethical Committee approval (04/Q2707/236 and 07/H0304/71).

Post-mortem formalin-fixed paraffin-embedded tissue from a different set of SAH ($n=7$) and control cases ($n=5$) was obtained from the brain bank, BRAIN UK (Research Ethical Committee approval 09/H0504/68). Control cases were matched for age and sex, did not die from neurological causes, and were selected carefully to exclude inflammatory, haemorrhagic or neurodegenerative pathology; these served as "external" controls. In SAH cases, regions of cerebral cortex with overlying blood and no overlying blood were selected for each case; the cortical areas with no overlying blood were chosen to act as additional "internal" controls (avoiding inter-individual variability). Sections were cut, rehydrated, microwaved in EDTA buffer for 25 min to retrieve antigen, incubated with anti-CD163 antibody (EDhu1, AbD Serotec, UK) at 1:1000 dilution for 90 min at room temperature, then with secondary antibody, followed by 0.05 % 3,3′-diaminobenzidine, and finally counterstained with haemotoxylin, dehydrated and mounted in DPX. Sections were stained in the same run. Images were digitally acquired using a camera mounted on a light microscope, at magnification ×20, and analysed on ImageJ (version 1.41, NIH US) to obtain a percentage protein load. Mann-Whitney test was used because the data was non-parametric (SPSS 19 software, SPSS Inc., US). Plots were generated in GraphPad Prism 6.

Results

Examination of the kinetics of CSF Hb levels showed that they rose progressively between days 1 and 4 after SAH (Fig. 1a). There was an additional rise in CSF Hb levels between day 4 and day 6, however the standard deviation on day 6 was very high. CSF haptoglobin levels rose sharply after SAH (Fig. 1b), reflecting spillage of blood-derived haptoglobin into the CSF during the acute bleed. This was followed by a steady decline in CSF haptoglobin, reflecting consumption during CD163-mediated scavenging of haptoglobin–Hb complexes. However depletion did not occur, indicating saturation and/or loss of membrane-bound CD163

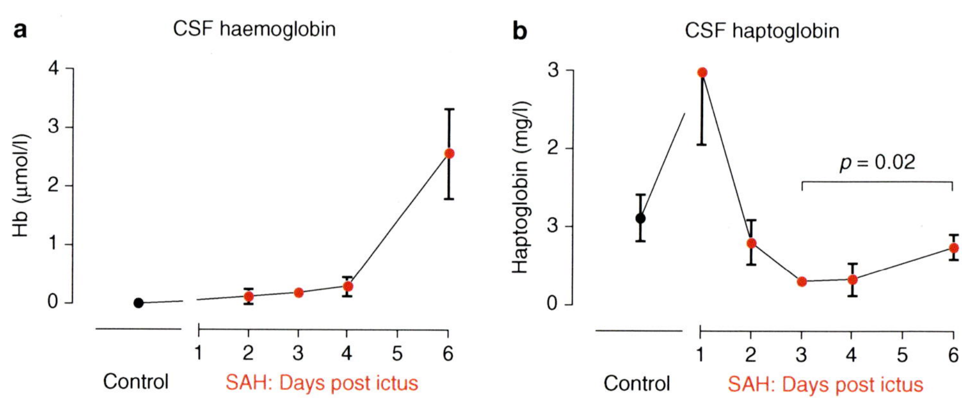

Fig. 1 The kinetics of Hb (**a**) and haptoglobin (**b**) levels in CSF after SAH

available for scavenging. Moreover, CSF haptoglobin levels started rising again on day 4, and there was a statistically significant difference between day 4 and day 6 CSF haptoglobin levels, indicating saturation of the CD163–haptoglobin system.

Our previous study had suggested intrathecal soluble CD163 shedding after SAH [6], which may partially explain the saturation of Hb–haptoglobin clearance via loss of membrane-bound CD163 sites available, if these are not replenished. We therefore proceeded to examine meningeal CD163 expression in post-mortem tissue after SAH and in control individuals. CD163 stained cells with the morphological appearance of meningeal (Fig. 2) and perivascular macrophages. SAH resulted in up-regulation of CD163 expression (Fig. 3a, two-fold, $p = 0.02$), in keeping with the pro-inflammatory nature of SAH. Interestingly, in meningeal areas with overlying blood, CD163 levels were lower versus areas without overlying blood (Fig. 3a, $p = 0.02$), approximating the levels seen in control cases. This was also observed after comparing meningeal areas with and without overlying blood from the same patients, to eliminate intra-individual variability (Fig. 3b, $p = 0.03$). No such difference was observed in the grey matter (ie perivascular CD163). CD163 meningeal staining is illustrated in Fig. 3.

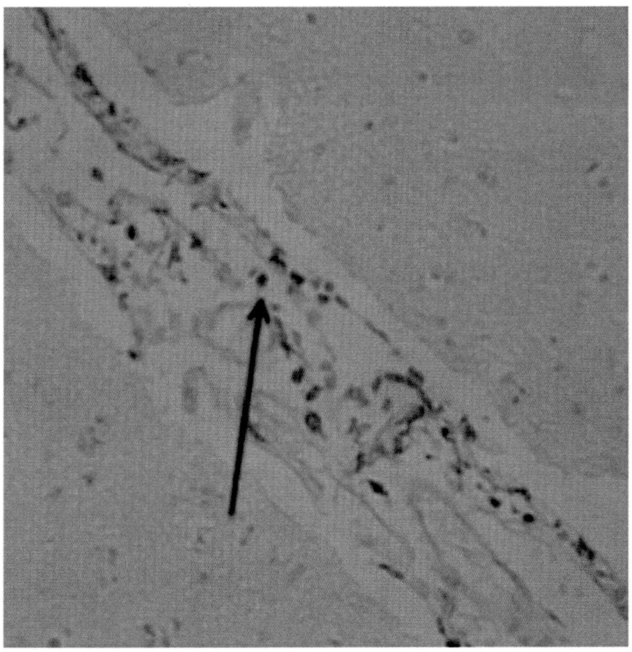

Fig. 2 CD163 immunohistochemical staining of meninges after SAH, counterstained with haemotoxylin, at magnification ×20. *Arrow* indicates CD163+ve meningeal macrophages (*brown*)

Discussion

In this kinetic study, we showed that CSF haptoglobin levels rise acutely after SAH as a consequence of the injection of blood into the subarachnoid space. Under normal circumstances, the CNS is deficient of haptoglobin, with the total Hb-binding capacity in the CSF being ×50,000 less than that of blood [6]. The automatic delivery of haptoglobin from serum to CSF during aneurysmal rupture may well protect against and help clear the Hb released during initial haemolysis. Haptoglobin binding to Hb prevents it from participating in toxic redox reactions [1] that damage blood vessels and neurones.

During extracranial haemolysis, haptoglobin never coexists with free uncomplexed Hb. This is because the affinity of membrane-bound CD163 to haptoglobin–Hb complexes is very high, and the total Hb-binding capacity of the body

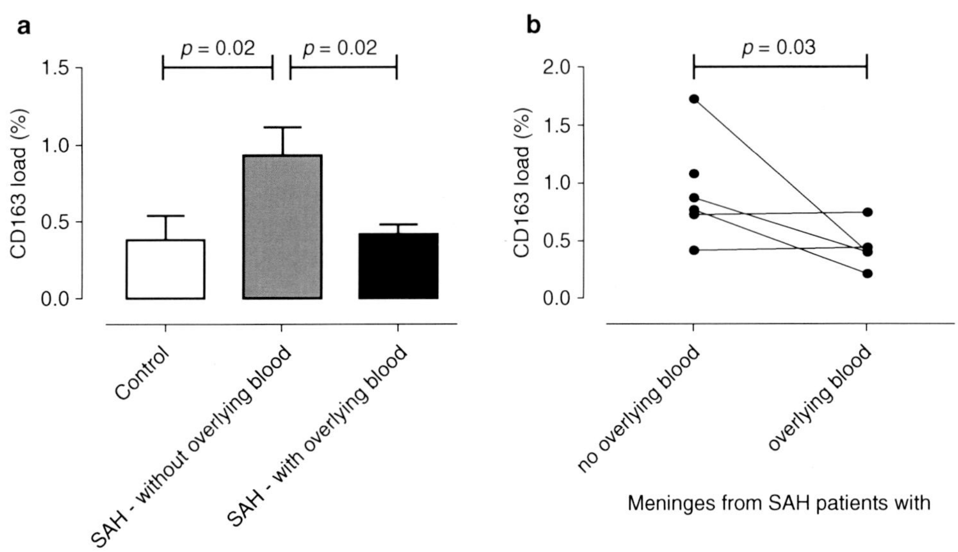

Fig. 3 The CD163 mean percentage protein load in the meninges from control and SAH patients (**a**). A pairwise comparison of CD163 in SAH meninges with or without overlying blood from the same cases is shown in (**b**)

is not limiting. We show that the situation is different during intracranial haemolysis. Not only does haptoglobin co-exist with Hb, but haptoglobin levels start rising between days 4 and 6. This is clear evidence of saturation of CD163-mediated uptake of haptoglobin–Hb complexes. Such saturation is likely to be of importance because CSF Hb levels rise further between days 4 and 6.

In this preliminary neuropathological study, we demonstrate that a potential mechanism for the persistence of haptoglobin despite high levels of Hb is the loss of membrane-bound CD163 sites available for scavenging haptoglobin–Hb complexes. Although meningeal CD163 up-regulation occurred after SAH, there was loss of CD163 in meningeal areas with overlying blood.

Replication of these findings in a larger number of cases in needed. CD163 is shed by the proteolytic action of ADAM17 expressed by the same macrophages. ADAM17 is a highly regulated enzyme, with at least two known naturally occurring inhibitors: TIMP3 (tissue inhibitor of metalloproteinase-3) and PDI (protein disulphide isomerase), and can adopt active and non-active conformational states [10, 11].

Conclusion

We demonstrate that haemoglobin levels rise gradually after SAH. Haptoglobin levels rise acutely with aneurysmal rupture as a result of injection of blood into the subarachnoid space. Although levels decline as haemoglobin scavenging occurs, complete depletion of haptoglobin does not occur and levels start rising again, indicating saturation of CD163 sites available for haptoglobin–haemoglobin clearance. Meningeal CD163 expression is upregulated after SAH, in keeping with a proinflammatory state. Further study is needed to dissect the mechanism of CD163 shedding after SAH because ADAM17 inhibition may be a potential therapeutic strategy.

Acknowledgements We thank the patients who were involved in this study. The Neuropathology Section (Department of Cellular Pathology, University Hospital Southampton NHS Foundation Trust) and the Histochemistry Research Unit and Biomedical Imaging Unit (Faculty of Medicine, University of Southampton) facilitated tissue processing, staining and analysis. We thank the staff of the Histochemistry Research Unit at the University of Southampton. Neil Bailey from BRAIN UK provided the tissue. This work was supported by funding from NIHR, Wellcome Trust and the MRC.

Conflicts of Interest Statement We declare that we have no conflict of interest.

References

1. Alayash AI, Andersen CB, Moestrup SK, Bulow L (2013) Haptoglobin: the hemoglobin detoxifier in plasma. Trends Biotechnol 31:2–3
2. Cardenas A, Moro MA, Leza JC, O'Shea E, Davalos A, Castillo J, Lorenzo P, Lizasoain I (2002) Upregulation of TACE/ADAM17 after ischemic preconditioning is involved in brain tolerance. J Cereb Blood Flow Metab 22:1297–1302
3. Etzerodt A, Maniecki MB, Moller K, Moller HJ, Moestrup SK (2010) Tumor necrosis factor alpha-converting enzyme (TACE/ADAM17) mediates ectodomain shedding of the scavenger receptor CD163. J Leukoc Biol 88:1201–1205
4. Fabriek BO, Van Haastert ES, Galea I, Polfliet MM, Dopp ED, Van Den Heuvel MM, Van Den Berg TK, De Groot CJ, Van Der Valk P, Dijkstra CD (2005) CD163-positive perivascular macrophages in the human CNS express molecules for antigen recognition and presentation. Glia 51:297–305
5. Galea I, Palin K, Newman TA, Van RN, Perry VH, Boche D (2005) Mannose receptor expression specifically reveals perivascular macrophages in normal, injured, and diseased mouse brain. Glia 49:375–384
6. Galea J, Cruickshank G, Teeling JL, Boche D, Garland P, Perry VH, Galea I (2012) The intrathecal CD163-haptoglobin-hemoglobin scavenging system in subarachnoid hemorrhage. J Neurochem 121:785–792
7. Hintz KA, Rassias AJ, Wardwell K, Moss ML, Morganelli PM, Pioli PA, Givan AL, Wallace PK, Yeager MP, Guyre PM (2002) Endotoxin induces rapid metalloproteinase-mediated shedding followed by up-regulation of the monocyte hemoglobin scavenger receptor CD163. J Leukoc Biol 72:711–717
8. Kristiansen M, Graversen JH, Jacobsen C, Sonne O, Hoffman HJ, Law SK, Moestrup SK (2001) Identification of the haemoglobin scavenger receptor. Nature 409:198–201
9. Macdonald RL, Weir BK (1991) A review of hemoglobin and the pathogenesis of cerebral vasospasm. Stroke 22:971–982
10. Murphy G (2008) The ADAMs: signalling scissors in the tumour microenvironment. Nat Rev Cancer 8:929–941
11. Willems SH, Tape CJ, Stanley PL, Taylor NA, Mills IG, Neal DE, McCafferty J, Murphy G (2010) Thiol isomerases negatively regulate the cellular shedding activity of ADAM17. Biochem J 428:439–450

Mild Exercise Reduces Cerebral Vasospasm After Aneurysm Subarachnoid Hemorrhage: A Retrospective Clinical Study and Correlation with Laboratory Investigation

Margaret A. Riordan, Michele Kyle, Christina Dedeo, Mark R. Villwock, Matthew Bauer, Mary Lou Vallano, and Eric M. Deshaies

Abstract Background: Aneurysmal subarachnoid hemorrhage (SAH) is a leading cause of death and disability and is often complicated by cerebral vasospasm (CV). Conventional management to prevent CV includes bedrest; however, inactivity places the patient at risk for nonneurological complications. We investigated the effect of mild exercise after SAH in clinical and laboratory settings. **Methods**: *Clinical*: Data from 80 patients with SAH were analyzed retrospectively. After aneurysms were secured, physical therapy was initiated as tolerated. CV and complications were compared by the timing of active physical therapy. *Laboratory*: 18 Rodents were divided into three groups: (1) control, (2) SAH without exercise, and (3) SAH plus mild exercise. On day 5, brainstems were removed and analyzed for the injury marker inducible nitric oxide synthase (iNOS). **Results**: *Clinical*: Mild exercise before day 4 significantly lowered the incidence of symptomatic CV compared with the nonexercised group. There was no difference in the incidence of additional complications based upon exercise. *Laboratory*: Staining for iNOS was significantly higher in the SAH group than the control group, but there was no difference between exercised and nonexercised SAH groups, confirming that exercise did not promote neuronal injury. **Conclusion**: Early mobilization significantly reduced clinical CV. The relationship should be studied further in a prospective trial with defined exercise regimens.

M.A. Riordan, MD • M. Kyle, BS • M.R. Villwock, MS • M. Bauer
Department of Neurosurgery, SUNY Upstate Medical University, Syracuse, NY, USA

C. Dedeo, BS • M.L. Vallano, PhD
Department of Neuroscience and Physiology, SUNY Upstate Medical University, Syracuse, NY, USA

E.M. Deshaies, MD (✉)
Department of Neurosurgery, SUNY Upstate Medical University, Syracuse, NY 13210, USA
e-mail: eric.m.deshaies@gmail.com

Keywords Aneurysm • Cerebral vasospasm • Early mobilization • Subarachnoid hemorrhage

Introduction

In the United States alone, nearly 30,000 people suffer from subarachnoid hemorrhage (SAH) after cerebral aneurysm rupture. Up to 70 % of the initial survivors are at risk for subsequent complications from cerebral vasospasm (CV). CV may be either mild and asymptomatic, or severe and resulting in delayed ischemic neurological deficits (DINDs) in 30–40 % of patients [9–11, 25, 37, 38]. The delayed onset after SAH makes CV an ideal target for preventative interventions [9, 18, 24, 26, 28, 38, 41].

Contemporary management of CV includes aneurysm sac occlusion followed by bedrest, triple-H (hypertension, hypervolemia, and hemodilution) therapy, and, although controversial, administration of potential neuroprotectant agents such as magnesium sulfate, nimodipine, statins, and enoxaparin. Each component is aimed at reducing the negative effects of CV by promoting cerebral blood flow (CBF) to prevent ischemia from hypoperfusion and microembolic infarcts. Although triple-H therapy was developed to minimize the effects of CV, it is not without medical complications, including cardiac failure, electrolyte abnormalities, cerebral edema, bleeding diatheses, and pulmonary edema [11, 19, 34]. Furthermore, only hypertension has been shown to be effective against DINDs, clearly demonstrating a need for further investigation into new therapies and management techniques for SAH [1, 4, 6, 10, 11, 19, 27, 34].

Stringent bedrest, which is frequently prescribed to prevent DINDs after the aneurysm has been secured, intuitively seems to counteract therapeutic efforts to optimize CBF. Bedrest and immobilization reduce cardiac return, decrease vascular tone, and increase venous pooling, all of which counteract the efforts of triple-H therapy and increase the risk of cardiopulmonary and venous complications.

DOI 10.1007/978-3-319-04981-6_10,

Randomized control trials have demonstrated that critically ill patients treated with early physical and occupational therapy had fewer adverse events associated with prolonged bedrest; however, these studies did not include SAH patients [31, 35]. In addition, similar studies have shown improved outcomes in patients with ischemic stroke who were mobilized early during their hospitalization [5, 14, 40] and demonstrated that changes in head position, passive range of motion, and mild exercise do not increase intracranial pressure or negatively impact CBF [6, 8, 17, 29]. These studies at the very least suggest that early physical therapy should be safe and may prove beneficial in patients with SAH. We took a two-targeted approach to investigating whether this is true, using both clinical and basic science venues. We hypothesized that early mobilization using mild exercise in patients with SAH (after their aneurysms had been secured) would not increase the incidence of CV. This hypothesis also was investigated further at the biomolecular level by engaging rodents in a mild exercise regimen after SAH that mimics the human clinical scenario [12, 20–22].

Materials and Methods

After obtaining approval from our Institutional Review Board, data was retrospectively collected from the charts of all aneurysm SAH patients who presented to our institution during a 3-year period (2009–2012) and who were treated by the same dual fellowship-trained cerebrovascular–endovascular neurosurgeon to minimize variability between physicians. Data collected from the charts are listed in Table 1. For purpose of analysis, a Fisher Grade (FG) 3+4 was assigned to patients with a FG 3 plus extensive intraventricular (IVH) or intraparenchymal (IPH) hemorrhage to distinguish them from a FG 4 implying extensive IVH and IPH without extensive SAH, such that FG 3+4 implies a SAH more severe than either FG 3 or FG 4 alone. This system is used at our institution to distinguish between those patients with extensive IPH or IVH who are at a low risk for CV (FG 4) according to Fisher's original reports and those with IVH or IPH at high risk for CV because of associated extensive SAH (FG 3+4) [13].

All of the patients were managed by our standard SAH protocol that included nimodipine, continuous intravenous magnesium sulfate infusion, and simvastatin at the time of admission and enoxaparin after securing the aneurysm. All aneurysms were secured with either surgical clip ligation or endovascular embolization by the senior author (EMD) within 24 h of admission. Deep venous thrombosis (DVT) prophylaxis was initiated immediately after admission using lower extremity sequential compression devices.

Table 1 Patient demographics

Characteristic	Number (%)
Male	29 (36)
Female	51 (64)
Hunt and Hess grade	
I	1 (1)
II	39 (49)
III	26 (32)
IV	12 (15)
V	2 (2)
Fisher grade	
0	4 (5)
1	4 (5)
2	4 (5)
3	21 (26)
3+4	23 (29)
4	24 (30)
Aneurysm location	
Anterior circulation	58 (73)
Posterior circulation	13 (16)
Multiple	9 (11)
Treatment	
Clip	29 (36)
Coil	51 (64)

Physical (PT) and occupational (OT) therapies were initiated within 24 h after the aneurysm was secured and patients were encouraged to ambulate with the nursing staff. The PT regimens were not standardized and activity was based on the functional ability of the patient. Functional ability and level of participation in therapy was divided into three categories: (1) *Mild Exercise with Ambulation*—ambulated whenever possible throughout the day plus participation in therapy sessions for 15–45 min daily, (2) *Mild Exercise without Ambulation*—out of bed and ambulation to chair only with participation in active range of motion (ROM) exercises, and (3) *Non-Exercised Control*—passive ROM exercises in all extremities and unable to participate in therapy sessions because of the severity of illness. Therapists and nurses would assist those who had difficulty with transferring out of bed, standing, and ROM exercises to ensure that they were exercised or had sufficient limb movement throughout the day.

For the purpose of statistical comparison, we categorized any patients from group 1 or 2 by the day they initiated active participation. Four groups were established: (1) initiation of active physical therapy before the vasospasm period (i.e., postbleed day (PBD)-4), (2) initiation before PBD-10, (3) initiation before PBD-20, and (4) no active participation in physical therapy throughout the first 20 days of hospitalization.

Daily bedside transcranial Doppler studies were used to monitor for CV, and CT-angiography and CT-perfusion were performed at admission before the onset of CV as a reference and then on PBDs 4, 6, and 10 with some variation if CV was suspected clinically; PBD 14 was also included if severe CV was present on PBD 10 before discharging the patient to rehabilitation or home. Aggressive intraarterial spasmolytic therapy was provided with spasmolytic agents or balloon angioplasty in symptomatic cases resistant to a maximum of 1 hour of standard medical management. Complications occurring during hospitalization were noted on the basis of discharge diagnoses noted in the discharge summary as well as consultation notes from specialty services.

Data were analyzed using SPSS Version 17 (IBM Corporation, Armonk, NY, USA). Categorical variables were compared using Fisher Exact Tests. Multivariate analysis was performed using forward stepwise binary logistic regression with symptomatic CV as the dependent variable. Categorical variables tested in the model included (1) FG $\geq$ 3, (2) Hunt Hess Score (HHS) $\geq$ 3, (3) active exercise initiation, and (4) endovascular treatment. Odds ratios and their 95 % confidence intervals were reported. Two-sided probability values were considered statistically significant for all analyses if $P < 0.05$.

Rodent SAH Model of Early Mobilization

All procedures involving the use of animals were in accordance with the *Guide for Care and Use of Laboratory Animals*, US Department of Health and Human Services, and approved by the Committee for the Humane Use of Animals of the university. The double-injection SAH rodent model for induction of basilar artery CV described by us previously was used for this study [12]. Briefly, 18 male Sprague-Dawley rats ranging from 250–300 g (Taconic Farms, Germantown, NY, USA) were equally divided into four groups: (1) *SAH Control*—cisternal injections of normothermic (37 °C) normal saline (0.9 % NaCl) as a substitute for the blood injections and no exercise; (2) *Exercised Control*—SAH, no exercise; (3) *Early Exercise*—SAH plus mild exercise 24 h after injections; and (4) *Late Exercise*—SAH plus mild exercise 48 h after injection. These groups were established to mimic the early and late mild exercise regimens seen clinically. We implemented a mild exercise regimen that did not induce a severe stress response reported in the more intense exercise regimens to minimize confounding variables in the model [30, 39]. A treadmill (IITC Life Science model 801) was used to engage the rats in a mild exercise regimen. All rats were familiarized with, but not exercised on, the treadmill daily for 3 days before the first surgery to minimize the potential psychological stressor of a new environment at the time of experimentation. Exercised animals ran at 10 m/min for 20 min each day (200 m/day) for 4 consecutive days; non-exercised animals were placed on a static treadmill using the same time parameters. All subjects were killed 5 days after the second cisternal injection and the brain tissues were fixed for tissue slicing [12, 23].

The cisternal double-injection SAH model specifically induces basilar artery CV; thus, we chose to analyze the brainstem for the injury marker, inducible nitric oxide synthase (iNOS) [3, 32]. Briefly, brainstem sections were incubated with primary iNOS antibody (Santa Cruz), rinsed in phosphate-buffered saline (PBS), and then incubated in 10 % normal donkey serum (NDS). Tissue was then incubated for 2 h with primary iNOS antibody (1:50 dilution). After primary antibody incubation, sections were washed in PBS and incubated with the secondary antibody Alexa Fluor 594 anti-rabbit (1:400 dilution). These sections were washed and incubated in Hoechst (1:1000 dilution) for nuclear staining. Sections were washed and cover slipped with Vectashield Mounting Media. Antibody fluorescence was visualized with a Nikon TE2000-U fluorescent microscope at 20×. Images were photographed using SPOT Advance imaging software. Photographs of brainstem tissue adjacent to the basilar artery were used to quantify iNOS-positive cells (20×). Fluorescing cells were counted in a predetermined rectangular section of brainstem tissue. These data were collected and statistical comparison between the groups was performed using Analysis of Variance (ANOVA) followed by Fisher's Protected Least Significant Difference (PLSD) or Tukey/Kramer post hoc test. A probability of ($P < 0.05$) was considered statistically significant.

Results

Eighty SAH patients met criteria to be included in this study and were all managed according to the standard SAH protocol described above. The mean age was 56.0 years with a female predominance (64 %), and the majority presented with a good to mildly impaired neurological examination (HHS of 2 or 3) and severe SAH (FG 3, 3+4). 51 patients (64 %) were treated with coil embolization and the rest were surgically clipped (Table 1). There was no difference in HHS ($P = 0.645$) or FG ($P = 0.335$) between surgically and endovascular treated patients, but as would be expected, there was a statistically significant difference in HHS ($P = 0.003$) between FG's. Of those with a FG $\geq$ 3, 57 % also had a HHS $\geq$ 3, in comparison to only 8 % of those with a FG < 3. Twenty-two patients from the mild exercise groups were able to ambulate or participate in active ROM therapy prior to PBD-4, an additional 20 patients began active therapy before PBD-10, and 9 patients began before PBD-20. The remaining 29 patients received passive ROM during the first 20 days of hospitalization (Table 2).

Table 2 Patient characteristics and outcome comparison by the timing of active physical therapy

	Day of active exercise initiation				
	≤3 (*n*=22)	4–9 (*n*=20)	10–19 (*n*=9)	≥20/none (*n*=29)	*P*
Male	6 (27.3 %)	9 (45.0 %)	5 (55.6 %)	9 (31.0 %)	0.366
Hunt-Hess ≥ 3	7 (31.8 %)	7 (35.0 %)	4 (44.4 %)	22 (75.9 %)	0.005[a]
Fisher grade ≥ 3	19 (86.4 %)	14 (70.0 %)	9 (100 %)	26 (89.7 %)	0.179
Endovascular aneurysm securement	18 (81.8 %)	12 (60.0 %)	6 (66.7 %)	15 (51.7 %)	0.158
Symptomatic cerebral vasospasm	3 (13.6 %)	7 (35.0 %)	4 (44.4 %)	16 (55.2 %)	0.019[b]
Radiographic cerebral vasospasm	14 (63.6 %)	11 (55.0 %)	6 (66.7 %)	18 (62.1 %)	0.917
Complications	8 (36.4 %)	9 (45.0 %)	5 (55.6 %)	12 (41.4 %)	0.795
Discharge disposition					
Home	17 (77.3 %)	10 (50.0 %)	4 (44.4 %)	8 (27.6 %)	0.005[c]
Rehabilitation	3 (13.6 %)	9 (45.0 %)	5 (55.6 %)	12 (41.4 %)	0.050[d]
Deceased	2 (9.1 %)	1 (5.0 %)	0 (0 %)	9 (31.0 %)	0.035[e]

[a]≤3 versus ≥20, *P*=0.002; 4–9 versus ≥20, *P*=0.007
[b]≤3 versus ≥20, *P*=0.003
[c]≤3 versus ≥20, *P*=0.001
[d]≤3 versus 4–9, *P*=0.040; ≤3 versus 10–19, *P*=0.027
[e]4–9 versus ≥20, *P*=0.007

Forty-seven patients (59 %) developed asymptomatic radiographic CV and 30 (38 %) developed symptomatic CV. Symptomatic CV was higher in patients presenting with FG 3, 3+4, and 4 (*P*=0.048), consistent with previous reports (2–4, 8–9, 12). Mild exercise before PBD-4 significantly lowered the incidence of symptomatic CV compared with patients who were not exercised (13.6 % vs 55.2 %, respectively; *P*=0.003). Patients who only received passive ROM therapy had a greater incidence of severe HHS in comparison with patients who began active therapy before PBD-10 (*P*=0.007) (Table 2). There was no difference in the incidence of FG ≥3 between groups (*P*=0.179).

The influence of FG, HHS, active exercise, and coiling on symptomatic CV was explored in multivariate analysis. This allows the impact of each variable to be assessed while controlling for confounding variables. Endovascular treatment of the aneurysm (*P*=0.647) and HHS ≥ 3 (*P*=0.637) were not significant predictors of symptomatic CV and were removed from the equation. Having a FG ≥ 3 was found to significantly increase the odds of symptomatic CV (*P*=0.046, OR=9.117, 95 % CI: 1.042–79.764). Lack of active exercise significantly increased the odds of symptomatic CV in comparison with exercise initiation before PBD-4 (*P*=0.004, OR=8.161, 95 % CI: 1.918–34.720).

Throughout the hospitalization, 4 patients (0.2 %) developed DVTs and 22 patients (27.5 %) developed pulmonary complications, including pneumonia and pleural effusions. Other complications noted in the discharge diagnoses included meningitis from external ventricular drainage (17 patients, 21 %), sacral decubitus ulcers (2 patients, 0.1 %), ischemic bowel (1 patient, 0.05 %), pancreatitis (1 patient, 0.05 %), cardiac dysfunction (2 patients, 0.1 %), and arterial embolism secondary to arterial line placement (1 patient, 0.05 %). There were significantly more complications in patients with a higher FG (*P*=0.003) and in those who were surgically clipped (*P*=0.018). There was not a significant difference in the number of complications based on the initiation of active physical therapy (*P*=0.795) (Table 2).

Laboratory Outcomes

Immunohistochemical staining demonstrated a significantly higher number of brainstem neurons staining with the injury marker, iNOS, in the SAH group than in the saline control (*P*<0.001) (Fig. 1). This confirmed that iNOS is a useful marker for detecting injury after SAH. There was no difference in iNOS staining between Exercised and Non-Exercised groups after SAH, suggesting that exercise did not increase injury markers (*P*>0.05).

Discussion

In healthy individuals, CBF remains relatively constant during mild-to-moderate exercise because cerebral autoregulatory mechanisms maintain a relatively constant CBF despite fluctuations in arterial pressure [7, 15, 28]. However, these

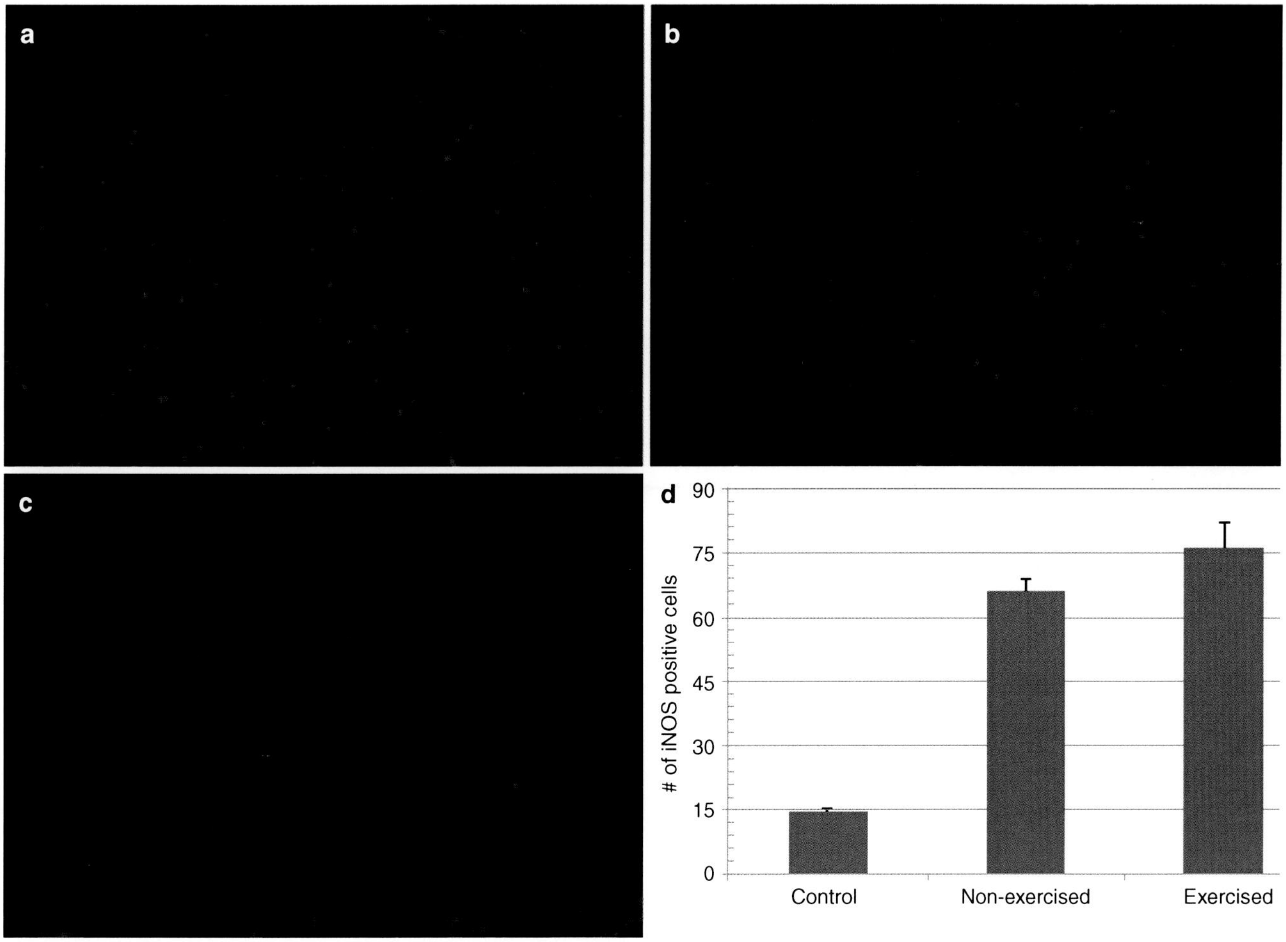

Fig. 1 Staining for the injury marker, inducible nitric oxide synthase (iNOS), in the brain stem. (**a**) Control, no blood injection or exercise, (**b**) subarachnoid hemorrhage without exercise, (**c**) subarachnoid hemorrhage with mild exercise, (**d**) histogram comparing the total number of iNOS-positive cells per group

autoregulatory mechanisms can be perturbed in critically ill patients.

Bedrest and triple-H therapy are commonly prescribed for SAH patients after securing the aneurysm in order to lower the risk of poor neurological outcomes from CV [27]. Bedrest and immobilization purportedly prevent exacerbation of already impaired autoregulation; thus preventing the rerouting of blood from the brain to the musculature during ambulation. However, immobility also reduces cardiac output, increases pulmonary complications, and results in venous stasis from pooling in the extremities at a time when increased cerebral oxygenation and blood flow are necessary.

It has been our standard of care to initiate exercise in SAH patients soon after they are able to participate, with the intent of minimizing the risk of complications associated with venous stasis, reduced cardiac output, and pulmonary dysfunction, but there have not been any prior studies evaluating whether mild exercise altered the natural history of CV in this patient population. Data have demonstrated that mobilization in ischemic stroke patients is not harmful and does not negatively impact intracranial pressure or CBF [5, 6, 8, 14, 17, 29, 40]. The primary purpose of this retrospective clinical study in conjunction with laboratory analysis was to test the hypothesis that mild early exercise does not increase the risk of CV or associated complications, nor does it increase molecular markers of neuronal injury.

Although our clinical results are limited by the retrospective nature of our data collection, the incidence of CV in those who exercised before 4 days of hospitalization was significantly lower than in the non-exercised group. A larger number of patients who were actively mobilized early during their recovery phase were less neurologically devastated and had lower HHS, as would be expected. To control for HHS, a multivariate analysis was performed. These results demonstrated that lack of active exercise raised the odds of symptomatic CV more than eightfold in comparison with patients who participated in active exercise before PBD-4. This illustrates that the beneficial effect of early exercise after aneurysm SAH was independent of HHS.

In this study, the incidence of pulmonary-related complications, such as pneumonia and pleural effusions, was 27 %, consistent with published rates and did not differ between exercised and non-exercised groups [19]. The incidence of DVT was 5 %, without a significant difference between groups; this may be attributed to our aggressive DVT prophylaxis protocol in all of these patients using Sequential Compression Devices, TED stockings, and subcutaneous enoxaparin. The incidence of DVTs in the published literature ranges from 1 to 50 % in critically ill and SAH patients [2, 3, 16, 33, 36].

To examine the effect that exercise may have at the tissue level in SAH patients, we used a rodent model we are familiar with and have published on previously to test for changes in the expression of the neuronal injury marker, iNOS. Brainstem tissue was chosen for molecular analysis because this model predominantly causes CV in the basilar artery; thus, we wanted to examine the effects of exercise in the tissue supplied by this parent artery. The number of iNOS-positive cells was significantly increased in the SAH group compared with saline-treated control animals, confirming that iNOS is a good marker of injury in this model [9]. Most importantly, no difference was found between the SAH groups, demonstrating that exercise did not exacerbate neuronal tissue damage. Although we would have liked to see reduced iNOS levels in the exercised group, it is important to confirm that no additional injury occurs with exercise; that has important clinical implications for exercised patients. A mild SAH model was intentionally chosen so that the rodents could easily be exercised on the treadmill. However, we may not see a difference in iNOS expression between groups because this model may represent only a mild form of brain injury from SAH compared with the endovascular perforation model, which may more closely mimic severe SAH in the clinical setting. Future studies looking for differences between exercised and non-exercised animals using other neuron-specific injury markers in this model and in the severe SAH endovascular perforation model may be of interest and more clinically relevant.

This study is retrospective in nature and is limited by accurate charting by clinicians and physical therapists to determine the nature and duration of exercise. The therapists did not follow a specific protocol design when treating SAH patients and could affect outcomes. Furthermore, nursing notes were not available for review, thus providing no documentation of additional mobilization that often occurs throughout the day. The data seen in this study; however, do suggest that a prospective study is warranted, using a standardized therapy regimen and collecting intracranial pressure (ICP) and CBF data so that these variables can also be investigated to determine whether they are affected by exercise. Additionally, laboratory studies further investigating the biochemical effects of exercise on brain tissue after SAH can be performed in both this mild SAH model and the more severe endovascular perforation model, using a spectrum of injury and inflammatory markers.

Conclusion

Early mobilization with mild exercise significantly reduced the odds of developing symptomatic cerebral vasospasm. These relationships need to be studied further in a prospective trial with defined exercise regimens that can be compared with changes in intracranial pressure (ICP) and cerebral blood flow (CBF). Additional investigation in the laboratory using mild and severe SAH models to more closely mimic the human scenario of SAH and expanding the spectrum of molecular injury markers examined may continue to support our early clinical findings. Identification of protective pathways in the SAH model could result in targeted intervention in the clinical arena.

Conflict of Interest Statement We declare that we have no conflict of interest.

References

1. Alaraj A, Charbel FT, Amin-Hanjani S (2009) Peri-operative measures for treatment and prevention of cerebral vasospasm following subarachnoid hemorrhage. Neurol Res 31(6): 651–659
2. Attia J, Ray JG, Cook DJ, Douketis J, Ginsberg JS, Geerts WH (2001) Deep vein thrombosis and its prevention in critically ill adults. Arch Intern Med 161(10):1268–1279
3. Ayer RE, Zhang JH (2008) The clinical significance of acute brain injury in subarachnoid hemorrhage and opportunity for intervention. Acta Neurochir Suppl 105:179–184
4. Barry C, Turner RJ, Corrigan F, Vink R (2012) New therapeutic approaches to subarachnoid hemorrhage. Expert Opin Investig Drugs 21(6):845–859
5. Bernhardt J, Dewey H, Thrift A, Collier J, Donnan G (2008) A very early rehabilitation trial for stroke (AVERT): phase II safety and feasibility. Stroke 39(2):390–396
6. Blissitt PA, Mitchell PH, Newell DW, Woods SL, Belza B (2006) Cerebrovascular dynamics with head-of-bed elevation in patients with mild or moderate vasospasm after aneurysmal subarachnoid hemorrhage. Am J Crit Care 15(2):206–216
7. Bowker TJ, Watton PN, Summers PE, Byrne JV, Ventikos Y (2010) Rest versus exercise hemodynamics for middle cerebral artery aneurysms: a computational study. AJNR Am J Neuroradiol 31(2):317–323
8. Brimioulle S, Moraine JJ, Norrenberg D, Kahn RJ (1997) Effects of positioning and exercise on intracranial pressure in a neurosurgical intensive care unit. Phys Ther 77(12):1682–1689
9. Caner B, Hou J, Altay O, Fuj M 2nd, Zhang JH (2012) Transition of research focus from vasospasm to early brain injury after subarachnoid hemorrhage. J Neurochem 123(Suppl 2): 12–21
10. Connolly ES Jr, Rabinstein AA, Carhuapoma JR et al (2012) Guidelines for the management of aneurysmal subarachnoid hemorrhage: a guideline for healthcare professionals from the American Heart Association/American Stroke Association. Stroke 43(6):1711–1737
11. Dankbaar JW, Slooter AJ, Rinkel GJ, van der Schaaf IC (2010) Effect of different components of triple-H therapy on cerebral perfusion in patients with aneurysmal subarachnoid haemorrhage: a systematic review. Crit Care 14(1):R23

12. Dudhani RV, Kyle M, Dedeo C, Riordan M, Deshaies EM (2013) A low mortality rat model to assess delayed cerebral vasospasm after experimental subarachnoid hemorrhage. J Vis Exp. doi:10.3791/4157
13. Fisher CM, Kistler JP, Davis JM (1980) Relation of cerebral vasospasm to subarachnoid hemorrhage visualized by computerized tomographic scanning. Neurosurgery 6(1):1–9
14. Ivey FM, Ryan AS, Hafer-Macko CE, Macko RF (2011) Improved cerebral vasomotor reactivity after exercise training in hemiparetic stroke survivors. Stroke 42(7):1994–2000
15. Jeong S-M, Shibata S, Levine BD, Zhang R (2012) Exercise plus volume loading prevents orthostatic intolerance but not reduction in cerebral blood flow velocity after bed rest. Am J Physiol Heart Circ Physiol 302(2):H489–H497
16. Khaldi A, Helo N, Schneck MJ, Origitano TC (2011) Venous thromboembolism: deep venous thrombosis and pulmonary embolism in a neurosurgical population. J Neurosurg 114(1):40–46
17. Koch SM, Fogarty S, Signorino C, Parmley L, Mehlhorn U (1996) Effect of passive range of motion on intracranial pressure in neurosurgical patients. J Crit Care 11(4):176–179
18. Lee KH, Lukovits T, Friedman JA (2006) "Triple-H" therapy for cerebral vasospasm following subarachnoid hemorrhage. Neurocrit Care 4(1):68–76
19. Lee K, Rincon F (2012) Pulmonary complications in patients with severe brain injury. Crit Care Res Pract 2012:207247
20. Lee J-Y, Sagher O, Keep R, Hua Y, Xi G (2009) Comparison of experimental rat models of early brain injury after subarachnoid hemorrhage. Neurosurgery 65(2):331–343
21. Lin C-L, Calisaneller T, Ukita N, Dumont AS, Kassell NF, Lee KS (2003) A murine model of subarachnoid hemorrhage-induced cerebral vasospasm. J Neurosci Methods 123(1):89–97
22. Marbacher S, Fandino J, Kitchen ND (2010) Standard intracranial in vivo animal models of delayed cerebral vasospasm. Br J Neurosurg 24(4):415–434
23. Matz P, Turner C, Weinstein PR, Massa SM, Panter SS, Sharp FR (1996) Heme-oxygenase-1 induction in glia throughout rat brain following experimental subarachnoid hemorrhage. Brain Res 713(1–2):211–222
24. Mindea SA, Yang BP, Bendok BR, Miller JW, Batjer HH (2006) Endovascular treatment strategies for cerebral vasospasm. Neurosurg Focus 21(3):E13
25. Mori T, Katayama Y, Igarashi T, Moro N, Kojima J, Hirayama T (2012) Is the circulating plasma volume sufficiently maintained? Fluid management of an aneurysmal subarachnoid hemorrhage in the acute phase. Neurol Res 34(10):1016–1019
26. Newell DW, Elliott JP, Eskridge JM, Winn HR (1999) Endovascular therapy for aneurysmal vasospasm. Crit Care Clin 15(4):685–699, v
27. Nibbelink DW, Torner JC, Henderson WG (1977) Intracranial aneurysms and subarachnoid hemorrhage – report on a randomized treatment study. IV-A. regulated bed rest. Stroke 8(2): 202–218
28. Ogoh S, Ainslie PN (2009) Cerebral blood flow during exercise: mechanisms of regulation. J Appl Physiol 107(5):1370–1380
29. Olkowski BF, Devine MA, Slotnick LE, Veznedaroglu E, Liebman KM, Arcaro ML, Binning MJ (2013) Safety and feasibility of an early mobilization program for patients with aneurysmal subarachnoid hemorrhage. Phys Ther 93(2):208–215
30. Park J-W, Bang M-S, Kwon B-S, Park Y-K, Kim D-W, Shon S-M, Jeong S-W, Lee D-K, Kim D-E (2010) Early treadmill training promotes motor function after hemorrhagic stroke in rats. Neurosci Lett 471(2):104–108
31. Pohlman MC, Schweickert WD, Pohlman AS et al (2010) Feasibility of physical and occupational therapy beginning from initiation of mechanical ventilation. Crit Care Med 38(11): 2089–2094
32. Prunell GF, Svendgaard N-A, Alkass K, Mathiesen T (2005) Inflammation in the brain after experimental subarachnoid hemorrhage. Neurosurgery 56(5):1082–1092
33. Ray WZ, Strom RG, Blackburn SL, Ashley WW, Sicard GA, Rich KM (2009) Incidence of deep venous thrombosis after subarachnoid hemorrhage. J Neurosurg 110(5):1010–1014
34. Romner B, Reinstrup P (2001) Triple H therapy after aneurysmal subarachnoid hemorrhage. A review. Acta Neurochir Suppl 77:237–241
35. Schweickert WD, Pohlman MC, Pohlman AS et al (2009) Early physical and occupational therapy in mechanically ventilated, critically ill patients: a randomised controlled trial. Lancet 373(9678):1874–1882
36. Shorr AF, Ramage AS (2001) Enoxaparin for thromboprophylaxis after major trauma: potential cost implications. Crit Care Med 29(9):1659–1665
37. Siironen J, Juvela S, Varis J, Porras M, Poussa K, Ilveskero S, Hernesniemi J, Lassila R (2003) No effect of enoxaparin on outcome of aneurysmal subarachnoid hemorrhage: a randomized, double-blind, placebo-controlled clinical trial. J Neurosurg 99(6):953–959
38. Smith TP, Enterline DS (2000) Endovascular treatment of cerebral vasospasm. J Vasc Interv Radiol 11(5):547–559
39. Soya H, Mukai A, Deocaris CC, Ohiwa N, Chang H, Nishijima T, Fujikawa T, Togashi K, Saito T (2007) Threshold-like pattern of neuronal activation in the hypothalamus during treadmill running: establishment of a minimum running stress (MRS) rat model. Neurosci Res 58(4):341–348
40. Sundseth A, Thommessen B, Rønning OM (2012) Outcome after mobilization within 24 hours of acute stroke: a randomized controlled trial. Stroke 43(9):2389–2394
41. Weyer GW, Nolan CP, Macdonald RL (2006) Evidence-based cerebral vasospasm management. Neurosurg Focus 21(3):E8

Time-Dependent Changes in Cerebrospinal Fluid Metal Ions Following Aneurysm Subarachnoid Hemorrhage and Their Association with Cerebral Vasospasm

Amit Singla, Mark R. Villwock, Margaret A. Riordan, David J. Padalino, and Eric M. Deshaies

Abstract Aneurysm subarachnoid hemorrhage affects 10 in 100,000 people annually, 40 % of whom will develop neurological deficits from ischemic stroke caused by cerebral vasospasm. Currently, the underlying mechanisms are uncertain. Metal ions are important modulators of neuronal electrophysiological conduction and smooth muscle cell activity, thereby potentially contributing to vasospasm. We hypothesized that metal ion concentrations in the cerebrospinal fluid (CSF) after aneurysm rupture would change over time and be associated with vasospasm. To test this hypothesis, for 21 days, we collected CSF from patients with aneurysmal rupture and subjected it to spectrometry to detect metals. A repeated measures analysis was performed to analyze concentration changes over time. Six of the seven patients with aneurysmal rupture experienced vasospasm, all resolving by day 14. Changes in Fe^{2+} and Zn^{2+} concentrations in the CSF paralleled the incidence of vasospasm in this study population. Na^{+}, Ca^{2+}, Mg^{2+}, and Cu^{2+} concentrations exhibited no statistically significant changes over time. In conclusion, Fe^{2+} concentration in the CSF was significantly elevated during days 7–10, whereas Zn^{2+} concentrations spiked shortly thereafter, during days 11–14. This suggests that Fe^{2+} may be related to the induction of vasospasm and Zn^{2+} may be a marker of early brain injury secondary to ischemic injury and inflammation.

Keywords Cerebral vasospasm • Cerebrospinal fluid • Metallomics • Subarachnoid hemorrhage • Zinc

A. Singla, MD • M.R. Villwock, MS • M.A. Riordan, MD
D.J. Padalino, MD • E.M. Deshaies, MD (✉)
Department of Neurosurgery,
SUNY Upstate Medical University,
Syracuse, NY 13210, USA
e-mail: eric.m.deshaies@gmail.com

Introduction

Aneurysm subarachnoid hemorrhage (SAH) occurs in 10 per 100,000 people annually [2, 19]. Contamination of the cerebrospinal fluid (CSF) with arterial blood from SAH bathes the cerebral arteries in a sea of plasma, toxic by-products from lysed red blood cells, and the biodegrading and inflammatory processes of white blood cells [15, 17]. By uncharacterized mechanisms, this toxic bath of blood products induces a delayed event called cerebral vasospasm (CV). CV is a diffusely occurring constriction of the intracranial arteries resulting in a narrowed arterial lumen, reducing cerebral blood flow (CBF) and oxygenation. Ultimately, CV can result in delayed ischemic neurological deficits (DINDs). A vasospasm-free window typically exists for 3 days after SAH, with the risk of CV beginning on posthemorrhage day (PHD) 4 and lasting for 21 days.

During this 2- to 3-week vasospasm period, approximately 70 % of patients with aneurysm SAH will develop radiographic evidence of CV [1, 6, 7, 24], 40 % of whom will develop DINDs resulting in permanent disability from early brain injury and ischemic stroke secondary to CV. Currently, there is no treatment for CV or its neurological sequelae; treatment is limited to symptom management. The triggering events of CV and associated early brain injury have not been identified and remain important for developing therapeutic interventions that mitigate these potentially devastating and lethal consequences of SAH.

Metal ions are necessary for electrophysiological signaling pathways of neurons and contraction of smooth muscle cells in cerebral arteries. In addition, they are vital to the activation and regulation of the resident immune cells of the central nervous system and inflammatory pathways. Therefore, we examined the time course and concentrations of specific metal ions in human CSF and serum plasma after aneurysm SAH. In so doing, we intend to develop neuroprotective

J. Fandino et al. (eds.), *Neurovascular Events After Subarachnoid Hemorrhage*, Acta Neurochirurgica Supplement, Vol. 120,
DOI 10.1007/978-3-319-04981-6_11,

strategies aimed at the regulation of metal ions, thereby amplifying protective cascades and reducing inhibitory and inflammatory factors that contribute to CV.

Methods

Sample Collection

Fourteen patients (7 with aneurysm SAH and 7 non-SAH control patients) presenting to our university and requiring external ventricular drainage were eligible and enrolled into this single-center prospective study in accordance with our institutional review board guidelines. In the SAH group, CSF was collected from an external ventricular drain (up to 10 cc/day) until the drain was removed, or until the 21st day (end of the vasospasm period), whichever came first. The control CSF was collected from patients presenting to our institution who needed CSF drainage and did not have blood in the subarachnoid space.

The CSF from both groups was centrifuged at 3,000 rpm for 10 min to remove cellular debris, then autoclaved before analysis. SAH samples were pooled into five time periods for each patient to see whether we could detect changes in the ion concentrations during the CV period: PHD 0–3, 4–6, 7–10, 11–14, and 15–21. These intervals were chosen based on the time periods at which the patients typically received routine computed tomography (CT)-angiography/CT-perfusion studies so that we could compare the CSF results directly to radiographic findings. The CSF from the control patients was pooled together for analysis to yield a homogenous sample for reference. Five- to ten-milliliter aliquots of CSF were subjected to inductively coupled plasma – mass spectrometry (ICP-MS) and inductively coupled plasma – optical emission spectrometry (ICP-OES) to identify the concentration of metal ions.

Mass Spectrophotometry for Metallomic Studies

Autoclaved samples were diluted fivefold with deionized water. Calibration standards were prepared from single-element standard solutions (VWR International, Bridgeport, PA and RICCA, Arlington, TX). A Perkin Elmer Elan DRCe ICP-MS (Perkin Elmer, Shelton, CT) fitted with a Meinhard Nebulizer (Meinhard Glass Products, Golden, CO) was connected to a glass cyclonic spray chamber for analysis of $65Cu^{2+}$ and $66Zn^{2+}$; Sc was used as internal standard. K^{+} (766.490 nm), Na^{+} (330.237 nm), Ca^{2+} (315.887 nm), Mg^{2+} (279.077 nm), and Fe^{2+} (259.939 nm) were analyzed with a Perkin Elmer OPTIMA 3300DV ICP-OES. The ICP-OES was fitted with an OpalMist Nebulizer and Tracey HF Spray Chamber (Glass Expansion, Pocasset, MA).

Serum Electrolyte Levels

The serum levels of Na^{+}, K^{+}, Ca^{2+}, and Mg^{2+} were routinely measured throughout the patient's hospital stay (SAH group only) in our clinical laboratory in accordance with its standard of care. The average concentration during each time period (PHD 0–3; 4–6; 7–10; 11–14; 15–21) was calculated and compared with the range for normal values (Na^{+}:133–145 mmol/L; K^{+}: 3.3–5.5 mmol/L; Mg^{2+}:0.65–1.05 mmol/L; Ca^{2+}: 8.4–10.2 mg/dL).

Statistics

Data were analyzed using SPSS Version 17 (IBM Corporation, Armonk NY, USA). A repeated measures one-way ANOVA with least significant difference multiple comparisons was performed to analyze concentration changes in the metals over time. P values less than 0.05 were considered significant for all analyses.

Results

CSF Metal Ion Concentrations

Six of the seven SAH patients experienced CV, ranging in onset from PHD 2 through PHD 10, and resolving by PHD 14. The greatest frequency of CV (five of seven patients) occurred during the time period from PHD 11 to 14 (Fig. 1). Seven metal ions were quantified in all sample sets: Na^{+}, K^{+}, Ca^{2+}, Mg^{2+}, Fe^{2+}, Cu^{2+}, and Zn^{2+}. The peak concentration of Fe^{2+} occurred during PHD 7–10 (27.85 μmol/L) and was significantly greater than PHD 0–3 ($P=0.033$), PHD 4–6 ($P=0.046$), and PHD 15–21 ($P=0.048$) (Fig. 2a). The peak concentration of Zn^{2+} occurred during PHD 11–14 (1.31 μmol/L) and was significantly greater than PHD 15–21 ($P=0.003$) (Fig. 2b). The highest average concentration of K^{+} occurred during PHD 15–21 (3.059 mmol/L), and was significantly greater than PHD 7–10 ($P=0.020$) (Fig. 2c). Na^{+}, Mg^{2+}, Ca^{2+}, and Cu^{2+} exhibited no statistically significant changes over time (Fig. 2d–g).

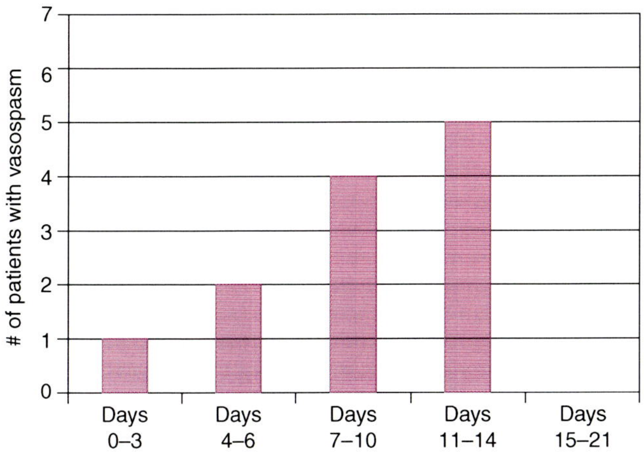

Fig. 1 Histogram of documented cerebral vasospasm. The greatest frequency of vasospasm was during days 11–14 (5 of 7 patients)

Serum Chemistry Values

The serum chemistry values of Na^+, K^+, Ca^{2+}, and Mg^{2+} were assessed until PHD 21. The average concentration of Na^+ and K^+ exhibited no deviation from the normal range throughout the entire time frame (Fig. 3a, b). However, there were significant fluctuations within these limits. The initial serum level for K^+ was significantly lower than PHD 7–10 ($P=0.048$). The serum level of Na during PHD 7–10 was significantly lower than PHD 0–3 ($P=0.002$) and PHD 4–6 ($P=0.009$). Mg^{2+} levels were above normal through PHD 14; peaking during PHD 4–6 (1.34 mmol/L) (Fig. 3c). The peak was significantly higher than the level recorded during PHD 15–21 ($P=0.024$). Lastly, Ca^{2+} levels were below normal through PHD 7, with the lowest concentration occurring during the first time period (8.0 mg/dL). Ca^{2+} levels returned to normal for PHD 7 through PHD 21 (Fig. 3d). The peak level during PHD 15–21 was significantly higher than during PHD 0–3 ($P=0.013$), PHD 4–6 ($P=0.003$), and PHD 11–14 ($P=0.024$).

Discussion

Blood products in the CSF after SAH are attributed to CV and early brain injury, but the mechanism remains elusive. The time between SAH and CV provides a unique window for therapeutic intervention. Proposed pathophysiological mechanisms of CV and early brain injury have included oxygen free radical (OFR) release from the degradation of hemoglobin in the CSF, an inflammatory response from blood products in the subarachnoid space, and lower levels of vasodilators such as carbon monoxide (CO) released by the degradation of hemoglobin by the enzyme, heme-oxygenase (HO)-1 [4, 9, 10, 26].

Knowledge of the metal ion composition of CSF and its association with CV may provide insight into the pathways that trigger vasospasm, thereby promoting the development of neuroprotective strategies. We demonstrated that two of the measured metal ions, Fe^{2+} and Zn^{2+}, change significantly over time and parallel the time course of radiographic and clinical CV. Thus, both of these ions may have important roles in the process of CV and, in the case of Zn^{2+}, may also be a marker of neuronal injury.

Changes in the CSF Fe^{2+} concentrations in this study paralleled the onset and resolution of CV seen in the SAH population. The red blood cells, released into the subarachnoid space after aneurysm rupture, lyse, releasing hemoglobin into the CSF. HO-1 degrades heme, releasing Fe^{2+} and the byproduct, CO. Fe^{2+} is responsible for a number of oxidative pathways that create OFRs, stimulating an inflammatory response as the iron is removed by the resident macrophage-like cells of the nervous system, called microglia [5, 27, 28, 30]. This inflammatory process can promote CV and neuron toxicity [15]. Interestingly, both Fe^{2+} and Zn^{2+} decreased during the final time period (PHD 15–21) of CV in parallel with the incidence of CV in this study population, further supporting their role in the pathophysiology of vasospasm.

Zinc CSF concentrations also paralleled the incidence of CV in this study, peaking just after those of Fe^{2+}. Zn^{2+} has many key roles in cellular metabolism, protein synthesis, and injury pathways, such as OFR formation, ATP-depletion, transcription factors (the zinc finger), and the initiation of glycolysis. Each of these roles is potentially important in the development of neuronal injury and CV [22, 23, 25]. Another potentially interesting role of Zn^{2+} in CV is as a competitive inhibitor of HO-1 when in the form of Zn^{2+} protoporphyrin-IX, a hemoglobin analog found in red blood cells [9, 30]. HO-1 has a higher affinity for hemoglobin than its Zn^{2+} analog, but its competitive inhibition of HO-1 can lower carbon monoxide production, a vasodilating gas molecule, thereby potentiating CV [4, 9, 10, 24, 26, 30]. Zn^{2+} is also involved with endothelial and smooth muscle cell ultrastructural composition and smooth muscle relaxation, each an important concept when considering the potential role of Zn^{2+} in CV pathways [20–22].

Whether Zn^{2+} is directly involved with CV as discussed above or represents a marker of neuronal injury is an important question. "Zinc neurons" have been described in the cortex. These neurons store Zn^{2+} in vesicles contained within the cell and have been shown to release Zn^{2+} during ischemia, a process called "zinc dumping" [11–14]. Thus, elevated Zn^{2+} levels may not only be seen because of its role in CV modulation, but also as a marker of a more subtle

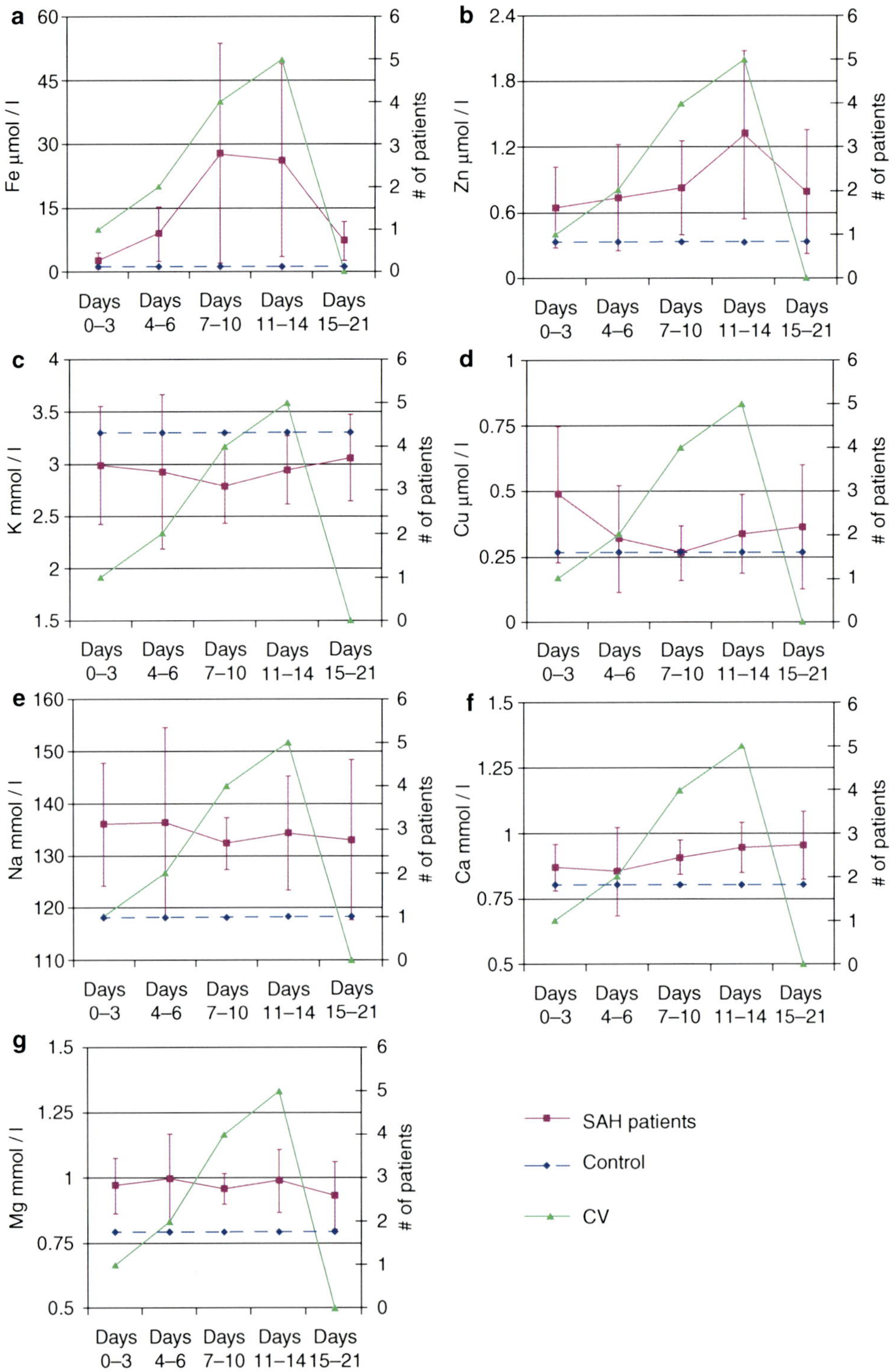

Fig. 2 Changes in the metal cation concentration in the cerebrospinal fluid of subarachnoid hemorrhage patients. The *horizontal dashed line* is the concentration of the metal cation in the control group (this was not collected over time and is plotted as a line for reference). The number of patients who experienced cerebral vasospasm during a given time period is plotted on the secondary axis. (**a**) Fe^{2+}, (**b**) Zn^{2+}, (**c**) K^{+}, (**d**) Cu^{2+}, (**e**) Na^{+}, (**f**) Ca^{2+}, (**g**) Mg^{2+}

ischemic process and cellular injury from CV occurring at the neuronal level. Lastly, Zn^{2+} plays an important role in immune modulation. The resident immune cells of the nervous system, microglia, are activated from a scavenging mode that is more benign to a more activated cytotoxic phenotype that releases OFRs and promotes inflammation [14, 16, 18, 24]. This proinflammatory role of Zn^{2+} may be an important target for antispasmotic therapy and neuroprotection in aneurysm SAH patients.

Although the concentrations of the cations Na^{+}, Cu^{2+}, Mg^{2+}, and Ca^{2+} in the CSF did not change significantly during the course of CV, they were different from control values.

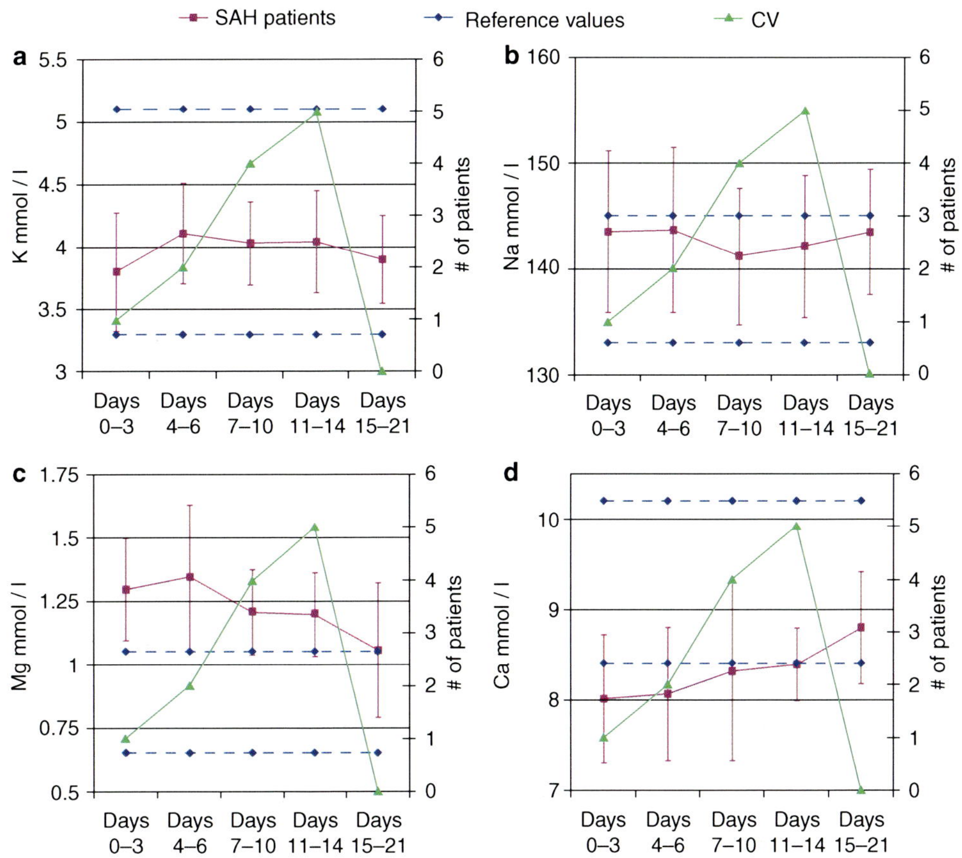

Fig. 3 Changes in the serum chemistry values for subarachnoid hemorrhage patients. The *horizontal dashed lines* represent the high and low limits of the normal range. The number of patients who experienced cerebral vasospasm during a given time period is plotted on the secondary axis. (**a**) K^+, (**b**) Na^+, (**c**) Mg^{2+}, (**d**) Ca^{2+}

This suggests that these metal ions likely reflect contamination of CSF space with serum plasma that entered the subarachnoid space during the initial aneurysm rupture, release of cytosolic contents from blood cells, and changes in the serum levels over the course of SAH treatment. The latter is particularly true for Na^+ and Mg^{2+} where patients are routinely placed on magnesium sulfate infusions intravenously for neuroprotection and, in selected cases, hypertonic 3 % sodium chloride solutions to maintain mild hypernatremia to reduce brain tissue swelling.

Serum Na^+ and K^+ concentrations were significantly lower early after SAH. Previous reports have demonstrated similar results and attribute this to cortisol release during the stress response [29]. Cortisol causes Na^+ and K^+ to be lost from the kidneys and, additionally, the K^+ to be taken in by cells from the extracellular space. This may explain the initial lower levels of these metal ions. Additionally, it is well known that the hypothalamic–pituitary axis malfunctions after SAH, seen clinically as the syndromes of inappropriate antidiuretic hormone secretion and cerebral salt wasting [8]; both causing hyponatremia. Serum magnesium levels are elevated above control levels in this study because magnesium sulfate continuous infusions are initiated as part of our standard of care because of data demonstrating its action as a neuroprotectant. Clinically, we aim to keep serum Mg^{2+} levels at 2.5–3.5 mEq/L. Lastly, serum Ca^{2+} levels were lowest early after SAH. It is uncertain whether this hypocalcemia is related to the stress response, the routine use of a calcium channel blocker (Nimotop) and $MgSO_4$ for neuroprotection, or some other undefined etiology [3]. Further evaluation of trends in serum Na^+, K^+, and Ca^{2+} levels in the setting of SAH seem warranted. Additionally, future studies looking at trends in serum Mg^{2+} concentrations in patients without magnesium sulfate infusions would be interesting to see whether there are any changes that occur over the course of CV, because smaller changes may not be measured when the patients are being administered Mg^{2+} infusions.

Conclusions

Metal ions are critical to the normal functioning and maintenance of cellular processes, biochemical reactions, inflammation, and electrical signaling pathways in the neurons and smooth muscle cells of the cerebral arteries.

Alterations in CSF Fe^{2+} and Zn^{2+} concentrations were found to parallel the incidence of CV in this study group throughout the duration of the vasospasm period, suggesting that they may have a critical role in the development and resolution of CV. Further investigation of the potential role metal ions may have in CV and early brain injury from ischemic insult is warranted. This could be further studied in the laboratory to elucidate the pathways involved in vasospasm and early brain injury after SAH, to target mechanisms for neuroprotection.

Acknowledgments The authors acknowledge Deb Driscoll and the SUNY College of Environmental Science and Forestry for the metallomics analysis. This study was not funded by any source.

Conflict of Interest Statement We declare that we have no conflict of interest.

References

1. Ayer RE, Zhang JH (2008) The clinical significance of acute brain injury in subarachnoid hemorrhage and opportunity for intervention. Acta Neurochir Suppl 105:179–184
2. Bederson JB, Connolly ES Jr, Batjer HH, Dacey RG, Dion JE, Diringer MN, Duldner JE Jr, Harbaugh RE, Patel AB, Rosenwasser RH (2009) Guidelines for the management of aneurysmal subarachnoid hemorrhage: a statement for healthcare professionals from a special writing group of the Stroke Council, American Heart Association. Stroke 40(3):994–1025
3. Van den Bergh WM, van de Water JMW, Hoff RG, Algra A, Rinkel GJE (2008) Calcium homeostasis during magnesium treatment in aneurysmal subarachnoid hemorrhage. Neurocrit Care 8(3): 413–417
4. Christova T, Diankova Z, Setchenska M (2000) Heme oxygenase–carbon monoxide signalling pathway as a physiological regulator of vascular smooth muscle cells. Acta Physiol Pharmacol Bulg 25(1):9–17
5. Connor JR, Cheepsunthorn P, Reid J, Radov LA (2002) Iron mediates gene expression in activated microglia. J Neurochem 81: 52–53
6. Deshaies EM, Boulos AS, Drazin D, Popp AJ (2009) Evidence-based pharmacotherapy for cerebral vasospasm. Neurol Res 31(6):615–620
7. Deshaies EM, Boulos AS, Popp AJ (2009) Peri-operative medical management of cerebral vasospasm. Neurol Res 31(6):644–650
8. Dooling E, Winkelman C (2004) Hyponatremia in the patient with subarachnoid hemorrhage. J Neurosci Nurs 36(3):130–135
9. Dulak J, Józkowicz A, Foresti R, Kasza A, Frick M, Huk I, Green CJ, Pachinger O, Weidinger F, Motterlini R (2002) Heme oxygenase activity modulates vascular endothelial growth factor synthesis in vascular smooth muscle cells. Antioxid Redox Signal 4(2):229–240
10. Durante W (2002) Carbon monoxide and bile pigments: surprising mediators of vascular function. Vasc Med 7(3):195–202
11. Frederickson CJ, Maret W, Cuajungco MP (2004) Zinc and excitotoxic brain injury: a new model. Neuroscientist 10(1):18–25
12. Frederickson CJ, Moncrieff DW (1994) Zinc-containing neurons. Biol Signals 3(3):127–139
13. Frederickson CJ, Suh SW, Silva D, Frederickson CJ, Thompson RB (2000) Importance of zinc in the central nervous system: the zinc-containing neuron. J Nutr 130(5S Suppl):1471S–1483S
14. Galasso SL, Dyck RH (2007) The role of zinc in cerebral ischemia. Mol Med 13(7–8):380–387
15. Goldstein L, Teng Z-P, Zeserson E, Patel M, Regan RF (2003) Hemin induces an iron-dependent, oxidative injury to human neuron-like cells. J Neurosci Res 73(1):113–121
16. Kaindl AM, Degos V, Peineau S et al (2012) Activation of microglial N-methyl-D-aspartate receptors triggers inflammation and neuronal cell death in the developing and mature brain. Ann Neurol 72(4):536–549
17. Kassell NF, Sasaki T, Colohan AR, Nazar G (1985) Cerebral vasospasm following aneurysmal subarachnoid hemorrhage. Stroke 16(4):562–572
18. Kauppinen TM, Higashi Y, Suh SW, Escartin C, Nagasawa K, Swanson RA (2008) Zinc triggers microglial activation. J Neurosci 28(22):5827–5835
19. King JT Jr (1997) Epidemiology of aneurysmal subarachnoid hemorrhage. Neuroimaging Clin N Am 7(4):659–668
20. Kusleikaite M, Stonkus S, Kusleika S (2003) The effect of zinc on endothelium-dependent relaxation of blood-vessels and on the ultrastructure of endothelial cells under immobilization stress. J Trace Elem Med Biol 17(3):193–198
21. Kusleikaite M, Stonkus S, Laukeviciene A, Kusleika G (2003) The significance of zinc for contractility of smooth muscles and ultrastructure of their microfilaments in case of hypodynamic stress. Medicina (Kaunas) 39(6):579–583
22. Labyntseva RD, Ul'ianenko TV, Kosterin SA (1998) Effect of heavy metal ions on superprecipitation and ATPase activity of uterine smooth muscle actomyosin activity. Ukr Biokhim Zh 70(2):71–77
23. Lemire J, Mailloux R, Appanna VD (2008) Zinc toxicity alters mitochondrial metabolism and leads to decreased ATP production in hepatocytes. J Appl Toxicol 28(2):175–182
24. Pluta RM (2005) Delayed cerebral vasospasm and nitric oxide: review, new hypothesis, and proposed treatment. Pharmacol Ther 105(1):23–56
25. Rudolf E (2007) Depletion of ATP and oxidative stress underlie zinc-induced cell injury. Acta Medica (Hradec Kralove) 50(1): 43–49
26. Siow RC, Sato H, Mann GE (1999) Heme oxygenase-carbon monoxide signalling pathway in atherosclerosis: anti-atherogenic actions of bilirubin and carbon monoxide? Cardiovasc Res 41(2): 385–394
27. Song D, Song Y, Hadziahmetovic M, Zhong Y, Dunaief JL (2012) Systemic administration of the iron chelator deferiprone protects against light-induced photoreceptor degeneration in the mouse retina. Free Radic Biol Med 53(1):64–71
28. Suttkus A, Rohn S, Jäger C, Arendt T, Morawski M (2012) Neuroprotection against iron-induced cell death by perineuronal nets – an in vivo analysis of oxidative stress. Am J Neurodegener Dis 1(2):122–129
29. Wong GKC, Poon WS, Chan MTV, Boet R, Gin T, Lam CW (2007) The effect of intravenous magnesium sulfate infusion on serum levels of sodium and potassium in patients with aneurysmal subarachnoid hemorrhage. Magnes Res 20(1):37–42
30. Yoshida T, Tanaka M, Sotomatsu A, Hirai S (1995) Activated microglia cause superoxide-mediated release of iron from ferritin. Neurosci Lett 190(1):21–24

Effects of Tenascin-C on Early Brain Injury After Subarachnoid Hemorrhage in Rats

Masato Shiba, Masashi Fujimoto, Fumio Kawakita, Kyoko Imanaka-Yoshida, Toshimichi Yoshida, Kenji Kanamaru, Waro Taki, and Hidenori Suzuki

Abstract *Background and Purpose:* We previously reported that tenascin-C (TNC), a matricellular protein, was involved in the pathogenesis of cerebral vasospasm after subarachnoid hemorrhage (SAH), but the role of TNC in early brain injury (EBI) is unknown. This study assessed whether inhibition of TNC upregulation in brain by imatinib mesylate (imatinib), an inhibitor of the tyrosine kinases of platelet-derived growth factor receptors, prevents EBI after experimental SAH.

Methods: Rats were assigned to sham, SAH plus vehicle, and SAH plus imatinib groups ($n=4$ per group). Imatinib (50 mg/kg body weight) was administered intraperitoneally to rats undergoing SAH by endovascular perforation, and EBI was evaluated using terminal deoxynucleotidyl transferase-mediated uridine 5-triphosphate-biotin nick end-labeling staining at 24 h after SAH. Imatinib-treated SAH rats were also treated by a cisternal injection of recombinant TNC.

Results: SAH upregulated TNC and caused EBI. Imatinib treatment suppressed both TNC upregulation and EBI at 24 h. Recombinant TNC reinduced EBI in imatinib-treated SAH rats.

Conclusions: TNC may be involved in the pathogenesis of EBI after SAH.

Keywords Tenascin-C • Early brain injury • Subarachnoid hemorrhage

M. Shiba, MD, PhD (✉) • M. Fujimoto, MD, PhD
F. Kawakita, MD • W. Taki, MD, PhD
Department of Neurosurgery, Mie University Graduate School of Medicine, 2-174 Edobashi, Tsu, Mie 514-8507, Japan
e-mail: mshiba@clin.medic.mie-u.ac.jp

K. Imanaka-Yoshida, MD, PhD • T. Yoshida, MD, PhD
Department of Pathology and Matrix Biology, Mie University Graduate School of Medicine, Tsu, Mie 514-8507, Japan

Research Center for Matrix Biology, Mie University Graduate School of Medicine, Tsu, Mie 514-8507, Japan

K. Kanamaru, MD, PhD
Department of Neurosurgery, Suzuka Kaisei Hospital, Suzuka, Japan

H. Suzuki, MD, PhD
Department of Neurosurgery, Mie University Graduate School of Medicine, 2-174 Edobashi, Tsu, Mie 514-8507, Japan

Research Center for Matrix Biology, Mie University Graduate School of Medicine, Tsu, Mie 514-8507, Japan

Introduction

Tenascin-C (TNC) is a matricellular protein in the family of nonstructural and secreted extracellular matrix proteins [7]. We recently reported that imatinib mesylate (imatinib), an inhibitor of the tyrosine kinases of platelet-derived growth factor (PDGF) receptors (PDGFRs), prevented cerebral vasospasm via inhibiting TNC expression [10]. It has also been reported that TNC was induced in serum and cerebrospinal fluid after subarachnoid hemorrhage (SAH) in a clinical setting, and associated with poor outcomes [12, 13]. However, recent research has demonstrated that cerebral vasospasm is not necessarily correlated with poor outcomes, and that treating early brain injury (EBI) is more important to improve outcomes after SAH [9]. In this study, thus, we examined whether inhibition of TNC by imatinib prevents EBI at 24 h after experimental SAH in rats.

Materials and Methods

All procedures were approved by the Animal Ethics Review Committee of Mie University, and were in accordance with the institution's Guidelines for Animal Experiments.

SAH Model and Study Protocol

We produced the endovascular filament perforation model of SAH in male adult Sprague-Dawley rats (age 8–9 weeks, 270–320 g; SLC, Hamamatsu, Japan) as previously described

J. Fandino et al. (eds.), *Neurovascular Events After Subarachnoid Hemorrhage*, Acta Neurochirurgica Supplement, Vol. 120,
DOI 10.1007/978-3-319-04981-6_12, © Springer International Publishing Switzerland 2015

[10]. In brief, rats were anesthetized by an intraperitoneal injection of 4 % chloral hydrate (10 ml/kg). Blood pressure and blood gases were measured via the left femoral artery. Rectal temperature was kept at 37 °C during surgery. After the left common carotid artery, external carotid artery, and internal carotid artery were exposed, a sharpened 4–0 monofilament nylon suture was advanced rostrally into the internal carotid artery from the external carotid artery stump until resistance was felt, and then it was pushed 3 mm farther to perforate the bifurcation of the anterior and middle cerebral arteries. Immediately after puncture, the suture was withdrawn into the external carotid artery stump, and the internal carotid artery was reperfused to produce SAH. Sham-operated rats underwent an identical procedure, except that the suture was withdrawn once resistance was felt, without puncture. After the animals were killed, high-resolution pictures of the base of the brain were taken for assessing the severity of SAH under ice cooling. The brain was stored in 10 % neutral buffered formalin for terminal deoxynucleotidyltransferase-mediated dUTP nick end-labeling (TUNEL) staining and immunohistochemistry.

First, 22 rats underwent endovascular perforation SAH or sham operation. After 30 min, the 12 surviving rats were randomly divided into three groups, and 50 mg/kg body weight of imatinib (Novartis, Basel, Switzerland) or vehicle (phosphate-buffered saline [PBS], 10 mL/kg) was injected intraperitoneally. We evaluated EBI at 24 h after surgery by TUNEL staining and immunohistochemical TNC staining.

Next, 2 μg of recombinant TNC or vehicle (PBS, 100 μL) was injected into the cisterna magna in rats. After 30 min, SAH was produced and SAH rats were treated with 50 mg/kg of imatinib as above. Randomization into either TNC- or vehicle-treated SAH–imatinib groups was continued until there were at least three animals per group. TUNEL staining was performed 24 h after SAH.

Severity of SAH

The severity of SAH was assessed in a blinded fashion as previously described [11]. In brief, the basal cistern was divided into six segments, and each segment was allotted a grade from 0 to 3, depending on the amount of SAH. The animals received a total score ranging from 0 to 18 by summing up the scores.

Intracisternal Infusion

Using a surgical microscope (Zeiss, Germany), the posterior cervical muscles were dissected through a suboccipital midline skin incision, and the atlanto-occipital membrane was exposed [14]. The membrane was penetrated by a 27-gauge needle. Sterile PBS vehicle (100 μL) or mouse recombinant TNC (murine myeloma cell line, NS0-derived, Gly23–Pro625, with a C-terminal 6-His tag, 2 μg in 100 μL; R&D Systems, Minneapolis, MN) was infused at a rate of 100 μL/min regardless of the animal's body weight at 30 min before surgery, as previously described [10]. The needle was removed 10 min after an infusion, and the pore was quickly plugged with oxidized cellulose.

TUNEL Staining

TUNEL staining was performed as previously described [2]. Four-micron-thick coronal sections at the level of bregma + 1.0 mm were cut using a microtome and were subjected to TUNEL staining with an in situ cell death detection kit (Roche Inc., Mannheim, Germany). Color reactions were developed in diaminobenzidine/hydrogen peroxide solution and the sections were counterstained with hematoxylin solution for light microscopic examination. Incubation with labeling solution without the enzyme served as a negative labeling control. The TUNEL-positive neurons were counted in 10 fields per case at × 400 magnification in the left frontal cortex and expressed as the mean number of TUNEL-positive neurons/mm^2 in a blinded manner.

Immunohistochemistry

Immunohistochemistry on formalin-fixed paraffin-embedded sections was performed as described previously [15]. After dewaxing and rehydration, the sections were treated with 3 % hydrogen peroxide for 10 min to block endogenous peroxidase activities, placed in 1 mmol ethylenediaminetetraacetic acid (pH 8.0) and heated in an autoclave at 121 °C for 1 min. The sections were then blocked with 5 % horse serum and incubated overnight at 4 °C with the mouse monoclonal anti-TNC antibody (1 μg/mL, Immuno-Biological Laboratories, Takasaki, Japan). They were subsequently incubated with biotinylated anti-mouse immunoglobulin (Vector Laboratories, Burlingame, CA) for 30 min and then with an avidin–biotin complex for 30 min at room temperature. Color reactions were developed in diaminobenzidine/hydrogen peroxide solution and the sections were counterstained with hematoxylin solution for light microscopic examination. Negative controls consisted of serial sections incubated with buffer alone instead of the primary antibody.

Statistics

The number of TUNEL-positive neurons was expressed as mean ± standard error of the mean (SEM), and one-way analysis of variance (ANOVA) with Tukey-Kramer *post hoc* tests was used as appropriate. $P < 0.05$ was considered significant.

Results

There were no significant differences in physiological parameters, severity of SAH, and mortality among the groups (data not shown). TUNEL-positive neurons were seen in the left frontal cortex at 24 h after SAH (Fig. 1). The imatinib treatment significantly prevented an increase in TUNEL-positive neurons at 24 h after SAH. Immunohistochemistry showed that TNC was increased in the neuropil mainly in the brain surface of the left frontal cortex. The imatinib treatment remarkably inhibited the immunoreactivity at 24 h (Fig. 2). Intracisternal infusions of recombinant TNC increased TUNEL-positive neurons in the left frontal cortex compared with the PBS-treated SAH–imatinib group (Fig. 3).

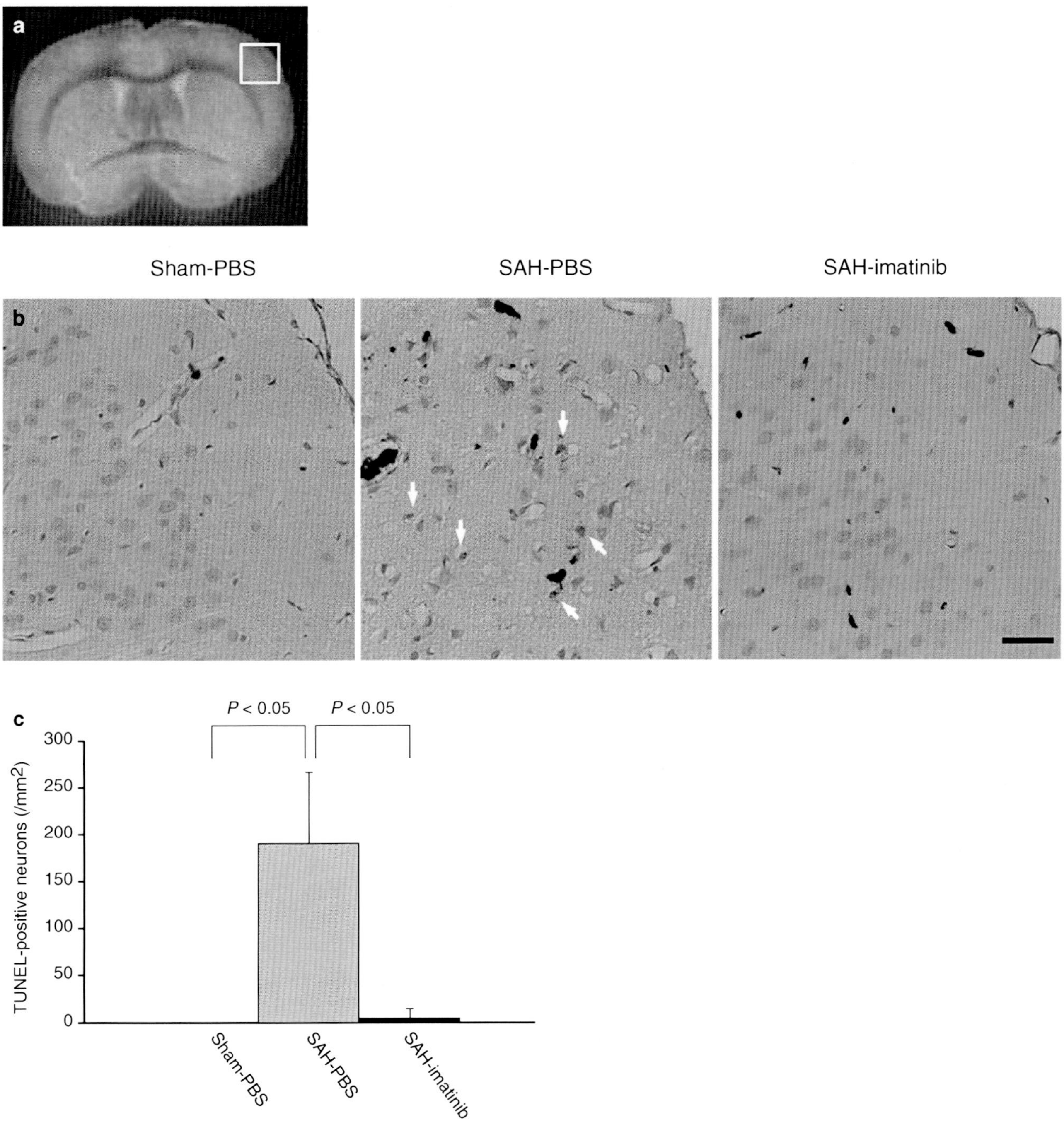

Fig. 1 Effects of imatinib treatment after SAH on EBI in the left frontal cortex at bregma + 1 mm. Representative SAH brain slice showing the left frontal cortex (**a**). Representative images showing TUNEL-positive neurons (*arrows*) (**b**) and quantitative analysis of TUNEL-positive neurons (**c**). *Sham-PBS* sham-operated rats treated with PBS, *SAH-PBS* SAH-imatinib, *SAH* rats treated with PBS or imatinib, *data* mean ± SEM, *P* value, ANOVA. $N = 4$ per group. Bar = 50 μm

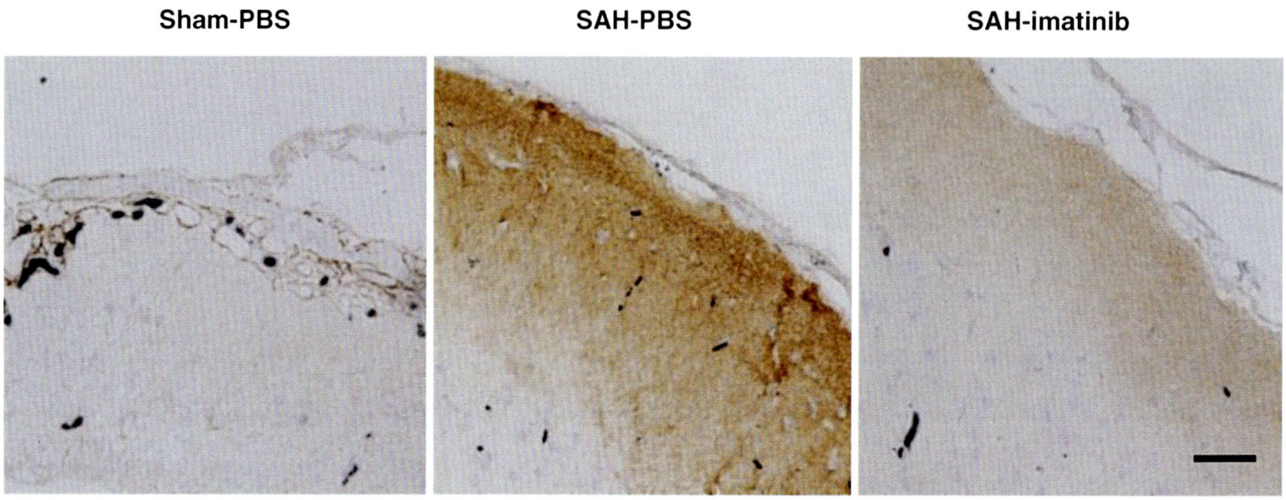

Fig. 2 Effects of imatinib treatment after SAH on immunohistochemical TNC staining in the left frontal cortex at bregma + 1 mm at 24 h after SAH. *Sham-PBS* sham-operated rats treated with PBS, *SAH-PBS* or *SAH-imatinib* SAH rats treated with PBS or imatinib, Bar = 50 μm

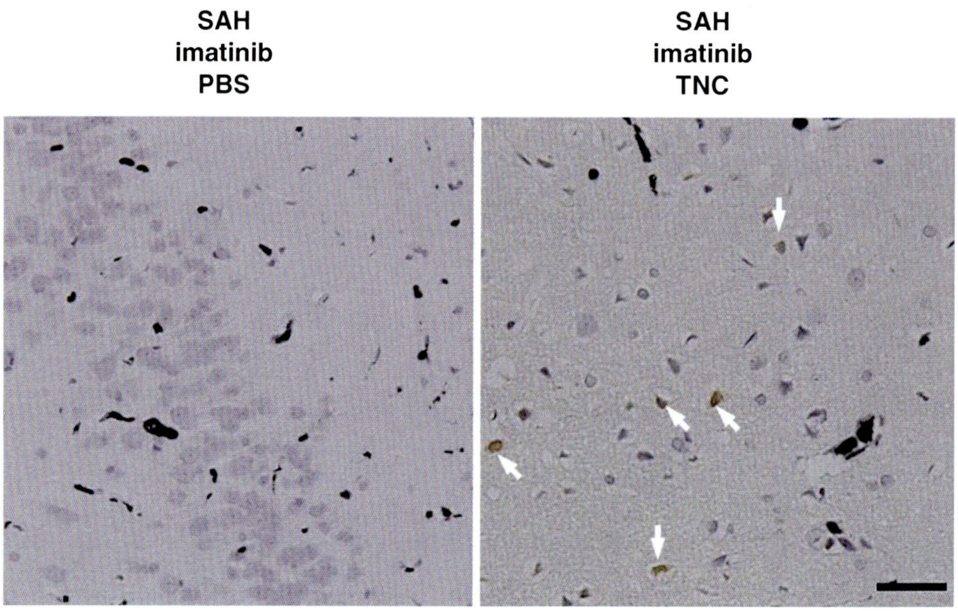

Fig. 3 Effects of intracisternal infusions of recombinant TNC on EBI in SAH rats treated with imatinib (*SAH-imatinib*) at 24 h after SAH. *SAH-imatinib-PBS* or *SAH-imatinib-TNC*, SAH-imatinib with a pre-SAH intracisternal infusion of PBS or TNC. *Arrows*, TUNEL-positive neurons. Bar = 50 μm

Discussion

In our recent study, TNC induced cerebral vasospasm after SAH via activating p38 and upregulating PDGFR-β; and imatinib prevented cerebral vasospasm via inhibiting TNC expression [10]. This study also showed that SAH upregulated TNC in the cerebral cortex with induction of TUNEL-positive neurons, and inhibition of TNC by imatinib decreased the number of TUNEL-positive neurons. Recombinant TNC injections reincreased TUNEL-positive neurons in SAH brain regardless of imatinib treatment. These findings suggested that TNC was involved in the pathogenesis of EBI after SAH.

TNC, a matricellular protein, is highly expressed in embryonic tissue during morphogenesis and sparsely expressed in the adult, but reappears in pathological states [3]. It has been reported that TNC can activate mitogen-activated protein kinases and some growth factor receptors, and can upregulate proinflammatory cytokines [8] and endothelin receptor type A [6]. By these means, TNC has multiple functions in the regulation of cell migration, proliferation, and apoptosis [5]. Apoptosis, inflammation, and endothelin-1 release play an important role in the mechanisms of EBI after SAH [9]. Thus, TNC may have a significant role in the pathophysiology of EBI after SAH, but the mechanisms to induce EBI remain unclear and need further studies to clarify the mechanisms.

After SAH, platelets activate and aggregate in the lumen of small cerebral vessels [9]. Luminal platelet aggregates activate and promote mechanisms that cause structural injury and functional deficits in small vessels, and devastate the already compromised brain. PDGF can induce TNC expression via the phosphoinositide 3-kinase/Akt pathway [4] and MAPK pathway [1]. In addition, our previous study suggested that PDGF-induced TNC may positively feedback on PDGFR activation via PDGFR upregulation and crosstalk signaling between receptors as well as upregulation of TNC itself, leading to MAPK activation and cerebral vasospasm after SAH [10]. Thus, PDGF-induced TNC signaling is suggested to be involved in the induction of EBI after SAH.

Recent research efforts moved to focus on clarifying the pathophysiology of EBI after SAH and on developing protective strategies against EBI to improve outcome after SAH [9]. Neuronal apoptosis is involved in the pathogenesis of EBI after SAH [2, 9]. This study showed that TNC may induce neuronal apoptosis, but further studies are needed to prove the underlying mechanisms.

Conclusion

TNC may play an important role in the pathogenesis of EBI after SAH. Further investigations are necessary to understand the mechanism behind how TNC affects EBI and to determine a new therapeutic approach against EBI for improving neurological outcome after SAH.

Acknowledgments We thank Ms. Chiduru Yamamoto (Department of Neurosurgery, Mie University Graduate School of Medicine) for her technical assistance.

This work was supported in part by a grant-in-aid for Scientific Research from the Japan Society for the Promotion of Science to Drs. Shiba and Suzuki.

Conflicts of Interest Statement We declare that we have no conflict of interest.

References

1. Chiquet M, Sarasa-Renedo A, Tunc-Civelek V (2004) Induction of tenascin-C by cyclic tensile strain versus growth factors: distinct contributions by Rho/ROCK and MAPK signaling pathways. Biochim Biophys Acta 1693:193–204
2. Hasegawa Y, Suzuki H, Altay O, Zhang JH (2011) Preservation of tropomyosin-related kinase B (TrkB) signaling by sodium orthovanadate attenuates early brain injury after subarachnoid hemorrhage in rats. Stroke 42:477–483
3. Imanaka-Yoshida K, Hiroe M, Yasutomi Y, Toyozaki T, Tsuchiya T, Noda N, Maki T, Nishikawa T, Sakakura T, Yoshida T (2002) Tenascin-C is a useful marker for disease activity in myocarditis. J Pathol 197:388–394
4. Jinnin M, Ihn H, Asano Y, Yamane K, Trojanowska M, Tamaki K (2006) Platelet derived growth factor induced tenascin-C transcription is phosphoinositide 3-kinase/Akt-dependent and mediated by Ets family transcription factors. J Cell Physiol 206:718–727
5. Jones PL, Jones FS (2000) Tenascin-C in development and disease: gene regulation and cell function. Matrix Biol 19: 581–596
6. Lange K, Kammerer M, Hegi ME, Grotegut S, Dittmann A, Huang W, Fluri E, Yip GW, Gotte M, Ruiz C, Orend G (2007) Endothelin receptor type B counteracts tenascin-C-induced endothelin receptor type A-dependent focal adhesion and actin stress fiber disorganization. Cancer Res 67:6163–6173
7. Matsui Y, Morimoto J, Uede T (2010) Role of matricellular proteins in cardiac tissue remodeling after myocardial infarction. World J Biol Chem 1:69–80
8. Midwood KS, Orend G (2009) The role of tenascin-C in tissue injury and tumorigenesis. J Cell Commun Signal 3:287–310
9. Sehba FA, Pluta RM, Zhang JH (2011) Metamorphosis of subarachnoid hemorrhage research: from delayed vasospasm to early brain injury. Mol Neurobiol 43:27–40
10. Shiba M, Suzuki H, Fujimoto M, Shimojo N, Imanaka-Yoshida K, Yoshida T, Kanamaru K, Matsushima S, Taki W (2012) Imatinib mesylate prevents cerebral vasospasm after subarachnoid hemorrhage via inhibiting tenascin-C expression in rats. Neurobiol Dis 46:172–179
11. Sugawara T, Ayer R, Jadhav V, Zhang JH (2008) A new grading system evaluating bleeding scale in filament perforation subarachnoid hemorrhage rat model. J Neurosci Methods 167: 327–334
12. Suzuki H, Kanamaru K, Shiba M, Fujimoto M, Imanaka-Yoshida K, Yoshida T, Taki W (2011) Cerebrospinal fluid tenascin-C in cerebral vasospasm after aneurysmal subarachnoid hemorrhage. J Neurosurg Anesthesiol 23:310–317
13. Suzuki H, Kanamaru K, Suzuki Y, Aimi Y, Matsubara N, Araki T, Takayasu M, Kinoshita N, Imanaka-Yoshida K, Yoshida T, Taki W (2010) Tenascin-C is induced in cerebral vasospasm after subarachnoid hemorrhage in rats and humans: a pilot study. Neurol Res 32:179–184
14. Suzuki H, Kanamaru K, Tsunoda H, Inada H, Kuroki M, Sun H, Waga S, Tanaka T (1999) Heme oxygenase-1 gene induction as an intrinsic regulation against delayed cerebral vasospasm in rats. J Clin Invest 104:59–66
15. Yatsushige H, Ostrowski RP, Tsubokawa T, Colohan A, Zhang JH (2007) Role of c-Jun N-terminal kinase in early brain injury after subarachnoid hemorrhage. J Neurosci Res 85:1436–1448

The Role of Erythropoietin in Aneurysmal Subarachnoid Haemorrhage: From Bench to Bedside

Giovanni Grasso, Michele Buemi, and Filippo Giambartino

Abstract Subarachnoid haemorrhage (SAH) caused by a ruptured aneurysm accounts for only 5 % of strokes, but occurs at a fairly young age and carries a poor prognosis. Delayed cerebral ischaemia (DCI) is an important cause of death and dependence after aneurysmal SAH. The current mainstay of preventing DCI is nimodipine and maintenance of normovolemia, but even with this strategy DCI occurs in a considerable proportion of patients.

Several drugs have been developed that have the potential to limit cerebral vasospasm and delayed ischaemic neurologic deficit, thus improving outcome for patients. However, although numerous agents can prevent arterial narrowing and/or block the excitatory cascade of events leading to ischaemic neuronal death in experimental conditions, there is still no pharmacologic agent that has been shown conclusively to improve the outcome in clinical practice.

Erythropoietin (EPO) is a well-known erythropoietic hormone recently found to exert neuroprotective properties and has been shown to reduce cerebral vasospasm and infarct volume after experimental SAH. In humans, although EPO treatment did not impact the overall incidence of vasospasm, it significantly reduced the incidence of severe vasospasm, the incidence of delayed ischaemic deficits with new cerebral infarcts, and the duration of impaired autoregulation. The current study provides new evidence for the potential benefit and relative safety of EPO for the treatment of SAH in humans. Future clinical trials will hopefully provide definite evidence whether EPO treatment is beneficial in SAH patients.

G. Grasso, MD, PhD (✉)
Department of Neurosurgery,
University of Palermo, Policlinico Universitario "Giaccone",
Via del Vespro 129, Palermo 90100, Italy
e-mail: giovanni.grasso@unipa.it

M. Buemi, MD
Department of Internal Medicine,
University of Messina, Messina, Italy

F. Giambartino, MD
Department of Anesthesiology,
University of Palermo, Palermo, Italy

Keywords Cerebral aneurysm • Erythropoietin • Subarachnoid hemorrhage

Subarachnoid haemorrhage (SAH) caused by ruptured aneurysm occurs in 700,000 individuals a year [5]. Although the mortality rate associated with the occurrence of SAH appears to have improved over the last 50 years, nearly half of all patients with an SAH will still die within 1 month of the initial bleeding [5]. Cerebral vasospasm (CVS) occurs in a majority of patients and is associated with poor outcome [46]; therefore it remains a prevalent complication following aneurysmal SAH (aSAH). The occurrence of secondary ischaemia and delayed ischaemic neurologic deficits (DINDs) are common sequelae in vasospasm and lead to poor long-term outcomes. The diagnosis and treatment of CVS is challenging because of the heterogeneity of presentation and ambiguous aetiology. An early, short-lived phase may occur immediately after SAH, and there may be a subsequent phase that is prolonged or chronic [47]. The delayed vasospasm, seen on angiograms in 40–70 % of patients with SAH in the second week after haemorrhage, seems to be most important clinically. Acute vasoconstriction, previously considered to be a laboratory observation, has also been strongly suspected in humans [7]. Both phases of vasospasm are considered to result from an abnormal constriction of the muscular layers of the cerebral vessels, and both have been considered the main cause of cerebral ischaemia after SAH. However, whether the two phases are independent or interactive with respect to the clinical course has not been settled. The cause of vasospasm, whether angiographic or clinical, is still a source of debate. The inflammatory response to SAH does appear to contribute to the aetiology of CVS, specifically the role of leukocytes in releasing oxyhaemoglobin after lysing extravasated erythrocytes in the subarachnoid space [13]. Platelet aggregation has also been indicated in the aetiology of CVS [38], indicating a link between a patient's Fisher grade upon presentation and the incidence of CVS.

J. Fandino et al. (eds.), *Neurovascular Events After Subarachnoid Hemorrhage*, Acta Neurochirurgica Supplement, Vol. 120,
DOI 10.1007/978-3-319-04981-6_13,

Effective interventions providing protection from CVS as well as improved outcomes after CVS have lagged behind the treatment of SAH.

Many controversies exist generally in the management of patients suffering aSAH and specifically in the prevention and/or the pharmacological treatment of aSAH-induced vasospasm. Scientific communities have put forth some interesting efforts of to create guidelines for the management of aSAH and the associated CVS [6, 17]. A general consensus exists only for the oral administration of nimodipine, a well-known calcium channel blocker, to all patients suffering from aSAH [15].

Recently, various therapies targeting cytokines have demonstrated some therapeutic efficacy in the management of CVS. Cytokines are proteins that are powerful mediators and regulators of immune responses and have also been implicated in the pathogenesis of CVS following aSAH. In this scenario, a large body of evidence has indicated the efficacy of the cytokine erythropoietin (EPO).

EPO, a 34-kD glycoprotein, is the primary hormone that regulates the differentiation and proliferation of immature erythroid cells [29]. EPO is present in the human body since intrauterine life. In the fetus EPO is produced by the liver until late gestation, when a switch is gradually initiated from the liver to the kidney and completed after birth [52]. Its production is regulated by hypoxia inducible factor-1 (HIF-1), which is in turn activated by various stressors, particularly hypoxia [19]. EPO exerts its function by binding with its receptor (EPOR). EPOR belongs to the cytokine receptor type I super family [48]. In the hematopoietic compartment, receptor activation follows after homodimerisation on EPO binding, which allows autophosphorylation of EPOR-associated Janus-tyrosine kinase-2 (JAK-2). JAK-2 activation leads to phosphorylation of several downstream signalling pathways, including Ras mitogen-activated protein kinase (MAPK), phosphatidylinositol 3-kinase [PI(3)K], and the transcription factor STAT5 (signal transducers and activators of transcription) [28]. In erythroblasts, the effect of EPO through EPOR activation is the inhibition of apoptosis, proliferation, and differentiation.

The hormone erythropoietin was cloned in 1985 and after that was rapidly used in clinical practice. Over the past several years, its recombinant form (rHuEPO) has greatly enhanced the management of anaemia of chronic renal failure and has substantially improved quality of life in dialysis patients.

Although EPO has been long known for its erythropoietic action, it was just a few years ago that its expression was described in the brain and spinal cord, and only then was it realised that human neurons and glia express both EPO and its receptor [16]. Furthermore, its hypoxic induction raised the possibility that EPO, synthesised by hypoxic astrocytes, may mediate the protective phenomenon of "preconditioning" in the nervous system [8], in which mild, non-injurious stress increases resistance to a subsequent stress. On these bases, EPO was assessed as a therapy for experimental brain ischaemia [8, 10] and for the first successful clinical trial in patients with ischaemic stroke [18, 22].

The mechanisms by which EPO acts as neuroprotectant are still a matter of controversy. An increasing amount of evidence suggests that EPOR activation following EPO binding inhibits neuronal apoptosis similarly to erythropoiesis [12]. Prevention of neuronal apoptosis involves the activation of JAK-2 and nuclear factor (NF)-κB signalling pathways [12]. In particular, it has been suggested that the binding of EPO to its receptor induces the activation of JAK-2, leading to activation of secondary signalling pathways that involve MAPK, PI3K and NF-κB. Phosphorylation of the inhibitor of NF-κB provides subsequent translocation of the transcription factor NF-κB from the cytoplasm to the nucleus and transcription of neuroprotective genes. Various in vitro studies have shown that signal transduction mediated by STAT5 can also be activated by the erythropoietin receptor to provide neuroprotection [32, 37] although in vivo evidence is still lacking. In addition, EPO also appears to prevent apoptotic injury through an Akt-dependent mechanism [4]. Among a variety of pathways to promote cell survival, Akt has been shown to block cellular apoptotic degradation through inhibition of glycogen synthase kinase (GSK)-3ß activity [9]. GSK-3ß is a well-known kinase that is involved in the signalling pathway of PC in the heart [44]; to play a significant role in the regulation of apoptosis in neurons [2], vascular smooth muscle cells [33] and cardiomyocytes [51] and to be suppressed by EPO [41].

EPO-mediated neuroprotection can include other possible triggering events such as maintenance of vascular autoregulation, as has been reported for experimental SAH [24, 42], neuronal protection from glutamate toxicity by activation of calcium channels [39], production of antioxidant enzymes in neurons [30], and neoangiogenesis, which improves blood flow and tissue oxygenation in the border zone of an ischaemic area [8].

Neuroprotection is a complex mechanism in which multiple forces operate to maintain the integrity of the central nervous system. Studies have demonstrated a neuroprotective action for EPO against various insults in different experimental models. In particular, in vitro studies with neurons or neuron-like cells have demonstrated a protective effect for EPO against several insults, such as serum deprivation, excitotoxicity and growth factor deprivation [35, 40]. Neuroprotective effects of EPO have been demonstrated in a large variety of animal models. In rodent models of ischaemic stroke, infarct volume was reduced [8, 10, 40] and functional outcome was improved [8]. Beneficial effects of EPO have been observed in animal models of traumatic brain and spinal cord injury [10, 12, 20, 34, 50]. Furthermore, EPO has been shown to reduce neuronal damage and improve functional outcome in animal models of multiple sclerosis, diabetic neuropathy and retinal disease [10].

Once recognised as having beneficial effects on hypoxic neural damage, the effects of EPO were assessed in several experimental models of brain and spinal cord injury [1, 8, 10, 11, 20, 21, 24, 40, 42], and EPO became a serious candidate for neuroprotection.

Our current study critically reviews the pertinent literature regarding the role of EPO in CVS following aSAH and encompasses reports from experimental findings through the first clinical evidence.

Experimental Data

Substantial evidence indicates that peripherally administered erythropoietin can protect against cerebrovascular dysfunction following experimental SAH [1, 14, 24, 27, 36, 53]. In this regard, our research group was the first to suggest the beneficial effect exerted by EPO during experimental SAH. Briefly, after experimental SAH was induced in rabbits, functional recovery and mortality rate following systemic rHuEPO administration was evaluated [11]. Interestingly, all EPO-treated animals survived, whereas 42.9 % of placebo-treated animals died within 72 h. An open-field test performed after SAH showed a better neurological outcome in rabbits treated with rHuEPO compared with untreated animals. These encouraging results led to a desire to further investigate the neuroprotective effect of rHuEPO on SAH in subsequent experimental studies. The efficacy of rHuEPO on acute cerebral ischaemia following experimental SAH in a rabbit model has been evaluated [1, 21]. Histological analysis performed 24 h following injury showed that treatment with rHuEPO resulted in a dramatic reduction in brain ischaemic damage [1]. Another important finding provided by the same study was the observation that the concentration of EPO in the cerebrospinal fluid (CSF) was significantly higher in the rHuEPO-treated animals; suggesting that systemically administered EPO can statistically increase the EPO concentration in CSF by crossing the blood–brain barrier (BBB). The manner in which rHuEPO administered peripherally acts in the central nervous system across the BBB was controversial until it was demonstrated that, after systemic administration, rHuEPO may be transported across the BBB by a specific receptor-mediated mechanism [10]. These results were confirmed by a subsequent study further investigating the neuroprotective role of systemically administered rHuEPO in a rabbit model of SAH [24]. Based on reports demonstrating that EPO enhances the NO system activity [3] and that receptors for EPO are expressed by brain endothelial cells [10, 49], the ability of exogenously administered EPO to exert a vascular effect and in particular to counteract the spastic response of the cerebral arteries during SAH was investigated. Through morphometric analysis of the basilar artery, it was observed that rHuEPO administration significantly reduced the vasoconstriction in SAH-treated animals compared with untreated animals that underwent SAH. Pathological findings also showed that EPO attenuated SAH-induced brain ischaemia thus supporting the previous results. Finally, an additional experiment confirmed the neuroprotective properties exerted by EPO by measuring the S-100 protein concentration in CSF of SAH-injured rabbits [25]. The S-100 protein is a calcium-binding protein known as a biological marker of the severity of brain injury. Changes in CSF and serum S-100 protein levels have been reported in patients with SAH, in whom a close correlation between increases in S-100 protein concentration and poor clinical course has been observed [26]. The findings of such a study indicated that high levels of S-100 protein were well correlated with mortality rate, neurological outcome, and ischaemic brain damage. Interestingly, animals treated with rHuEPO were found to have significantly lower levels of S-100 protein in their CSF, no deaths, favourable neurological outcome, and significant protection against brain ischaemic damage. Subsequent experimental studies [14, 36, 42, 53] confirmed the role of EPO during experimental SAH and expanded the available findings on this topic, leading to clinical trials.

Clinical Data

Despite the large body of experimental evidence, few clinical observations propose a direct effect of EPO in neurological diseases. Springborg and collaborators reported the first double-blinded clinical trial on rHuEPO in patients after SAH [43]. Briefly, 73 patients with computed tomography (CT)-verified spontaneous SAH were randomised to treatment with either intravenous rHuEPO (500 U/kg/day) or placebo for 3 days. The primary endpoint was the Glasgow Outcome Score (GOS) at 6 months. Multiple parameters were recorded such as Fisher scale and World Federation of Neurosurgical Societies criteria, neurologic status, daily transcranial Doppler measurements, CSF levels of S-100 protein, neuron-specific enolase, and EPO, CSF:serum albumin ratios to evaluate BBB integrity. Based on their data, the authors were not able to draw any definitive conclusions, which they attributed to a small sample size, in part caused by patient exclusion. Beneficial effects of EPO in patients with SAH cannot be excluded or concluded on the basis of such a study.

In a phase-II randomised, double-blind, placebo-controlled clinical trial, Tseng et al. evaluated the potential role of intravenous EPO administration in patients suffering from aSAH [45]. Eighty patients with aSAH were randomised to receive placebo or 90,000 U EPO during the course of 48 h. Transcranial Doppler ultrasonography was used to assess vasospasm incidence, duration, and severity as well as impairment of autoregulation. DINDs and outcomes at discharge and at 6 months were also recorded. Trial medications were given within 1.7 ± 1.5 days of SAH. They found that EPO decreased the incidence of severe vasospasm in a statistically significant fashion from 27.5 to 7.5 %, whereas the occurrence of delayed ischaemic deficit was reduced from 40.0 to 7.5 %. They postulated that EPO reduced delayed cerebral ischaemia (DCI) secondary to aSAH by decreasing the frequency and severity of the observed vasospasm and also by shortening the time span of impaired cerebral autoregulation [45].

Although the data coming from preclinical and clinical studies suggest new avenues in this field, some issues should be carefully considered. First, the safety of recombinant human EPO administration in the setting of SAH should be considered. It must be taken into account that all of the information available at present regarding the safety of recombinant human EPO in humans comes from its non-neurologic use. The logical extension of these arguments is that translating such information from recombinant human EPO-treated anaemic patients to SAH-affected patients can be misleading, because interactions and influences between recombinant human EPO and different physiologic variables, as well as with common drugs taken by patients with SAH, are unknown. Second, although recombinant human EPO is usually a well-tolerated drug, several lines of evidence have shown that therapy with recombinant EPO can result in hypertension, hypertensive encephalopathy, accelerated atherosclerosis, seizures, and thrombotic/vascular events. In these pioneering clinical studies, no adverse effects during the EPO treatment have been reported. These findings, however, should be cautionary because these results are related to a short-term treatment and low EPO dosage. In this regard, in preclinical studies we have provided evidence that recombinant human EPO treatment at a dose of 1,000 IU/kg, administered every 8 h, is effective in reducing CVS, ischaemic brain damage, and significantly capable of improving neurologic outcome [23]. The dose used in the clinical setting is the lowest dose known to be effective after SAH. However, it can be argued that the unfavourable results from the first clinical trial [43] and the weak findings of the second clinical study [45] can be related to the small dose used and frequency of administration. In this regard, it is well known that vasospasm and cerebral ischaemia after aSAH follow a time course completely different when considering humans and animals. In preclinical studies, EPO has been considered effective at a dose starting from 400 IU to 1,000 IU/kg with a duration of 24–72 h [24]. In humans, although evidence has shown that there may be an early, short-lived phase that occurs immediately after SAH and a subsequent phase that is prolonged or chronic, the delayed vasospasm, seen on angiograms in 40–70 % of patients with SAH in the second week after haemorrhage, appears clinically to be most important. Consequently, there is a rationale for starting and continuing neuroprotection for at least 14 days after SAH onset to achieve stronger effects.

Future Directions

It should be considered, at present, that all phase III trials using neuroprotective drugs have failed to demonstrate efficacy and the lesson learned suggests that great optimism can lead to very early clinical investigations mainly driven by wishful thinking, undertaken without much detailed information. For this reason additional studies must be carried out to assess the safety of EPO in the setting of this new clinical application, optimal tolerated dosages, therapeutic time window, and duration of therapy. Furthermore, increased blood viscosity and possible thrombotic events seem to be the major complications after prolonged EPO treatment. Accordingly, the new EPO-derived drugs without erythropoietic effects [31], developed and experimentally tested with efficacy at present, should be further investigated to tailor successful future clinical trials.

Although the value of EPO therapy for the treatment of CVS in humans remains debatable, EPO still plays a role in the course and eventual treatment of this disease. These studies also may indicate a different role for CVS in mortality and morbidity following SAH. There may be other causes of DCI or DIND that are not directly related to vasospasm, and research into alternative aetiologies, and to how those alternative aetiologies may confound investigations into EPO is warranted.

Conclusion

Although the value of EPO therapy for the treatment of CVS in humans remains debatable, EPO still plays a role in the course and eventual treatment of this disease. These studies also may indicate a different role for CVS in mortality and morbidity following SAH. There may be other causes of DCI or DIND that are not directly related to vasospasm, and research into alternative aetiologies, and to how those alternative aetiologies may confound investigations into EPO is warranted.

Conflict of Interest Statement We declare that we have no conflict of interest.

References

1. Alafaci C, Salpietro F, Grasso G, Sfacteria A, Passalacqua M, Morabito A, Tripodo E, Calapai G, Buemi M, Tomasello F (2000) Effect of recombinant human erythropoietin on cerebral ischemia following experimental subarachnoid hemorrhage. Eur J Pharmacol 406:219–225

2. Alvarez G, Munoz-Montano J, Satrustegui J, Avila J, Bogonez E, Diaz-Nido J (1999) Lithium protects cultured neurons against beta-amyloid-induced neurodegeneration. FEBS Lett 453:260–264
3. Banerjee D, Rodriguez M, Nag M, Adamson JW (2000) Exposure of endothelial cells to recombinant human erythropoietin induces nitric oxide synthase activity. Kidney Int 57:1895–1904
4. Bao H, Jacobs-Helber SM, Lawson AE, Penta K, Wickrema A, Sawyer ST (1999) Protein kinase B (c-Akt), phosphatidylinositol 3-kinase, and STAT5 are activated by erythropoietin (EPO) in HCD57 erythroid cells but are constitutively active in an EPO-independent, apoptosis-resistant subclone (HCD57-SREI cells). Blood 93:3757–3773
5. Barry C, Turner RJ, Corrigan F, Vink R (2012) New therapeutic approaches to subarachnoid hemorrhage. Expert Opin Investig Drugs 21:845–859
6. Bederson JB, Connolly ES Jr, Batjer HH, Dacey RG, Dion JE, Diringer MN, Duldner JE Jr, Harbaugh RE, Patel AB, Rosenwasser RH (2009) Guidelines for the management of aneurysmal subarachnoid hemorrhage: a statement for healthcare professionals from a special writing group of the Stroke Council, American Heart Association. Stroke 40:994–1025
7. Bederson JB, Levy AL, Ding WH, Kahn R, DiPerna CA, Jenkins AL 3rd, Vallabhajosyula P (1998) Acute vasoconstriction after subarachnoid hemorrhage. Neurosurgery 42:352–360; discussion 360–362
8. Bernaudin M, Marti HH, Roussel S, Divoux D, Nouvelot A, MacKenzie ET, Petit E (1999) A potential role for erythropoietin in focal permanent cerebral ischemia in mice. J Cereb Blood Flow Metab 19:643–651
9. Bhat R, Shanley J, Correll M, Fieles W, Keith R, Scott C, Lee CM (2000) Regulation and localization of tyrosine216 phosphorylation of glycogen synthase kinase-3beta in cellular and animal models of neuronal regeneration. Proc Natl Acad Sci U S A 97:11074–11079
10. Brines ML, Ghezzi P, Keenan S, Agnello D, de Lanerolle NC, Cerami C, Itri LM, Cerami A (2000) Erythropoietin crosses the blood-brain barrier to protect against experimental brain injury. Proc Natl Acad Sci U S A 97:10526–10531
11. Buemi M, Grasso G, Corica F, Calapai G, Maria Salpietro F, Casuscelli T, Sfacteria A, Aloisi C, Concetta A, Sturiale A, Frisina N, Tomasello F (2000) In vivo evidence that erythropoietin has a neuroprotective effect during subarachnoid hemorrhage. Eur J Pharmacol 392:31–34 [In Process Citation]
12. Celik M, Gokmen N, Erbayraktar S, Akhisaroglu M, Konakc S, Ulukus C, Genc S, Genc K, Sagiroglu E, Cerami A, Brines M (2002) Erythropoietin prevents motor neuron apoptosis and neurologic disability in experimental spinal cord ischemic injury. Proc Natl Acad Sci U S A 99:2258–2263
13. Chaichana KL, Pradilla G, Huang J, Tamargo RJ (2010) Role of inflammation (leukocyte-endothelial cell interactions) in vasospasm after subarachnoid hemorrhage. World Neurosurg 73:22–41
14. Chen G, Zhang S, Shi J, Ai J, Hang C (2009) Effects of recombinant human erythropoietin (rhEPO) on JAK2/STAT3 pathway and endothelial apoptosis in the rabbit basilar artery after subarachnoid hemorrhage. Cytokine 45:162–168
15. Connolly ES Jr, Rabinstein AA, Carhuapoma JR, Derdeyn CP, Dion J, Higashida RT, Hoh BL, Kirkness CJ, Naidech AM, Ogilvy CS, Patel AB, Thompson BG, Vespa P, American Heart Association Stroke Council, Council on Cardiovascular Radiology and Intervention, Council on Cardiovascular Nursing, Council on Cardiovascular Surgery and Anesthesia, Council on Clinical Cardiology (2012) Guidelines for the management of aneurysmal subarachnoid hemorrhage: a guideline for healthcare professionals from the American Heart Association/American Stroke Association. Stroke 43:1711–1737
16. Digicaylioglu M, Bichet S, Marti HH, Wenger RH, Rivas LA, Bauer C, Gassmann M (1995) Localization of specific erythropoietin binding sites in defined areas of the mouse brain. Proc Natl Acad Sci U S A 92:3717–3720
17. Diringer MN, Bleck TP, Claude Hemphill J 3rd, Menon D, Shutter L, Vespa P, Bruder N, Connolly ES Jr, Citerio G, Gress D, Hanggi D, Hoh BL, Lanzino G, Le Roux P, Rabinstein A, Schmutzhard E, Stocchetti N, Suarez JI, Treggiari M, Tseng MY, Vergouwen MD, Wolf S, Zipfel G (2011) Critical care management of patients following aneurysmal subarachnoid hemorrhage: recommendations from the Neurocritical Care Society's Multidisciplinary Consensus Conference. Neurocrit Care 15:211–240
18. Ehrenreich H, Hasselblatt M, Dembowski C, Cepek L, Lewczuk P, Stiefel M, Rustenbeck HH, Breiter N, Jacob S, Knerlich F, Bohn M, Poser W, Ruther E, Kochen M, Gefeller O, Gleiter C, Wessel TC, De Ryck M, Itri L, Prange H, Cerami A, Brines M, Siren AL (2002) Erythropoietin therapy for acute stroke is both safe and beneficial. Mol Med 8:495–505
19. Goldberg MA, Dunning SP, Bunn HF (1988) Regulation of the erythropoietin gene: evidence that the oxygen sensor is a heme protein. Science 242:1412–1415
20. Gorio A, Gokmen N, Erbayraktar S, Yilmaz O, Madaschi L, Cichetti C, Di Giulio AM, Vardar E, Cerami A, Brines M (2002) Recombinant human erythropoietin counteracts secondary injury and markedly enhances neurological recovery from experimental spinal cord trauma. Proc Natl Acad Sci U S A 99:9450–9455
21. Grasso G (2001) Neuroprotective effect of recombinant human erythropoietin in experimental subarachnoid hemorrhage. J Neurosurg Sci 45:7–14
22. Grasso G (2003) Erythropoiesis and neuroprotection: two sides of the same coin? Lancet Neurol 2:332
23. Grasso G (2004) An overview of new pharmacological treatments for cerebrovascular dysfunction after experimental subarachnoid hemorrhage. Brain Res Brain Res Rev 44:49–63
24. Grasso G, Buemi M, Alafaci C, Sfacteria A, Passalacqua M, Sturiale A, Calapai G, De Vico G, Piedimonte G, Salpietro FM, Tomasello F (2002) Beneficial effects of systemic administration of recombinant human erythropoietin in rabbits subjected to subarachnoid hemorrhage. Proc Natl Acad Sci U S A 99:5627–5631
25. Grasso G, Passalacqua M, Sfacteria A, Conti A, Morabito A, Mazzullo G, De VG, Buemi M, Macri B, Tomasello F (2002) Does administration of recombinant human erythropoietin attenuate the increase of S-100 protein observed in cerebrospinal fluid after experimental subarachnoid hemorrhage? J Neurosurg 96:565–570
26. Hardemark HG, Almqvist O, Johansson T, Pahlman S, Persson L (1989) S-100 protein in cerebrospinal fluid after aneurysmal subarachnoid haemorrhage: relation to functional outcome, late CT and SPECT changes, and signs of higher cortical dysfunction. Acta Neurochir (Wien) 99:135–144
27. Helbok R, Shaker E, Beer R, Chemelli A, Sojer M, Sohm F, Broessner G, Lackner P, Beck M, Zangerle A, Pfausler B, Thome C, Schmutzhard E (2012) High dose erythropoietin increases brain tissue oxygen tension in severe vasospasm after subarachnoid hemorrhage. BMC Neurol 12:32
28. Ihle JN, Witthuhn B, Tang B, Yi T, Quelle FW (1994) Cytokine receptors and signal transduction. Baillieres Clin Haematol 7:17–48
29. Jelkmann W (1994) Biology of erythropoietin. Clin Investig 72:3–10
30. Koshimura K, Murakami Y, Sohmiya M, Tanaka J, Kato Y (1999) Effects of erythropoietin on neuronal activity. J Neurochem 72:2565–2572
31. Leist M, Ghezzi P, Grasso G, Bianchi R, Villa P, Fratelli M, Savino C, Bianchi M, Nielsen J, Gerwien J, Kallunki P, Larsen AK, Helboe L, Christensen S, Pedersen LO, Nielsen M, Torup L, Sager T, Sfacteria A, Erbayraktar S, Erbayraktar Z, Gokmen N, Yilmaz O, Cerami-Hand C, Xie QW, Coleman T, Cerami A, Brines M (2004) Derivatives of erythropoietin that are tissue protective but not erythropoietic. Science 305:239–242
32. Li K, Miller C, Hegde S, Wojchowski D (2003) Roles for an Epo receptor Tyr-343 Stat5 pathway in proliferative co-signaling with kit. J Biol Chem 278:40702–40709

33. Loberg RD, Vesely E, Brosius F (2002) Enhanced glycogen synthase kinase-3beta activity mediates hypoxia-induced apoptosis of vascular smooth muscle cells and is prevented by glucose transport and metabolism. J Biol Chem 277:41667–41673
34. Lu D, Mahmood A, Qu C, Goussev A, Schallert T, Chopp M (2005) Erythropoietin enhances neurogenesis and restores spatial memory in rats after traumatic brain injury. J Neurotrauma 22:1011–1017
35. Morishita E, Masuda S, Nagao M, Yasuda Y, Sasaki R (1997) Erythropoietin receptor is expressed in rat hippocampal and cerebral cortical neurons, and erythropoietin prevents in vitro glutamate-induced neuronal death. Neuroscience 76:105–116
36. Murphy AM, Xenocostas A, Pakkiri P, Lee TY (2008) Hemodynamic effects of recombinant human erythropoietin on the central nervous system after subarachnoid hemorrhage: reduction of microcirculatory impairment and functional deficits in a rabbit model. J Neurosurg 109:1155–1164
37. Pajonk F, Weil A, Sommer A, Suwinski R, Henke M (2004) The erythropoietin-receptor pathway modulates survival of cancer cells. Oncogene 23:8987–8991
38. Pyne GJ, Cadoux-Hudson TA, Clark JF (2003) Platelets play an essential role in the aetiology of cerebral vasospasm after subarachnoid haemorrhage. Med Hypotheses 60:525–530
39. Sakanaka M, Wen TC, Matsuda S, Masuda S, Morishita E, Nagao M, Sasaki R (1998) In vivo evidence that erythropoietin protects neurons from ischemic damage. Proc Natl Acad Sci U S A 95:4635–4640
40. Siren AL, Fratelli M, Brines M, Goemans C, Casagrande S, Lewczuk P, Keenan S, Gleiter C, Pasquali C, Capobianco A, Mennini T, Heumann R, Cerami A, Ehrenreich H, Ghezzi P (2001) Erythropoietin prevents neuronal apoptosis after cerebral ischemia and metabolic stress. Proc Natl Acad Sci U S A 98:4044–4049
41. Somervaille TC, Linch DC, Khwaja A (2001) Growth factor withdrawal from primary human erythroid progenitors induces apoptosis through a pathway involving glycogen synthase kinase-3 and Bax. Blood 98:1374–1381
42. Springborg JB, Ma X, Rochat P, Knudsen GM, Amtorp O, Paulson OB, Juhler M, Olsen NV (2002) A single subcutaneous bolus of erythropoietin normalizes cerebral blood flow autoregulation after subarachnoid haemorrhage in rats. Br J Pharmacol 135:823–829
43. Springborg JB, Moller C, Gideon P, Jorgensen OS, Juhler M, Olsen NV (2007) Erythropoietin in patients with aneurysmal subarachnoid haemorrhage: a double blind randomised clinical trial. Acta Neurochir 149:1089–1101; discussion 1101
44. Tong H, Imahashi K, Steenbergen C, Murphy E (2002) Phosphorylation of glycogen synthase kinase-3 during preconditioning through a phosphatidylinositol-3-kinase–dependent pathway is cardioprotective. Circ Res 90:377–379
45. Tseng MY, Hutchinson PJ, Richards HK, Czosnyka M, Pickard JD, Erber WN, Brown S, Kirkpatrick PJ (2009) Acute systemic erythropoietin therapy to reduce delayed ischemic deficits following aneurysmal subarachnoid hemorrhage: a Phase II randomized, double-blind, placebo-controlled trial. Clinical article. J Neurosurg 111:171–180
46. Vergouwen MD, Ilodigwe D, Macdonald RL (2011) Cerebral infarction after subarachnoid hemorrhage contributes to poor outcome by vasospasm-dependent and -independent effects. Stroke 42:924–929
47. Weir B, Grace M, Hansen J, Rothberg C (1978) Time course of vasospasm in man. J Neurosurg 48:173–178
48. Wojchowski DM, Gregory RC, Miller CP, Pandit AK, Pircher TJ (1999) Signal transduction in the erythropoietin receptor system. Exp Cell Res 253:143–156
49. Yamaji R, Okada T, Moriya M, Naito M, Tsuruo T, Miyatake K, Nakano Y (1996) Brain capillary endothelial cells express two forms of erythropoietin receptor mRNA. Eur J Biochem 239:494–500
50. Yatsiv I, Grigoriadis N, Simeonidou C, Stahel P, Schmidt O, Alexandrovitch A, Tsenter J, Shohami E (2005) Erythropoietin is neuroprotective, improves functional recovery, and reduces neuronal apoptosis and inflammation in a rodent model of experimental closed head injury. FASEB J 19:1701–1703
51. Yin H, Chao L, Chao J (2004) Adrenomedullin protects against myocardial apoptosis after ischemia/reperfusion through activation of Akt-GSK signaling. Hypertension 43:109–116
52. Zanjani ED, Gordon AS, Wong KK, McLaurin WD (1969) The renal erythropoietic factor (REF). X. The question of species and class specificity. Proc Soc Exp Biol Med 131:1095–1098
53. Zhang J, Zhu Y, Zhou D, Wang Z, Chen G (2010) Recombinant human erythropoietin (rhEPO) alleviates early brain injury following subarachnoid hemorrhage in rats: possible involvement of Nrf2-ARE pathway. Cytokine 52:252–257

Valproic Acid Treatment After Experimental Subarachnoid Hemorrhage

Michael K. Tso, Elliot Lass, Jinglu Ai, and R. Loch Macdonald

Abstract *Introduction*: Subarachnoid hemorrhage (SAH) can result in significant brain injury. Valproic acid (VPA), a widely-used anti-epileptic drug, was investigated as a possible neuroprotective drug in a prechiasmatic injection model of SAH in mice.

Methods: Mice were randomized to the following experimental groups: SAH, SAH + VPA, Sham, and Sham + VPA. VPA (400 mg/kg) or saline was administered within 30 min of SAH induction and every 12 h thereafter for 48 h. Neurobehavioral assessments using the modified Garcia Score were conducted at 24 and 48 h. Brain injury was assessed at 48 h with fluoro-jade b and caspase-3/NeuN histo- and immunohistochemistry. Vasospasm was assessed in the MCA branches using hematoxylin & eosin histology.

Results: SAH mice treated with VPA appeared to have improved neurobehavioral assessments at both 24 and 48 h compared to untreated SAH mice. VPA treatment in SAH mice also significantly decreased the number of degenerating neurons on fluoro-jade b staining. In VPA-treated SAH mice, there was a trend toward a decrease in the number of apoptotic neurons on caspase-3/NeuN immunohistochemistry. VPA did not significantly affect vasospasm.

Conclusion: This study demonstrated that VPA improves neurological outcome and decreases brain injury in a mouse model of SAH.

Keywords Subarachnoid hemorrhage • Valproic acid • Neuroprotection • Brain injury • Mouse • Prechiasmatic injection model

Introduction

Subarachnoid hemorrhage (SAH) remains associated with high morbidity and mortality [7]. Patients with aneurysmal SAH may develop angiographic vasospasm and delayed cerebral ischemia (DCI) [3]. A multi-center randomized clinical trial has not shown improvement in neurologic outcome despite ameliorating the delayed large artery vasospasm [5]. New therapies are needed.

Valproic acid (VPA) is a branched short-chain fatty acid that crosses the blood-brain barrier (BBB) easily and has an established safety profile [1]. It is used clinically for seizure control, bipolar affective disorder, neuropathic pain and migraine headache [1]. Pre-clinical studies have demonstrated neuroprotective effects in rodent models of traumatic brain injury and ischemic stroke [2, 4, 6]. Currently, no studies have investigated the impact of VPA on brain injury after experimental SAH. This study investigates VPA as a potential neuroprotective agent in a mouse model of SAH. Because it crosses the BBB easily and has a well-established safety profile in other neurological conditions, VPA is an attractive drug to study given the potential to test it in SAH clinical trials.

M.K. Tso, MD
Division of Neurosurgery, Labatt Family Centre of Excellence in Brain Injury and Trauma Research, Keenan Research Centre of the Li KaShing Shing Knowledge Institute of St. Michael's Hospital, 30 Bond St., Toronto, ON M5B 1W8, Canada

Institute of Medical Science, University of Toronto, Toronto, ON Canada

E. Lass, BSc • J. Ai, MD, PhD • R.L. Macdonald, MD, PhD (✉)
Division of Neurosurgery, Labatt Family Centre of Excellence in Brain Injury and Trauma Research, Keenan Research Centre of the Li KaShing Knowledge Institute of St. Michael's Hospital, 30 Bond St., Toronto, ON M5B 1W8, Canada
e-mail: macdonaldlo@smh.ca

J. Fandino et al. (eds.), *Neurovascular Events After Subarachnoid Hemorrhage*, Acta Neurochirurgica Supplement, Vol. 120, DOI 10.1007/978-3-319-04981-6_14, © Springer International Publishing Switzerland 2015

Materials and Methods

Experimental Design

This study received approval from the institutional Animal Care Committee. Four experimental groups were planned: mice with SAH induction ($n=8$), mice with SAH induction and treated with VPA ($n=8$), sham mice ($n=4$), and sham mice treated with VPA ($n=4$). Mice were randomized to one of the four groups.

SAH Model

C57BL/6 J male mice (Jackson Laboratory, Bar Harbor, ME), 8–10 weeks old and weighing 20–25 g, were used. The prechiasmatic injection model of SAH was used and has been described previously [8]. Mice were anesthetized with 3 % isoflurane and maintained with 1.5 l of oxygen via orotracheal delivery. Body temperature was measured by rectal temperature probe and maintained at 37.0° Celsius by a homeothermic heating pad (Harvard Apparatus, Holliston, MA). The head of each mouse was immobilized in a stereotactic frame. A midline incision was made and a burr hole was created 4.5 mm anterior to the bregma and slightly off the midline. Laser flow Doppler (BLT21, Transonics Systems, New York City, NY) was used to measure cerebral blood flow (CBF). A 27-gauge spinal needle was advanced through the burr hole at a 37.5° cranial to caudal angle in the sagittal plane and the tip positioned in the subarachnoid space. SAH mice received 80 μL of donor littermate arterial blood injected over 10 s. Sham mice had needle placement without injection of blood. Mice were treated with 400 mg/kg of VPA (Sigma-Aldrich, St. Louis, MO.) or 0.9 % NaCl (VPA vehicle) via intraperitoneal injection within 30 min after the procedure and every 12 h thereafter for 48 h. The experimenter was blinded to the identity of these injections. All mice received routine post-operative subcutaneous injections of buprenorphine (Sigma-Aldrich, St. Louis, MO), 0.1 mg/kg, at the time of SAH induction and every 12 h for 48 h.

Two days after SAH induction, the mice were anesthetized with ketamine (10 mg/kg) and xylazine (4 mg/kg) and underwent transcardial perfusion with 4 % paraformaldehyde (PFA) in phosphate buffer at physiological blood pressure (80–100 mmHg by sphygmomanometer). Brains were extracted and fixed in PFA for 24 h. Brain cuts were performed as previously described followed by paraffin embedding [8]. Five μm sections were sliced with a microtome (Leica, Wetzlar, Germany) and placed on glass slides.

Neurobehavioral Assessment: Modified Garcia Score

The modified Garcia Score is an acute neurobehavioral assessment developed for the endovascular perforation rodent model of SAH [10]. The global assessment consists of 6 domains – spontaneous activity, spontaneous movement of all 4 limbs, forepaw outstretching, climbing, body proprioception, and response to vibrissae touch. The maximum score is 18, indicative of normal mouse behavior. Behavioral assessments were performed at 24 and 48 h after SAH induction by 2 observers blinded to the experimental group allocation.

Brain Injury Assessment: Fluoro-Jade b and Caspase-3/NeuN Immunohistochemistry

Fluoro-jade b (Histo-Chem Inc., Jefferson, Arkansas) was used as marker of neuronal injury and degeneration [9]. The specimen slides were deparaffinized and rehydrated. Slides were placed in 0.06 % potassium permanganate (Sigma-Aldrich, St. Louis, MO) solution for 15 min. After rinsing in deionized water, the slides were then placed in 0.001 % fluoro-jade b solution for 30 min. The slides were then washed, dried, cleared in xylene and cover-slipped with non-aqueous mounting media DPX (Sigma-Aldrich, St. Louis, MO).

Caspase-3/NeuN immunohistochemistry was used to label apoptotic neurons. Specimen slides were placed in heated antigen retrieval solution and then 0.3 % Triton X-100 solution for 60 min. Slides were then incubated with 10 % normal goat serum in 1 % bovine serum albumin for 30 min. The primary antibodies used were rabbit anti-active caspase 3 (1:300, BD Pharmingen, Franklin Lakes, NJ) and mouse anti-NeuN (1:200, Invitrogen, Carlsbad, CA). The secondary antibodies used were goat anti-rabbit alexa fluor 488 (1:1,000, Invitrogen, Carlsbad, CA) and goat anti-mouse alexa fluor 568 (1:1,000, Invitrogen, Carlsbad, CA). Slides were cover-slipped with aqueous mounting medium and sealed with nail polish.

Coronal brain slices of both fluoro-jade b and caspase-3/NeuN slides were viewed with an Olympus upright microscope. Positively-labeled cells were counted throughout the entire coronal brain slice. Counts were made in a blinded manner by 2 observers.

Vasospasm Assessment: Hematoxylin & Eosin Staining

Slides were deparaffinized and rehydrated, followed by staining by hematoxylin and eosin. Slides were cover-slipped with Permount mounting medium (Sigma-Aldrich, St. Louis, MO) and viewed with an Olympus upright microscope. Slide pictures were taken of parasagittal brain sections, looking at the middle cerebral artery (MCA) branches. Vasospasm was assessed by calculating the ratio of the MCA branch lumen diameter to the MCA branch vessel wall thickness, as measured by Image J (NIH, Bethesda, MD). The lumen diameter was estimated by dividing the free-hand drawn inner lumen circumference by π. A smaller lumen diameter to wall thickness ratio is indicative of more severe vasospasm. Measurements were made in a blinded manner.

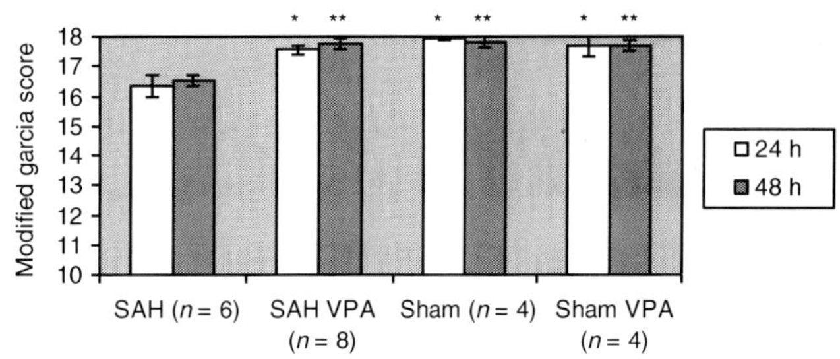

Fig. 1 Modified Garcia Score at 24 and 48 h (maximum score of 18). The SAH group had significantly lower modified Garcia Scores at both 24 and 48 h compared to the other three experimental groups. *$p<0.05$ compared with SAH group at 24 h. **$p<0.05$ compared with SAH group at 48 h. Error bars indicate standard error

Statistical Analysis

Results were expressed as means with standard errors. Comparisons between the four experimental groups were determined using one-way analysis of variance (ANOVA) with Holm-Sidak *post-hoc* analysis. Student's *t*-test was used for comparisons between 2 groups. The significance level was set at $p<0.05$.

Results

Intraoperative Cerebral Blood Flow

Intraoperative CBF measurements revealed no significant changes from baseline after needle insertion in the Sham and Sham + VPA groups (data not shown). In both the SAH and SAH + VPA groups, CBF dropped to 5–10 % of baseline after SAH induction and recovered to 70–80 % of baseline after 10 min (data not shown).

Mortality

Two mice in the SAH group died several minutes after SAH induction. Hence, only 6 mice in the SAH group are included in the neurobehavioral and histological assessments. There were no mortalities in the SAH + VPA, Sham, and Sham + VPA groups ($n=8$ each). The overall mortality rate after SAH induction was 12.5 % (2 out of 16 mice).

Improved Neurological Outcome with Valproic Acid Treatment

At both 24 and 48 h after SAH induction, mice in the SAH + VPA group had significantly higher modified Garcia Scores compared with mice in the SAH group (Fig. 1). Also, the SAH group had significantly lower neurological scores compared to the Sham and Sham + VPA groups at both time points. There were no significant differences in the modified Garcia Score at both time points between Sham and Sham + VPA groups. Finally, there were no significant changes in neurological scores between 24 and 48 h within each experimental group.

Decreased Histological Evidence of Brain Injury with Valproic Acid Treatment

SAH mice treated with VPA had significantly less brain injury compared with untreated SAH mice, as measured by the number of fluoro-jade b positive cells on coronal brain sections (Fig. 2a). Also, the SAH group had significantly more fluoro-jade b positive cells compared to the Sham and Sham + VPA groups. There were no significant differences in the number of fluoro-jade b positive cells between Sham and Sham + VPA groups. ANOVA statistical analysis revealed that there were significant differences in the number of caspase-3 positive neurons between experimental groups ($p=0.04$). However, after correcting for multiple statistical

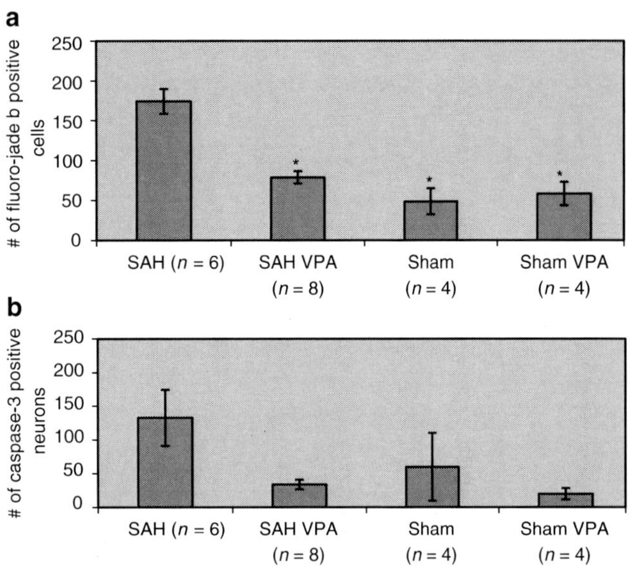

Fig. 2 Histological assessment of brain injury at 48 h. (**a**) Counts on coronal brain sections of fluoro-jade b positive cells. The SAH group had decreased number of fluoro-jade b positive cells compared with all the other experimental groups. (**b**) Counts on coronal brain sections of Caspase-3 positive neurons co-immunostained with NeuN. After correcting for multiple statistical comparisons, there was only a trend toward decreased number of Caspase-3 positive neurons in the SAH+VPA group compared with the SAH group. $*p<0.05$ compared with SAH group. Error bars indicate standard error

comparisons, there was only a trend toward decreased number of caspase-3 positive neurons in the SAH+VPA group compared with the SAH group ($p=0.01$) (Fig. 2b).

Vasospasm Unaffected by Valproic Acid Treatment

Mice in the SAH and SAH+VPA groups had significantly increased large-vessel vasospasm on histology compared with Sham or Sham+VPA groups (Fig. 3). However there was no significant difference in vasospasm between SAH mice treated with VPA and untreated SAH mice. Also, there was no difference in vasospasm between Sham and Sham+VPA groups.

Discussion

This preliminary study demonstrated that administration of VPA in the acute setting resulted in improved neurobehavioral outcomes and decreased histological evidence of brain injury in a prechiasmatic injection model of SAH in mice. Large-vessel vasospasm was not affected by VPA and

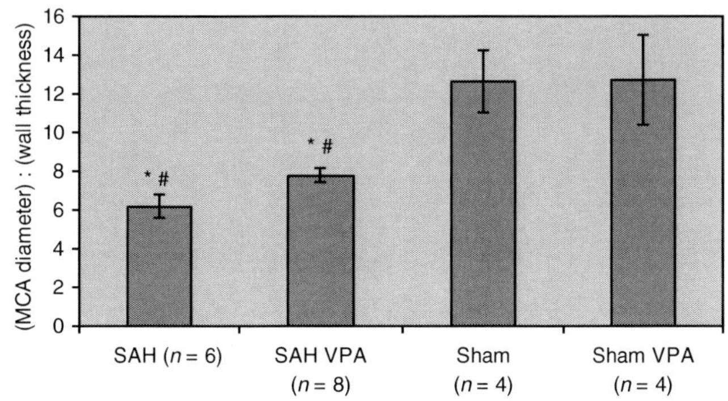

Fig. 3 Histological assessment of vasospasm. There was no significant difference in the degree of vasospasm between SAH and SAH+VPA groups. There was significantly more vasospasm in SAH and SAH+VPA groups compared with Sham and Sham+VPA groups. $*p<0.05$ compared with Sham group. $\#p<0.05$ compared with Sham+VPA group. Error bars indicate standard error

therefore may not mediate the neuroprotective effect of VPA, although it was only measured at one time after the SAH. Because molecular studies were not performed in this study, it is not clear by which mechanism VPA decreases brain injury. In a rat model of transient focal cerebral ischemia, the investigators have suggested that VPA is neuroprotective as a result of upregulation of heat shock proteins and inhibition of histone deacetylases (HDAC) [6]. Through its inhibition of HDAC1, VPA can increase histone acetylation resulting in a relaxed chromatin configuration and an increase in overall gene transcription [1]. The increased gene expression, with some genes possibly related to neuronal survival, may explain the improved neurological outcome and decreased brain injury after SAH induction. VPA may also reduce excitotoxic damage in the neurons through its inhibition of GABA degradation [1].

VPA is an attractive drug to study in the context of neuroprotection in SAH patients. First, it has already been administered in SAH patients, although VPA has not been prospectively studied in this patient population. It is a small molecule drug that is known to cross the blood brain barrier [1]. Also, VPA has a known safety profile due to its widespread use over many decades for other clinical conditions and it is readily available on the market.

Limitations in this study include the lack of serum VPA measurements. It is possible some mice may have serum concentrations of VPA outside of the therapeutic range, although a neuroprotective effect was still found in this study. Intracranial pressure (ICP) monitoring and mean arterial pressure monitoring were not utilized during SAH induction. Also, it is unclear how much of the brain injury is a result of the transient global cerebral ischemia from the initial increased ICP and how much is a result of the effect of blood in the subarachnoid space.

Further studies will need to investigate other measures of cognition, such as using the Morris Water Maze for assessment of spatial memory. Although the 48 h time point was used in this study, it would be appropriate to determine if this neuroprotective effect is sustained at later time points. Finally, molecular studies are needed to elucidate the mechanism by which VPA confers its neuroprotective effect.

Conclusion

This study demonstrated that VPA treatment improved neurological outcomes and decreased brain injury on immunohistochemistry in a prechiasmatic injection model of SAH in mice. Although further studies are needed, VPA appears to be promising as a treatment to improve neurological outcome after SAH.

Acknowledgments We would like to thank Hoyee Wan and Josephine D'Abbondanza for demonstrating the techniques used in this study. We would also like to thank Jeremy Zung for his assistance with the neurobehavioral assessments.

Financial Disclosure MT receives funding from the Vanier Canada Graduate Scholarship, Canadian Institutes of Health Research, Neurosurgery Research and Education Foundation, and the Joint Cerebrovascular Section of the American Association of Neurological Surgeons and the Congress of Neurological Surgeons. MT received travel funds from the Canadian Stroke Network and the University of Toronto School of Graduate Studies. RLM receives grant support from the Brain Aneurysm Foundation, Heart and Stroke Foundation of Canada, and is a stockholder of Edge Therapeutics. RLM is a consultant for Actelion Pharmaceuticals and Chief Scientific Officer of Edge Therapeutics.

Conflict of Interest Statement We declare that we have no conflict of interest.

References

1. Chateauvieux S, Morceau F, Dicato M, Diederich M (2010) Molecular and therapeutic potential and toxicity of valproic acid. J Biomed Biotechnol. doi:10.1155/2010/479364
2. Dash PK, Orsi SA, Zhang M, Grill RJ, Pati S, Zhao J, Moore AN (2010) Valproate administered after traumatic brain injury provides neuroprotection and improves cognitive function in rats. PLoS One. doi:10.1371/journal.pone.0011383
3. Etminan N, Vergouwen MD, Ilodigwe D, Macdonald RL (2011) Effect of pharmaceutical treatment on vasospasm, delayed cerebral ischemia, and clinical outcome in patients with aneurysmal subarachnoid hemorrhage: a systematic review and meta-analysis. J Cereb Blood Flow Metab 31:1443–1451
4. Kim HJ, Rowe M, Ren M, Hong JS, Chen PS, Chuang DM (2007) Histone deacetylase inhibitors exhibit anti-inflammatory and neuroprotective effects in a rat permanent ischemic model of stroke: multiple mechanisms of action. J Pharmacol Exp Ther 321: 892–901
5. Macdonald RL, Higashida RT, Keller E, Mayer SA, Molyneux A, Raabe A, Vajkoczy P, Wanke I, Bach D, Frey A, Marr A, Roux S, Kassell N (2011) Clazosentan, an endothelin receptor antagonist, in patients with aneurysmal subarachnoid haemorrhage undergoing surgical clipping: a randomised, double-blind, placebo-controlled phase 3 trial (CONSCIOUS-2). Lancet Neurol 10: 618–625
6. Ren M, Leng Y, Jeong M, Leeds PR, Chuang DM (2004) Valproic acid reduces brain damage induced by transient focal cerebral ischemia in rats: potential roles of histone deacetylase inhibition and heat shock protein induction. J Neurochem 89:1358–1367
7. Rinkel GJ, Algra A (2011) Long-term outcomes of patients with aneurysmal subarachnoid haemorrhage. Lancet Neurol 10: 349–356
8. Sabri M, Jeon H, Ai J, Tariq A, Shang X, Chen G, Macdonald RL (2009) Anterior circulation mouse model of subarachnoid hemorrhage. Brain Res 1295:179–185
9. Schmued LC, Hopkins KJ (2000) Fluoro-Jade B: a high affinity fluorescent marker for the localization of neuronal degeneration. Brain Res 874:123–130
10. Sherchan P, Lekic T, Suzuki H, Hasegawa Y, Rolland W, Duris K, Zhan Y, Tang J, Zhang JH (2011) Minocycline improves functional outcomes, memory deficits, and histopathology after endovascular perforation-induced subarachnoid hemorrhage in rats. J Neurotrauma 28:2503–2512

Macro- and Microcirculatory Disturbance

SAH-Induced MMP Activation and K_V Current Suppression is Mediated Via Both ROS-Dependent and ROS-Independent Mechanisms

Masayo Koide and George C. Wellman

Abstract Voltage-gated potassium (K_V) channels regulate cerebral artery tone and have been implicated in subarachnoid hemorrhage (SAH)-induced pathologies. Here, we examined whether matrix metalloprotease (MMP) activation contributes to SAH-induced K_V current suppression and cerebral artery constriction via activation of epidermal growth factor receptors (EGFRs). Using patch clamp electrophysiology, we observed that K_V currents were selectively decreased in cerebral artery myocytes isolated from SAH model rabbits. Consistent with involvement of enhanced MMP and EGFR activity in SAH-induced K_V current suppression, we found that: (1) oxyhemoglobin (OxyHb) and/or the exogenous EGFR ligand, heparin-binding EGF-like growth factor (HB-EGF), failed to induce further K_V current suppression after SAH and (2) gelatin zymography detected significantly higher MMP-2 activity after SAH. The removal of reactive oxygen species (ROS) by combined treatment with superoxide dismutase (SOD) and catalase partially inhibited OxyHb-induced K_V current suppression. However, these agents had little effect on OxyHb-induced MMP-2 activation. Interestingly, in the presence of a broad-spectrum MMP inhibitor (GM6001), OxyHb failed to cause K_V current suppression. These data suggest that OxyHb suppresses K_V currents through both ROS-dependent and ROS-independent pathways involving MMP activation. The ROS-independent pathway involves activation of MMP-2, whereas the ROS-dependent pathway involves activation of a second unidentified MMP or ADAM (a disintegrin and metalloprotease domain).

Keywords K^+ channels • Heparin-binding EGF-like growth factor (HB-EGF) • Parenchymal arteriole • Patch clamp • Vascular smooth muscle • Vasospasm

M. Koide, PhD (✉) • G.C. Wellman
Department of Pharmacology, University of Vermont College of Medicine, 89 Beaumont Avenue, Burlington, VT, USA
e-mail: masayo.koide@uvm.edu

Introduction

Subarachnoid hemorrhage (SAH) following cerebral aneurysm rupture is associated with substantial morbidity and mortality and existing therapeutic options have limited efficacy. A major contributor to poor outcome is delayed cerebral ischemia (DCI) manifesting 4–10 days after aneurysm rupture. Despite decades of study, mechanisms contributing to SAH-induced DCI remain controversial. Factors contributing to the development of DCI after SAH may include early brain injury, cortical spreading depression, disruption of the blood-brain barrier, activation of inflammatory pathways, and enhanced constriction of brain surface arteries/arterioles and intracerebral arterioles [5, 8, 16–18].

The membrane potential of cerebral artery myocytes is a key regulator of vascular diameter, with membrane potential depolarization leading to an increase in the open-state probability of voltage-dependent Ca^{2+} channels, enhanced Ca^{2+} entry, and vasoconstriction [15]. Studies using intracellular microelectrodes to measure smooth muscle membrane potential in intact cerebral arteries have found enhanced membrane potential depolarization concomitant with enhanced constriction in tissue from SAH model animals [6, 16, 22]. Voltage-gated potassium (K_V) channels play an important role in the regulation of smooth muscle membrane potential and arterial diameter with decreased K_V channel activity leading to membrane potential depolarization [1, 3, 4]. Evidence indicates that K_V current suppression contributes to enhanced membrane potential depolarization and constriction of cerebral arteries isolated from SAH model animals [7, 11, 20, 22]. Further, we have previously demonstrated that acute application of the blood component oxyhemoglobin (OxyHb) leads to matrix metalloprotease (MMP) activation, shedding of heparin-binding epidermal growth factor (EGF)-like growth factor (HB-EGF), epidermal growth factor receptor (EGFR) activation, and K_V channel suppression via internalization [11]. However, the mechanism underlying OxyHb-induced MMP activation and HB-EGF shedding is unclear. The objec-

DOI 10.1007/978-3-319-04981-6_15,

tive of this study was to examine the contribution of reactive oxygen species (ROS) on enhanced MMP activity and K_V current suppression in cerebral artery myocytes after SAH.

Materials and Methods

Rabbit Double-Hemorrhage SAH Model

As previously described, two injections of unheparinized autologous arterial blood (3 mL) were delivered via the cistern magna onto the brain surface of anesthetized rabbits at an interval of 48 h [7, 8, 10]. Five days after the initial surgery, rabbits were euthanized and posterior cerebral and cerebellar arteries (100–200-μm diameter) were isolated from the brain surface for in vitro studies. All experiments were conducted in accordance with The Guide for the Care and Use of Laboratory Animals (NIH Pub. No. 85-23, revised 1996) and followed protocols approved by the Institutional Animal Care and Use Committee of the University of Vermont.

Artery Diameter Measurements

Freshly isolated arteries were cannulated and pressurized to 60 mmHg, superfused with artificial cerebrospinal fluid (aCSF) and diameter measurements obtained using video edge-detection equipment [8, 16]. Constriction (tone) is expressed as percent decrease from maximum diameter obtained using Ca^{2+}-free aCSF with 100 μM diltiazem and 1 μM forskolin.

Patch Clamp Electrophysiology

Whole-cell K^+ currents were measured using the conventional whole-cell configuration of the patch-clamp technique [7, 10, 11]. Outward currents were elicited by 800-ms depolarizing voltage steps from a holding potential of −70 to +50 mV [7, 11]. The bath solution contained (in mM): 134 NaCl, 6 KCl, 1 $MgCl_2$, 0.1 $CaCl_2$, 10 glucose, and 10 HEPES (pH 7.4). Patch pipettes (3–5 MΩ) were filled with an internal solution that contained (in mM): 87 potassium aspartate, 20 KCl, 1 $CaCl_2$, 1 $MgCl_2$, 10 HEPES, 10 EGTA, and 25 KOH (pH 7.2). Inwardly rectifying K^+ (K_{IR}) channel currents were measured as 100-μM barium-sensitive currents using voltage ramps from −100 to +40 mV [23]. For K_{IR} recordings, the bath solution contained (in mM): 140 KCl, 1 $MgCl_2$, 0.1 $CaCl_2$, 10 glucose, and 10 HEPES (pH 7.4) and the patch pipette contained (in mM): 87 potassium aspartate, 20 KCl, 1 $CaCl_2$, 1 $MgCl_2$, 10 HEPES, 10 EGTA, and 25 KOH (pH 7.2). For all recordings, cell capacitance was not different between groups (control: 10.9±0.4 pF, $n=37$; SAH: 11.3±0.3 pF, $n=30$). Current density was calculated by dividing the K^+ current by the cell capacitance.

Zymography

MMP activity was measured using gelatin zymography [11]. Cerebral arteries were homogenized in gel loading buffer (100 mM Tris, 2 % SDS and 20 % glycerol). Lysate (15 μg protein, quantified by Bradford assay) was applied to a 10 % polyacrylamide gel copolymerized with the MMP2/9 substrate, gelatin (1 mg/mL). After electrophoresis, the gel was rinsed overnight then incubated at 37 °C for 20 h to allow gelatinolytic activity. The gel was stained with Coomassie Brilliant Blue and MMP activity was detected as unstained bands against the background of the blue-stained gelatin [11].

PCR

Expression of mRNA was examined by semi-quantitative RT-PCR [9]. Total RNA was extracted from intact cerebral arteries, and converted into cDNA. Amplification of cDNA was performed using Taq DNA polymerase (GenScript) and primers for MMP-2 (forward: 5′-CCG TGT GAA GTA TGG CAA TG-3′, reverse: 5′-CGT AGA GCT CTT GAA TGC CC-3′). Band intensity in the linear range of amplification was normalized to band intensity for 18S ribosomal RNA.

Statistical Analysis

Data are expressed as mean±SEM with n representing the number of cells or samples per group. Student's paired or unpaired *t*-test were used to determine statistical significance at the level of $P<0.05$ (*) or $P<0.01$ (**).

Results

Selective Suppression of K_V Channel Function After SAH Involves EGF Receptor Activation

Whole-cell voltage-dependent and inwardly rectifying K^+ currents were examined in cerebral artery myocytes freshly isolated from control and SAH model rabbits

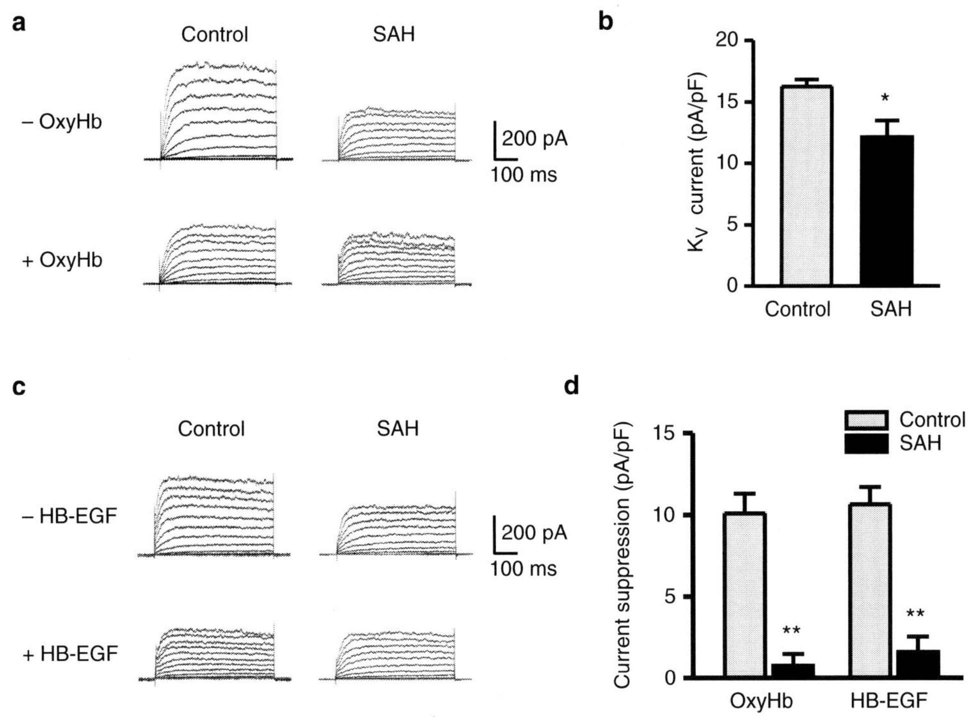

Fig. 1 OxyHb and HB-EGF suppressed K_V currents of cerebral artery myocytes from control animals but not from SAH model animals. (**a**) Example of whole-cell K^+ currents before and after 10 min application of OxyHb (10 μM) to cerebral artery myocytes isolated from control and SAH model animals. (**b**) Summary of 4-AP-sensitive K_V currents obtained from control ($n=6$) and SAH model ($n=4$) animals. (**c**) Examples of whole-cell K^+ currents before and after 10 min application of HB-EGF (30 ng/ml) to cerebral artery myocytes isolated from control and SAH model animals. (**d**) Summary data demonstrating that OxyHb and HB-EGF significantly suppressed K_V currents in cerebral artery myocytes from control, but not SAH model animals. OxyHb treatment: control $n=7$, SAH $n=4$; HB-EGF treatment: control $n=6$, SAH $n=5$. $^{**}P<0.01$ vs control, unpaired Student's t-test

using the conventional whole-cell configuration of the patch-clamp technique. Whole-cell voltage-dependent K^+ currents were measured during 10-mV voltage steps from a holding potential of −70 mV and represent the combined activity of large-conductance Ca^{2+}-activated (BK) and voltage-gated (K_V) K^+ channels. As illustrated in Fig. 1a, the current amplitude of whole-cell composite K^+ currents was reduced in cerebral artery myocytes from SAH model animals. To separate BK and K_V currents, selective blockers of BK channels (paxilline, 1 μM) and K_V channels (4-aminopyridine, 4-AP, 10 mM) were applied to myocytes isolated from control and SAH model animals. The current densities of paxilline-sensitive BK currents were similar in myocytes isolated from both groups; controls: 6.5 ± 0.7 pA/pF at +50 mV ($n=6$) and SAH: 5.6 ± 0.6 pA/pF at +50 mV ($n=4$). In marked contrast, 4-AP-sensitive K_V currents were significantly decreased in myocytes from SAH animals (12.1 ± 1.4 pA/pF at +50 mV, $n=4$) compared with myocytes from control animals (16.3 ± 0.6 pA/pF at +50 mV, $n=6$) (Fig. 1b). Inwardly rectifying K^+ (K_{IR}) channel currents, determined as inward currents sensitive to 100 μM Ba^{2+} using voltage ramps from −100 to +40 mV, were not significantly different between groups. For example, Ba^{2+}- sensitive current densities at −100 mV were -5.4 ± 0.9 pA/pF and -5.2 ± 0.6 pA/pF in myocytes from control ($n=24$) and SAH ($n=23$) animals, respectively. This data demonstrates that K_V currents are selectively suppressed in cerebral artery myocytes from SAH model rabbits. Consistent with SAH-induced K_V current suppression, constrictions to 4-AP (10 mM) were significantly reduced in arteries isolated from SAH (17.4 ± 3.7 % decrease in diameter, $n=4$) model animals compared with control (38.9 ± 6.2 % decrease in diameter, $n=4$) animals.

Our previous work has demonstrated that acute application of the blood component OxyHb decreased K_V currents in cerebral artery myocytes through a mechanism involving HB-EGF shedding and EGFR activation [11]. As with this previous work, OxyHb decreased K_V currents in myocytes isolated from control animals. However, OxyHb failed to reduce K_V currents obtained from SAH animals (Fig. 1a, d); indicating that acute application of OxyHb and 4-day exposure of subarachnoid blood in vivo may work through a common mechanism to decrease K_V channel activity. Further, exogenous application of HB-EGF mimicked the actions of acute application of OxyHb, causing a reduction in K_V

currents in myocytes obtained from control, but not SAH model animals (Fig. 1c, d). This data suggests SAH-induced K_V suppression involves HB-EGF shedding and EGFR activation in a manner similar to that caused by OxyHb.

MMP-2 Activity Is Enhanced in Cerebral Arteries from SAH Model Animals

The matrix metalloprotease subtype, MMP-2, has been implicated in HB-EGF shedding and mesenteric artery constriction [12]. In addition, our previous work has demonstrated that OxyHb increases MMP-2 activity in cerebral artery homogenates from control animals [11]. To examine if increased MMP-2 activity may be involved in SAH-induced HB-EGF shedding and K_V current suppression, zymography using the MMP-2 substrate gelatin was performed using cerebral artery homogenates from control and SAH model animals. Gelatin zymography from cerebral artery homogenates produced a single 65-kDa band similar to commercially purified MMP-2 (Fig. 2a). Interestingly, MMP-2 band intensity was significantly greater in homogenates from SAH model animals (Fig. 2b, c). Although MMP-2 activity was increased after SAH, mRNA levels of MMP-2 were similar in cerebral arteries from control and SAH model animals (Fig. 2d). This data demonstrates that MMP-2 activity, but not expression, is increased in cerebral arteries after SAH in a manner similar to that observed with acute application of OxyHb.

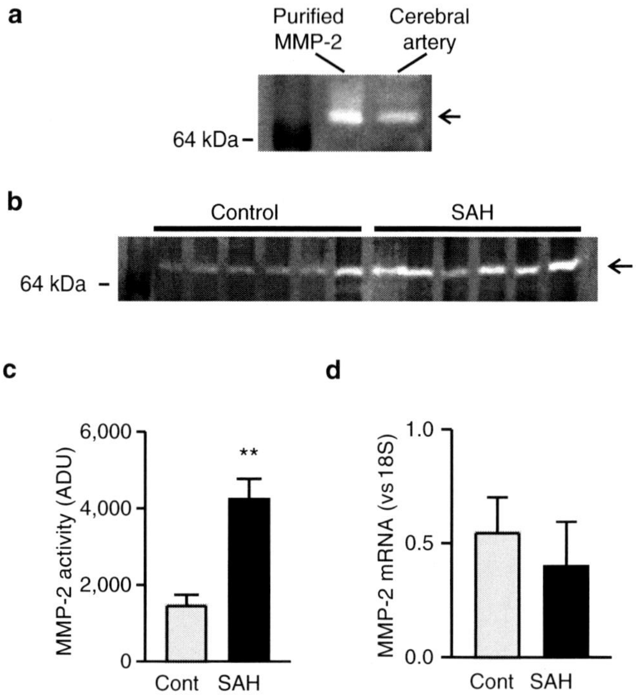

Fig. 2 MMP-2 activity is enhanced in cerebral arteries from SAH model animals. (**a**) Gelatin zymography demonstrating activity of commercially purified MMP-2 and cerebral artery homogenate from a control animal. (**b**) Gelatin zymography demonstrating enhanced MMP-2 activity in homogenates obtained from SAH model animals. (**c**) Summary data showing significantly greater MMP-2 activity in cerebral artery homogenates from SAH model animals compared with cerebral artery homogenates from unoperated control animals ($n=8$ for each). (**d**) Summary data demonstrating that MMP-2 mRNA levels are similar in cerebral artery homogenates obtained from control and SAH model animals ($n=7$ for each). $^{**}P<0.01$ vs control, unpaired Student's *t*-test

Oxyhemoglobin Activates MMPs and Suppresses K_V Currents Via ROS-Dependent and ROS-Independent Pathways

To examine whether reactive oxygen species (ROS) such as super oxide anions (O_2^-) contribute to increased MMP activity caused by OxyHb, studies were performed in cerebral artery myocytes from control animals using a combination of superoxide dismutase and catalase. Superoxide dismutase catalyzes the conversion of super oxide anions (O_2^-) into oxygen (O_2) and hydrogen peroxide (H_2O_2), whereas catalase converts H_2O_2 to H_2O and O_2. The combination of superoxide dismutase (150 U/mL) and catalase (500 U/mL) decreased OxyHb-induced K_V suppression by approximately 40 % (Fig. 3a, b). In comparison, the broad-spectrum MMP inhibitor, GM6001 (10 μM), caused a substantially greater decrease in OxyHb-induced K_V suppression of nearly 80 %. These findings suggest that ROS partially mediates OxyHb-induced K_V suppression; however, ROS-independent MMP activation also contributes to suppression of K_V currents by OxyHb. Further, as illustrated in Fig. 3c, OxyHb-induced MMP-2 activity was not altered by superoxide dismutase and catalase. These findings indicate that both ROS-dependent and ROS-independent MMP activation contribute to OxyHb-induced K_V current suppression and that OxyHb increases MMP-2 activity independently of ROS generation.

Discussion

The present study indicates that in vivo administration of subarachnoid blood or acute ex vivo application of OxyHb act via multiple pathways that converge to induce HB-EGF shedding and K_V current suppression in cerebral artery myocytes. We provide evidence that one of these pathways involves activation of MMP-2 via a mechanism independent of ROS generation and that a second pathway involves ROS-dependent activation of a matrix metalloprotease (MMP) or a disintegrin metalloprotease (ADAM) distinct from MMP-2. The combination of these ROS-dependent and ROS-independent mechanisms and the resultant shedding

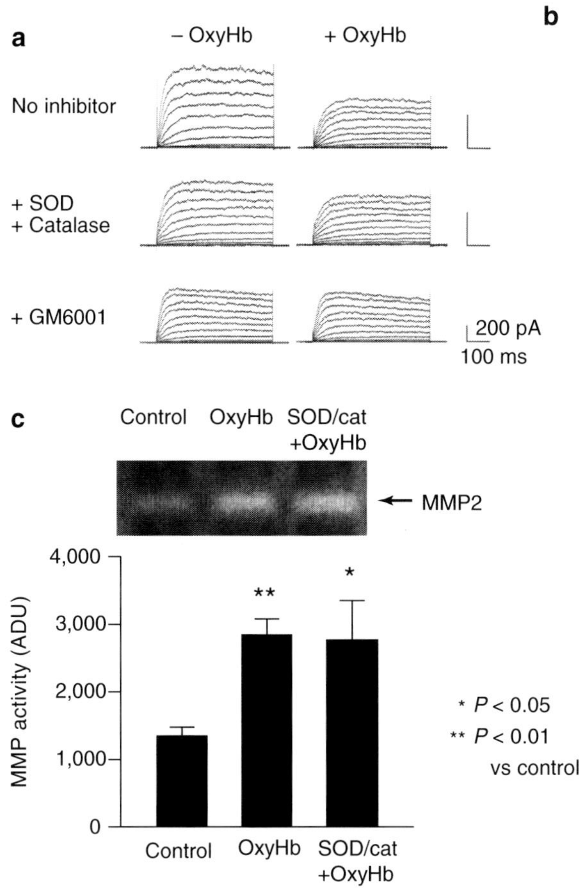

Fig. 3 ROS-dependent and ROS-independent MMP activation and K_V suppression caused by exogenous OxyHb. (**a**) Representative K_V current suppression. (**a**) Representative K_V current recordings demonstrating the ability of the free radical scavengers superoxide dismutase (SOD) and catalase or the MMP inhibitor, GM6001 to reduce OxyHb-induced K_V current suppression. (**b**) Summary data demonstrating that GM6001 caused a greater inhibition of OxyHb-induced K_V current suppression than SOD/catalase. $^{*}P<0.05$; $^{**}P<0.01$ SOD/catalase and GM6001 on OxyHb-induced K_V suppression ($n=7$); §$P<0.05$ GM6001 ($n=5$) vs. SOD/catalase treatment on OxyHb-induced K_V suppression ($n=5$). ANOVA followed by Tukey test. (**c**) Representative gel and summary of zymography data demonstrating that SOD/catalase treatment did not prevent OxyHb-induced MMP-2 activation. $^{*}P<0.05$; $^{**}P<0.01$ versus control. (Control: $n=8$, OxyHb: $n=8$, SOD/cat+OxyHb: $n=4$) ANOVA followed by Tukey test

of HB-EGF and EGFR activation account for the selective suppression of K_V channels in cerebral artery myocytes from SAH model animals.

Our observation that OxyHb does not cause additional suppression of K_V currents in myocytes isolated from SAH model animals indicates that OxyHb is the blood component largely responsible for reduced K_V currents leading to enhanced cerebral artery constriction after SAH. Consistent with this concept, both OxyHb and subarachnoid blood suppress K_V currents through a pathway involving MMP activation, HB-EGR shedding, and EGFR activation. Our present findings also indicate that OxyHb activates at least two distinct MMPs or ADAMs responsible for HB-EGF shedding—MMP-2 and an unidentified additional MMP/ADAM. It also appears that ROS are involved in the activation of the unidentified MMP/ADAM, but not MMP-2. The oxidation of OxyHb to methemoglobin releases O_2^- and secondarily leads to the production of hydroxyl radicals [14, 21]. Other studies [2, 13, 19] have demonstrated that these ROS can increase activity and expression of MMPs, including MMP-2. However in the present study, super oxide dismutase and catalase, scavengers of O_2^- and H_2O_2, did not prevent OxyHb-induced stimulation of MMP-2 activity (Fig. 3). This finding indicates that OxyHb can also act independently of ROS to enhance MMP-2 activity. Future studies are needed to determine the mechanism of ROS-independent MMP-2 activation and to determine the identity of additional MMPs/ADAMs involved in OxyHb-induced K_V current suppression.

Conclusions

Enhanced cerebral artery constriction represents one component of the multifactorial and interrelated series of pathological events leading to DCI in patients after aneurysmal SAH.

Our data indicate that OxyHb contributes to SAH-induced cerebral artery constriction via activation of multiple MMPs/ADAM, leading to HB-EGF shedding and K_V current suppression in cerebral artery myocytes. Evidence is also provided that ROS-dependent and ROS-independent pathways are involved in OxyHb-induced MMP activation. These findings suggest that SAH-induced MMP/ADAM activation may play an important role in the development of DCI after SAH and represent a new target for therapies to alleviate the detrimental consequences of cerebral aneurysm rupture.

Acknowledgments This work was supported by the Totman Trust for Medical Research, the Peter Martin Brain Aneurysm Endowment, the National Institutes of Health (NIH) (P01 HL095488, R01 HL078983, and R01 HL078983-05S1) and the American Heart Association (0725837T). The authors acknowledge the use and assistance of the University of Vermont Neuroscience COBRE molecular biology core facility.

Conflict of Interest Statement We declare that we have no conflict of interest.

References

1. Albarwani S, Nemetz LT, Madden JA, Tobin AA, England SK, Pratt PF, Rusch NJ (2003) Voltage-gated K^+ channels in rat small cerebral arteries: molecular identity of the functional channels. J Physiol 551:751–763
2. Ali MA, Kandasamy AD, Fan X, Schulz R (2013) Hydrogen peroxide-induced necrotic cell death in cardiomyocytes is independent of matrix metalloproteinase-2. Toxicol In Vitro 27:1686–1692
3. Amberg GC, Santana LF (2006) K_V2 channels oppose myogenic constriction of rat cerebral arteries. Am J Physiol Cell Physiol 291:C348–C356
4. Chen TT, Luykenaar KD, Walsh EJ, Walsh MP, Cole WC (2006) Key role of K_V1 channels in vasoregulation. Circ Res 99:53–60
5. Dreier JP (2011) The role of spreading depression, spreading depolarization and spreading ischemia in neurological disease. Nat Med 17:439–447
6. Harder DR, Dernbach P, Waters A (1987) Possible cellular mechanism for cerebral vasospasm after experimental subarachnoid hemorrhage in the dog. J Clin Invest 80:875–880
7. Ishiguro M, Morielli AD, Zvarova K, Tranmer BI, Penar PL, Wellman GC (2006) Oxyhemoglobin-induced suppression of voltage-dependent K^+ channels in cerebral arteries by enhanced tyrosine kinase activity. Circ Res 99:1252–1260
8. Ishiguro M, Puryear CB, Bisson E, Saundry CM, Nathan DJ, Russell SR, Tranmer BI, Wellman GC (2002) Enhanced myogenic tone in cerebral arteries from a rabbit model of subarachnoid hemorrhage. Am J Physiol Heart Circ Physiol 283:H2217–H2225
9. Koide M, Bonev AD, Nelson MT, Wellman GC (2012) Inversion of neurovascular coupling by subarachnoid blood depends on large-conductance Ca^{2+}-activated K^+ (BK) channels. Proc Natl Acad Sci U S A 109:E1387–E1395
10. Koide M, Nystoriak MA, Krishnamoorthy G, O'Connor KP, Bonev AD, Nelson MT, Wellman GC (2011) Reduced Ca^{2+} spark activity after subarachnoid hemorrhage disables BK channel control of cerebral artery tone. J Cereb Blood Flow Metab 31:3–16
11. Koide M, Penar PL, Tranmer BI, Wellman GC (2007) Heparin-binding EGF-like growth factor mediates oxyhemoglobin-induced suppression of voltage-dependent potassium channels in rabbit cerebral artery myocytes. Am J Physiol Heart Circ Physiol 293:H1750–H1759
12. Lucchesi PA, Sabri A, Belmadani S, Matrougui K (2004) Involvement of metalloproteinases 2/9 in epidermal growth factor receptor transactivation in pressure-induced myogenic tone in mouse mesenteric resistance arteries. Circulation 110:3587–3593
13. Martinez-Lemus LA, Zhao G, Galinanes EL, Boone M (2011) Inward remodeling of resistance arteries requires reactive oxygen species-dependent activation of matrix metalloproteinases. Am J Physiol Heart Circ Physiol 300:H2005–H2015
14. Misra HP, Fridovich I (1972) The generation of superoxide radical during the autoxidation of hemoglobin. J Biol Chem 247: 6960–6962
15. Nelson MT, Patlak JB, Worley JF, Standen NB (1990) Calcium channels, potassium channels, and voltage dependence of arterial smooth muscle tone. Am J Physiol 259:C3–C18
16. Nystoriak MA, O'Connor KP, Sonkusare SK, Brayden JE, Nelson MT, Wellman GC (2011) Fundamental increase in pressure-dependent constriction of brain parenchymal arterioles from subarachnoid hemorrhage model rats due to membrane depolarization. Am J Physiol Heart Circ Physiol 300:H803–H812
17. Pluta RM, Hansen-Schwartz J, Dreier J, Vajkoczy P, Macdonald RL, Nishizawa S, Kasuya H, Wellman G, Keller E, Zauner A, Dorsch N, Clark J, Ono S, Kiris T, Leroux P, Zhang JH (2009) Cerebral vasospasm following subarachnoid hemorrhage: time for a new world of thought. Neurol Res 31:151–158
18. Sehba FA, Bederson JB (2006) Mechanisms of acute brain injury after subarachnoid hemorrhage. Neurol Res 28:381–398
19. Siwik DA, Pagano PJ, Colucci WS (2001) Oxidative stress regulates collagen synthesis and matrix metalloproteinase activity in cardiac fibroblasts. Am J Physiol Cell Physiol 280:C53–C60
20. Sobey CG, Faraci FM (1998) Subarachnoid haemorrhage: what happens to the cerebral arteries? Clin Exp Pharmacol Physiol 25:867–876
21. Steele JA, Stockbridge N, Maljkovic G, Weir B (1991) Free radicals mediate actions of oxyhemoglobin on cerebrovascular smooth muscle cells. Circ Res 68:416–423
22. Wellman GC (2006) Ion channels and calcium signaling in cerebral arteries following subarachnoid hemorrhage. Neurol Res 28:690–702
23. Zaritsky JJ, Eckman DM, Wellman GC, Nelson MT, Schwarz TL (2000) Targeted disruption of Kir2.1 and Kir2.2 genes reveals the essential role of the inwardly rectifying K^+ current in K^+-mediated vasodilation. Circ Res 87:160–166

Mechanisms Underlying Increased Vascular Smooth Muscle Contractility in the Rabbit Basilar Artery Following Subarachnoid Hemorrhage

Yuichiro Kikkawa, Katsuharu Kameda, Satoshi Matsuo, Ryota Kurogi, Akira Nakamizo, Masahiro Mizoguchi, and Tomio Sasaki

Abstract Increased vascular contractility plays an important role in the development of cerebral vasospasm following subarachnoid hemorrhage (SAH). Here, we summarize our current knowledge regarding molecular mechanisms that contribute to increased smooth muscle contractility of rabbit basilar artery following SAH. Our studies demonstrated that upregulation of receptor expression, impairment of feedback regulation of receptor activity, and enhancement of myofilament Ca^{2+} sensitization might lead to increased smooth muscle contractility following SAH.

Keywords Vascular smooth muscle • Subarachnoid hemorrhage • Cerebral vasospasm • Basilar artery • Rabbit

Introduction

The mechanism of cerebral vasospasm following subarachnoid hemorrhage (SAH) can be attributed to either increased production of spasmogens or increased vascular contractility [8]. The contractile response of the cerebral arteries to various putative spasmogens including endothelin (ET)-1 [6], thrombin [14], platelet-derived growth factor [13], thromboxane A2 [18], and sphingosine 1-phosphate [19] have been demonstrated to be enhanced in the animal SAH model. These spasmogens may not only act as a vasoconstrictor but also cause alteration of vascular reactivity. The increase in vascular contractility may result from either endothelial dysfunction or an increase in smooth muscle contractility [10, 17]. This increased vascular contractility is suggested to play a fundamental role in the delayed onset of cerebral vasospasm. Here, we report some new findings regarding the mechanism underlying the increased smooth muscle contractility of rabbit basilar artery following SAH.

Upregulation of Receptor Expression in the Rabbit Basilar Artery Following SAH

Contractile responses to agonists were investigated using basilar arterial strips without endothelium that were isolated from the rabbit cisterna magna double-injection SAH model. Thrombin levels at even 10 U/ml in the basilar artery in the control model induced only a small contraction, whereas contractions were significantly enhanced at a lower concentration in the SAH model [11, 14]. Enhanced contractile response was also observed with an agonist peptide for the thrombin receptor after SAH [14]. Consistent with the increased contractile response to thrombin, expression of the thrombin receptor, proteinase-activated receptor 1 (PAR_1), was upregulated 5 and 7 days after SAH [14]. Intrathecal administration of a selective PAR_1 antagonist prevented both the upregulation of PAR_1 expression and enhancement of the contractile response to thrombin [7]. This suggests that thrombin-mediated activation of PAR_1 plays a critical role in upregulating the expression of PAR_1 itself, thereby enhancing the contractile response to thrombin after SAH. A similar enhancement of the contractility was also observed with platelet-derived growth factor, phenylephrine, and ET-1, but not for high K^+-depolarization or phorbol ester [11, 14]. The expression of PAR_1, α1-adrenoceptor, and ET_A receptor has also been found to be up-regulated after SAH [11]. On the basis of these findings, receptor upregulation is suggested to play an important role in the increased vascular reactivity to agonists.

Y. Kikkawa, MD, PhD (✉) • K. Kameda, MD, PhD
S. Matsuo, MD • R. Kurogi, MD • A. Nakamizo, MD, PhD
M. Mizoguchi, MD, PhD • T. Sasaki, MD, PhD
Department of Neurosurgery, Graduate School of Medical Sciences, Kyushu University, 3-1-1 Maidashi, Higashi-ku, Fukuoka 812-8582, Japan
e-mail: ykikkawa@ns.med.kyushu-u.ac.jp

J. Fandino et al. (eds.), *Neurovascular Events After Subarachnoid Hemorrhage*, Acta Neurochirurgica Supplement, Vol. 120,
DOI 10.1007/978-3-319-04981-6_16,

Impairment of the Feedback Regulation of Receptor Activity in the Rabbit Basilar Artery Following SAH

Contractile responses to agonists usually diminish during persistent or repetitive stimulation with agonists. These phenomena are referred to as desensitization or tachyphylaxis, respectively, and represent an important physiological feedback mechanism that protects against both acute and chronic receptor overstimulation [15, 20]. In actuality, the mechanism of receptor desensitization is impaired under various pathological conditions, such as hypoxia, cancer, and diabetes [1, 3, 4]. Thus, the attenuation of contractile responses through desensitization or tachyphylaxis may help to prevent the development of cerebral vasospasm.

In the control model, the agonist stimulation of rabbit basilar artery with ET-1, thrombin, and phenylephrine induced a transient contraction that reached a peak and then gradually declined to the significantly lower level [11]. This attenuation of the contractile response after persistent receptor stimulation is consistent with desensitization. On the other hand, the transient contractile response was converted to a sustained response in the SAH model [11]. A similar conversion of contractility following SAH was also observed for stimulations with angiotensin II or vasopressin [9]. This means that receptor desensitization was impaired after SAH. The conversion of the transient response to the sustained response was also observed with cytosolic Ca^{2+} concentration ($[Ca^{2+}]_i$) and myosin light chain (MLC) phosphorylation [11]. Furthermore, when the artery was consecutively stimulated with PAR_1-activating peptide, phenylephrine, angiotensin II, or vasopressin, the response to the second stimulus was significantly reduced in the control model. This attenuation of the contractile response to the second stimulation is consistent with tachyphylaxis. On the other hand, the contractile response to the second stimulation was well preserved in the SAH model [9, 11]. This means that tachyphylaxis was impaired after SAH. These observations suggest that, after SAH, the feedback regulation mechanisms of the receptor-mediated contraction, such as desensitization or tachyphylaxis, were impaired upstream of the Ca^{2+} signal, and presumably at the receptor level, thereby causing a sustained contraction and persistent response to the second stimulation.

The impaired feedback regulation may cause a significant influence on the contractile effect of thrombin because of the unique activation mechanism of PAR_1. The activation of PAR_1 by thrombin is initiated by proteolytic cleavage of the N-terminal region, which covers the region that acts as a tethered ligand and activates the receptor [2]. Feedback regulation therefore plays an important role in terminating the activity of the proteolytically activated PAR_1. In the SAH model, thrombin-induced sustained contraction was found to persist even after terminating the thrombin stimulation [11]. Trypsin is known to remove the ligand region of PAR_1, thereby converting the active conformation of PAR_1 to the inactive conformation [16]. The addition of trypsin during the thrombin-induced sustained contraction completely inhibited the contraction [11]. Furthermore, an inhibitor of the Gαq protein also inhibited the thrombin-induced sustained contraction in the SAH model [11]. These observations therefore suggest that the persistent contraction is associated with the persistent activation of PAR_1, and that the feedback inactivation of PAR_1 is impaired following SAH. The Gαq inhibitor also inhibited the sustained phase of the contraction induced by ET-1 and phenylephrine [11]. These findings suggest that impairment of the feedback regulation of the receptor activity is not limited to PAR_1, but also extends to other receptors. This general impairment of the receptor inactivation may explain the enhanced contractility to the various agonists that is observed following SAH.

The mechanism underlying the impairment of receptor desensitization has yet to be elucidated. In SAH, thrombin inactivation by argatroban prevented the enhancement of the contractile response to the PAR_1 agonist, whereas it did not prevent the impaired receptor desensitization [9]. On the other hand, a combination of argatroban and vitamin C or tempol prevented both the enhancement of the contractile response and impaired receptor desensitization, which suggests that oxidative stress is responsible for the impairment of receptor desensitization [9]. Use of the thiobarbituric acid reactive substances assay demonstrated that the level of oxidative stress in the brain tissues just beneath the basilar artery in the SAH model was significantly higher than that observed in the control brain [9]. This previous study also examined the effect of treatments using argatroban and anti-oxidative agents on the contractile response to three agonists, angiotensin II, prostaglandin F (PGF) 2α, and vasopressin. The results revealed that the angiotensin II receptor was the most strongly influenced by the desensitization mechanism, and the PGF2α receptor was the least affected [9]. Thus, these findings suggested that oxidative stress plays an important role in the impairment of receptor desensitization following SAH.

Enhancement of Myofilament Ca^{2+} Sensitization in the Rabbit Basilar Artery Following SAH

In the contraction of the vascular smooth muscle, the extent of tension development changes depending on the type of the contractile stimulus when the same amount of $[Ca^{2+}]_i$ elevation is given to each contraction. When a greater contraction is produced for a given elevation of $[Ca^{2+}]_i$, this phenomenon is referred to as "Ca^{2+} sensitization of the contractile apparatus" or as "an increase in the Ca^{2+} sensitivity" [5]. Vascular smooth muscle contraction is regulated by MLC phosphorylation, which is determined by the balance between the activities of the MLC phosphorylation and dephosphorylation [5]. MLC is dephosphorylated by the action of the MLC phosphatase (MLCP). The increase in the Ca^{2+} sensitivity is caused by a decrease in the MLCP activity, which is regulated by the inhibitory effect of both the phosphorylation of the myosin phosphatase target subunit 1 (MYPT1) and the inhibitory protein, 17-kDa PKC-potentiated inhibitory protein of type 1 protein phosphatase (CPI-17) [5]. The agonist stimulation causes the phosphorylation of MYPT1 and/or CPI-17 through the activation of the Rho-associated coiled-coil kinase (ROCK) and/or protein kinase C (PKC), resulting in an increase in the Ca^{2+} sensitivity.

Use of α-toxin-permeabilized preparations allows the direct evaluation of the extent of the myofilament Ca^{2+} sensitization. In α-toxin-permeabilized preparations, GTPγS, a non-hydrolyzable GTP analog that is known to directly activate G proteins by skipping the receptor-mediated activation, induces a transient response in the control model. However, in the SAH model, it induces a sustained response [11]. This suggests that the feedback regulation that occurs at the step that regulates the myofilament Ca^{2+} sensitivity is also impaired following SAH. The Ca^{2+}-sensitizing effect of ET-1 has been additionally investigated using α-toxin-permeabilized preparations. ET-1 induced enhanced and prolonged contraction in the SAH model, suggesting that the ET-1-induced Ca^{2+} sensitization is potentiated after SAH [12]. ET-1-induced Ca^{2+} sensitization became less sensitive to inhibitors of ROCK and PKC following SAH [12]. In the SAH model, expressions of PKCα, ROCK2, CPI-17, and MYPT1 were upregulated, and there was an elevation of the basal level of the phosphorylation of CPI-17 and MYPT1 [12]. Furthermore, ET-1 induced enhanced and prolonged phosphorylation of MYPT1 at both T696 and T853 in the SAH model [12]. Based on these results, it was suggested that the increased expression and activity of PKCα, ROCK2, CPI-17, and MYPT1 underlie the enhanced and prolonged Ca^{2+} sensitization induced by agonist stimulation, thereby contributing to the increased vascular contractility following SAH. However, the mechanism of upregulation and activation of these molecules remains to be elucidated.

Conclusion

Our recent studies demonstrated that the expression of various receptors was upregulated, the feedback regulation of the receptor activity was impaired, and the myofilament Ca^{2+} sensitization was enhanced in the rabbit basilar artery following SAH. Our findings suggest that these actions contribute to the increased vascular smooth muscle contractility to various spasmogens, and that they therefore play a fundamental role in the development of cerebral vasospasm following SAH.

Acknowledgment This research was supported by JSPS KAKENHI (Grant Numbers 24791510, 25670624 and 26462164).

Conflict of Interest Statement We declare that we have no conflict of interest.

References

1. Booden MA, Eckert LB, Der CJ, Trejo J (2004) Persistent signaling by dysregulated thrombin receptor trafficking promotes breast carcinoma cell invasion. Mol Cell Biol 24:1990–1999
2. Coughlin SR (2000) Thrombin signalling and protease-activated receptors. Nature 407:258–264
3. Endo K, Matsumoto T, Kobayashi T, Kasuya Y, Kamata K (2005) Diabetes-related changes in contractile responses of stomach fundus to endothelin-1 in streptozotocin-induced diabetic rats. J Smooth Muscle Res 41:35–47
4. Hinton M, Gutsol A, Dakshinamurti S (2007) Thromboxane hypersensitivity in hypoxic pulmonary artery myocytes: altered TP receptor localization and kinetics. Am J Physiol Lung Cell Mol Physiol 292:L654–L663
5. Hirano K (2007) Current topics in the regulatory mechanism underlying the Ca^{2+} sensitization of the contractile apparatus in vascular smooth muscle. J Pharmacol Sci 104:109–115
6. Ide K, Yamakawa K, Nakagomi T, Sasaki T, Saito I, Kurihara H, Yosizumi M, Yazaki Y, Takakura K (1989) The role of endothelin in the pathogenesis of vasospasm following subarachnoid haemorrhage. Neurol Res 11:101–104
7. Kai Y, Hirano K, Maeda Y, Nishimura J, Sasaki T, Kanaide H (2007) Prevention of the hypercontractile response to thrombin by proteinase-activated receptor-1 antagonist in subarachnoid hemorrhage. Stroke 38:3259–3265
8. Kai Y, Maeda Y, Sasaki T, Kanaide H, Hirano K (2008) Basic and translational research on proteinase-activated receptors: the role of thrombin receptor in cerebral vasospasm in subarachnoid hemorrhage. J Pharmacol Sci 108:426–432
9. Kameda K, Kikkawa Y, Hirano M, Matsuo S, Sasaki T, Hirano K (2012) Combined argatroban and anti-oxidative agents prevents increased vascular contractility to thrombin and other ligands after subarachnoid hemorrhage. Br J Pharmacol 165:106–119. doi:10.1111/j.1476-5381.2011.01485.x
10. Kassell NF, Sasaki T, Colohan AR, Nazar G (1985) Cerebral vasospasm following aneurysmal subarachnoid hemorrhage. Stroke 16:562–572
11. Kikkawa Y, Kameda K, Hirano M, Sasaki T, Hirano K (2010) Impaired feedback regulation of the receptor activity and the myofilament Ca^{2+} sensitivity contributes to increased vascular reactiveness after subarachnoid hemorrhage. J Cereb Blood Flow Metab 30:1637–1650
12. Kikkawa Y, Matsuo S, Kameda K, Hirano M, Nakamizo A, Sasaki T, Hirano K (2012) Mechanisms underlying potentiation of endothelin-1-induced myofilament Ca^{2+} sensitization after subarachnoid hemorrhage. J Cereb Blood Flow Metab 32: 341–352

13. Maeda Y, Hirano K, Hirano M, Kikkawa Y, Kameda K, Sasaki T, Kanaide H (2009) Enhanced contractile response of the basilar artery to platelet-derived growth factor in subarachnoid hemorrhage. Stroke 40:591–596
14. Maeda Y, Hirano K, Kai Y, Hirano M, Suzuki SO, Sasaki T, Kanaide H (2007) Up-regulation of proteinase-activated receptor 1 and increased contractile responses to thrombin after subarachnoid haemorrhage. Br J Pharmacol 152:1131–1139
15. Miasiro N, Paiva AC (1990) Homologous desensitization of the effects of endothelin on rabbit aorta rings and on cultured rat aorta smooth muscle cells. Eur J Pharmacol 179:151–158
16. Nakayama T, Hirano K, Shintani Y, Nishimura J, Nakatsuka A, Kuga H, Takahashi S, Kanaide H (2003) Unproductive cleavage and the inactivation of protease-activated receptor-1 by trypsin in vascular endothelial cells. Br J Pharmacol 138:121–130
17. Sasaki T, Kassell NF, Yamashita M, Fujiwara S, Zuccarello M (1985) Barrier disruption in the major cerebral arteries following experimental subarachnoid hemorrhage. J Neurosurg 63:433–440
18. Sasaki T, Wakai S, Asano T, Takakura K, Sano K (1982) Prevention of cerebral vasospasm after SAH with a thromboxane synthetase inhibitor, OKY-1581. J Neurosurg 57:74–82
19. Tosaka M, Okajima F, Hashiba Y, Saito N, Nagano T, Watanabe T, Kimura T, Sasaki T (2001) Sphingosine 1-phosphate contracts canine basilar arteries in vitro and in vivo: possible role in pathogenesis of cerebral vasospasm. Stroke 32:2913–2919
20. Trejo J (2003) Protease-activated receptors: new concepts in regulation of G protein-coupled receptor signaling and trafficking. J Pharmacol Exp Ther 307:437–442

Vasoconstrictive Effect of Tenascin-C on Cerebral Arteries in Rats

Masashi Fujimoto, Masato Shiba, Fumihiro Kawakita, Naoshi Shimojo, Kyoko Imanaka-Yoshida, Toshimichi Yoshida, Kenji Kanamaru, Waro Taki, and Hidenori Suzuki

Abstract *Background and purpose*: The authors have reported that tenascin-C (TNC), a matricellular protein, is induced after subarachnoid hemorrhage (SAH), associated with cerebral vasospasm. In this study, we examined whether TNC alone causes cerebral vasospasm-like constriction of the intracranial internal carotid arteries (ICAs) in rats, focusing on the p38 mitogen-activated protein kinase (MAPK)-mediated mechanisms.

Methods: First, we injected 10 μg of TNC into the cisterna magna of healthy rats and studied morphologically whether TNC caused constriction of the left ICA at 24–72 h after administration. Second, we examined the effect of SB203580 (a p38 MAPK inhibitor) on the vessel diameter of the left ICA in healthy rats at 24 h. Third, we evaluated the effect of SB203580 on TNC-induced constriction of the left ICA in healthy rats at 24 h.

Results: TNC significantly induced cerebral vasospasm-like angiographic constriction of the left ICAs, which continued at least for 72 h. SB203580 itself had no effect on the diameter of normal ICAs, but abolished the TNC-induced vasoconstrictive effect on the left ICA.

Conclusion: These findings show that TNC causes left ICA constriction via activation of p38 MAPK, resembling post-SAH vasospasm, and suggest the possible involvement of TNC in the pathogenesis of cerebral vasospasm.

Keywords Tenascin-C • Cerebral vasospasm • Subarachnoid hemorrhage • p38 MAPK

M. Fujimoto, MD, PhD (✉) • M. Shiba, MD, PhD
F. Kawakita, MD • W. Taki, MD, PhD
Department of Neurosurgery, Mie University Graduate School of Medicine, 2-174 Edobashi, Tsu, Mie 514-8507, Japan
e-mail: masa0416@clin.medic.mie-u.ac.jp

N. Shimojo, PhD
Department of Pathology and Matrix Biology, Mie University Graduate School of Medicine, 2-174 Edobashi, Tsu, Mie 514-8507, Japan

K. Imanaka-Yoshida, MD, PhD • T. Yoshida, MD, PhD
Department of Pathology and Matrix Biology, Mie University Graduate School of Medicine, 2-174 Edobashi, Tsu, Mie 514-8507, Japan

Research Center for Matrix Biology, Mie University Graduate School of Medicine, 2-174 Edobashi, Tsu, Mie 514-8507, Japan

K. Kanamaru, MD, PhD
Department of Neurosurgery, Suzuka Kaisei Hospital, 112-1 Kokufu, Suzuka, Mie 513-8505, Japan

H. Suzuki, MD, PhD
Department of Neurosurgery, Mie University Graduate School of Medicine, 2-174 Edobashi, Tsu, Mie 514-8507, Japan

Research Center for Matrix Biology, Mie University Graduate School of Medicine, 2-174 Edobashi, Tsu, Mie 514-8507, Japan

Introduction

Cerebral vasospasm after subarachnoid hemorrhage (SAH) remains a major cause of morbidity and mortality [8]. Despite considerable research effort, the mechanism underlying the development of cerebral vasospasm remains poorly understood [1]. Tenascin-C (TNC) is a matricellular protein, which are nonstructural and secreted extracellular matrix proteins. TNC is induced in many diseases and has proinflammatory effects [2]. Recently, we reported that TNC was expressed in the spastic cerebral artery wall in a rat SAH model [5, 6]. Furthermore, inhibition of post-SAH upregulation of TNC by imatinib mesylate prevented cerebral vasospasm in rats, associated with inactivation of p38 mitogen-activated protein kinase (MAPK) [5]. In addition, a cisternal injection of recombinant TNC aggravated post-SAH vasospasm with activation of p38 MAPK in rats. Thus, we hypothesized that TNC causes cerebral vasospasm through p38 MAPK activation. The aims of this study were to examine whether TNC in

J. Fandino et al. (eds.), *Neurovascular Events After Subarachnoid Hemorrhage*, Acta Neurochirurgica Supplement, Vol. 120,
DOI 10.1007/978-3-319-04981-6_17,

the subarachnoid space can generate constriction of cerebral arteries similar to vasospasm that occurs after SAH, and if the mechanisms involve p38 MAPK.

Materials and Methods

All procedures were approved by the Animal Ethics Review Committee of Mie University, and were carried out in accordance with the institution's Guidelines for Animal Experiments.

Intracisternal Injection and Study Protocol

Male Sprague-Dawley rats (age, 8–9 weeks; weight, 270–320 g; SLC, Hamamatsu, Japan) were anesthetized by an intraperitoneal injection of 4 % chloral hydrate (10 mL/kg) and allowed to breathe spontaneously. Blood pressure and blood gas were measured via the right femoral artery. Rectal temperature was kept at 37 °C during surgery. Using a surgical microscope (Zeiss, Germany), a midline occipitocervical skin incision was performed and the suboccipital muscles were dissected to reveal the arch of the atlas, the occipital bone, and the atlanto-occipital membrane. With a 27-gauge needle, the atlanto-occipital membrane was tapped carefully into the cisterna magna. Injection of drug or vehicle was performed over a 10-min period, after which the needle was withdrawn, the pore was quickly plugged with oxidized cellulose, and the wound was sutured [5].

First, phosphate-buffered saline (PBS) or TNC (10 μg) were administered randomly to 30 healthy rats. The effects of TNC on cerebral arteries were evaluated using neurobehavioral tests; India-ink angiography at 24, 48, and 72 h; and histopathological study at 24 h.

Second, PBS or SB203580 (p38 MAPK inhibitor, 3.8 μg; Wako Pure Chemical, Osaka, Japan) were administered randomly to eight healthy rats. The effects of SB203580 on cerebral arteries were evaluated using neurobehavioral tests and India-ink angiography at 24 h.

Third, TNC or TNC plus SB203580 were administered randomly to ten healthy rats. The effects of SB203580 on vasoconstriction by TNC were evaluated using neurobehavioral tests, India-ink angiography, and histopathological study at 24 h.

TNC Preparation

TNC was purified from culture supernatant of the U-251MG glioma cell line by ammonium sulfate precipitation, Sephacryl S-500 gel filtration, Mono Q ion-exchange chromatography, and using a hydroxyapatite column [11]. Purified TNC was extensively dialyzed against Ca^{2+}, Mg^{2+}-free Dulbecco's PBS, and passed through a 0.2-μm membrane filter.

Neurobehavioral Test

Neurological impairments were blindly evaluated using two methods [5]. Neurological scores (3–18) were assessed by summing up six test scores (spontaneous activity; spontaneous movement of four limbs; forepaw outstretching; climbing; body proprioception; and response to whisker stimulation). Beam balance test investigated the animal's ability to walk on a narrow wooden beam (2.25-cm diameter and columnar) for 60 s: four points, walking ≥20 cm; three points, walking ≥10 cm but <20 cm; two points, walking ≥10 cm but falling; one point, walking <10 cm; and zero points, falling with walking <10 cm. The mean score of three consecutive trials with 5-min intervals was calculated.

India-Ink Angiography

India-ink angiography was performed as previously reported [5]. The ascending aorta was cannulated with a blunted 16-gauge needle attached to flexible plastic tubing, which was connected to a pressure transducer (Nihon Kohden Co., Tokyo, Japan) and a syringe on an automatic infusion pump. After an incision was made in the right atrium to allow the outflow of perfusion solutions, 100 mL of PBS, 15 min of 10 % formalin, and 10 min of 3.5 % gelatin–India ink solution were infused through the closed circuit at 60–80 mmHg. The rat was refrigerated at 4 °C for 24 h to allow gelatin solidification. The brains were harvested and high-resolution pictures of the circle of Willis were taken with a scale. The brain was stored in 10 % neutral buffered formalin for histopathological study. An experienced researcher who was unaware of the treatment groups measured the smallest lumen diameter in the left intracranial internal carotid artery (ICA) three times using Image J software (National Institutes of Health, Bethesda, MD) and determined a mean value.

Histopathological Study

The left intracranial ICA was embedded in paraffin and cut into 3-μm-thick sections vertically to the axis. After hematoxylin and eosin (HE) staining, the morphology of the left intracranial ICA was examined under a light microscope.

Statistics

Neurological and beam balance scores were expressed as median ±25th–75th percentiles, and were analyzed using Mann–Whitney *U* tests. The diameter of ICA was expressed as mean ± standard error of the mean, and unpaired *t* tests were used to compare the values between the groups. $P<0.05$ was considered significant.

Results

Effects of TNC on the Left ICA in Rats

Comparisons of physiological parameters and neurological scores were not significantly different between the PBS and TNC groups (data not shown). TNC constricted the intracranial ICA and the effect continued at least for 72 h (unpaired *t* tests; Fig. 1a, b). HE staining confirmed TNC-induced severe vasoconstriction characterized by corrugation of the internal elastic lamina and constriction of the smooth muscle cells similar to observed with the cerebral vasospasm that occurs after SAH (Fig. 1c).

Effects of p38 MAPK Inhibitor on TNC-Induced Contraction of the Left ICA in Rats

SB203580 itself had no effects on the vessel diameter of the untreated left ICAs in rats (Fig. 2). In the TNC plus SB203580 group, the vessel diameter of the intracranial ICA was significantly greater than that in the TNC-only group at 24 h after injection (unpaired *t* tests; Fig. 3a). In histological examination of the intracranial ICA, vasoconstriction was observed in the TNC-only group, but was abolished in the SB203580-treated groups (Fig. 3b).

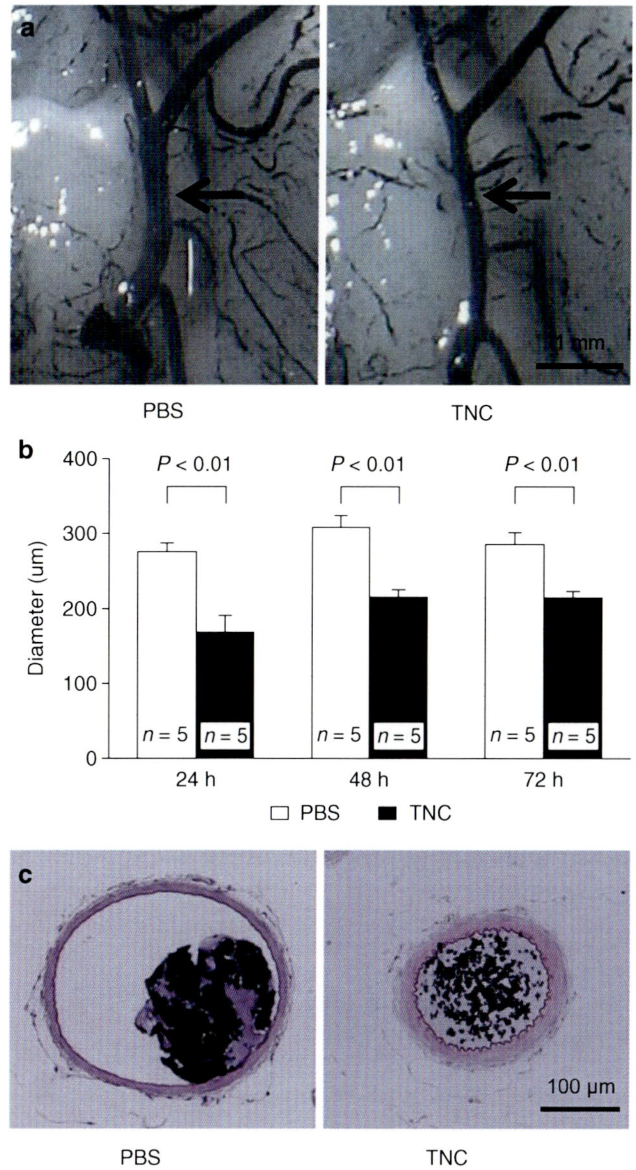

Fig. 1 Effects of TNC on cerebral arteries during the 72-h observation period. (**a**) Representative India-ink angiograms 24 h after injection; *arrow*, left internal carotid artery (ICA). (**b**) Vessel diameter of left intracranial ICA at 24, 48, and 72 h after injection. Data are expressed as mean ± standard error of the mean; *P* value, unpaired *t* tests. (**c**) Hematoxylin and eosin staining of the left intracranial ICA

Discussion

The main findings of this study are as follows: (1) an intracisternal injection of TNC caused constriction of the rat intracranial ICA at least for 72 h; and (2) SB203580, a p38 MAPK inhibitor, abolished the vasoconstriction induced by TNC.

TNC, a matricellular protein, is highly expressed during embryogenesis and is absent or much reduced in normal adult tissue, but reappears in many diseases including cancer, chronic inflammation, and tissue injury. TNC is induced by cytokines, growth factors, mechanical stress, and hypoxia, and exerts diverse functions through direct binding to cell surface receptors and other matrix proteins [2].

MAPKs including p38 MAPK are present in vascular smooth muscle cells and considered likely modulators of prolonged smooth muscle contraction through caldesmon, calponin, and heat shock protein 27 [7]. In cerebral vasospasm after SAH, Pan et al. [3] reported that phosphorylated p38 MAPK in the rabbit basilar arteries was expressed at significantly higher levels in the SAH group than in the control group, and SB20350 attenuated vasospasm associated with

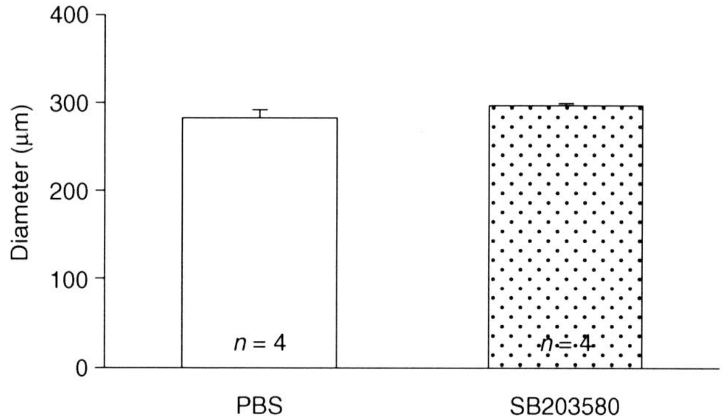

Fig. 2 Effects of p38 MAPK inhibitor on normal cerebral arteries at 24 h after injection. Vessel diameter of the left intracranial internal carotid artery. Data are expressed as mean ± standard error of the mean. No significant difference is seen between the two groups

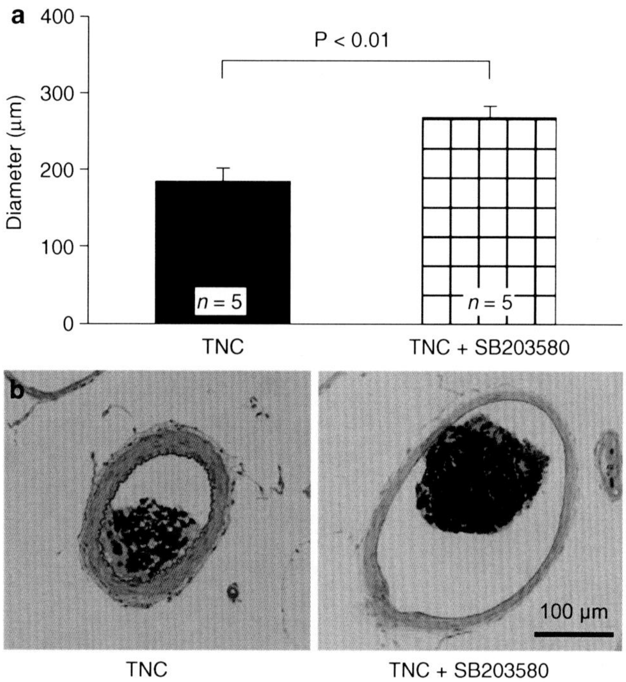

Fig. 3 Effects of p38 MAPK inhibitors on TNC-induced cerebral arterial constriction at 24 h after injection. (**a**) Vessel diameter of the left intracranial internal carotid artery (ICA). Data are expressed as mean ± standard error of the mean; *P* value, unpaired *t* tests. (**b**) Hematoxylin and eosin staining of the left intracranial ICA

decreased expression of phosphorylated p38 MAPK in the basilar arteries.

TNC has been found to activate MAPK signaling [4]. Wang et al. [9] reported that integrin β3, TNC, phosphorylated p38 MAPK, and urokinase-type plasminogen activator (uPA) were expressed in breast invasive ductal carcinoma, and expression of phosphorylated p38 MAPK and uPA in MDA-MB-231 breast cancer cells decreased after the addition of integrin β3 antibody and TNC antibody. In addition, interestingly, not only TNC does influence intracellular MAPK activation, but MAPKs also regulate TNC transcription and deposition [10]. Our previous experimental study showed that expression of TNC and phosphorylated p38 MAPK increased in the spastic cerebral artery wall in a rat SAH model, and that inhibition of post-SAH upregulation of TNC by imatinib mesylate prevented cerebral vasospasm associated with inactivation of p38 MAPK. In this study, TNC constricted rat intracranial ICA and activated p38 MAPK in the constricted artery wall. Taken together, TNC may play an important role in post-SAH vasospasm development by p38 MAPK activation.

Conclusion

We demonstrated that TNC induced prolonged cerebral arterial constriction, possibly through activation of p38 MAPK. TNC may be involved in the pathogenesis of cerebral vasospasm.

Acknowledgements We thank Ms. Chiduru Yamamoto (Department of Neurosurgery, Mie University Graduate School of Medicine) for her technical assistance. This work was supported in part by a Grant-in-Aid for Scientific Research from the Japan Society for the Promotion of Science to Dr. Suzuki.

Conflict of Interest Statement We declare that we have no conflict of interest.

References

1. Kern M, Lam MM, Knuckey NW, Lind CR (2009) Statins may not protect against vasospasm in subarachnoid haemorrhage. J Clin Neurosci 16:527–530
2. Midwood KS, Hussenet T, Langlois B, Orend G (2011) Advances in tenascin-C biology. Cell Mol Life Sci 68:3175–3199
3. Pan YX, Chen KF, Lin YX, Wu W, Zhou XM, Zhang XS, Zhang X, Shi JX (2013) Intracisternal administration of SB203580, a p38 mitogen-activated protein kinase inhibitor, attenuates cerebral vasospasm via inhibition of tumor-necrosis factor-α. J Clin Neurosci 20:726–730
4. Ruiz C, Huang W, Hegi ME, Lange K, Hamou MF, Fluri E, Oakeley EJ, Chiquet-Ehrismann R, Orend G (2004) Growth promoting signaling by tenascin-C. Cancer Res 64:7377–7385
5. Shiba M, Suzuki H, Fujimoto M, Shimojo N, Imanaka-Yoshida K, Yoshida T, Kanamaru K, Matsushima S, Taki W (2012) Imatinib mesylate prevents cerebral vasospasm after subarachnoid hemorrhage via inhibiting tenascin-C expression in rats. Neurobiol Dis 46:172–179
6. Suzuki H, Kanamaru K, Suzuki Y, Aimi Y, Matsubara N, Araki T, Takayasu M, Kinoshita N, Imanaka-Yoshida K, Yoshida T, Taki W (2010) Tenascin-C is induced in cerebral vasospasm after

subarachnoid hemorrhage in rats and humans: a pilot study. Neurol Res 32:179–184

7. Suzuki H, Hasegawa Y, Kanamaru K, Zhang JH (2011) Mitogen-activated protein kinases in cerebral vasospasm after subarachnoid hemorrhage: a review. Acta Neurochir Suppl 110:133–139
8. Taki W, Sakai N, Suzuki H, PRESAT group (2011) Determinants of poor outcome following aneurysmal subarachnoid hemorrhage when both clipping and coiling are available: Prospective Registry of Subarachnoid Aneurysms Treatment (PRESAT) in Japan. World Neurosurg 76:437–445
9. Wang R, Li ZQ, Han X, Li BL, Mi XY, Sun LM, Song M, Han YC, Zhao Y, Wang EH (2010) Integrin β3 and its ligand regulate the expression of uPA through p38 MAPK in breast cancer. APMIS 118:909–917
10. Yang Y, Dang D, Mogi S, Ramos DM (2004) Tenascin-C deposition requires beta3 integrin and Src. Biochem Biophys Res Commun 322:935–942
11. Yoshida T, Yoshimura E, Numata H, Sakakura Y, Sakakura T (1999) Involvement of tenascin-C in proliferation and migration of laryngeal carcinoma cells. Virchows Arch 435:496–500

Early Identification of Brain Tissue at Risk for Delayed Cerebral Ischemia After Aneurysmal Subarachnoid Hemorrhage

Leodante da Costa, Joseph Fisher, David J. Mikulis, Michael Tymianski, and Jorn Fierstra

Abstract *Background*: Delayed cerebral ischemia (DCI) continues to be a major cause of morbidity and mortality in patients with aneurysmal subarachnoid hemorrhage (aSAH) because it can only be diagnosed after the onset of clinical symptoms, contributing to poor clinical outcomes and huge use of clinical resources. We hypothesized that early disturbances in cerebrovascular reactivity, noninvasively measured with functional MRI+CO_2, can be a sensitive marker of brain tissue at risk for DCI.

Methods: Functional MRI exam as soon as possible after the initial bleed and after surgical treatment of the aneurysm was performed in five patients. The functional MRI exam consisted of spatial cerebrovascular reactivity measurements by the blood oxygenation level-dependent (BOLD) response to a standardized carbon dioxide challenge.

Results: Of the three patients who later developed DCI, two had abnormal functional MRI study results. The two patients without DCI had normal MRI results. Brain areas with impaired cerebrovascular reactivity on the functional MRI examination demonstrated a spatial correspondence between impaired cerebrovascular reactivity and the onset of DCI.

Conclusions: In this feasibility study, functional MRI measurements of cerebrovascular reactivity showed a spatial correspondence between impaired cerebrovascular reactivity and the onset of DCI in patients with aSAH.

Keywords Aneurysmal subarachnoid hemorrhage • BOLD-MRI • Cerebrovascular reactivity • Delayed cerebral ischemia

Introduction

Delayed cerebral ischemia (DCI) continues to be a major cause of morbidity and mortality in patients with aneurysmal subarachnoid hemorrhage (aSAH) [1]. Its incidence and impact on outcomes has not decreased significantly in the last half century, despite major advances in intracranial aneurysm treatment. Clinical signs and invasive imaging are resource intensive but poorly predictive of DCI [2]. Vasospasm of the larger cerebral arteries has been long considered the causative mechanism but that has recently been challenged because substantive research efforts could not confirm this mechanism to be solely responsible. The current hypothesis is that dysregulation of vascular tone may actually occur at the level of the microcirculation, which cannot be visualised by catheter angiography, the gold standard diagnostic test for major intracranial vessel vasospasm. Currently, DCI can only be diagnosed after onset of clinical symptoms, contributing to poor clinical outcomes despite intense and costly use of clinical resources [1]. Availability of a test that could identify vascular territories at risk for DCI might improve patients' clinical outcome in two important ways. First, prediction of vascular territories at risk for

L. da Costa, MD (✉)
Division of Neurosurgery, Department of Surgery, Sunnybrook Hospital, Sunnybrook Health Sciences Centre, University of Toronto, 2075 Bayview Avenue, Room A1-37, Toronto, ON, Canada

Department of Medical Imaging, Sunnybrook Hospital, University of Toronto, Toronto, ON, Canada
e-mail: leo.dacosta@sunnybrook.ca

J. Fisher, MD
Department of Anesthesia, Toronto General Hospital and University Health Network, University of Toronto, Toronto, ON, Canada

D.J. Mikulis, MD
Division of Neuroradiology, Toronto Western Hospital and University Health Network, University of Toronto, Toronto, ON, Canada

M. Tymianski, MD PhD
Division of Neurosurgery, Toronto Western Hospital and University Health Network, University of Toronto, Toronto, ON, Canada

J. Fierstra, MD PhD
Department of Neurosurgery, University Hospital Zürich, Zürich, Switzerland

J. Fandino et al. (eds.), *Neurovascular Events After Subarachnoid Hemorrhage*, Acta Neurochirurgica Supplement, Vol. 120,
DOI 10.1007/978-3-319-04981-6_18,

vasospasm can provide a window for prophylactic treatment. Second, it can shorten the requirements for ICU monitoring and costly and potentially harmful invasive tests and/or treatments might be avoided, not only benefitting the patients but also the healthcare system as a whole.

With this feasibility study, we aimed to identify a sensitive imaging marker to detect brain tissue at risk for DCI before symptoms occur. We hypothesized that early disturbances in cerebrovascular reactivity, noninvasively measured with functional MRI + CO_2, can be a sensitive spatial marker of brain tissue at risk for DCI.

Materials and Methods

Subjects

The local institutional ethics research committee approved the study protocol. The entire study protocol was reviewed with every subject and/or substitute decision maker before informed consent was obtained. For the purposes of this study, vasospasm is defined as documented radiological narrowing of a large vessel in the circle of Willis, compared with previous imaging, and DCI is defined as the neurological deficit that sometimes can be related to this finding.

Five nonconsecutive patients with aSAH, as confirmed by computed tomography (CT) and CT angiography (CTA), were enrolled in this case series. Patient enrollment was nonconsecutive because of limitations imposed by the severity of the disease. We elected to enroll only patients in good clinical condition and we used strict inclusion and exclusion criteria (Table 18.1). The test at this stage requires some (although minimal) collaboration, and patients who were too confused or somnolent were not enrolled. MRI examination was performed as soon as possible after hemorrhage, once the aneurysm was secured and the patient's clinical condition stable. The patients' clinical characteristics at presentation and demographics are shown in Table 18.2.

Table 18.1 Inclusion and exclusion criteria

Inclusion criteria	Exclusion criteria
Age ≥ 18 years old	Nonaneurysmal hemorrhage
Confirmed aSAH	Unstable clinical condition
Aneurysm secured (clipping or coiling)	Aneurysm not secured (clipping or coiling)
WFNS grade 1 or 2	Poor clinical grade (WFNS grade ≥ 3)
	Acute or chronic respiratory condition
	Untreated hydrocephalus
	Confusion, agitation
	Vasospasm on recent imaging

Imaging Protocol and Data Analysis

MR imaging was performed on a 3.0-T scanner (Signa; GE Healthcare, Milwaukee, WI) using an eight-channel phased-array head coil. Functional MRI-based blood oxygen level-dependent (BOLD) volumes were acquired during CO_2 challenge using a model-based prospective end-tidal targeting (MPET) algorithm [3] with the RespirAct™ (Thornhill Research Inc, Toronto, Canada). The technique has been described in greater detail elsewhere [4]. During the acquisition of the BOLD sequences, subjects' $P_{ET}CO_2$ levels were set to 40 mmHg for 2 min (step 1), 45 mmHg for 2 min (step 2), and then back to 40 mmHg (step 3). The fraction of inspired oxygen (FiO_2) was kept at 100 %.

To obtain the cerebrovascular reactivity (CVR) maps, from the tidal pCO_2 waveforms generated by the RespirAct™, the end-tidal points were manually selected, generating end-tidal CO_2 waveforms. MR and $P_{ET}CO_2$ data was imported into the software AFNI (Analysis of Functional Neuroimaging). The first raw images of each BOLD-MRI acquisition were reviewed and the first three volumes discarded to allow for magnetization equilibration. To correct for motion, up to 9 (of 72) volumes in which there was appreciable change in head position between the anatomical acquisition and the BOLD-MRI acquisition were excluded before generating maps of CVR. To account for the artifact generated by coils and clips, the source images were evaluated for signal loss when examining the CVR maps to identify regions where the CVR maps were valid and where they were unreliable. A linear slope of best fit approximated the percentage of BOLD signal change

Table 18.2 Demographics and clinical characteristics at presentation and type of treatment

CASE #	Age	Sex	WFNS grade	Fisher grade	Aneurysm treatment
1	42	Male	I	II	Coil
2	57	Male	II	III	Coil
3	61	Male	II	III	Clipping
4	43	Female	II	III	Coil
5	42	Female	II	IV	Coil

per mmHg change in end-tidal CO_2. Confidence of this fit was assessed with an r-value (Pearson product–moment correlation coefficient). CVR maps were generated by least-squares fitting of the BOLD-MRI signal waveform to the $P_{ET}CO_2$ waveform on a voxel-by-voxel basis. From the fitted data, percentage MRI signal change per mmHg $P_{ET}CO_2$ change on a voxel-by-voxel basis was calculated (= CVR index).

Results

We recruited 3 men and 2 women, mean age 49 (range 42–61) years. World Federation of Neurological Surgeons (WFNS) and Fisher grades are shown in Table 18.1. Despite the severity of their illness, good quality anatomical and functional images were obtained in all patients. No harmful events related to the MRI examination or CO_2 challenges were observed. CVR studies were obtained between 1 and 8 days after SAH (average 3.6 days). Three patients were scanned within 72 h after onset of the SAH, 1 patient at day 4, and 1 patient at day 8. All patients were in stable neurological condition, without clinical evidence of DCI before and during the MRI exam. Initial imaging before or during aneurysm treatment and repeated cerebrovascular imaging at the time of the CVR test showed no evidence of vasospasm.

Imaging results and clinical findings are shown in Table 18.2. As mentioned, the initial imaging showed no vasospasm in any patient. Delayed imaging showed vasospasm in four patients (80 %), three (60 %) of whom had DCI of varying severity. CVR–MRI test results were considered abnormal in two patients, and both developed DCI. One of these patients had a minor stroke documented in a follow-up MRI, 9 days after hemorrhage in the same territory (severely abnormal CVR suggestive of paradoxical flow with hypercapnia, the "steal phenomenon"). A third patient with a normal CVR-MRI result had DCI. This patient developed progressive confusion and decreased level of consciousness and was taken to the interventional suite for balloon angioplasty. Interestingly, despite the patient's neurological deterioration, the angiogram demonstrated mild-to-moderate vasospasm in the anterior circulation but no significant spasm in the posterior fossa, site of the aneurysm. Another patient with a normal CVR result had radiological evidence of vasospasm in routine follow-up imaging but no DCI. No mortality occurred in this series.

Illustrative Case

A 57-year-old man presented with sudden headache associated with nausea and vomiting. His WFNS scale was I. A head CT scan revealed a diffuse SAH, Fisher grade III. His medical history revealed daily smoking but was unremarkable otherwise. CT angiography revealed a large left paraclinoid internal carotid artery aneurysm that was treated with endovascular coiling. The BOLD-MRI CVR test was obtained 36 h after SAH, 12 h after the coiling (Fig. 1a). It demonstrated impaired cerebrovascular reserve in the medial temporal and frontal lobes bilaterally, but without signs of vasospasm on the MR angiogram (MRA) and no ischemic stroke. The patient was monitored according to the protocol for SAH and 8 days later he presented with speech difficulties and increased confusion. Triple-H therapy (hypertension, hypervolemia, and hemodilution) was initiated and another MRA was obtained, showing significant vasospasm in both the middle cerebral artery (MCA) and anterior cerebral artery (ACA) territories and an acute stroke in the mesial left temporal lobe (Fig. 1b, c). The patient responded to Triple-H therapy and eventually made a good recovery despite the stroke. The vascular territories in which the vasospasm and DCI occurred had a good spatial correlation with the vascular territories that exhibited impaired CVR days before the onset of DCI.

Discussion

Our small pilot study shows that functional MRI and CO_2 challenge are possible in the acute setting after aSAH. BOLD-MRI, with its high spatial resolution, will improve the understanding of the pathophysiological changes affecting the mechanisms for control of cerebral blood flow and might help to identify vascular territories that are at risk for developing DCI very early after aSAH, before clinical symptoms occur.

Impaired cerebrovascular reactivity has been related to poor clinical grade and prediction of vasospasm in a small series of SAH using transcranial Doppler ultrasound [5, 6]. We hypothesized that early disturbances in CO_2 reactivity could be used as a marker to identify patients and vascular territories at risk for DCI. Although our series is small, with BOLD-MRI in combination with precise control and prospective targeting of $P_{ET}CO_2$, we were able to obtain spatial CVR measurements before the onset of angiographic vasospasm or DCI that seemed to correlate well with the vascular territories that later developed DCI, before the symptoms occurred. MRI provides very good anatomical information, and functional MRI with CO_2 challenge could help to identify a subgroup of patients who would benefit from prophylactic balloon angioplasty and to perhaps target therapies that were more aggressive.

Another common stimulus used to test reactivity is acetazolamide, a carbon anhydrase inhibitor. It is known to cause

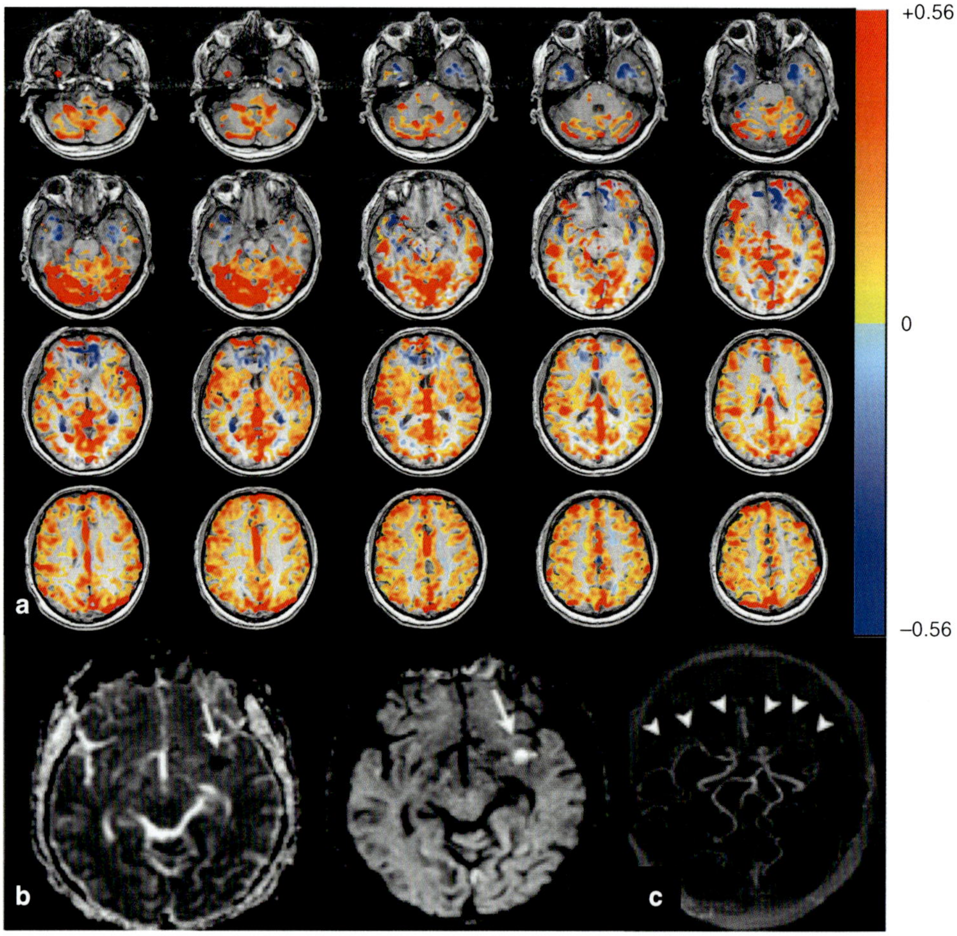

Fig. 1 Illustrative case. BOLD-MRI cerebrovascular reserve map (**a**) obtained 36 h after SAH for the same patient. Note the *blue regions* (color coded after data acquisition to indicate impaired cerebrovascular reserve) in the mesial temporal and frontal lobes bilaterally, suggesting loss of cerebrovascular reserve to CO_2 challenge. Apparent diffusion coefficient (ADC) and diffusion-weighted imaging (DWI) MR images (**b**) obtained on day 8 after SAH showing a small stroke in the left mesial temporal lobe. In the MRA performed at the same time (**c**), note the severe spasm in the anterior cerebral and middle cerebral arteries territory, corresponding to the CVR map changes

vasodilation and is applied widely. Acetazolamide has the advantage of not requiring any patient collaboration, which was a major advantage over CO_2 when using previous methods of control. However, it might increase intracranial pressure, and it cannot be easily terminated if the patient becomes uncomfortable. Acetazolamide also requires intravenous injection and reaches its maximum effect in 12–20 min. Timing the MRI acquisition with the peak of action can be difficult. Measurements performed outside of this window might not be reflective of true CVR, and it is not possible to ensure that images are acquired when similar levels of drug bioavailability are present. When acetazolamide and CO_2 methods are compared, the correlation between results using acetazolamide and hypercapnia is high [7]. Based on our extensive experience with CO_2 manipulation in reactivity testing, we think that our method provides precise CO_2 stimuli, and has a very short duration of action and an exceptional safety profile.

In this case series, two patients with impaired CVR study results developed DCI in the same vascular territory, and, most interestingly, the intensity of cerebrovascular reactivity impairment correlated with the severity of the deficit and therapeutic requirements. Being able to "grade" reactivity could be very useful and could be used to identify areas where induction of a vasodilatory stimulus leads to a reduction in blood flow. Although BOLD-MRI CVR testing is not a quantitative assessment of cerebral blood flow, a good correlation between the percentage of BOLD signal change and blood flow has been demonstrated [8].

We had one case in which the CVR result was reported as normal but the patient still developed DCI related to vasospasm in the posterior circulation. We think that this was cause by one of the major limitations of the BOLD-MRI CVR technique as it stands, poor signal-to-noise ratio and susceptibility artifact in the posterior fossa, altering the BOLD acquisitions and possibly explaining why no abnormality was detected.

Study Limitations

Although this case series suggests an interesting possible relationship between early disturbances in cerebrovascular reactivity to CO_2 after SAH and DCI, we recognize that no strong conclusion can be drawn from such small numbers.

Also, a single test was performed, and no information is available regarding temporal changes in CVR after SAH or regarding the relationship of these changes to clinical symptoms and outcome, obviously important points. Current methodology allows only for patients in spontaneous ventilation to be studied. The MRI study requires some degree of patient collaboration and can be cumbersome in critically ill patients, making repeat tests difficult to obtain. Another problem is that the studies were obtained at different days after hemorrhage, and temporary changes or abnormalities may have been lost or overlooked. Despite the differences in time from SAH, no evidence of vasospasm was seen on the MRAs performed at the same time of the BOLD-MRI CVR, and, therefore, established spasm cannot be the cause for the impaired CVR. Another limitation is the presence of artifacts close to the bones in the skull base. Unfortunately, we are still unable to correct for susceptibility artifacts near the base of the skull, and, thus, CVR in these regions cannot be assessed with our current method. This limitation is taken into account during clinical interpretation of the CVR maps.

Conclusions

In conclusion, we show that BOLD-MRI in combination with a CO_2 challenge is feasible in this difficult study population and may function as a tool to identify tissue at risk for delayed ischemia after SAH. In this small series, early disturbances in CO_2 reactivity demonstrated using BOLD-MRI seem to have good anatomical correlation with areas of future ischemic events. Even acknowledging that no definitive conclusion can be drawn from such a small case series, our findings are interesting and may open a new venue for investigation of vasospasm and delayed ischemic neurological deficits related to SAH using MRI. Despite the limitations of the study, we thnk that, in larger series, the method will prove to be more predictive than current available strategies.

Conflict of Interest Statement We declare that we have no conflict of interest.

References

1. Suarez JI, Tarr RW, Selman WR (2006) Aneurysmal subarachnoid hemorrhage. N Engl J Med 354:387–396
2. Weyer GW, Nolan CP, Macdonald RL (2006) Evidence-based cerebral vasospasm management. Neurosurg Focus 21:E8
3. Slessarev M, Han J, Mardimae A, Prisman E, Preiss D, Volgyesi G, Ansel C, Duffin J, Fisher JA (2007) Prospective targeting and control of end-tidal CO2 and O2 concentrations. J Physiol 581:1207–1219
4. Vesely A, Sasano H, Volgyesi G, Somogyi R, Tesler J, Fedorko L, Grynspan J, Crawley A, Fisher JA, Mikulus D (2001) MRI mapping of cerebrovascular reactivity using square wave changes in end-tidal PCO2. Magn Reson Med 45:1011–1013
5. Aaslid R, Huber P, Nornes H (1984) Evaluation of cerebrovascular spasm with transcranial Doppler ultrasound. J Neurosurg 60:37–41
6. Carrera E, Kurtz P, Badjatia N (2010) Cerebrovascular carbon dioxide reactivity and delayed cerebral ischemia after subarachnoid hemorrhage. Arch Neurol 67:434–439
7. Ringelstein EB, Sievers C, Ecker S, Schneider PA, Otis SM (1988) Noninvasive assessment of CO2-induced cerebral vasomotor response in normal individuals and patients with internal carotid artery occlusions. Stroke 19:963–969
8. Mandell D, Han J, Poublanc J, Crawley A, Stainsby J, Fisher J, Mikulis D (2008) Mapping cerebrovascular reactivity using BOLD MRI in patients with arterial steno-occlusive disease: comparison with arterial spin labeling MRI. Stroke 39:2021–2028

Activation of TRPV4 Channels Does Not Mediate Inversion of Neurovascular Coupling After SAH

Masayo Koide and George C. Wellman

Abstract Neurovascular coupling (NVC) allows increased blood flow to metabolically active neurons and involves the Ca^{2+}-dependent release of vasodilator influences by astrocyte endfeet that encase parenchymal arterioles. We previously reported inversion of NVC from dilation to constriction in brain slices from subarachnoid hemorrhage (SAH) model rats. Corresponding to NVC inversion, there was a marked increase in the amplitude of spontaneous Ca^{2+} oscillations in astrocyte endfeet. Calcium-permeable transient receptor potential vanilloid (TRPV)-4 channels have been reported in astrocyte endfeet, and activators of these channels enhance Ca^{2+} oscillations in healthy animals. Here, we examined the role of TRPV4 channels in the development of high-amplitude spontaneous Ca^{2+} oscillations in astrocyte endfeet and the inversion of neurovascular coupling after SAH. Treatment of brain slices with the TRPV4 channel antagonist, HC-067047 (10 μM), did not alter the amplitude of spontaneous Ca^{2+} oscillations after SAH. In addition, HC-067047 did not inhibit or change SAH-induced inversion of neurovascular coupling. In summary, TRPV4 channels do not appear to be involved in the inversion of neurovascular coupling after SAH. Further studies examining the impact of SAH on additional Ca^{2+} signaling pathways in astrocytes are likely to reveal valuable insights into new therapeutic strategies to advance SAH treatments.

Keywords Subarachnoid hemorrhage • Neurovascular coupling • Astrocytes • Ca^{2+} oscillation • Transient receptor potential channels • TRPV4

M. Koide, PhD (✉) • G.C. Wellman
Department of Pharmacology, University of Vermont College of Medicine, 89 Beaumont Avenue, Burlington, VT, USA
e-mail: masayo.koide@uvm.edu

Introduction

Neurovascular coupling (NVC) forms the basis of functional hyperemia and ensures adequate delivery of oxygen and nutrients to active neurons. This neurally evoked vasodilation matches blood flow to task-dependent increases in regional brain function and involves the coordinated activity of neurons, astrocytes, and intracerebral (parenchymal) arterioles. Under physiological conditions, neurovascular coupling involves (1) neuronal activation and release of the neurotransmitter, glutamate; (2) activation of metabotropic glutamate receptors (mGluRs) on astrocyte processes leading to a wave of elevated Ca^{2+} in astrocytes caused by activation of inositol triphosphate (IP_3) receptors (IP_3Rs); and (3) Ca^{2+}-dependent release of vasodilatory signals by astrocyte endfeet that encase parenchymal arterioles [8, 23, 25]. A number of pathologies, such as Alzheimer's disease, ischemic stroke, and hypertension, impair neurovascular coupling [11]. We recently demonstrated a fundamental change in the polarity of the neurovascular response in brain slices from subarachnoid hemorrhage (SAH) animals [12–14]. We found that neuronal activation of similar intensity has the opposite effect in brain slices from SAH animals, causing vasoconstriction rather than the vasodilation observed in control and sham-operated animals. Local vasoconstriction in response to neuronal activity after SAH could potentially restrict blood flow, compromise neuronal viability, and contribute to the development of delayed cerebral ischemic injury that manifests in humans several days after cerebral aneurysm rupture [24].

Our previous findings also indicate that increased amplitude of spontaneous Ca^{2+} oscillations in astrocyte endfeet after SAH is a key determinant in the inversion of neurovascular coupling [12]. However, the molecular mechanism leading to enhancement of these endfoot Ca^{2+} events

J. Fandino et al. (eds.), *Neurovascular Events After Subarachnoid Hemorrhage*, Acta Neurochirurgica Supplement, Vol. 120,
DOI 10.1007/978-3-319-04981-6_19, © Springer International Publishing Switzerland 2015

is presently unclear. Increased activity of transient receptor potential vanilloid (TRPV)-4 channels, a subtype of Ca^{2+}-permeable ion channels within the transient receptor potential (TRP) channel family [18], is one potential contributor to enhanced endfoot Ca^{2+} signaling after SAH. TRPV4 channels are located on the plasma membrane of cortical astrocytes [3] and evidence indicates that a synthetic activator of these channels can increase the amplitude of spontaneous Ca^{2+} oscillations in astrocyte endfeet encompassing parenchymal arterioles of healthy mice [6]. Therefore, the goal of the present study was to examine the role of TRPV4 channels in the SAH-induced increased amplitude of spontaneous Ca^{2+} events and the inversion of neurovascular coupling observed in brain slices obtained from SAH model rats. Our present findings indicate that TRPV4 channel activity does not contribute to altered astrocyte Ca^{2+} signaling or the inversion of neurovascular coupling that occurs after SAH.

Materials and Methods

Rat SAH Model

Using a surgical approach, two injections of autologous unheparinized arterial blood (500 μL) were made 24 h apart into the cisterna magna of anesthetized Sprague-Dawley (male, 10–12 week old) rats. After each injection, animals were placed head down at a 45° angle for 20 min before recovery from anesthesia, as previously described [12, 19]. Animals were euthanized 4 days after the first injection, and cortical brain slices (160-μm-thick coronal sections, middle cerebral artery territory) were prepared using a vibratome. All experiments were conducted in accordance with The Guide for the Care and Use of Laboratory Animals (NIH Pub. No. 85–23, revised 1996) and followed protocols approved by the Institutional Animal Care and Use Committee of the University of Vermont.

Brain Slice Studies

Brain slices were loaded for 1 h at 29 °C with the Ca^{2+} indicator dye, Fluo-4-AM (10 μM) and 0.05 % pluronic acid in artificial cerebrospinal fluid (aCSF) containing (in mM): 122 NaCl, 3 KCl, 18 $NaHCO_3$, 1.25 NaH_2PO_4, 1 $MgCl_2$, 2 $CaCl_2$, and 5 glucose aerated with 5 % CO_2 and 95 % O_2. For simultaneous measurements of astrocyte endfoot Ca^{2+} and parenchymal arteriolar diameter, brain slices were superfused at 37 °C with aCSF (aerated with 5 % CO_2/95 % O_2, pH ~7.35) containing 100 nM of the thromboxane analog, U46619. Similar experimental findings were obtained when brain slices were superfused with aCSF aerated with 5 % CO_2, 20 % O_2, and 75 % N_2 (Koide and Wellman, unpublished observations). Astrocyte endfoot Ca^{2+} was measured using a BioRad Radiance multiphoton imaging system coupled to a Chameleon Ti:Sapphire laser (Coherent) and an Olympus BX51WI upright microscope [10, 12]. Fluo-4 was excited at 820 nm and fluorescence emission was collected using a 575/150-nm bandpass filter. Calcium concentrations in astrocyte endfeet were determined using the maximal fluorescence (F_{max}) method [10, 15]. Arteriole diameter images were simultaneously acquired using infrared–differential interference contrast (IR-DIC) microscopy. Arteriolar diameter was determined by averaging measurements obtained from three points along the length of the vessel on the same image and are expressed as percent change from the diameter recorded from the first image of the recording. For induction of neuronal activation, electrical field stimulation (EFS; 50 Hz; 0.3-ms alternating square pulse; 3-s duration) was applied using a pair of platinum wires.

Statistical Analysis

Data are expressed as mean ± SEM with n representing the number of recordings per group. Student's paired *t*-test was used to determine statistical significance at the level of $P<0.05$.

Results

Inhibition of TRPV4 Channels Does Not Alter the Amplitude of Spontaneous Ca^{2+} Oscillations in Astrocyte Endfeet After SAH

SAH causes a marked increase in the amplitude of spontaneous Ca^{2+} oscillations leading to inversion of neurovascular coupling [12, 14]. However, the underlying mechanism responsible for the enhancement of this Ca^{2+} signaling modality after SAH is currently unclear. A recent study by Dunn et al. [6] found that the synthetic activator of TRPV4 channels, GSK 1016790A, increased the amplitude of spontaneous Ca^{2+} oscillations in endfeet imaged in brain slices from control mice. To examine whether SAH causes an increase in endfoot TRPV4 channel activity, studies were performed using the TRPV4 antagonist, HC-067047. In the absence of this compound, the amplitude of spontaneous endfoot Ca^{2+} events was 474.5 ± 20.0 nM ($n=13$ endfeet from four animals) (Fig. 1a, b) in brain slices from SAH model animals. These measurements are in agreement with our previous work, with peak amplitudes approximately 100 nM higher than spontaneous Ca^{2+} events recorded in

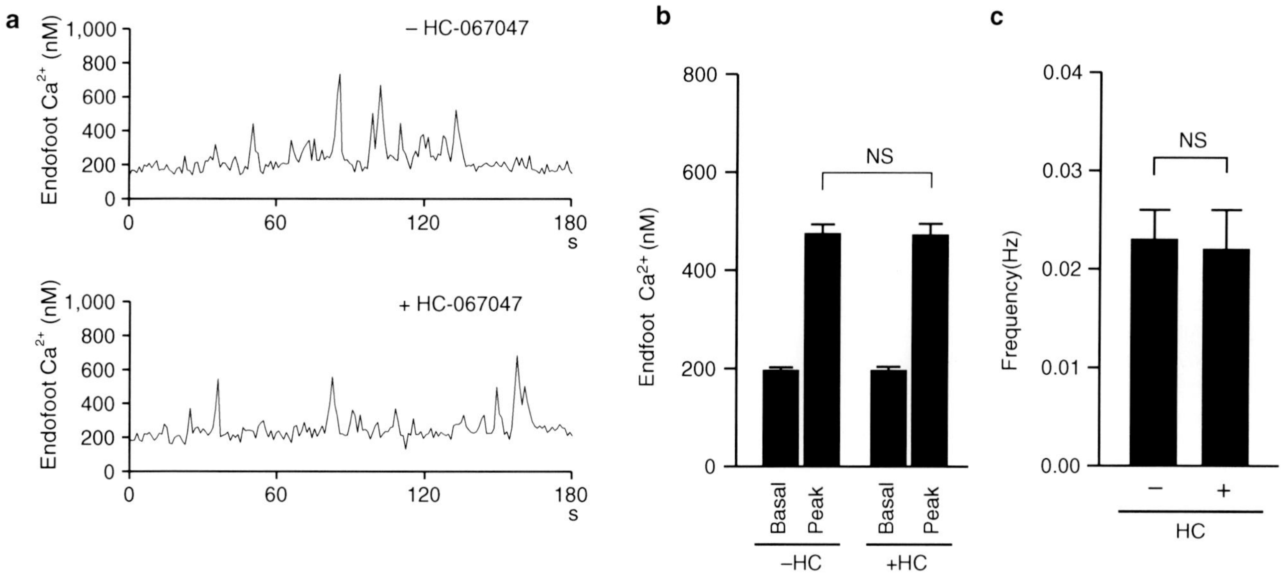

Fig. 1 TRPV4 inhibition does not alter the amplitude or frequency of spontaneous Ca^{2+} events in astrocyte endfeet after SAH. (**a**) Spontaneous Ca^{2+} oscillations recorded from 1.2 × 1.2-μm regions of interest placed on distinct astrocyte endfeet in a brain slice from one SAH animal in the absence (*upper trace*) and presence (*lower trace*) of the TRPV4 antagonist HC-067047 (10 μM). (**b**) Summary data of endfoot Ca^{2+} levels in the absence and presence of HC-067047 (10 μM) obtained from brain slices of SAH model rats. The term *peak* represents the average maximum Ca^{2+} concentration measured during individual spontaneous Ca^{2+} oscillations. (**c**) Summary data of the frequency of spontaneous Ca^{2+} oscillations ± HC-067047 (10 μM) obtained from 4-min recordings using brain slices from SAH model rats. For panels (**b**, **c**), recordings were made from 13 endfeet in four brain slices from four animals. NS, not statistically significant ($P > 0.05$), using paired Student's t-test

endfeet from control animals. Incubation of brain slices from SAH animals with HC-067047 (10 μM for 25 min) did not alter basal levels of Ca^{2+} (−HC-067047: 195.0 ± 7.1 nM; +HC-067047: 195.3 ± 8.5 nM; $n = 13$ endfeet from four brain slices) measured during the interval between spontaneous events (Fig. 1b). HC-067047 also did not change the frequency of these spontaneous Ca^{2+} events (Fig. 1c). Further, as illustrated in Fig. 1a and b, HC-067047 did not alter the amplitude of spontaneous Ca^{2+} events (+HC-067047: 471.7 ± 23.7 nM, $n = 13$ endfeet from four animals) in brain slices from SAH model animals. This data demonstrates that TRPV4 channel activity does not contribute to the enhanced amplitude of spontaneous Ca^{2+} events that occur in astrocyte endfeet after SAH.

TRPV4 Channels Do Not Mediate SAH-Induced Inversion of Neurovascular Coupling

To examine the impact of TRPV4 channels on SAH-induced inversion of neurovascular coupling, electrical field simulation (EFS) was used to induce neuronal action potentials in brain slices from SAH animals. Consistent with our previous studies [12, 13], EFS resulted in an increase in endfoot Ca^{2+} from a resting level of 169.6 ± 8.6 nM to a peak of 348.9 ± 33.0 nM ($n = 5$) (Fig. 2a, c). Associated with this EFS-induced increase in Ca^{2+}, parenchymal arterioles encased by these endfeet constricted by 21.2 ± 4.3 % (Fig. 2a, b). This vasoconstriction in response to neuronal activation after SAH represents an inversion of the physiological vasodilation observed in brain slices from healthy control animals [8, 12, 25]. Incubation of brain slices with the TRPV4 channel antagonist, HC-067047 (10 μM), did not alter EFS-evoked increases in endfoot Ca^{2+} (peak Ca^{2+} after EFS: 330 ± 30.5 nM) or the magnitude of ensuing vasoconstriction (18.6 ± 3.1 % decrease in diameter) (Fig. 2a–c). These findings indicate that TRPV4 channels do not alter EFS-induced increases in endfoot Ca^{2+} or SAH-induced inversion of neurovascular coupling.

Discussion

Neurovascular coupling is an important physiological process enabling increased local blood flow to metabolically active regions of the brain. Recent evidence indicates that subarachnoid blood causes a fundamental change in NVC that could lead to pathological decreases in blood flow,

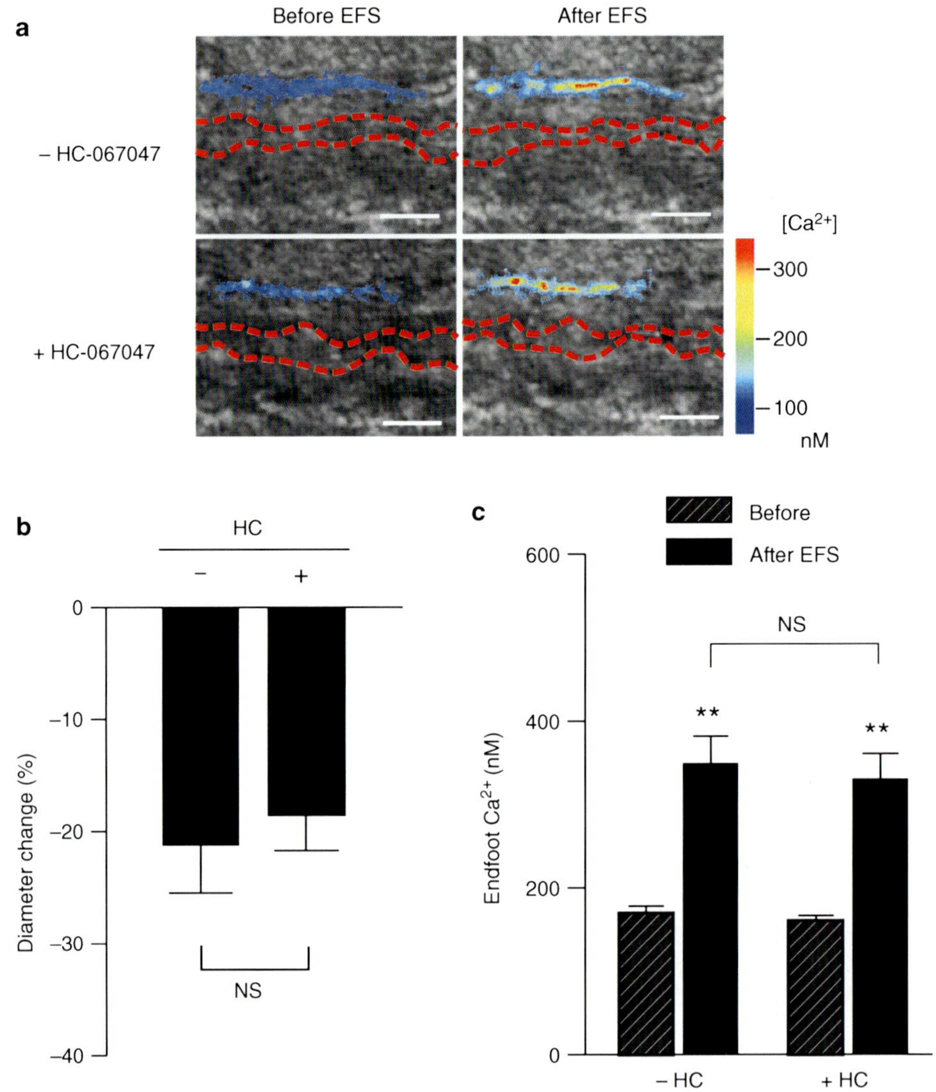

Fig. 2 TRPV4 channel inhibition does not influence SAH-induced inversion of neurovascular coupling. Parenchymal arteriolar diameter and astrocyte endfoot Ca^{2+} concentration were simultaneously measured using two-photon imaging and infrared–differential interference contrast (IR-DIC) microscopy. (**a**) IR-DIC images in the absence (*upper panels*) and in the presence (*lower panels*) of the TRPV4 antagonist HC-067047 (10 μM) obtained from brain slices of SAH model rats. *Red dashes* outline the intraluminal diameter of parenchymal arterioles using IR-DIC microscopy. Overlapping pseudocolor-mapped endfoot Ca^{2+} levels were obtained using the fluorescent Ca^{2+} indicator Fluo-4 and two-photon imaging. Scale bars, 10 μm. (**b**, **c**) Summary of EFS-evoked changes in arteriolar diameter (**b**) and astrocytic endfoot Ca^{2+} (**c**) obtained from SAH ($n=5$ brain slices from three animals) model rats in the presence and absence of HC-067047. *NS* not statistically significant ($P>0.05$), –HC-067047 vs + HC-067047, using paired Student's *t*-test. $^{**}P<0.001$, before vs after EFS, using ANOVA followed by Tukey test

rather than the "normal" physiological increases in blood flow associated with localized, task-dependent increases in neuronal activity. Altered Ca^{2+} signaling in astrocyte endfeet, in the form of high-amplitude spontaneous Ca^{2+} oscillations, are responsible for this SAH-induced inversion of neurovascular coupling. In this present study, we hypothesized that enhanced Ca^{2+} entry via TRPV4 channels contributes to the increased amplitude of spontaneous Ca^{2+} events observed in astrocyte endfeet after SAH. However, this does not appear to be the case, because pharmacological inhibition of TRPV4 channels did not alter endfoot Ca^{2+} signaling or the inversion of neurovascular coupling in brain slices from SAH model animals.

Astrocytes exhibit a diverse array of Ca^{2+} signaling events, including nerve-evoked propagating Ca^{2+} transients [8, 13, 25], spontaneous intracellular and intercellular propagating Ca^{2+} waves [7, 22], and nonpropagating spontaneous Ca^{2+} oscillations that can occur in either the cell body or in cell processes such as endfeet wrapping around intracerebral blood vessels [13, 17, 20]. Our recent evidence demonstrates that a marked elevation in the amplitude of spontaneous Ca^{2+} oscillations in endfeet rather than changes in nerve-evoked astrocyte Ca^{2+} signaling underlie inversion of neurovascular coupling after SAH [12]. In brain slices from SAH animals, high-amplitude Ca^{2+} oscillations in endfeet lead to increased K^+ efflux into the perivascular space via increased activity of large-conductance Ca^{2+}-activated K^+ (BK) channels. This increase in basal extracellular K^+ when summed with nerve-evoked astrocyte K^+ efflux elevates extracellular K^+ in the microenvironment surrounding parenchymal arterioles above the constriction threshold, leading to a polarity change in the neurovascular response from vasodilation to vasoconstriction.

In astrocytes from healthy animals, spontaneous Ca^{2+} oscillations reflect the release of Ca^{2+} stored in endoplasmic reticulum through activation of IP_3-sensitive Ca^{2+} release channels (i.e., IP_3 receptors) and occur independently from neuronal activity or mGluR activation [17, 20]. The activity of IP_3 receptors is bimodally regulated by cytoplasmic Ca^{2+}, with moderate increases in Ca^{2+} leading to an increase in IP_3 receptor activation [9]. Thus, although requiring release of Ca^{2+} from intracellular stores, the amplitude of these spontaneous Ca^{2+} events in endfeet can be modulated by Ca^{2+} entering the cell through the plasma membrane. For example, Ca^{2+}-permeable TRPV4 channels are present on astrocyte processes [3, 4], and activation of these channels caused an increase in the amplitude of spontaneous Ca^{2+} events in endfeet of brain slices prepared from healthy mice [6]. In addition, TRPV4 expression and function is upregulated in hippocampal astrocytes after cerebral ischemia [4]. However, our present data indicates that Ca^{2+} entry via TRPV4 channels does not contribute to the increase in amplitude of endfoot Ca^{2+} events occurring in SAH model animals. The present study does not exclude the possibility that Ca^{2+} entry through other TRP family members is upregulated in astrocytes after SAH. Although evidence suggests that normal native astrocytes do not express voltage-dependent Ca^{2+} channels, it is also possible that expression of these channels is upregulated in astrocytes after SAH. Alternatively, an increase in IP_3 levels or other Ca^{2+}-independent mechanisms leading to enhanced IP_3 receptor activity may underlie the increase in the amplitude of spontaneous Ca^{2+} events in endfeet after SAH. Altered astrocyte Ca^{2+} signaling has been reported to occur in brain pathologies other than SAH, such as Alzheimer's disease, ischemia/hypoxia, and epilepsy [2, 4, 5, 23]. Further, reactive astrogliosis and microglia activation have also been associated with multiple forms of brain injuries, including SAH [16, 21]. It has been postulated that Ca^{2+} oscillations in activated astrocytes may result in gliotransmitter release starting a cascade of events leading to excitotoxicity and brain damage [1]. Presently, the relationship between induction of reactive astrogliosis and the enhancement of astrocyte Ca^{2+} signaling is unclear and requires further investigation.

Conclusions

The inversion of neurovascular coupling from vasodilation to vasoconstriction represents a pathological response after SAH and is a likely contributor to the poor outcome observed in SAH patients. Increased amplitude of spontaneously occurring Ca^{2+} oscillations underlying this SAH-induced inversion of neurovascular coupling are not affected by antagonism of TRPV4 ion channels. Thus, future studies are required to elucidate the underlying mechanisms of the pathological changes in astrocyte Ca^{2+} signaling after SAH and pinpoint specific blood components involved in this response. A greater understanding of this pathway is likely to reveal new therapeutic targets that could benefit patients suffering from SAH.

Acknowledgments This work was supported by the Totman Trust for Medical Research, the Peter Martin Brain Aneurysm Endowment, and the NIH (P01 HL095488, R01 HL078983 and R01 HL078983-05S1). The authors also acknowledge the use and assistance of the University of Vermont Neuroscience COBRE imaging core facility (NIH P30 GM103498 and S10 OD 010583) and input from Drs. Mark T. Nelson and Kathryn M. Dunn.

Conflict of Interest Statement We declare that we have no conflict of interest.

References

1. Agulhon C, Sun MY, Murphy T, Myers T, Lauderdale K, Fiacco TA (2012) Calcium signaling and gliotransmission in normal vs. reactive astrocytes. Front Pharmacol 3:139
2. Balazsi G, Cornell-Bell AH, Moss F (2003) Increased phase synchronization of spontaneous calcium oscillations in epileptic human versus normal rat astrocyte cultures. Chaos 13:515–518
3. Benfenati V, Amiry-Moghaddam M, Caprini M, Mylonakou MN, Rapisarda C, Ottersen OP, Ferroni S (2007) Expression and functional characterization of transient receptor potential vanilloid-related channel 4 (TRPV4) in rat cortical astrocytes. Neuroscience 148:876–892
4. Butenko O, Dzamba D, Benesova J, Honsa P, Benfenati V, Rusnakova V, Ferroni S, Anderova M (2012) The increased activity of TRPV4 channel in the astrocytes of the adult rat hippocampus after cerebral hypoxia/ischemia. PLoS One 7:e39959
5. Ding S, Wang T, Cui W, Haydon PG (2009) Photothrombosis ischemia stimulates a sustained astrocytic Ca^{2+} signaling in vivo. Glia 57:767–776
6. Dunn KM, Hill-Eubanks DC, Liedtke WB, Nelson MT (2013) TRPV4 channels stimulate Ca^{2+}-induced Ca^{2+} release in astrocytic endfeet and amplify neurovascular coupling responses. Proc Natl Acad Sci U S A 110:6157–6162
7. Fiacco TA, McCarthy KD (2006) Astrocyte calcium elevations: properties, propagation, and effects on brain signaling. Glia 54:676–690
8. Filosa JA, Bonev AD, Straub SV, Meredith AL, Wilkerson MK, Aldrich RW, Nelson MT (2006) Local potassium signaling couples neuronal activity to vasodilation in the brain. Nat Neurosci 9: 1397–1403
9. Foskett JK, White C, Cheung KH, Mak DO (2007) Inositol trisphosphate receptor Ca^{2+} release channels. Physiol Rev 87: 593–658
10. Girouard H, Bonev AD, Hannah RM, Meredith A, Aldrich RW, Nelson MT (2010) Astrocytic endfoot Ca^{2+} and BK channels determine both arteriolar dilation and constriction. Proc Natl Acad Sci U S A 107:3811–3816
11. Girouard H, Iadecola C (2006) Neurovascular coupling in the normal brain and in hypertension, stroke, and Alzheimer disease. J Appl Physiol 100:328–335
12. Koide M, Bonev AD, Nelson MT, Wellman GC (2012) Inversion of neurovascular coupling by subarachnoid blood depends on large-conductance Ca^{2+}-activated K^+ (BK) channels. Proc Natl Acad Sci U S A 109:E1387–E1395

13. Koide M, Bonev AD, Nelson MT, Wellman GC (2013) Subarachnoid blood converts neurally evoked vasodilation to vasoconstriction in rat brain cortex. Acta Neurochir Suppl 115:167–171
14. Koide M, Sukhotinsky I, Ayata C, Wellman GC (2013) Subarachnoid hemorrhage, spreading depolarizations and impaired neurovascular coupling. Stroke Res Treat 2013:819340
15. Maravall M, Mainen ZF, Sabatini BL, Svoboda K (2000) Estimating intracellular calcium concentrations and buffering without wavelength ratioing. Biophys J 78:2655–2667
16. Murakami K, Koide M, Dumont TM, Russell SR, Tranmer BI, Wellman GC (2011) Subarachnoid hemorrhage induces gliosis and increased expression of the pro-inflammatory cytokine high mobility group box 1 protein. Transl Stroke Res 2:72–79
17. Nett WJ, Oloff SH, McCarthy KD (2002) Hippocampal astrocytes in situ exhibit calcium oscillations that occur independent of neuronal activity. J Neurophysiol 87:528–537
18. Nilius B, Vriens J, Prenen J, Droogmans G, Voets T (2004) TRPV4 calcium entry channel: a paradigm for gating diversity. Am J Physiol Cell Physiol 286:C195–C205
19. Nystoriak MA, O'Connor KP, Sonkusare SK, Brayden JE, Nelson MT, Wellman GC (2011) Fundamental increase in pressure-dependent constriction of brain parenchymal arterioles from subarachnoid hemorrhage model rats due to membrane depolarization. Am J Physiol Heart Circ Physiol 300:H803–H812
20. Parri HR, Crunelli V (2003) The role of Ca^{2+} in the generation of spontaneous astrocytic Ca^{2+} oscillations. Neuroscience 120:979–992
21. Pekny M, Nilsson M (2005) Astrocyte activation and reactive gliosis. Glia 50:427–434
22. Scemes E, Giaume C (2006) Astrocyte calcium waves: what they are and what they do. Glia 54:716–725
23. Takano T, Tian GF, Peng W, Lou N, Libionka W, Han X, Nedergaard M (2006) Astrocyte-mediated control of cerebral blood flow. Nat Neurosci 9:260–267
24. Vergouwen MD, Vermeulen M, van Gijn J, Rinkel GJ, Wijdicks EF, Muizelaar JP, Mendelow AD, Juvela S, Yonas H, Terbrugge KG, Macdonald RL, Diringer MN, Broderick JP, Dreier JP, Roos YB (2010) Definition of delayed cerebral ischemia after aneurysmal subarachnoid hemorrhage as an outcome event in clinical trials and observational studies: proposal of a multidisciplinary research group. Stroke 41:2391–2395
25. Zonta M, Angulo MC, Gobbo S, Rosengarten B, Hossmann KA, Pozzan T, Carmignoto G (2003) Neuron-to-astrocyte signaling is central to the dynamic control of brain microcirculation. Nat Neurosci 6:43–50

Tenascin-C Is a Possible Mediator Between Initial Brain Injury and Vasospasm-Related and -Unrelated Delayed Cerebral Ischemia After Aneurysmal Subarachnoid Hemorrhage

Hidenori Suzuki, Kenji Kanamaru, Masato Shiba, Masashi Fujimoto, Fumio Kawakita, Kyoko Imanaka-Yoshida, Toshimichi Yoshida, and Waro Taki

Abstract *Introduction*: Tenascin-C (TNC), a matricellular protein, exerts diverse functions, including tissue remodeling and apoptosis, and is induced in cerebrospinal fluid (CSF) after aneurysmal subarachnoid hemorrhage (SAH). The purpose of this study was to examine the relationships among CSF TNC levels, initial brain injury, delayed cerebral ischemia (DCI), and vasospasm after SAH.

Methods: CSF TNC levels were measured in 30 patients with aneurysmal SAH of Fisher computed tomography (CT) group III who were treated microsurgically or endovascularly with CSF drainage within 24 h of SAH. Admission World Federation of Neurosurgical Societies (WFNS) grade was supposed to indicate the severity of initial brain injury. Cerebral vasospasm was defined as narrowed (≥25 %) cerebral arteries demonstrated by angiography. DCI was defined as any neurological deterioration presumed related to ischemia that persisted for ≥1 h.

Results: Higher CSF TNC levels were correlated with worse admission WFNS grades. Vasospasm was aggravated with higher TNC levels. DCI occurred regardless of the degree of vasospasm but was associated with TNC induction. Multivariate analyses showed that higher TNC levels and vasospasm were independent predictors of DCI occurrence.

Conclusions: SAH (initial brain injury) that is more severe induces more TNC, which may cause the subsequent development of both vasospasm and vasospasm-unrelated secondary brain injury, leading to DCI.

Keywords Cerebral vasospasm • Cerebrospinal fluid • Delayed cerebral ischemia • Extracellular matrix • Initial brain injury • Subarachnoid hemorrhage • Tenascin-C

Introduction

Tenascin-C (TNC) is one of the matricellular proteins, which are a class of nonstructural and secreted extracellular matrix proteins that exert diverse functions, including tissue remodeling and apoptosis through direct binding to cell surface receptors, other matrix proteins, and soluble extracellular factors such as growth factors and cytokines [8, 9]. It was reported that TNC was induced in cerebrospinal fluid (CSF) and serum after aneurysmal subarachnoid hemorrhage (SAH), which was associated with the occurrence of vasospasm, shunt-dependent hydrocephalus, and poor outcome [15–18]. Experimental studies also showed that TNC caused cerebral vasospasm in rats [5, 12, 16]. However, the clinical significance of measuring TNC levels remains unclear. Accumulated evidence suggests that the primary cause of poor outcome after SAH is not only cerebral vasospasm, but also early brain injury [1]. Therefore, in this study, we examined the relationships among TNC levels in CSF, initial brain injury, delayed cerebral ischemia (DCI), and vasospasm after aneurysmal SAH.

H. Suzuki, MD, PhD (✉)
Department of Neurosurgery, Mie University Graduate School of Medicine, 2-174 Edobashi, Tsu, Mie 514-8507, Japan

Research Center for Matrix Biology, Mie University Graduate School of Medicine, Tsu, Mie Japan
e-mail: suzuki02@clin.medic.mie-u.ac.jp

K. Kanamaru, MD, PhD
Department of Neurosurgery, Suzuka Kaisei Hospital, Suzuka, Japan

M. Shiba, MD, PhD • M. Fujimoto, MD, PhD • F. Kawakita, MD
W. Taki, MD, PhD
Department of Neurosurgery, Mie University Graduate School of Medicine, 2-174 Edobashi, Tsu, Mie 514-8507, Japan

K. Imanaka-Yoshida, MD, PhD • T. Yoshida, MD, PhD
Department of Pathology and Matrix Biology, Mie University Graduate School of Medicine, Tsu, Mie Japan

Research Center for Matrix Biology, Mie University Graduate School of Medicine, Tsu, Mie Japan

J. Fandino et al. (eds.), *Neurovascular Events After Subarachnoid Hemorrhage*, Acta Neurochirurgica Supplement, Vol. 120, DOI 10.1007/978-3-319-04981-6_20, © Springer International Publishing Switzerland 2015

Materials and Methods

Patient Population

The present study was approved by the ethical committee of our institute and was performed in accordance with institutional guidelines. Appropriate informed consent was obtained from all patients or their relatives.

The subjects of this study were 30 consecutive patients (7 men and 23 women), 40–83 years of age (mean 62.6 ± 2.4 years) who met the following inclusion criteria: ≥20 years of age at onset, SAH classified as Fisher group III on admission computed tomography (CT) scans [4], saccular aneurysm as the cause of SAH confirmed on digital subtraction angiography (DSA), aneurysmal obliteration by clipping or coiling within 24 h after onset, and subsequent insertion of cisternal or spinal drainage tubes according to the preference of the attending neurosurgeons. Excluded from the study were patients who demonstrated any angiographic or surgical complications, as well as individuals with inflammatory, malignant, or other diseases that can affect TNC metabolism. Cases of acute hydrocephalus treated with ventricular drainage were also excluded, because impaired CSF dynamics in these patients may influence the measured TNC levels. World Federation of Neurosurgical Societies (WFNS) SAH scores on admission were evaluated in 2 patients as grade I, in 11 patients as grade II, in 4 patients as grade III, in 7 patients as grade IV, and in 6 patients as grade V [3]. The locations of the ruptured aneurysms were the internal carotid artery in 12 patients, anterior communicating artery in 9 patients, middle cerebral artery in 7 patients, and basilar tip in 2 patients.

After angiographic confirmation of the aneurysm, surgical clipping (23 patients) or endovascular coiling (7 patients) of the lesion was performed within 24 h of the initial onset. A cisternal drainage tube was placed in the basal cistern after surgical clipping, and a spinal drainage tube was put in place after endovascular coiling to promote SAH clearance. The drainage was continued for 7–14 days, and the volume of drained CSF was maintained at 150–250 mL/day by changing the height of the drainage siphon. All patients received intravenous fasudil hydrochloride (Asahi Kasei Pharma, Tokyo, Japan) from 1 day after surgery to 14 days after SAH. Additional treatments were included to maintain normovolemia; prevent meningitis, pneumonia, and hypoxia; and correct anemia and hypoproteinemia. Transcranial Doppler (TCD) was performed daily, and DSA was performed when the clinical findings or blood velocity as measured by TCD indicated vasospasm. CT scanning was performed to evaluate all instances of clinical deterioration. DCI was treated with hypertensive hypervolemic therapy and/or endovascular therapy (intraarterial fasudil hydrochloride infusions or angioplasty) if the cause was severe vasospasm.

Definitions of Initial Brain Injury, DCI, and Vasospasm

Admission WFNS grade was used to indicate the severity of initial brain injury. Cerebral vasospasm was defined as narrowed cerebral arteries (a 25 % or greater reduction in the baseline vessel diameter: none, <25 %; mild, 25–50 %; severe, ≥50 %) demonstrated by DSA [5], which was performed at Days 6–8 or at the onset of clinical symptoms. DCI indicated any neurological deterioration (e.g., hemiparesis, aphasia, altered consciousness) presumed related to ischemia that persisted for longer than an hour, after exclusion of other potential causes of clinical deterioration, such as hydrocephalus, rebleeding, or seizures [19]. The clinical outcome was evaluated 3 months after onset using the Glasgow Outcome Scale [7]. All clinical assessments were carried out without knowledge of TNC levels.

Measurement of TNC

CSF samples were serially obtained via a cisternal or spinal drain on Days 1–3, 4–6, 7–9, and 10–14 after onset. Control samples were obtained from eight patients with unruptured cerebral aneurysms at craniotomy for the surgical clipping. All samples were centrifuged for 5 min at 3,000 × g, and supernatants were stored at −30 °C until assayed. Concentrations of TNC were determined using a commercially available detection kit (IBL, Takasaki, Japan), as previously reported [15].

Statistical Analysis

Data were reported as a mean ± standard error, and unpaired *t* test and one-way analysis of variance (ANOVA) with Bonferroni *post hoc* tests were used as appropriate. Correlation between two variables was evaluated using Spearman's rank correlation coefficient. The impact of each variable on DCI occurrence was determined by multivariate unconditional logistic regression analyses using the dichotomous status (presence or absence) as the dependent variable. All variables were considered independent variables regardless of the significance on univariate analysis, although only the variable with the smallest probability value was used as a candidate variable among similar clinical variables that were intercorrelated. Adjusted odds ratios with 95 % confidence intervals were calculated and independence of variables was tested using the likelihood ratio test on reduced models. A probability value less than 0.05 was considered significant.

Results

TNC Levels in the CSF

TNC was not detected in control patients (<1.5 ng/mL). TNC levels peaked at Days 1–3 post-SAH, and decreased with time. TNC levels were not significantly different between CSF samples obtained from cisternal and spinal drains.

Admission WFNS Grade (Initial Brain Injury) Versus TNC Levels in the CSF

TNC levels were higher as WFNS grades on admission were worse. A significant correlation was observed between CSF TNC levels and admission WFNS grades at Days 1–9 (Fig. 1).

DCI or Vasospasm Versus TNC Levels in the CSF

DCI occurred in 14 patients: Day 5, $n=1$; Day 6, $n=5$; Day 7, $n=3$; Day 8, $n=1$; Day 9, $n=3$; and Day 10, $n=1$. Patients with DCI had significantly higher TNC levels compared with those without DCI at Days 1–6 (Fig. 2a). DSA was performed in 22 patients, and severe vasospasm was associated with significantly higher TNC levels compared with mild or no vasospasm at Days 1–6 (Fig. 2b). Patients with poor outcomes (severe disability, persistent vegetative state and death; $n=10$) also had significantly higher TNC levels than patients with good outcomes (good recovery and moderate disability; $n=20$) at Days 1–3 ($P=0.002$), 4–6 ($P<0.0001$), and 7–9 ($P=0.023$; unpaired t test).

CSF TNC Levels Stratified by DCI and Vasospasm

When CSF TNC levels at Days 1–6 were evaluated for each DCI–vasospasm bracket, patients with DCI had significantly higher TNC levels than those with no DCI in both mild and severe vasospasm (Fig. 3).

On multivariate analyses, higher TNC levels in the CSF at Days 1–6 (continuous variable; odds ratio, 1.070; 95 % confidence interval, 1.032–1.109; $P<0.001$) and cerebral (angiographic) vasospasm (odds ratio, 4.352; 95 % confidence interval, 1.095–17.301; $P=0.037$) significantly predicted DCI occurrence, when age, sex, WFNS grade on admission, aneurysm location, treatment modality, angiographic vasospasm, and TNC levels in CSF at Days 1–6 were used in the analyses.

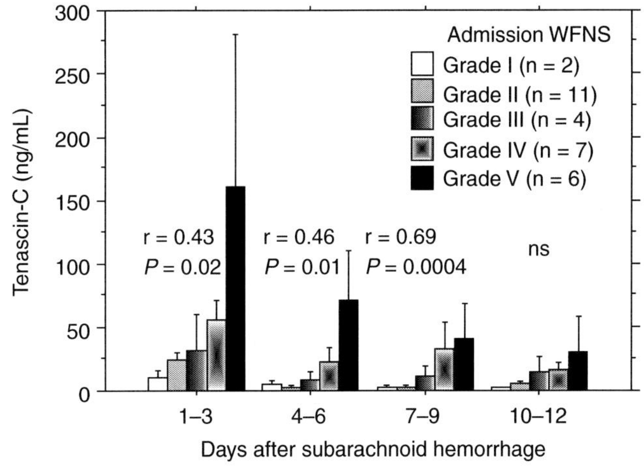

Fig. 1 Relationships between tenascin-C levels in the cerebrospinal fluid and World Federation of Neurosurgical Societies (*WFNS*) grade on admission. *Bars*, means ± standard errors of the means, *r* Spearman's rank correlation coefficient, *ns* not significant

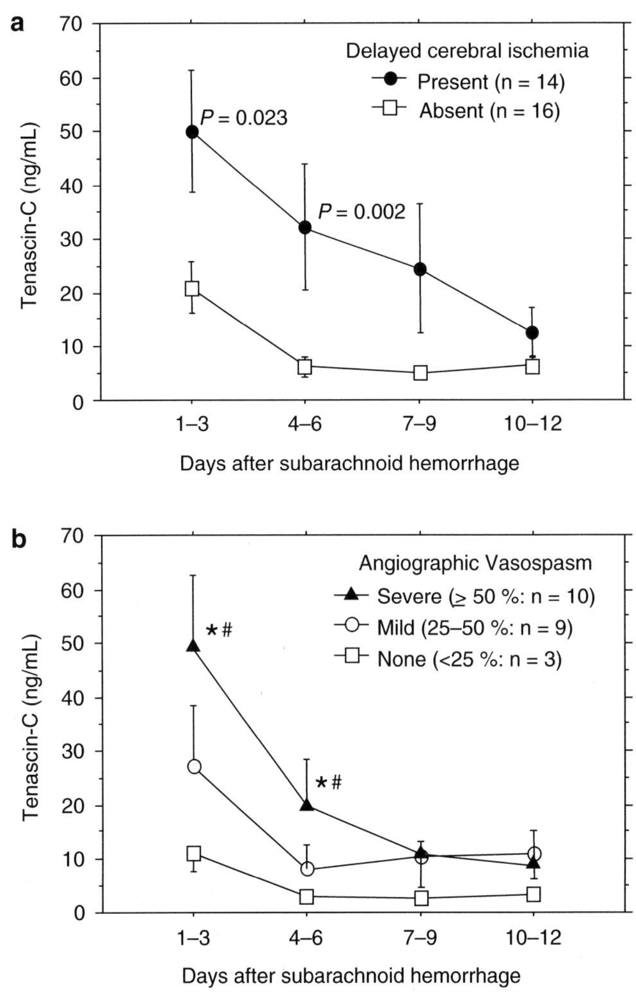

Fig. 2 Relationships between tenascin-C levels in the cerebrospinal fluid and delayed cerebral ischemia (**a**) or cerebral vasospasm (**b**). *Bars*, means ± standard errors of the means, *P* values in (**a**), unpaired *t* test; significantly different from the values in patients with no vasospasm (*$P=0.031$, ANOVA); significantly different from the values in patients with mild vasospasm ($^{\#}P=0.042$, ANOVA)

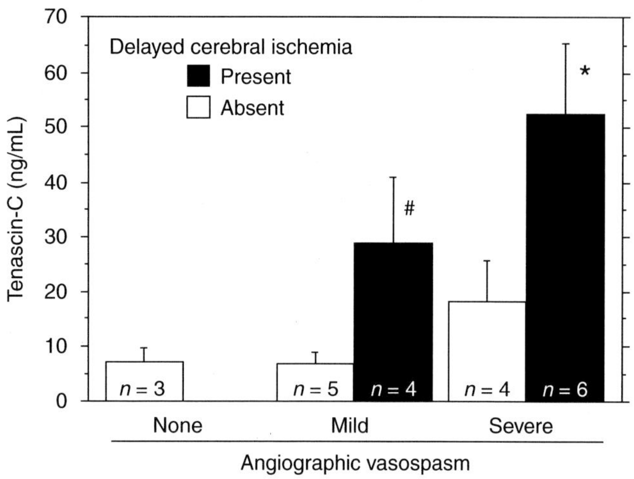

Fig. 3 Tenascin-C levels in the cerebrospinal fluid at Days 1–6 after subarachnoid hemorrhage stratified by delayed cerebral ischemia (DCI) and cerebral vasospasm (severe, ≥50 %; mild, 25–50 %; none, <25 %). *Bars*, means ± standard errors of the means; significantly different from the values in patients with severe vasospasm but no DCI (*P=0.011, ANOVA); significantly different from the values in patients with mild vasospasm but no DCI (#P=0.028, ANOVA)

Discussion

The novel findings in this study are as follows: (1) SAH or initial brain injury that is more severe induces more TNC, which may cause vasospasm and DCI separately or simultaneously; (2) severe vasospasm may cause DCI with more TNC induction; and (3) DCI may occur without severe vasospasm, but by vasospasm-unrelated causes with TNC induction. These findings support recent research efforts that focus on clarifying the pathophysiology of post-SAH early brain injury as well as vasospasm, and on developing protective strategies against them to improve outcome after SAH.

The expression of TNC, a matricellular protein, is extremely limited in healthy adult tissues, but is induced rapidly (within several hours), ectopically, and profusely by inflammatory or noxious stimuli and disappears with their removal [2]. A previous clinical study reported that higher CSF TNC levels were associated with the development of vasospasm [15], and this study suggested that TNC induction also caused vasospasm-unrelated secondary brain injury, which is supposed to be early brain injury. Although these studies suggest that CSF TNC may be a useful biomarker to quickly diagnose or predict the development of vasospasm and DCI, whether TNC can be a therapeutic target to prevent or treat vasospasm and/or DCI is undetermined.

TNC activates mitogen-activated protein kinase (MAPK) [5, 12], which may cause both vasospasm and early brain injury after SAH [13, 14]. TNC may also stimulate synthesis of proinflammatory cytokines and growth factors, and promote their signaling pathways to MAPK activation via enhancing crosstalk signaling between receptors [6, 10]. Our recent experimental study demonstrated that imatinib mesylate, an inhibitor of the tyrosine kinases of platelet-derived growth factor receptors, suppressed TNC induction and MAPK activation, and prevented both cerebral vasospasm and neurological impairments after SAH in rats [12]. However, we cannot exclude the possibility that imatinib mesylate exerted protective effects via mechanisms other than TNC suppression. Because there are neither inhibitors nor neutralizing antibodies specific for TNC, TNC knockout mice would be useful to demonstrate the exact functional role of TNC in vasospasm or early brain injury after SAH [11].

In conclusion, this study shows that TNC, a matricellular protein, in the CSF potentially causes both vasospasm and vasospasm-unrelated delayed brain injury. Further clinical as well as experimental investigations may prove that TNC provides a novel therapeutic approach against both vasospasm-related and vasospasm-unrelated DCI.

Acknowledgments and Funding This work was supported in part by a grant-in-aid for Scientific Research from Japan Society for the Promotion of Science and Mie Society for the Promotion of Medical Research to Dr. Suzuki.

Conflict of Interest Statement We declare that we have no conflict of interest.

References

1. Ayer R, Zhang J (2010) Connecting the early brain injury of aneurysmal subarachnoid hemorrhage to clinical practice. Turk Neurosurg 20:159–166
2. Chiquet-Ehrismann R, Chiquet M (2003) Tenascins: regulation and putative functions during pathological stress. J Pathol 200:488–499
3. Drake CG (1988) Report of World Federation of Neurological Surgeons Committee on a universal subarachnoid hemorrhage grading scale. J Neurosurg 68:985–986
4. Fisher CM, Kistler JP, Davis JM (1980) Relation of cerebral vasospasm to subarachnoid hemorrhage visualized by computerized tomographic scanning. Neurosurgery 6:1–9
5. Fujimoto M, Suzuki H, Shiba M, Shimojo N, Imanaka-Yoshida K, Yoshida T, Kanamaru K, Matsushima S, Taki W (2013) Tenascin-C induces prolonged constriction of cerebral arteries in rats. Neurobiol Dis 55:104–109
6. Ishigaki T, Imanaka-Yoshida K, Shimojo N, Matsushima S, Taki W, Yoshida T (2011) Tenascin-C enhances crosstalk signaling of integrin αvβ3/PDGFR-β complex by SRC recruitment promoting PDGF-induced proliferation and migration in smooth muscle cells. J Cell Physiol 226:2617–2624
7. Jennett B, Bond M (1975) Assessment of outcome after severe brain damage. Lancet 1:480–484
8. Jones PL, Jones FS (2000) Tenascin-C in development and disease: gene regulation and cell function. Matrix Biol 19:581–596
9. Matsui Y, Morimoto J, Uede T (2010) Role of matricellular proteins in cardiac tissue remodeling after myocardial infarction. World J Biol Chem 1:69–80

10. Midwood K, Sacre S, Piccinini AM, Inglis J, Trebaul A, Chan E, Drexler S, Sofat N, Kashiwagi M, Orend G, Brennan F, Foxwell B (2009) Tenascin-C is an endogenous activator of toll-like receptor 4 that is essential for maintaining inflammation in arthritic joint disease. Nat Med 15:774–780
11. Nishioka T, Onishi K, Shimojo N, Nagano Y, Matsusaka H, Ikeuchi M, Ide T, Tsutsui H, Hiroe M, Yoshida T, Imanaka-Yoshida K (2010) Tenascin-C may aggravate left ventricular remodeling and function after myocardial infarction in mice. Am J Physiol Heart Circ Physiol 298:H1072–H1078
12. Shiba M, Suzuki H, Fujimoto M, Shimojo N, Imanaka-Yoshida K, Yoshida T, Kanamaru K, Matsushima S, Taki W (2012) Imatinib mesylate prevents cerebral vasospasm after subarachnoid hemorrhage via inhibiting tenascin-C expression in rats. Neurobiol Dis 46:172–179
13. Suzuki H, Hasegawa Y, Kanamaru K, Zhang JH (2010) Mechanisms of osteopontin-induced stabilization of blood–brain barrier disruption after subarachnoid hemorrhage in rats. Stroke 41:1783–1790
14. Suzuki H, Hasegawa Y, Kanamaru K, Zhang JH (2011) Mitogen-activated protein kinases in cerebral vasospasm after subarachnoid hemorrhage: a review. Acta Neurochir Suppl 110:133–139
15. Suzuki H, Kanamaru K, Shiba M, Fujimoto M, Imanaka-Yoshida K, Yoshida T, Taki W (2011) Cerebrospinal fluid tenascin-C in cerebral vasospasm after aneurysmal subarachnoid hemorrhage. J Neurosurg Anesthesiol 23:310–317
16. Suzuki H, Kanamaru K, Suzuki Y, Aimi Y, Matsubara N, Araki T, Takayasu M, Kinoshita N, Imanaka-Yoshida K, Yoshida T, Taki W (2010) Tenascin-C is induced in cerebral vasospasm after subarachnoid hemorrhage in rats and humans: a pilot study. Neurol Res 32:179–184
17. Suzuki H, Kanamaru K, Suzuki Y, Aimi Y, Matsubara N, Araki T, Takayasu M, Takeuchi T, Okada K, Kinoshita N, Imanaka-Yoshida K, Yoshida T, Taki W (2008) Possible role of tenascin-C in cerebral vasospasm after aneurysmal subarachnoid hemorrhage. Acta Neurochir Suppl 104:179–182
18. Suzuki H, Kinoshita N, Imanaka-Yoshida K, Yoshida T, Taki W (2008) Cerebrospinal fluid tenascin-C increases preceding the development of chronic shunt-dependent hydrocephalus after subarachnoid hemorrhage. Stroke 39:1610–1612
19. Vergouwen MDI, Vermeulen M, van Gijn J, Rinkel GJE, Wijdicks EF, Muizelaar JP, Mendelow AD, Juvela S, Yonas H, Terbrugge KG, Macdonald RL, Diringer MN, Broderick JP, Dreier JP, Roos YBWEM (2010) Definition of delayed cerebral ischemia after aneurysmal subarachnoid hemorrhage as an outcome event in clinical trials and observational studies. Proposal of a Multidisciplinary Research Group. Stroke 41:2391–2395

Pathophysiology of DIND

Characteristics of Patients Without Neuropsychological Deficits Following Aneurysmal Subarachnoid Haemorrhage

Martin N. Stienen, Rahel Weisshaupt, Javier Fandino, Gerhard Hildebrandt, Aline Studerus-Germann, and Bawarjan Schatlo

Abstract *Background*: Previous studies have shown that the incidence of neuropsychological deficits (NPD) after aneurysmal subarachnoid haemorrhage (aSAH) is high despite excellent outcome evaluated by traditional neurological grading scales. The aim of this study was to elucidate the clinical characteristics in patients presenting with aSAH who had a good clinical outcome without NPD.

Methods: Files of patients treated for aSAH between January 2009 and August 2012 at the neurovascular centres of the Kantonsspital St. Gallen (KSSG) and Kantonsspital Aarau (KSA), respectively, were reviewed. Neuropsychological outcome was assessed by an experienced, independent neuropsychologist. Patients were graded as regular, or as having minimal-, moderate-, or severe disability according to normative population data.

Results: A total of 92 patients (35 men and 57 women) with a mean age of 51.4 ± 11.6 years were analysed. Eight of 92 patients (8.7 %) had no NPD at follow-up. Patients without NPD were admitted with lower median WFNS (1.00 vs. 2.00; $p=0.011$) and Fisher grades (2.00 vs. 3.00; $p=0.001$). They were equally distributed between clipping and coiling (four patients each). No patient with regular neuropsychological outcome displayed chronic hydrocephalus ($p=0.019$) or developed delayed cerebral ischaemia (DCI) during the hospital course ($p=0.100$). Five patients were graded as modified Rankin Scale (mRS) 0 and three patients as mRS 1 at discharge.

Conclusion: Patients without NPD after aSAH are likely to present with mild admission scores, develop neither chronic hydrocephalus nor DCI. In this series the aneurysm occlusion modality did not influence the cognitive outcome.

Keywords Subarachnoid haemorrhage • Cognitive impairment Aneurysm • Neuropsychological outcome • Hydrocephalus Outcome

Introduction

Aneurysmal subarachnoid haemorrhage (aSAH) carries a high risk of immediate mortality and significant long-term morbidity. It usually occurs at younger patient age than ischaemic stroke and therefore often affects employed patients before retirement [2]. Increasing understanding of the pathophysiological implications of aSAH and patient management that is more aggressive has led to higher survival rates [4]. Thus, the current focus has shifted towards improvement of the patient's long-term functional outcome [8].

In addition to neurological disability, neuropsychological deficits (NPD) account for significant mid- and long-term disability in aSAH survivors [1, 3, 9, 10]. Even in patients with otherwise good or excellent neurological outcome according to the Glasgow Outcome Scale (GOS), NPD in one or more cognitive domains could be detected in up to 60 % of patients [6, 7]. Although NPD negatively influence

M.N. Stienen, MD (✉) • G. Hildebrandt, MD
Department of Neurosurgery, Kantonsspital St.Gallen, Rorschacher Str. 95, 9007 St.Gallen, Switzerland
e-mail: mnstienen@gmail.com

R. Weisshaupt, MSc
Neuropsychology Unit, Department of Neurology, Kantonsspital Aarau, Aarau, Switzerland

J. Fandino, MD • B. Schatlo, MD
Department of Neurosurgery, Kantonsspital Aarau, Aarau, Switzerland

A. Studerus-Germann, MSc
Neuropsychology Unit, Department of Neurology, Kantonsspital St.Gallen, St. Gallen, Switzerland

J. Fandino et al. (eds.), *Neurovascular Events After Subarachnoid Hemorrhage*, Acta Neurochirurgica Supplement, Vol. 120, DOI 10.1007/978-3-319-04981-6_21, © Springer International Publishing Switzerland 2015

the ability of affected patients to lead an independent life and return to work, this important aspect of patient outcome has only sporadically been addressed in clinical research. As recently pointed out, the neuropsychological aspects of patient outcome are largely underreported in current clinical studies on aSAH [11]. It remains impossible today to predict whether a patient will experience neuropsychological constraint after the haemorrhage. The aim of this study therefore was to identify clinical characteristics that may predict or be associated with the absence of NPD in patients following aSAH.

Materials and Methods

This retrospective two-centre cohort study analysed aSAH patients who were treated at the Kantonsspital St. Gallen (KSSG) or Aarau (KSA) between January 2009 and August 2012, respectively. Both local ethical committees consented to the study protocol. In every patient, an aneurysm responsible for the haemorrhage was detected by either digital subtraction angiography or CT angiography.

Acute hydrocephalus was defined as impaired consciousness at admission with CT evidence of ventricular dilatation and was treated with ventriculostomy (external ventricular drainage (EVD)) or a lumbar drain. Chronic hydrocephalus was suspected if patients worsened >2 points on the Glasgow coma Scale (GCS) in combination with progressive ventricular dilatation after clamping of the EVD. Chronic hydrocephalus was treated by shunt surgery.

Cerebral vasospasm (CVS) was defined as mean blood flow velocity (Vmean) >140 cm/s or increase in Vmean >50 cm/s/24 h or as a Lindegaard-Index >3 in transcranial Doppler sonography or diagnosis was confirmed with CT angiography or digital subtraction angiography. DCI was defined as occurrence of focal neurological impairment, a decrease of at least 2 points on the GCS after excluding other causes (hydrocephalus, electrolyte disturbance, epilepsy, infection), or as the occurrence of new cerebral infarctions not related to the aneurysm treatment on imaging at discharge as a surrogate marker [12]. CVS was treated by oral nimodipine, induced arterial hypertension and normovolemia; patients with DCI received endovascular angioplasty (PTA) or chemical vessel dilution, if feasible and the treatment was regarded meaningful by the treating neurosurgeons and neuroradiologists.

Neurological outcome was evaluated at hospital discharge using the modified Rankin scale (mRS; 0–6). Favourable outcome was defined as mRS 0–2 and morbidity as mRS 3–5 [10]. Only surviving patients with available full neuropsychological assessment by an independent neuropsychologist were selected for analysis. The test battery was applied considering the patients' individual pre-morbid level of workload and social activities and accounted for the following cognitive domains: (1) memory; (2) attention; (3) executive function; (4) visual perception and construction; (5) language/calculation; and (6) behaviour. Patients were graded as regular, or as having minimal-, moderate- or severe disability by an experienced neuropsychologist according to normative population data.

The software used for the statistical analysis was SPSS 18.0 and Graph Pad Prism 5.0c. Probability values (p-value) <0.05 were considered statistically significant.

Results

In total, data from 92 patients (35 men and 57 women) with a mean age of 51.4 ± 11.6 years (± SD) were analysed. The median admission scores were 14.00 (GCS), 2.00 (WFNS) and 3.00 (Fisher). Detailed information on patient and aneurysm-related parameters of the respective study groups are depicted in Table 1.

Table 2 shows information on the clinical course and the treatment performed in patients of both study groups. Acute hydrocephalus requiring CSF diversion was associated with neuropsychological morbidity after discharge ($p=0.009$). Aneurysm occlusion was performed within 72 h after haemorrhage, whenever feasible. A total of 58 aneurysms were clipped and 36 aneurysms were occluded using endovascular techniques (including 34 coiling procedures; one stent-assisted coiling and one aneurysm was primarily stented). Patients without NPD were distributed equally between the two modalities of aneurysm therapy ($p=0.706$). No patient with regular neuropsychological outcome required shunt surgery for chronic hydrocephalus ($p=0.019$). Two of 12 patients who required decompressive hemicraniectomy (DHC) for elevated intracranial pressure (ICP) refractory to maximal conservative therapy showed no NPD at the follow-up ($p=0.590$). Patients without NPD showed a tendency towards a lower rate of CVS (12.5 vs. 45.2 %; $p=0.131$) and none developed DCI (0 vs. 33.3 %; $p=0.100$). Patients with regular neuropsychological outcome were discharged significantly earlier than patients with cognitive constraint ($p<0.001$).

An overview of the outcomes is provided in Table 3. Overall neurological outcome according to the mRS was 1.00 (median), with better results in the group without NPD ($p=0.001$). In general, 100 % of patients without NPD and 75 % of patients with NPD had a good outcome (mRS 0–2) at discharge. Rates of neurological deficits were similar between the study groups. Of 84 patients (91.3 %) who developed NPD, these were graded minimal in 29 patients (34.5 %), moderate in 32 patients (38.1 %) and severe in 23 patients (27.4 %). The domains affected most were attention, memory and executive functions (Table 3).

Table 1 Baseline patient and aneurysm characteristics of the study groups

	Patients without NPD	Patients with NPD	*p* value
Age			
Mean value (years ± SD)	51.9 ± 11.8	51.4 ± 11.6	$p=0.718^a$
Women/men ratio	1:1	1.7:1	$p=0.705^b$
Admission scores			
GCS (median)	15.00	14.00	$p=0.012^a$
WFNS (median)	1.00	2.00	$p=0.011^a$
Fisher (median)	2.00	3.00	$p=0.001^a$
Aneurysm bearing artery			
Acom + ACA	3 (37.5 %)	38 (45.2 %)	
MCA	2 (25.0 %)	22 (26.2 %)	
ICA + Pcom	3 (37.5 %)	14 (16.7 %)	
Vertebrobasilar	–	10 (11.9 %)	
Aneurysm location			$p=0.591^b$
Anterior circulation	8 (100 %)	74 (88.1 %)	
Posterior circulation	–	10 (11.9 %)	
Aneurysm size			
Mean value (mm ± SD)	6.3 ± 2.0	6.5 ± 2.6	$p=0.817^a$

ACA anterior cerebral artery, *Acom* anterior communicating artery, *GCS* Glasgow Coma Scale, *ICA* internal cerebral artery, *MCA* medial cerebral artery, *NPD* neuropsychological deficit, *Pcom* posterior communicating artery, *SD* standard deviation, *WFNS* World Federation of Neurological Surgeons grading scale

[a]Two-tailed Mann–Whitney tests were used for analysis

[b]Two-tailed Fisher tests were used for analysis

Table 2 Information on the clinical course and the treatment performed in patients of both study groups

	Patients without NPD	Patients with NPD	*p* value
ICP – therapy/CSF – diversion			
EVD/lumbar drain placement	1 (12.5 %)	52 (61.9 %)	$p=0.009^a$
Shunt placement	–	38 (45.2 %)	$p=0.019^a$
DHC	2 (25.0 %)	10 (11.9 %)	$p=0.590^a$
Aneurysm treatment			$p=0.706^a$
Microsurgical clipping	4 (50.0 %)	54 (64.3 %)	
Endovascular therapy*	4 (50.0 %)	32 (9 %)	
None	–	–	
Timing of occlusion therapy			
Mean value (days from SAH ± SD)	4.5 ± 4.5	3.8 ± 5.7	$p=0.445^b$
Mean value (days from admission ± SD)	1.6 ± 1.6	2.0 ± 3.6	$p=0.821^b$
Treatment ≤ 72 h after haemorrhage	5 (62.5 %)	60 (71.4 %)	$p=0.688^a$
CVS	1 (12.5 %)	38 (45.2 %)	$p=0.131^a$
DCI	–	28 (33.3 %)	$p=0.100^a$
Duration of hospital stay			
Mean value (days ± SD)	12.6 ± 4.9	24.3 ± 11.1	$p<0.001^b$

CSF cerebrospinal fluid, *CVS* cerebral vasospasm, *DCI* delayed cerebral ischaemia, *DHC* decompressive hemicraniectomy, *EVD* external ventricular drainage, *ICP* intracranial pressure, *NPD* neuropsychological deficit, *SAH* subarachnoid haemorrhage, *SD* standard deviation

[a]Two-tailed Fisher tests were used for analysis

[b]Two-tailed Mann–Whitney tests were used for analysis

*Including 34 coiling procedures; one stent-assisted coiling and one aneurysm was primarily stented

Table 3 Neurological outcome at discharge and neuropsychological outcome after discharge of patients of the study groups

	Patients without NPD	Patients with NPD	*p* value
mRS[a]			
Median value	0.00	1.00	$p=0.001$[b]
Patients with good outcome (mRS 0–2)	8 (100 %)	63 (75 %)	$p=0.200$[c]
Patients with bad outcome (mRS 3–5)	–	18 (21.4 %)	
mRS not assessed	–	3 (3.6 %)	
Focal neurological deficit	1 (12.5 %)	26 (31 %)	$p=0.428$[c]
Neuropsychological deficit			
None/regular assessment	8 (100 %)	–	
Minimal	–	29 (34.5 %)	
Moderate	–	32 (38.1 %)	
Severe	–	23 (27.4 %)	
Affected neurocognitive domains			
Attention	–	69 (82.1 %)	
Memory	–	64 (76.2 %)	
Executive functions	–	63 (75.0 %)	
Language/calculation	–	26 (31.0 %)	
Visuoconstructive abilities	–	24 (28.6 %)	
Behaviour	–	23 (27.4 %)	
Time between aneurysm occlusion to neuropsychological assessment			
Mean value (days ± SD)	72.5 ± 43.2	70.2 ± 69.4	$p=0.308$[b]

mRS modified Rankin Scale, *NPD* neuropsychological deficit, *SD* standard deviation
[a]Missing data present: mRS was not assessed at discharge in three patients with NPD
[b]Two-tailed Mann–Whitney tests were used for analysis
[c]Two-tailed Fisher tests were used for analysis

Discussion

In this cohort, we demonstrate that patients after aSAH without NPD and good neurocognitive outcome presented with initial mild admission scores on the GCS, WFNS and Fisher scale, developed no chronic hydrocephalus and did not experience DCI. Patients with regular cognitive outcome in our series were discharged twice as fast as compared with patients with neuropsychological constraint.

Interestingly, important factors used in daily clinical routine for patient evaluation, such as age, gender, aneurysm localization and size did not differ between patients with and without NPD, as evident from Table 1. Likewise, our data identified two patients in the group of patients with regular neurocognitive examination who received DHC during the hospital course. Therefore, excellent functional outcome is possible even in patients who are at least intermittently critically ill and have to undergo a "rescue therapy" for elevated ICP irresponsive to maximal conservative treatment.

Although controversies regarding the two major aneurysm treatment modalities remain [1, 5], our data suggest equal chances for good cognitive recovery of treated patients with both techniques ($p=0.706$). An excellent neuropsychological outcome was achieved in the four patients in each group.

Even though this was a retrospective data collection, all of the factors introducing potential bias (e.g. age, gender, time between aSAH and aneurysm occlusion therapy, and time between surgery and neuropsychological assessment) did not significantly differ between the study groups. The low rate of patients with regular cognitive outcome inevitably led to heterogeneous group sizes. Thus, our series might be underpowered to detect statistical differences of further parameters, if any existed. It would be necessary to study a larger patient sample to address this issue. Lastly, our cohort was subject to a strong selection bias. Only surviving patients with available full neurocognitive assessment were included, which is likely to explain the remarkably good neurological outcomes according to the mRS at discharge. Therefore, our results must be interpreted with caution. Still, the overall consistent and plausible results suggest that the generated data are stable and it is appropriate to generalise the results to the clinical setting for a selected subgroup of aSAH patients.

Conclusion

Patients without NPD after aSAH are likely to present with mild admission scores, develop no chronic hydrocephalus and to be spared from DCI. In this series the aneurysm occlusion modality did not influence the cognitive outcome.

Conflict of Interest Statement We declare that we have no conflict of interest.

References

1. Al-Khindi T, Macdonald RL, Schweizer TA (2010) Cognitive and functional outcome after aneurysmal subarachnoid hemorrhage. Stroke 41:e519–e536
2. Bederson JB, Connolly ES Jr, Batjer HH, Dacey RG, Dion JE, Diringer MN, Duldner JE Jr, Harbaugh RE, Patel AB, Rosenwasser RH, American Heart A (2009) Guidelines for the management of aneurysmal subarachnoid hemorrhage: a statement for healthcare professionals from a special writing group of the Stroke Council, American Heart Association. Stroke 40:994–1025
3. Chahal N, Barker-Collo S, Feigin V (2011) Cognitive and functional outcomes of 5-year subarachnoid haemorrhage survivors: comparison to matched healthy controls. Neuroepidemiology 37:31–38
4. Dorhout Mees SM, Rinkel GJ, Feigin VL, Algra A, van den Bergh WM, Vermeulen M, van Gijn J (2007) Calcium antagonists for aneurysmal subarachnoid haemorrhage. Cochrane Database Syst Rev:2007 Jul 18;(3):CD000277. PMID 17636626
5. Fontanella M, Perozzo P, Ursone R, Garbossa D, Bergui M (2003) Neuropsychological assessment after microsurgical clipping or endovascular treatment for anterior communicating artery aneurysm. Acta Neurochir (Wien) 145:867–872; discussion 872
6. Fung C, Beck J, Lauber L, Muri R, Raabe A, Nyffeler T (2012) Clinical assessment of deficits after SAH: hasty neurosurgeons and accurate neurologists. J Neurol 259:2198–2201
7. Hutter BO, Gilsbach JM (1993) Which neuropsychological deficits are hidden behind a good outcome (Glasgow = I) after aneurysmal subarachnoid hemorrhage? Neurosurgery 33:999–1005; discussion 1005–6
8. Macdonald RL, Cusimano MD, Etminan N, Hanggi D, Hasan D, Ilodigwe D, Jaja B, Lantigua H, Le Roux P, Lo B, Louffat-Olivares A, Mayer S, Molyneux A, Quinn A, Schweizer TA, Schenk T, Spears J, Todd M, Torner J, Vergouwen MD, Wong GK, Sahit C (2013) Subarachnoid Hemorrhage International Trialists data repository (SAHIT). World Neurosurg 79:418–422
9. Preiss M, Netuka D, Koblihova J, Bernardova L, Charvat F, Kratochvilova D, Benes V (2012) Quality of life 1 year after aneurysmal subarachnoid hemorrhage in good outcome patients treated by clipping or coiling. J Neurol Surg A Cent Eur Neurosurg 73:217–223
10. Seule MA, Stienen MN, Gautschi OP, Richter H, Desbiolles L, Leschka S, Hildebrandt G (2012) Surgical treatment of unruptured intracranial aneurysms in a low-volume hospital – outcome and review of literature. Clin Neurol Neurosurg 114:668–672
11. Stienen MN, Weisshaupt R, Fandino J, Fung C, Keller E, Hildebrandt G, Studerus-Germann A, Muri R, Gutbrod K, Blasi S, Monsch AU, Brugger P, Mondadori C, Sailer M, Bijlenga P, Schaller K, Schatlo B, on behalf of the Swiss SOS study group (2013) Current practice in neuropsychological outcome reporting after aneurysmal subarachnoid haemorrhage. Acta Neurochir (Wien) 155:2045–2051
12. Vergouwen MD, Vermeulen M, van Gijn J, Rinkel GJ, Wijdicks EF, Muizelaar JP, Mendelow AD, Juvela S, Yonas H, Terbrugge KG, Macdonald RL, Diringer MN, Broderick JP, Dreier JP, Roos YB (2010) Definition of delayed cerebral ischemia after aneurysmal subarachnoid hemorrhage as an outcome event in clinical trials and observational studies: proposal of a multidisciplinary research group. Stroke 41:2391–2395

Nitric Oxide Synthases: Three Pieces to the Puzzle?

Mohammed Sabri Attia, Eliott Lass, and R. Loch Macdonald

Abstract Subarachnoid hemorrhage remains to be a devastating diagnosis in this day and age, with very few effective interventions. Rising evidence is now pointing towards the marked importance of secondary complications after the hemorrhage, and its active role in morbidity and mortality of this stroke. This review will focus on the role of Nitric Oxide Synthases (NOSes) the role they play in the pathogenesis of SAH.

Keywords Subarachnoid haemorrhage • SAH • Nitric Oxide Synthases • NO • eNOS • iNOS • nNOS • EBI • Secondary complications

Introduction

Recent research and rising evidence are now pointing to the importance of secondary complications of subarachnoid hemorrhage (SAH), and their role in poor outcome after SAH [10, 18]. More specifically, rising interest is now dedicated toward early brain injury (EBI), or parenchymal, vascular, and microcirculatory damage or dysfunction that occurs the first 24–48 h of the hemorrhagic onset [37, 38]. It remains unclear what secondary complications belong to EBI or are of delayed onset; however, what is becoming clearer is that perhaps mechanistic dysfunction in EBI may predispose the brain to a number of observed secondary complications, such as microcirculatory spasm and microthrombosis, early and delayed neuronal injury, and oxidative and nitrosative parenchymal damage [8, 26, 29, 35, 37, 38].

One of the common and recurring mechanistic themes in SAH research is the importance of nitric oxide (NO) as a vasodilatory and antithrombotic agent that is of value in maintaining physiological homeostasis in the brain [1, 21, 24]. Much research has been dedicated to observing the importance of NO, but few papers exist that focus on nitric oxide synthases (NOSes) and their potential role after SAH [19, 20, 23, 26, 30, 40]. In this review paper, we discuss and highlight the importance and role of NOSes and NO in the pathogenesis of SAH.

A number of theories have been proposed for microthromboembolism, apoptosis, and large vessel vasospasm after SAH, one of which is the unbalanced production of NO coupled with its scavenging and reduced bioavailability [34, 39]. NO is a potent gaseous diffusible free radical that is synthesized by a number of cells; by macrophages, neurons, and glial cells, and largely by endothelial cells. The molecule is synthesized enzymatically and non-enzymatically in the human body. Three known enzymes are responsible for the synthesis of NO, three NOS isoforms: neuronal NOS (nNOS), endothelial NOS (eNOS), and inducible NOS (iNOS). It is debated that eNOS in endothelial cells produces most of the NO responsible for vascular homeostasis, because it is produced via endothelial cells. NO produced by eNOS in endothelial cells is thought to regulate vascular

M.S. Attia, MSc • E. Lass, BSc
Division of Neurosurgery, St. Michael's Hospital, 30 Bond Street, Toronto, ON M5B 1W8, Canada

Labatt Family Centre of Excellence in Brain Injury and Trauma Research, Keenan Research Centre, Li Ka Shing Knowledge Institute of St. Michael's Hospital, Toronto, ON Canada

R.L. Macdonald, MD, PhD (✉)
Division of Neurosurgery, St. Michael's Hospital, 30 Bond Street, Toronto, ON M5B 1W8, Canada

Labatt Family Centre of Excellence in Brain Injury and Trauma Research, Keenan Research Centre, Li Ka Shing Knowledge Institute of St. Michael's Hospital, Toronto, ON Canada

Department of Surgery, Institute of Medical Science, University of Toronto, Toronto, ON Canada
e-mail: macdonaldlo@smh.ca

Disclosures M. Sabri Attia and E. Lass have no disclosures. R. L. Macdonald receives grant support from the Physicians Services Incorporated Foundation, Brain Aneurysm Foundation, Canadian Stroke Network, and the Heart and Stroke Foundation of Ontario. R.L. Macdonald is a consultant for Actelion Pharmaceuticals and Chief Scientific Officer of Edge Therapeutics, Inc.

J. Fandino et al. (eds.), *Neurovascular Events After Subarachnoid Hemorrhage*, Acta Neurochirurgica Supplement, Vol. 120, DOI 10.1007/978-3-319-04981-6_22, © Springer International Publishing Switzerland 2015

tone, modulate thrombosis, regulate smooth muscle division, and confer antiinflammatory properties [11, 12]. A number of papers have briefly touched on the differential roles of NOSes after SAH, but have not yet properly investigated their role and outcome; our laboratory has also focused mainly on eNOS after SAH.

iNOS: To Induce or not to Induce? That Is the Question

iNOS is the one of the three isoforms that generates NO in a calcium-independent fashion and, despite its low abundance in the brain, it has been documented to generate the largest amount of NO and has been implicated to be involved with inflammatory conditions and mediation of oxidative stress [15]. Because of its dependence on calcium, once iNOS is expressed, it can produce copious amounts of NO for sustained periods and is only limited by cofactors and substrate availability [15]. Oxidative stress linked to iNOS is mediated largely via lipid peroxidation, DNA damage, inhibition, and damage of mitochondrial structures and enzymes [15]. INOS has been studied in relation to SAH in a number of animal models, and the exact role of iNOS in the pathogenesis of SAH is still unclear.

Some reports point to the possible deleterious role of iNOS after SAH, and how the enzyme may indeed drive or exacerbate pathogenesis and injury after hemorrhagic insult. Work by Suzuki et al. demonstrated that a blood by-product, Hemin, may indeed activate iNOS and subsequent pathways. Work by this team demonstrated that the overactivation of INOS resulted in the overdevelopment of NO, leading to nitrosative stress and peroxynitrite formation [32, 33]. This increased oxidative burden was linked to damaged smooth muscle cells in the vasculature and may cause a predisposition to a number of vascular complications observed after SAH. Furthermore, work by Sayama et al. demonstrated that iNOS activation and deleterious effects may be part of the EBI cascade of events [32, 33]. The team reported that there was an overexpression of iNOS mRNA in the basal pia 24 h after experimental SAH. iNOS expression was heightened in polymorphonuclear cells and mononuclear cells and in cells throughout the CNS 24 h after SAH. The group concluded that overactivation of iNOS resulted in the overproduction of free radicals and detectable lipid peroxidation, which correlated with the degree of MCA vasospastic burden.

Aminoguanidine (AG), an iNOS specific inhibitor, was used to help inhibit iNOS in an experimental SAH model. Fukada et al. demonstrated that AG inhibition of iNOS resulted in a significant reduction in endothelial and smooth muscle cell damage, which resulted in subsequent reduction in aneurysm formation in a model of aneurysm induction [9]. Reducing shear stress via Batroxobin (defibronyltic) reduced iNOS overexpression and vascular "overstimulation," which was shown to be protective and reduced aneurysm rupture. Transgenic manipulation in experimental models of SAH also indicated a possible deleterious role of iNOS after SAH induction. Work by Saito demonstrated that mice that overexpress CuZn-SOD (an iNOS inhibitor) had significantly reduced vasospasm. The degree of vasospasm correlated directly with the amount of iNOS mRNA and protein expression. Additionally, the team reported that reactive oxygen species directly activate iNOS and may explain the trigger and exacerbation of complications after SAH [31].

Work by Lin et al. demonstrated that vasospasm after SAH may be driven at least partially by the observed upregulation of iNOS after the onset of hemorrhage. In the model reported by this group, animals demonstrated reductions in eNOS levels and significant upregulation of iNOS expression. The group then used adenosine A1 receptor agonists that partially prevented vasospasm and resulted in a significant reduction in eNOS expression. However, the agonists were not successful at reducing iNOS expression, which allowed the group to conclude that continued upregulation of iNOS may play a major role in vasospasm. Similarly, the use of 17beta-estrogen in male rats before experimental SAH reduced vasospasm significantly. 17beta-Estrogen was found to reduce the expression of iNOS mRNA and protein expression, and this reduction in iNOS bioavailability was linked to the reduction of iNOS, indicating a possible deleterious role of iNOS [16, 17].

Despite the many reports and studies that point toward a deleterious nature of iNOS after SAH, a few studies report a neutral and possibly beneficial role of iNOS and its oxidative properties after SAH. Inhibiting iNOS with P-toluenesulfonate after SAH conferred no attenuation of blood-brain barrier (BBB) damage, cerebral edema, or delayed neuronal apoptosis. Inhibiting iNOS did not improve outcome or neurological score after SAH, indicating that although it might be a pathological player, it may not be the biggest or most pertinent target [41].

Work by Vellimana et al. focused on studying the differential expression of all three NOSes after experimental SAH under preconditioning or non-preconditioning situations. The study reported that preconditioning resulted in a more favorable outcome after SAH, and only eNOS demonstrated an increase in expression and was considered likely be protective when preconditioning was provided. Both nNOS and iNOS were deemed to not play a major protective role after SAH [40].

Work by our group focused on using simvastatin as an acute treatment and as prophylaxis in experimental mice in SAH. Simvastatin was observed to reduce the expression of iNOS when given prophylactically, but when administered after the induction of SAH, iNOS expression remained elevated after 48 h of induction. Despite the sustained increased expression in the post-SAH treatment group, animals still demonstrated reduced vasospasm, apoptosis, and microthromboembolism, indicating that iNOS may be a minor player in the pathogenesis of SAH in this particular model [30].

INOS has been reported to possibly confer protective effects, solely based on its proximity and expression in the vascular walls after SAH. Work by Pluta et al. postulated that because Hemin (a blood by-product) is readily available after SAH and is also an activator of iNOS, there should be an increased amount of iNOS expression and activation around the vicinity of hemorrhage. Pluta et al. postulated that iNOS may be a source of NO after SAH because of the involvement of macrophages after SAH, specifically in and around the endothelium of large- and middle-sized vessels. This expression of NO and overabundance of iNOS expression may help alleviate SAH-induced vasospasm [22].

nNOS: The Dark Horse

In a primate model of SAH, nNOS expression was found to be markedly reduced and correlated greatly with the degree of vasospastic burden. SAH induction was associated with reduced staining of nNOS in the vascular adventitia in animals with significant vasospasm. These findings point toward the possible protective role of nNOS, and indicate that NO synthesized by nNOS may indeed be important in the homeostatic modulation of vascular tone in large- and middle-sized vessels [25].

Work by Sehba et al. demonstrated that following experimental SAH there was a heightened measurable expression of nNOS in neurons and the microvasculature. nNOS expression and concentration was significantly increased in the SAH group alone. The heightened expression of nNOS was deemed to be a protective response caused by acute stress and decreased cerebral blood flow, and likely driven to introduce increased expression of NO to reverse any pathological consequences of the hemorrhage [36].

nNOS involvement and protective role could also be a major player in the formation and rupture of aneurysms. Experimental aneurysms were induced in mice and the role of eNOS and nNOS was assessed. eNOS knock-out (KO) mice demonstrated a compensatory upregulation of nNOS expression in the walls of cerebral aneurysms. Interestingly, introducing aneurysms in eNOS and nNOS KO mice resulted in an increase in the amount of aneurysms present, with evidence of late-stage aneurysm formation. Double KO animals demonstrated a significantly increased amount of macrophage (the main cell mediators of inflammation) infiltration, vascular degradation, and progression to aneurysmal rupture. These findings point to the possible protective role of nNOS in maintaining the integrity and structural stability of cerebral aneurysms [2].

Recent work by our lab focused on understanding the role of NOSes after SAH. We reported that nNOS was upregulated in eNOS KO SAH mice, and likely to have been upregulated for compensatory purposes and possible protective expression of NO under pathological conditions such as SAH, where oxidative stress is a major player of pathogenesis [27].

eNOS: The Double-Edged Sword

The other well-studied, perhaps most-studied, constitutive NOS isoform is eNOS. It is usually found in endothelial cells, and often responsible for generating NO that is used for protective homeostatic functions such as endogenous anti-microthrombosis, vasomotor regulation, and smooth muscle growth modulation. eNOS has been the target of several research studies pertaining to SAH because of its involvement in vascular regulation, possible role in middle/large vessel vasospasm, and physiological expression in the brain. Several studies focused on the measurement of and detecting levels of eNOS after SAH, and debated its possible protective, deleterious, or even neutral role.

eNOS has been repeatedly shown to be upregulated after SAH, possibly because of the shear stress introduced by large vessel vasospasm that stimulates endothelial cells to generate more eNOS as a protective physiological response [4]. Indeed, subjecting endothelial cells to shear stress in culture resulted in eNOS mRNA levels to rise, making the vasospasm theory of eNOS upregulation plausible. Work by Jung et al. demonstrated the opposite, that eNOS upregulation maybe futile because of the upregulation and increased expressions of endogenous inhibitors of NOS such as asymmetric dimethylarginine (ADMA) [14]. The study reported that ADMA concentrations correlated positively with the degree of angiographic vasospasm in patients with SAH, which would mean that eNOS levels are reduced, or, on the other hand, may stimulate a positive feedback for further eNOS expression [14].

eNOS is responsible for the production of NO in and around vessels; however, recent evidence suggests that NO might not be the only molecule produced by eNOS. Under normal physiological conditions, eNOS maintains a regulated connection between its homodimers to allow for proper electron flow, which assists in the production of NO from the ferrous–dioxygen complex. It was demonstrated that, under oxidative environments or stress, there is a reduction of NOS cofactors such as tetrahydrobiopterin (BH_4)

and L-arginine in addition to the oxidization of the ferrous–dioxygen complex. These two mechanisms may result in the dimer breaking down or in an allosteric shift that alters the flow of electrons through both dimers. This mechanistic breakdown of the structural dimers of eNOS results in the production of superoxides instead of NO [6, 7]. This mechanism is of particular importance in SAH, a pathology associated with a substantial amount of introduced oxidative stress. The overproduction of O^{2-} may also result in eventual interaction with the limited NO that is available, producing ONOO−, which further oxidizes cofactors such as BH_4 and feeds into a loop of further destruction of eNOS enzyme. Peroxynitrites carry on to produce nitrotyrosine deposits and result in lipid peroxidation and cellular damage, contributing greatly to the apoptotic burden seen after SAH [26].

Pluta et al. reported that blood products found in the subarachnoid space may actually scavenge the pool of NO available and produce endogenous inhibitors of eNOS, resulting in a substantial reduction in vasodilator production and possibly a cause of large vessel vasospasm after SAH. Reports demonstrated that diminished endothelium vasodilatation correlates with the degree of angiographic vasospasm after SAH to post-SAH reductions in CBF [13, 22]. Diminished eNOS activity is associated with a reduced outcome after SAH and associated with increased brain injury after ischemia [3].

Work in our laboratory focused on identifying and understanding the role of eNOS after SAH in an experimental model in mice. We found that SAH resulted in a specific upregulation of dysfunction eNOS, characterized with uncoupling of the eNOS dimer and oxidation of the ferrous–dioxygen complex, releasing its balancing zinc core. This uncoupling resulted in the upregulation of O^{2-} production, reduced NO bioavailability, and increased peroxynitrite and nitrotyrosine deposits in the parenchyma. This mechanism of eNOS dysfunction was hypothesized to be one of the main culprits behind secondary complications that arise in this model; complications such as delayed neuronal injury (DND), microthrombosis, and parenchymal oxidative stress [26, 27].

We used a number of therapeutic interventions to observe whether eNOS upregulation pharmacologically can attenuate any of the observed secondary complications. Work in our laboratory and by McGirt et al. demonstrated that using simvatstain to upregulate eNOS, enhance NO production, and scavenge superoxide production ameliorated a substantial amount of the secondary complications caused by SAH [19, 30]. Intriguingly, using clazosentan, an endothelin-1 receptor antagonist, to reverse large vessel vasospasm improved mortality and large vessel vasospasm; however, animals still demonstrated secondary complications and evidence of eNOS dysfunction [5, 28].

Alternatively, experimental preconditioning of animals subjected to SAH demonstrated a protective upregulation of eNOS in comparison with other NOS isoforms, resulting in a favorable outcome. Only eNOS was deemed protective when animals were preconditioned, and nNOS and iNOS expression remained normal in SAH animals subjected to preconditioning before SAH. These findings indicate that perhaps, under the correct physiological criteria and environment, eNOS can be primed to remain or become protective in a hemorrhagic insult [40].

It remains unclear how eNOS truly contributes to the pathogenesis after SAH in both humans and experimental models; however, work in our laboratory strongly indicates that eNOS can be both beneficial and deleterious, depending on the environment of expression. Further research is warranted to understand the true interaction between subarachnoid blood and eNOS and whether eNOS uncoupling is one of the major pathways in the pathogenesis of SAH.

Conclusion

Focus should be given and distributed equally to all NOS isoforms to truly understand the physiological response to the pathogenesis of SAH. NO production, depletion, and its function as a vasodilator have been repeatedly emphasized in SAH research, highlighting its continued importance. Further research should be dedicated along the spectrum of NO synthesis from mRNA transcript of NOSes to NO as a potent dilator, to truly understand how NOSes contribute to the complex multifaceted pathogenesis of SAH.

Conflict of Interest Statement We declare that we have no conflict of interest.

References

1. Afshar JK, Pluta RM, Boock RJ, Thompson BG, Oldfield EH (1995) Effect of intracarotid nitric oxide on primate cerebral vasospasm after subarachnoid hemorrhage. J Neurosurg 83:118–122
2. Aoki T, Nishimura M, Kataoka H, Ishibashi R, Nozaki K, Miyamoto S (2011) Complementary inhibition of cerebral aneurysm formation by eNOS and nNOS. Lab Invest 91:619–626
3. Atochin DN, Wang A, Liu VW, Critchlow JD, Dantas AP, Looft-Wilson R, Murata T, Salomone S, Shin HK, Ayata C, Moskowitz MA, Michel T, Sessa WC, Huang PL (2007) The phosphorylation state of eNOS modulates vascular reactivity and outcome of cerebral ischemia in vivo. J Clin Invest 117:1961–1967
4. Black SM, Fineman JR, Steinhorn RH, Bristow J, Soifer SJ (1998) Increased endothelial NOS in lambs with increased pulmonary blood flow and pulmonary hypertension. Am J Physiol 275: H1643–H1651
5. Chen G, Tariq A, Ai J, Sabri M, Jeon HJ, Tang EJ, Lakovic K, Wan H, Macdonald RL (2011) Different effects of clazosentan on consequences of subarachnoid hemorrhage in rats. Brain Res1392:132–139
6. Forstermann U (2006) Janus-faced role of endothelial NO synthase in vascular disease: uncoupling of oxygen reduction from NO

synthesis and its pharmacological reversal. Biol Chem 387: 1521–1533

7. Forstermann U, Munzel T (2006) Endothelial nitric oxide synthase in vascular disease: from marvel to menace. Circulation 113:1708–1714
8. Friedrich V, Flores R, Sehba FA (2012) Cell death starts early after subarachnoid hemorrhage. Neurosci Lett 512:6–11
9. Fukuda S, Hashimoto N, Naritomi H, Nagata I, Nozaki K, Kondo S, Kurino M, Kikuchi H (2000) Prevention of rat cerebral aneurysm formation by inhibition of nitric oxide synthase. Circulation 101:2532–2538
10. Hansen-Schwartz J, Vajkoczy P, Macdonald RL, Pluta RM, Zhang JH (2007) Cerebral vasospasm: looking beyond vasoconstriction. Trends Pharmacol Sci 28:252–256
11. Hashiguchi A, Yano S, Morioka M, Hamada J, Shirasaki Y, Kochi M, Fukunaga K (2004) The post-ischemic administration of 3-[2-[4-(3-chloro-2-methylphenyl)-1-piperazinyl]ethyl]-5,6-dimethoxy-1-(4-imidazo lylmethyl)-1H-indazole dihydrochloride 3.5 hydrate (DY-9760e), a novel calmodulin antagonist, prevents delayed neuronal death in gerbil hippocampus. J Pharmacol Sci 96:65–72
12. Hashiguchi A, Yano S, Morioka M, Hamada J, Ushio Y, Takeuchi Y, Fukunaga K (2004) Up-regulation of endothelial nitric oxide synthase via phosphatidylinositol 3-kinase pathway contributes to ischemic tolerance in the CA1 subfield of gerbil hippocampus. J Cereb Blood Flow Metab 24:271–279
13. Hino A, Tokuyama Y, Weir B, Takeda J, Yano H, Bell GI, Macdonald RL (1996) Changes in endothelial nitric oxide synthase mRNA during vasospasm after subarachnoid hemorrhage in monkeys. Neurosurgery 39:562–567
14. Jung CS, Iuliano BA, Harvey-White J, Espey MG, Oldfield EH, Pluta RM (2004) Association between cerebrospinal fluid levels of asymmetric dimethyl-L-arginine, an endogenous inhibitor of endothelial nitric oxide synthase, and cerebral vasospasm in a primate model of subarachnoid hemorrhage. J Neurosurg 101:836–842
15. Kroncke KD, Fehsel K, Kolb-Bachofen V (1998) Inducible nitric oxide synthase in human diseases. Clin Exp Immunol 113:147–156
16. Lin CL, Shih HC, Dumont AS, Kassell NF, Lieu AS, Su YF, Hwong SL, Hsu C (2006) The effect of 17beta-estradiol in attenuating experimental subarachnoid hemorrhage-induced cerebral vasospasm. J Neurosurg 104:298–304
17. Lin CL, Su YF, Dumont AS, Shih HC, Lieu AS, Howng SL, Lee KS, Kwan AL (2006) The effect of an adenosine A1 receptor agonist in the treatment of experimental subarachnoid hemorrhage-induced cerebrovasospasm. Acta Neurochir (Wien) 148:873–879
18. Macdonald RL, Pluta RM, Zhang JH (2007) Cerebral vasospasm after subarachnoid hemorrhage: the emerging revolution. Nat Clin Pract Neurol 3:256–263
19. McGirt MJ, Lynch JR, Parra A, Sheng H, Pearlstein RD, Laskowitz DT, Pelligrino DA, Warner DS (2002) Simvastatin increases endothelial nitric oxide synthase and ameliorates cerebral vasospasm resulting from subarachnoid hemorrhage. Stroke 33:2950–2956
20. Osuka K, Watanabe Y, Takagi T, Usuda N, Atsuzawa K, Yoshida J, Takayasu M (2008) Activation of endothelial nitric oxide synthase following spinal cord injury in mice. Neurosci Lett 436:265–268
21. Pluta RM (2005) Delayed cerebral vasospasm and nitric oxide: review, new hypothesis, and proposed treatment. Pharmacol Ther 105:23–56
22. Pluta RM (2006) Dysfunction of nitric oxide synthases as a cause and therapeutic target in delayed cerebral vasospasm after SAH. Neurol Res 28:730–737
23. Pluta RM (2008) Dysfunction of nitric oxide synthases as a cause and therapeutic target in delayed cerebral vasospasm after SAH. Acta Neurochir Suppl 104:139–147
24. Pluta RM, Dejam A, Grimes G, Gladwin MT, Oldfield EH (2005) Nitrite infusions to prevent delayed cerebral vasospasm in a primate model of subarachnoid hemorrhage. JAMA 293:1477–1484
25. Pluta RM, Thompson BG, Dawson TM, Snyder SH, Boock RJ, Oldfield EH (1996) Loss of nitric oxide synthase immunoreactivity in cerebral vasospasm. J Neurosurg 84:648–654
26. Sabri M, Ai J, Knight B, Tariq A, Jeon H, Shang X, Marsden PA, Loch MR (2011) Uncoupling of endothelial nitric oxide synthase after experimental subarachnoid hemorrhage. J Cereb Blood Flow Metab 31:190–199
27. Sabri M, Ai J, Lass E, D'abbondanza J, Macdonald RL (2013) Genetic elimination of eNOS reduces secondary complications of experimental subarachnoid hemorrhage. J Cereb Blood Flow Metab 33:1008–1014
28. Sabri M, Ai J, Macdonald RL (2011) Dissociation of vasospasm and secondary effects of experimental subarachnoid hemorrhage by clazosentan. Stroke 42:1454–1460
29. Sabri M, Ai J, Macdonald RL (2011) Nitric oxide related pathophysiological changes following subarachnoid haemorrhage. Acta Neurochir Suppl 110:105–109
30. Sabri M, Ai J, Marsden PA, Macdonald RL (2011) Simvastatin re-couples dysfunctional endothelial nitric oxide synthase in experimental subarachnoid hemorrhage. PLoS One 6:e17062
31. Saito A, Kamii H, Kato I, Takasawa S, Kondo T, Chan PH, Okamoto H, Yoshimoto T (2001) Transgenic CuZn-superoxide dismutase inhibits NO synthase induction in experimental subarachnoid hemorrhage. Stroke 32:1652–1657
32. Sayama T, Suzuki S, Fukui M (1998) Expression of inducible nitric oxide synthase in rats following subarachnoid hemorrhage. Neurol Res 20:79–84
33. Sayama T, Suzuki S, Fukui M (1999) Role of inducible nitric oxide synthase in the cerebral vasospasm after subarachnoid hemorrhage in rats. Neurol Res 21:293–298
34. Schwartz AY, Sehba FA, Bederson JB (2000) Decreased nitric oxide availability contributes to acute cerebral ischemia after subarachnoid hemorrhage. Neurosurgery 47:208–214
35. Sehba FA, Bederson JB (2011) Nitric oxide in early brain injury after subarachnoid hemorrhage. Acta Neurochir Suppl 110:99–103
36. Sehba FA, Chereshnev I, Maayani S, Friedrich V Jr, Bederson JB (2004) Nitric oxide synthase in acute alteration of nitric oxide levels after subarachnoid hemorrhage. Neurosurgery 55:671–677
37. Sehba FA, Friedrich V (2011) Early micro vascular changes after subarachnoid hemorrhage. Acta Neurochir Suppl 110:49–55
38. Sehba FA, Pluta RM, Zhang JH (2011) Metamorphosis of subarachnoid hemorrhage research: from delayed vasospasm to early brain injury. Mol Neurobiol 43:27–40
39. Sehba FA, Schwartz AY, Chereshnev I, Bederson JB (2000) Acute decrease in cerebral nitric oxide levels after subarachnoid hemorrhage. J Cereb Blood Flow Metab 20:604–611
40. Vellimana AK, Milner E, Azad TD, Harries MD, Zhou ML, Gidday JM, Han BH, Zipfel GJ (2011) Endothelial nitric oxide synthase mediates endogenous protection against subarachnoid hemorrhage-induced cerebral vasospasm. Stroke 42:776–782
41. Yatsushige H, Calvert JW, Cahill J, Zhang JH (2006) Limited role of inducible nitric oxide synthase in blood–brain barrier function after experimental subarachnoid hemorrhage. J Neurotrauma 23:1874–1882

How Spreading Depolarization Can Be the Pathophysiological Correlate of Both Migraine Aura and Stroke

Jens P. Dreier, Clemens Reiffurth, Johannes Woitzik, Jed A. Hartings, Christoph Drenckhahn, Claudia Windler, Alon Friedman, Brian MacVicar, and Oscar Herreras for the COSBID study group

Abstract The term spreading depolarization describes a mechanism of abrupt, massive ion translocation between neurons and the interstitial space, which leads to a cytotoxic edema in the gray matter of the brain. In energy-compromised tissue, spreading depolarization is preceded by a nonspreading silencing (depression of spontaneous activity) because of a neuronal hyperpolarization. By contrast, in tissue that is not energy compromised, spreading depolarization is accompanied by a spreading silencing (spreading depression) of spontaneous activity caused by a depolarization block. It is assumed that the nonspreading silencing translates into the initial clinical symptoms of ischemic stroke and the spreading silencing (spreading depression) into the symptoms of migraine aura. In energy-compromised tissue, spreading depolarization facilitates neuronal death, whereas, in healthy tissue, it is relatively innocuous. Therapies targeting spreading depolarization in metabolically compromised tissue may potentially treat conditions of acute cerebral injury such as aneurysmal subarachnoid hemorrhage.

Keywords Aneurysmal subarachnoid hemorrhage • Spreading depression • Delayed cerebral ischemia

Introduction

Spreading depolarization is characterized by (1) extensive breakdown of transmembrane ion gradients [16, 35], (2) extreme shunting of neuronal membrane resistance [2], and (3) transient neuronal swelling with dendritic spine distortion [31, 37]. In 1945, the Brazilian neurophysiologist

J.P. Dreier (✉)
Center for Stroke Research Berlin, Charité University Medicine Berlin, Campus Charité Mitte, Charitéplatz 1, 10117 Berlin, Germany

Department of Neurology, Charité University Medicine Berlin, 10117, Berlin, Germany

Department of Experimental Neurology, Charité University Medicine Berlin, 10117, Berlin, Germany
e-mail: jens.dreier@charite.de

C. Reiffurth
Department of Experimental Neurology, Charité University Medicine Berlin, 10117 Berlin, Germany

Center for Stroke Research Berlin, Charité University Medicine Berlin, Campus Charité Mitte, Charitéplatz 1, 10117, Berlin, Germany

J. Woitzik
Department of Neurosurgery, Charité University Medicine Berlin, 10117 Berlin, Germany

Center for Stroke Research Berlin, Charité University Medicine Berlin, Campus Charité Mitte, Charitéplatz 1, 10117, Berlin, Germany

J.A. Hartings
Department of Neurosurgery, University of Cincinnati, Cincinnati, OH, USA

C. Drenckhahn
Department of Neurology, Charité University Medicine Berlin, 10117 Berlin, Germany

Center for Stroke Research Berlin, Charité University Medicine Berlin, Campus Charité Mitte, Charitéplatz 1, 10117, Berlin, Germany

C. Windler
Center for Stroke Research Berlin, Charité University Medicine Berlin, Campus Charité Mitte, Charitéplatz 1, 10117 Berlin, Germany

A. Friedman
Department of Physiogy, Zlotowski Center for Neuroscience, Ben-Gurion University of the Negev, Beer-Sheva, Israel

Department of Neurobiology, Zlotowski Center for Neuroscience, Ben-Gurion University of the Negev, Beer-Sheva, Israel

B. MacVicar
Brain Research Centre, University of British Columbia, Vancouver, BC, Canada

Department of Psychiatry, University of British Columbia, Vancouver, BC, Canada

O. Herreras
Department of Systems Neuroscience, Cajal Institute-CSIC, Madrid, Spain

J. Fandino et al. (eds.), *Neurovascular Events After Subarachnoid Hemorrhage*, Acta Neurochirurgica Supplement, Vol. 120,
DOI 10.1007/978-3-319-04981-6_23, © Springer International Publishing Switzerland 2015

Aristides Leão proposed that spreading depolarization is the pathophysiological correlate of the migraine aura [22], and, in 1947, he linked migraine aura and stroke to spreading depolarization as their common mechanism [21].

Spreading Depolarization may Be a Common Mechanism of Migraine Aura and Stroke Although Their Clinical Symptoms Are Different

Most neurologists today agree that spreading depolarization is likely the pathophysiological correlate of the migraine aura [30] and contributes to the cellular injury in stroke even though migraine aura and stroke typically have different medical histories. This applies particularly to the temporal pattern of the initial symptoms and to the fact that migraine with aura is usually a harmless disease in contrast to stroke [17]. It is therefore counterintuitive that spreading depolarization is a mechanism of stroke, which initiates and facilitates neuronal injury in energy-depleted tissue, and, on the other hand, can be the pathophysiological correlate of the migraine aura. However, Leão provided a plausible explanation for this paradox when he discovered that the energy state of the tissue determines both (1) the duration of the spreading depolarization and (2) the depression (silencing) pattern of spontaneous activity that accompanies the depolarization. The two major types of silencing of spontaneous activity which can co-occur with spreading depolarization are nonspreading depression and spreading depression of spontaneous activity [21]. Nonspreading depression describes a sudden silencing of spontaneous activity that is simultaneously observed in different brain regions wherever brain perfusion drops below ~20 ml/100 g/min [12]. When spreading depolarization develops in such electrically silent tissue, it cannot cause spreading depression of activity because the spontaneous activity has already ceased.

But, unless spreading depolarization is preceded by arrest of spontaneous activity, it initiates spreading depression of activity because the near-complete depolarization is above the inactivation threshold for the action potential-generating ion channels [13]. Spreading depression of activity thus requires a grossly intact energy supply in stark contrast to nonspreading depression of activity. Thus, both spreading and nonspreading depression of activity can occur in stroke where there is a gradient of energy depletion from the core to adjacent watershed and healthy regions of cortex. In the ischemic core, where nonspreading depression of activity has already developed, spreading depolarizations are ignited and propagate into adjacent tissue with preserved spontaneous activity, which is then depressed in a spreading manner.

Nonspreading depression of activity caused by occlusion of blood flow is assumed to be the pathophysiological correlate of the sudden and simultaneous neurological deficits of transitory ischemic attacks, nonmigrainous stroke, and cardiac arrest. The spreading depression of spreading depolarization that occurs in these conditions may have additional clinical correlates, but these would be subtle and difficult to detect on a baseline of obtundation and major widespread deficits [6]. In contrast, the creeping neurological deficits of migraine aura and migrainous stroke are obvious to patients and clinicians in the context of intact neurologic function and are thought to be mediated by the spreading depression of brain electrical activity. Thus, the depression patterns caused by disruption of energy supply and by spreading depolarization determine the clinical symptoms of these diseases. The existing energy supply, such as the level of perfusion [5] and the level of blood glucose [15], for example, largely determine whether spreading depolarization initiates a countdown to neuronal death. The tissue fate is reflected by the duration of spreading depolarization, because neuronal survival depends on rapid repolarization, which is energy dependent. Notably, if, in experiments, spreading depolarization is markedly prolonged by other means than energy shortage, for example, by a long-lasting artificial increase in the baseline potassium concentration, neurons will eventually also die although the energy supply is normal. However, under such conditions, the time period from the onset of spreading depolarization to the neuronal death will be longer than under conditions of energy depletion [5]. For a more comprehensive account of the signals in relation to migrainous stroke, we refer the reader to a former review [4].

Processes Leading Up to Spreading Depolarization: Potential Targets for Therapeutic Intervention

The abrupt near-complete breakdown of neuronal ion homeostasis characterizes spreading depolarization. Spreading depolarization could contribute significantly to the higher vulnerability of neurons to ischemic stress compared with other cells of the body. This raises important questions: (1) which neuron-specific channels and processes in the membrane are large enough to allow for such a rapid influx of cations and water and (2) might it be possible to block them pharmacologically to protect the cells and delay the cell death?

The experimental study of the membrane channels participating in spreading depolarization has been hindered by their mixed contribution and the heterogeneous subcellular distribution over the anatomy of neurons. Of note, the channels that contribute to the initiation or propagation of spreading depolarization could be different from the major carriers of electric charge during the sustained phase of depolarization. Thus, the massive ion translocation across the membrane occurs during the first 2–3 s, in close time association to the initial DC shift. Thereafter, the ions remain stable at this new plateau or drift slightly [11, 16], indicating that conditions close to a new steady state have been achieved. Channels contributing to initiation of spreading depolarization may include voltage-gated cation channels and *N*-methyl-D-aspartate (NMDA) receptor-controlled channels [1, 8, 10, 19, 20, 25, 38]. Nevertheless, the question of which channels contribute specifically to the initiation or propagation processes seems to depend largely on the conditions present immediately before the spreading depolarization. This is reflected by the notion that the propagation of spreading depolarization can be blocked by NMDA receptor antagonists in healthy, naïve tissue [8, 20, 25], whereas this is not possible under hypoxic or ischemic conditions [1, 10, 19, 26] or when the baseline extracellular potassium concentration is artificially increased [28].

The process of massive ion translocation is even less understood than the processes of initiation or propagation. In a pioneering study, a large voltage-independent current was identified using whole-cell recordings during ongoing spreading depolarization [3]. The large voltage-independent current flows inward through membrane channels that stay open during spreading depolarization and are mostly localized in dendritic regions [2]. A wealth of pharmacological data has not singled out one membrane channel that is involved but it has pointed to a combination [29]. In a realistic neuron model aiming to replicate the subcellular changes of membrane resistance during spreading depolarization, it was found that in addition to standard potassium-, sodium-, and glutamate-mediated conductances, the initial opening and gradual closing of an as yet undetermined large conductance is required [24]. So far there are no hints regarding the nature of such spreading depolarization-specific conductance. It may be a known channel with modified kinetics produced by the severe chemical changes imposed during spreading depolarization, or it may be a totally different channel. New families of neuron membrane channels are being discovered. Among possible candidates, gap junction hemichannels have a variable pore aperture that would permit the passage of common ions. However, although gap junction blockers halt spreading depolarization in some experimental settings [18], they do not in others [27, 33]. In a similar fashion to that described for gap junctions, pannexin hemichannels could contribute as major carriers of electric charge during spreading depolarization [32]; interestingly, recent evidence also points to a role for pannenxins in the release of factors triggering pain after spreading depolarization [14]. Other putative candidates are transient receptor potential (TRP) channels [23] and tandem pore domain potassium (2PK) channels [7], but their distribution and kinetics are largely unknown. It is therefore not yet possible to analyze their contribution in the realistic neuron model. Finally, low calcium-activated cation channels are possible candidates [9, 36], because they are gated by external calcium reduction and appear to be voltage independent, two conditions found during spreading depolarization. Last but not least, the caveat must be added that space clamp problems associated with voltage-clamping central nervous system neurons [34] mean that a number of voltage-dependent channels expressed on distal dendrites cannot be completely excluded as contributors, including NMDA receptor-controlled channels.

Conclusion

Spreading depolarization is an important phenomenon of cerebral pathology. Notably, it occurs in patients with stroke including subarachnoid hemorrhage. Its pharmacology is very complex as it changes with the conditions under which it occurs.

Acknowledgments This work was supported by grants of the Deutsche Forschungsgemeinschaft (DFG DR 323/6-1) and the Bundesministerium für Bildung und Forschung (Center for Stroke Research Berlin, 01 EO 0801; Bernstein Center for Computational Neuroscience Berlin 01GQ1001C B2) to Dr. Dreier; the German Israeli Foundation (GIF No. 124/2008) to Dr. Friedman and Dr. Dreier; the ERA-NET NEURON (01EW1212) to Dr. MacVicar, Dr. Friedman, and Dr. Dreier; DFG DR 323/5-1 to Dr. Friedman, Dr. Woitzik and Dr. Dreier; DFG WO 1704/1-1 to Dr. Woitzik; and US Army CDMRP PH/TBI research program to Dr. Hartings.

Conflict of Interest Statement We declare that we have no conflict of interest.

References

1. Aitken PG, Balestrino M, Somjen GG (1988) NMDA antagonists: lack of protective effect against hypoxic damage in CA1 region of hippocampal slices. Neurosci Lett 89:187–192
2. Canals S, Makarova I, Lopez-Aguado L, Largo C, Ibarz JM, Herreras O (2005) Longitudinal depolarization gradients along the somatodendritic axis of CA1 pyramidal cells: a novel feature of spreading depression. J Neurophysiol 94:943–951
3. Czeh G, Aitken PG, Somjen GG (1993) Membrane currents in CA1 pyramidal cells during spreading depression (SD) and SD-like hypoxic depolarization. Brain Res 632:195–208
4. Dreier JP (2011) The role of spreading depression, spreading depolarization and spreading ischemia in neurological disease. Nat Med 17:439–447
5. Dreier JP, Victorov IV, Petzold GC, Major S, Windmuller O, Fernandez-Klett F, Kandasamy M, Dirnagl U, Priller J (2013) Electrochemical failure of the brain cortex is more deleterious when it is accompanied by low perfusion. Stroke 44:490–496
6. Dreier JP, Woitzik J, Fabricius M, Bhatia R, Major S, Drenckhahn C, Lehmann TN, Sarrafzadeh A, Willumsen L, Hartings JA, Sakowitz OW, Seemann JH, Thieme A, Lauritzen M, Strong AJ

(2006) Delayed ischaemic neurological deficits after subarachnoid haemorrhage are associated with clusters of spreading depolarizations. Brain 129:3224–3237
7. Gabriel A, Abdallah M, Yost CS, Winegar BD, Kindler CH (2002) Localization of the tandem pore domain K+ channel KCNK5 (TASK-2) in the rat central nervous system. Brain Res Mol Brain Res 98:153–163
8. Gorelova NA, Koroleva VI, Amemori T, Pavlik V, Bures J (1987) Ketamine blockade of cortical spreading depression in rats. Electroencephalogr Clin Neurophysiol 66:440–447
9. Hablitz JJ, Heinemann U, Lux HD (1986) Step reductions in extracellular Ca2+ activate a transient inward current in chick dorsal root ganglion cells. Biophys J 50:753–757
10. Hernandez-Caceres J, Macias-Gonzalez R, Brozek G, Bures J (1987) Systemic ketamine blocks cortical spreading depression but does not delay the onset of terminal anoxic depolarization in rats. Brain Res 437:360–364
11. Herreras O, Somjen GG (1993) Analysis of potential shifts associated with recurrent spreading depression and prolonged unstable spreading depression induced by microdialysis of elevated K+ in hippocampus of anesthetized rats. Brain Res 610:283–294
12. Hossmann KA (1994) Viability thresholds and the penumbra of focal ischemia. Ann Neurol 36:557–565
13. Kager H, Wadman WJ, Somjen GG (2002) Conditions for the triggering of spreading depression studied with computer simulations. J Neurophysiol 88:2700–2712
14. Karatas H, Erdener SE, Gursoy-Ozdemir Y, Lule S, Eren-Kocak E, Sen ZD, Dalkara T (2013) Spreading depression triggers headache by activating neuronal Panx1 channels. Science 339: 1092–1095
15. Kraig RP, Chesler M (1990) Astrocytic acidosis in hyperglycemic and complete ischemia. J Cereb Blood Flow Metab 10:104–114
16. Kraig RP, Nicholson C (1978) Extracellular ionic variations during spreading depression. Neuroscience 3:1045–1059
17. Kurth T, Chabriat H, Bousser MG (2012) Migraine and stroke: a complex association with clinical implications. Lancet Neurol 11:92–100
18. Largo C, Tombaugh GC, Aitken PG, Herreras O, Somjen GG (1997) Heptanol but not fluoroacetate prevents the propagation of spreading depression in rat hippocampal slices. J Neurophysiol 77:9–16
19. Lauritzen M, Hansen AJ (1992) The effect of glutamate receptor blockade on anoxic depolarization and cortical spreading depression. J Cereb Blood Flow Metab 12:223–229
20. Lauritzen M, Rice ME, Okada Y, Nicholson C (1988) Quisqualate, kainate and NMDA can initiate spreading depression in the turtle cerebellum. Brain Res 475:317–327
21. Leão AAP (1947) Further observations on the spreading depression of activity in the cerebral cortex. J Neurophysiol 10:409–414
22. Leão AAP, Morison RS (1945) Propagation of spreading cortical depression. J Neurophysiol 8:33–45
23. Lipski J, Park TI, Li D, Lee SC, Trevarton AJ, Chung KK, Freestone PS, Bai JZ (2006) Involvement of TRP-like channels in the acute ischemic response of hippocampal CA1 neurons in brain slices. Brain Res 1077:187–199
24. Makarova J, Ibarz JM, Canals S, Herreras O (2007) A steady-state model of spreading depression predicts the importance of an unknown conductance in specific dendritic domains. Biophys J 92:4216–4232
25. Marrannes R, Willems R, De Prins E, Wauquier A (1988) Evidence for a role of the N-methyl-D-aspartate (NMDA) receptor in cortical spreading depression in the rat. Brain Res 457:226–240
26. Muller M, Somjen GG (1998) Inhibition of major cationic inward currents prevents spreading depression-like hypoxic depolarization in rat hippocampal tissue slices. Brain Res 812:1–13
27. Peters O, Schipke CG, Hashimoto Y, Kettenmann H (2003) Different mechanisms promote astrocyte Ca2+ waves and spreading depression in the mouse neocortex. J Neurosci 23:9888–9896
28. Petzold GC, Windmuller O, Haack S, Major S, Buchheim K, Megow D, Gabriel S, Lehmann TN, Drenckhahn C, Peters O, Meierkord H, Heinemann U, Dirnagl U, Dreier JP (2005) Increased extracellular K+ concentration reduces the efficacy of N-methyl-D-aspartate receptor antagonists to block spreading depression-like depolarizations and spreading ischemia. Stroke 36:1270–1277
29. Somjen GG (2001) Mechanisms of spreading depression and hypoxic spreading depression-like depolarization. Physiol Rev 81:1065–1096
30. Sprenger T, Goadsby PJ (2009) Migraine pathogenesis and state of pharmacological treatment options. BMC Med 7:71
31. Takano T, Tian GF, Peng W, Lou N, Lovatt D, Hansen AJ, Kasischke KA, Nedergaard M (2007) Cortical spreading depression causes and coincides with tissue hypoxia. Nat Neurosci 10:754–762
32. Thompson RJ, Zhou N, MacVicar BA (2006) Ischemia opens neuronal gap junction hemichannels. Science 312:924–927
33. Vilagi I, Klapka N, Luhmann HJ (2001) Optical recording of spreading depression in rat neocortical slices. Brain Res 898: 288–296
34. Williams SR, Mitchell SJ (2008) Direct measurement of somatic voltage clamp errors in central neurons. Nat Neurosci 11:790–798
35. Windmuller O, Lindauer U, Foddis M, Einhaupl KM, Dirnagl U, Heinemann U, Dreier JP (2005) Ion changes in spreading ischaemia induce rat middle cerebral artery constriction in the absence of NO. Brain 128:2042–2051
36. Xiong Z, Lu W, MacDonald JF (1997) Extracellular calcium sensed by a novel cation channel in hippocampal neurons. Proc Natl Acad Sci U S A 94:7012–7017
37. Zhou N, Gordon GR, Feighan D, MacVicar BA (2010) Transient swelling, acidification, and mitochondrial depolarization occurs in neurons but not astrocytes during spreading depression. Cereb Cortex 20:2614–2624
38. Zhou N, Rungta RL, Malik A, Han H, Wu DC, Macvicar BA (2013) Regenerative glutamate release by presynaptic NMDA receptors contributes to spreading depression. J Cereb Blood Flow Metab 33:1582–1594

Estrogen Induces Nitric Oxide Production Via Nitric Oxide Synthase Activation in Endothelial Cells

Edin Nevzati, Maziar Shafighi, Kamran D. Bakhtian, Hannes Treiber, Javier Fandino, and Ali Reza Fathi

Abstract *Introduction*: 17β-estradiol (E2) has been found to induce vasodilation in the cardiovascular system and at physiological levels, resulting in prevention of cerebral vasospasm following subarachnoid hemorrhage (SAH) in animal models. The goal of this study was to analyze the cellular mechanism of nitric oxide (NO) production and its relation to E2, in vitro in brain and peripheral endothelial cells.

Methods: Human umbilical endothelial cells (HUVEC) and brain endothelial cells (bEnd.3) were treated with estradiol (E2, 0.1, 10, 100, and 1,000 nM), and supernatant was collected at 0, 5, 15, 30, 60, and 120 min for nitric oxide metabolome (nitrite, NO_2) measurements. Cells were also treated with E2 in the presence of 1400W, a potent eNOS inhibitor, and ICI, an antagonist of estradiol receptors (ERs). Effects of E2 on eNOS protein expression were assessed with Western blot analysis.

Results: E2 significantly increased NO_2 levels irrespective of its concentration in both cell lines by 35 % and 42 % ($p<0.05$). The addition of an E2 antagonist, ICI (10 μM), prevented the E2-induced increases in NO_2 levels (11 % $p>0.05$). The combination of E2 (10 nM) and a NOS inhibitor (1400W, 5 μM) inhibited NO_2 increases in addition (4 %, $p>0.05$). E2 induced increases in eNOS protein levels and phosphorylated eNOS (eNOS^p).

Conclusions: This study indicates that E2 induces NO level increases in cerebral and peripheral endothelial cells in vitro via eNOS activation and through E2 receptor-mediated mechanisms. Further in vivo studies are warranted to evaluate the therapeutic value of estrogen for the treatment of SAH-induced vasospasm.

Keywords Subarachnoid hemorrhage • Nitrogen monoxide • Estrogens • Nitric oxide synthase

Introduction

As part of a complex pathophysiology itself, cerebral vasospasm has multiple causal factors. One such factor is deprivation of nitric oxide (NO) in the vicinity of brain vessels as a result of nitric oxide synthase (NOS) dysfunction [20] and scavenging of NO by deoxyhemoglobin [15]. Considerable research has been carried out that investigates the enhancement of perivascular NO concentration after SAH and prevention or reversal of vasospasm. The positive effect of NO donors on vessel diameter is known; their impact on overall clinical outcome is still uncertain, however [6].

In addition to the ischemic neuroprotection qualities of E2 [22], physiological levels of this female sex hormone have been shown to reduce mortality and secondary ischemic damage [27] and also prevent cerebral vasospasm following SAH in animal models [13]. E2 has been found to induce vasodilation in the cardiovascular system by increasing NO production [10, 25]. This paper discusses possible E2-triggered molecular pathways associated with cellular mechanisms of NO production. We report on our preliminary in vitro results in endothelial cells.

Materials and Methods

Cell Cultures

Primary cultures of human umbilical vein endothelial cells (HUVECs), immortalized mouse brain endothelial cells (bEnd.3), and cell culture reagents were obtained from

E. Nevzati, MD • J. Fandino, MD • A.R. Fathi, MD (✉)
Department of Neurosurgery, Kantonsspital Aarau, Aarau, Switzerland
e-mail: ali-reza.fathi@ksa.ch

M. Shafighi, MD
Department of Plastic, Reconstructive and Hand Surgery, University Hospital, Inselspital, University of Bern, Bern, Switzerland

K.D. Bakhtian, MS • H. Treiber, MD
Surgical Neurology Branch, National Institute of Neurological Disorders and Stroke, National Institutes of Health, Bethesda, MD, USA

J. Fandino et al. (eds.), *Neurovascular Events After Subarachnoid Hemorrhage*, Acta Neurochirurgica Supplement, Vol. 120, DOI 10.1007/978-3-319-04981-6_24,

Lonza (Walkersville, MD, USA). E2, ICI-hydrochloride (an E2 receptor antagonist) and 1400W (an NOS inhibitor) dihydrochloride were purchased from Sigma-Aldrich Corp. (St. Louis, MO, USA). HUVECs were cultured in endothelial growth medium (EGM) and bEnd.3 cells in Dulbecco's Modified Eagle Medium (DMEM) and 10 % fetal bovine serum (FBS) according to the manufacturer's directions in a humidified incubator with 5 % CO_2 at 37 °C. Subconfluent cells were harvested and seeded at a density of 2,500–5,000 cells/cm^2 in six-well culture plates with EGM. At a confluency of approximately 75–80 %, cells were washed twice with HEPES-buffered saline solution (HEPES-BSS) and treated with drugs or vehicle.

Study Design

To evaluate the impact of E2 on eNOS activity and consequently NO production, bEnd.3 cells were treated with three different concentrations of E2 (0.1, 10, and 1,000 nM) and HUVECs were additionally treated with 100 nM E2. Supernatant was collected at 0, 5, 15, 30, 60, and 120 min. For measurement of NO_2 concentration, 300 μL of the supernatant was placed on ice in each corresponding well. Because of the very short half-life of NO (few milliseconds), measuring its NO_2 metabolome is a more reliable indicator of NO production. Endothelial cells were also treated for 2 h with all concentrations of E2 in the presence of 1400W (50 μM), a potent NOS inhibitor. To evaluate whether the E2-induced NO release is mediated via estradiol receptors (ERs), we used ICI (100 nM), an antagonist of ERs. To verify the presence of eNOS in the cells and to assess the effects of E2 on eNOS expression, Western blot analyses were performed after cells were treated for 2 h in the presence or absence of E2.

NO Metabolome Measurements

Levels of NO_2 in cell supernatant were measured using a chemiluminescence technique (Sievers Model 280i NO analyzer, Boulder, CO) as described by MacArthur et al. [14].

Protein Preparation and Immunoblot Analysis

HUVECs and bEnd.3 cells were maintained in growth medium according to the manufacturer's protocol (Lonza, Walkersville, MD, USA). Total cell protein content was extracted using RIPA lysis buffer (Thermo Scientific, Waltham, MA). The quantity of protein was determined in the supernatant solution using a Bio-Rad Protein Assay Kit. Proteins were separated by NuPAGE 4–12 % Bis-Tris gel (Invitrogen, Carlsbad, CA) and transferred to polyvinylidenfluoride (PVDF) membranes (Invitrogen, Carlsbad, CA). Membranes were blocked in 5 % nonfat dry milk and probed with primary antibody. Antibodies used for this study were eNOS (1:1,000; BD Biosciences, San Diego, CA), antibodies against phosphorylated eNOS (Ser 1177; Cell Signaling 10 Technology, Beverly, MA), and beta-actin (1:2,000, Santa Cruz Biotechnology, Santa Cruz, CA). Gel blot quantification was performed using the gel analysis tool in Image J software (Version 1.42q, National Institutes of Health, Bethesda, MD).

Statistical Analysis

Statistical analysis was performed by the two-tailed Student's *t*-test. Significance was defined as a value of $p<0.05$. Calculations were made with the software SPSS 11.5 Windows (© SPSS Inc., Chicago, IL, USA). Data are expressed as mean ± SD.

Results

The effects of E2 on NO production in HUVEC and bEnd.3 cell lines are shown in Fig. 1. E2 induced significant NO_2 levels regardless of its concentration in supernatant (0.1, 10, and 1,000 nM) in both HUVEC and bEnd.3 cell lines. Levels increased compared with baseline by 35 and 42 %, respectively ($p<0.05$). The addition of an E2 antagonist (ICI, 10 μM) to E2 prevented the E2-induced increases in NO_2 levels (11 % $p>0.05$), maintaining them at the same level as controls. This indicates that activation of NO production in endothelial cells is an E2R-mediated outcome. The combination of E2 (10 nM) and a NOS inhibitor (1,400 W, 10 μM) suppressed NO_2 increases in both cell lines (4 %, $p>0.05$), indicating that NOS is involved in the E2-mediated enzymatic mechanism of generating NO.

eNOS expression was detectable in cell lysates (Fig. 2). E2 induced increases in eNOS protein levels at concentrations of 1,000 nM, suggesting that E2 controls NO production by transcriptional activation of eNOS. There was no effect on eNOS protein expression at 10 nM, but increased levels of NO_2 were detected, implying that there is posttranscriptional activation of eNOS at this concentration. This fact is supported by elevated levels of phosphorylated eNOS (eNOS^p) after E2 treatment (Fig. 3).

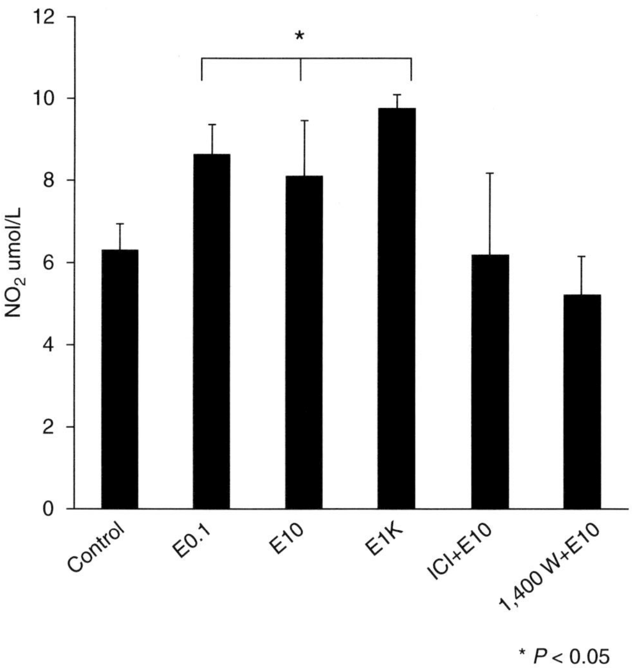

Fig. 1 The effect of various concentrations of E2 on NO production in bEnd.3 cells after 2 h of treatment. Nitrite (NO_2; a metabolite) was measured as a marker for NO production. There is a significant increase with all three E2 concentrations (0.1, 10, and 1,000 nM) when compared with the control cell population ($p<0.05$). However, there is no significant difference within the applied E2 concentrations. Addition of ICI (100 nM, inhibitor of ER) as well as 1400W (10 μM, antagonist of NOS) significantly inhibited the E2-induced NO production ($p<0.05$)

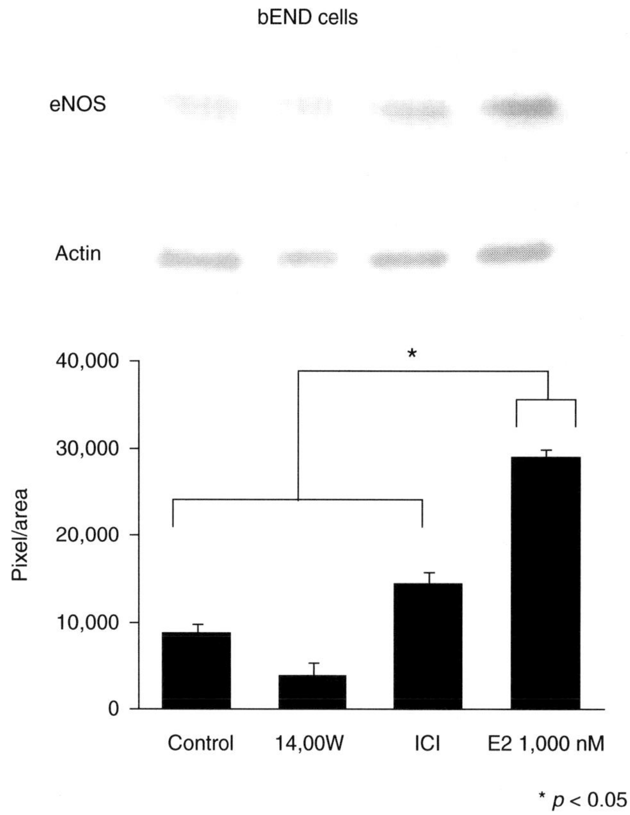

Fig. 2 (*Upper part*) Western blot analysis of eNOS expression in control bEnd.3 cells, bEnd.3 cells treated with 1400W, ICI, and E2 concentrations at 1,000 nM after 2 h of treatment. (*Lower part*) Quantitative Western blot gel analysis. The *y*-axis shows mean ($n=3$ measurements) pixel per area calculated with NIH Image J software. Error bars are standard deviations ($p<0.05$)

Discussion

This study indicates that E2 induces NO level increases in cerebral and peripheral endothelial cells in vitro via eNOS activation and through E2-receptor mediated mechanisms. This is presumably mediated through activation of eNOS by Akt-dependent phosphorylation and via transcriptional activation of eNOS.

NOS Subtypes and E2 Receptors

Among the three different NOS types, there are two consecutive Ca^{2+}/calmodulin-dependent isoforms; namely neuronal NOS (nNOS) and endothelial NOS (eNOS). nNOS is widely distributed in the central nervous system, where NO production occurs via activation of nNOS in neural cells [21, 23]. eNOS is distributed throughout the cardiovascular system, including cerebrovascular tissue, where its activity leads to NO production in endothelial cells [16, 19]. Shear stress to blood vessels [5] and E2 [3] are two of the few agonists that can activate eNOS in a Ca^{2+}-independent manner. Phosphorylation of human eNOS at Serine^{1177} results in enhanced eNOS activity and increased NO release [5, 9]. The inducible NOS (iNOS) is a Ca^{2+}/calmodulin-independent isoform and is mainly expressed in activated immune cells, including microglia of the brain [17].

Currently, three different types of E2 receptors (ER) are known, namely ERα, ERβ, and a G-protein-coupled receptor, GPR30/GPER. ERα and ERβ act as ligand-dependent nuclear transcriptional factors; ERα also possesses ligand-independent activity. These two nuclear transcriptional factor ER receptors share a high homology in the regions that bind DNA and can form heterodimers. All three receptors are found in the brain and play important roles in neuroprotection, though the role of ERα appears most prominent [22]. Classically, the sex hormone estrogen exerts its effects by modifying gene expression [2, 12]. However, it has been shown that ERα mediates rapid, nongenomic effects in human endothelial cells by activating eNOS, suggestive of a process that does not involve the nuclear effects of the hormone [4]. These effects, mediated by estrogens, are too rapid to be elicited by protein synthesis and are not blocked by inhibitors of transcription. This novel activity

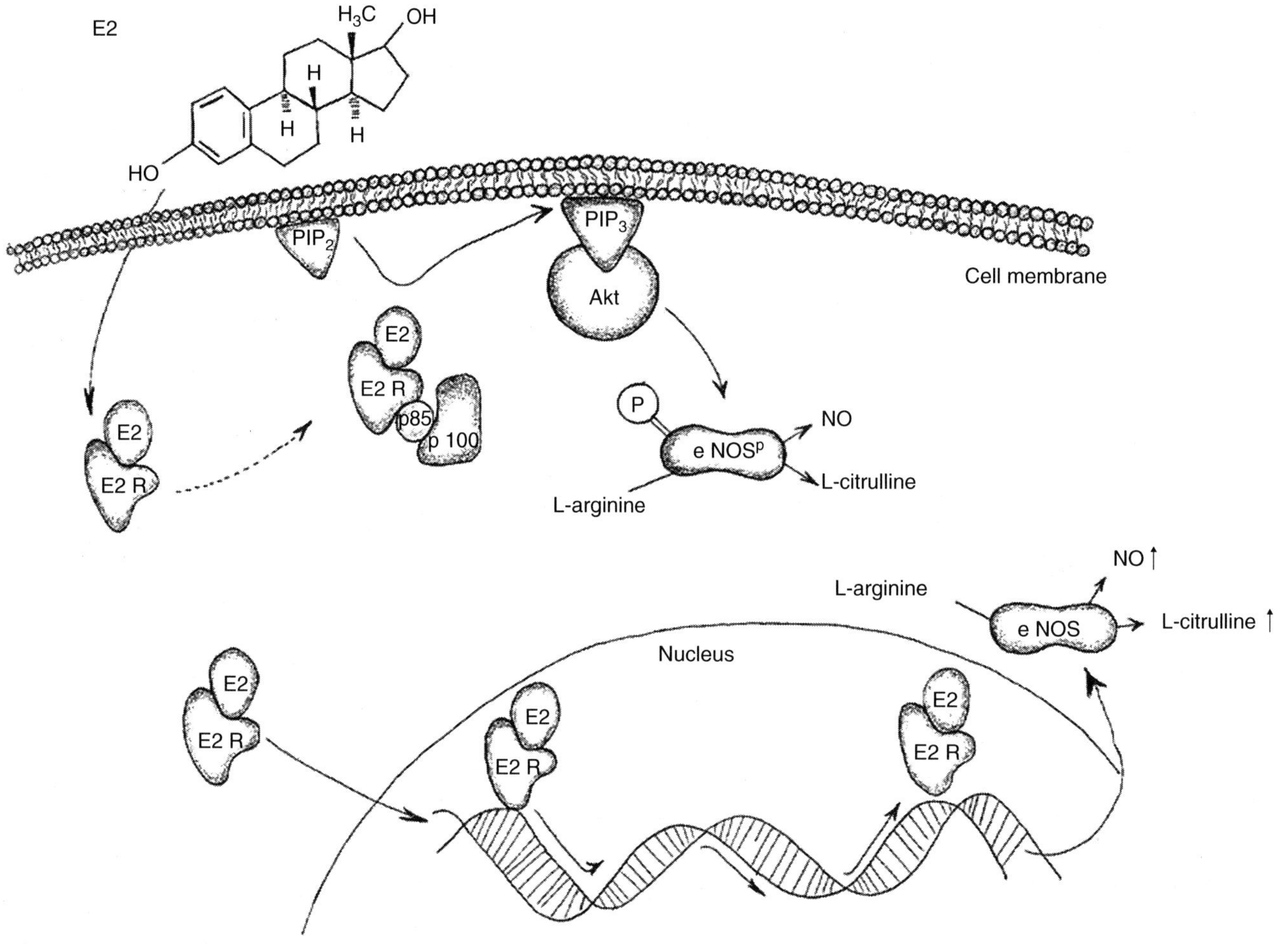

Fig. 3 Schematic illustration of postulated E2 effect in bEnd.3 cells. E2 binds to its receptor E2R. One pathway to increases NO production is by activation of phosphatidylinositol 3-OH kinase (PI3K). PI3K is a heterodimeric phosphoinositide kinase consisting of a regulatory (p85) and catalytic subunit (p100). E2R binds to the catalytic subunit of PI3K and leads to the production of phosphatidylinositol 3-phosphate (PIP3), which, in turn, activates the serine–threonine protein kinase B (Akt). Akt leads to a rapid activation an eNOS, accomplished through phosphorylation at serine[1177]. Another pathway of E2 is through directly enhancing gene expression of eNOS. This, in turn, enhances intracellular protein levels of eNOS in bEnd.3 and increases NO production

has promoted the search for alternative signaling mechanisms and led to the term "nongenomic" actions of E2 or membrane-initiated steroid signaling (MISS). Hynes et al. were able to show that E2 leads to eNOS activation via the phosphatidylinositol 3-OH kinase (PI3K)– serine–threonine protein kinase B (Akt) pathway [11]. Further, it was shown that ERα couples with the regulatory subunit of the lipid kinase, PI3K, activating the catalytic subunit and increasing intracellular production of phosphoinositides (PI) [24]. PI3K is a heterodimeric phosphoinositide kinase consisting of a regulatory and catalytic subunit [1]. PI3K transfers the signaling cascade to intracellular protein kinases by phosphorylation of phosphatidylinositol at the D-3 position, which, in turn, acts as a lipid-mediated second messenger. Akt is one of the principle targets of this cascade. Many of the downstream effects of PI3K are mediated by activated Akt, including rapid eNOS activation, accomplished through eNOS phosphorylation at serine[1177] [5, 9].

bEnd.3 cells express both isoforms (ERα and ERβ) of the estrogen receptor [18], therefore we chose Fulvestrant (ICI) to completely block the ERs, which, in turn, inhibited E2-triggered NO production. E2 led to a significant increase of NO_2 in bEnd.3 and HUVECs by increasing eNOS protein levels and also increased levels of eNOS[P]. Because the administration of a potent eNOS inhibitor (1400W) inhibited the increase of NO_2 levels in bEnd.3 cells, we assume that E2 has a direct effect on eNOS in these cells. It has been shown that E2 increases the expression of NOS [26]. Aside from the increased protein expression induced by E2 in both cell lines in our study, we postulate that increased levels of eNOS[P] are activated by Akt-mediated pathways. Both cell lines revealed similar molecular effects after estrogen treatment, suggesting that brain and peripheral endothelial responses to E2 have similar outcomes.

Relation to Vasospasm and DIND After SAH

Cerebral vasospasm itself as part of a complex pathophysiology has multiple causal factors. One such factor is deprivation of nitric oxide (NO) in the vicinity of brain vessels as a result of nitric oxide synthase (NOS) dysfunction [20] and scavenging of NO by deoxyhemoglobin [15]. Enhanced perivascular NO concentration has been shown to prevent or reverse vasospasm [7, 8]. Administration of NO donors may lead to several systemic adverse effects, including development of drug tolerance, systemic hypotension, rebound phenomenon, and brain edema [6]. To avoid these side effects, direct activation of eNOS, and thus increasing endogenous NO levels, has emerged as a promising research direction. E2 has been shown to reduce mortality and secondary ischemic damage [27] and prevent cerebral vasospasm following SAH in animal models [13]. The results of our in vitro study demonstrate the direct effect of E2 in brain endothelial cells by activating eNOS and raising NO levels by transcriptional and posttranscriptional mechanisms, warranting further confirmation in future in vivo studies.

Conflict of Interest Statement None of the authors has any conflict of interest.

References

1. Carpenter CL, Duckworth BC, Auger KR, Cohen B, Schaffhausen BS, Cantley LC (1990) Purification and characterization of phosphoinositide 3-kinase from rat liver. J Biol Chem 265:19704–19711
2. Carson-Jurica MA, Schrader WT, O'Malley BW (1990) Steroid receptor family: structure and functions. Endocr Rev 11:201–220
3. Caulin-Glaser T, Garcia-Cardena G, Sarrel P, Sessa WC, Bender JR (1997) 17 beta-estradiol regulation of human endothelial cell basal nitric oxide release, independent of cytosolic Ca^{2+} mobilization. Circ Res 81:885–892
4. Chen Z, Yuhanna IS, Galcheva-Gargova Z, Karas RH, Mendelsohn ME, Shaul PW (1999) Estrogen receptor alpha mediates the nongenomic activation of endothelial nitric oxide synthase by estrogen. J Clin Invest 103:401–406
5. Dimmeler S, Fleming I, Fisslthaler B, Hermann C, Busse R, Zeiher AM (1999) Activation of nitric oxide synthase in endothelial cells by Akt-dependent phosphorylation. Nature 399:601–605
6. Fathi AR, Bakhtian KD, Pluta RM (2011) The role of nitric oxide donors in treating cerebral vasospasm after subarachnoid hemorrhage. Acta Neurochir Suppl 110:93–97
7. Fathi AR, Marbacher S, Graupner T, Wehrli F, Jakob SM, Schroth G, Fandino J (2011) Continuous intrathecal glyceryl trinitrate prevents delayed cerebral vasospasm in the single-SAH rabbit model in vivo. Acta Neurochir (Wien) 153:1669–1675; discussion 1675
8. Fathi AR, Pluta RM, Bakhtian KD, Qi M, Lonser RR (2011) Reversal of cerebral vasospasm via intravenous sodium nitrite after subarachnoid hemorrhage in primates. J Neurosurg 115:1213–1220
9. Fulton D, Gratton JP, McCabe TJ, Fontana J, Fujio Y, Walsh K, Franke TF, Papapetropoulos A, Sessa WC (1999) Regulation of endothelium-derived nitric oxide production by the protein kinase Akt. Nature 399:597–601
10. Guo X, Razandi M, Pedram A, Kassab G, Levin ER (2005) Estrogen induces vascular wall dilation: mediation through kinase signaling to nitric oxide and estrogen receptors alpha and beta. J Biol Chem 280:19704–19710
11. Haynes MP, Sinha D, Russell KS, Collinge M, Fulton D, Morales-Ruiz M, Sessa WC, Bender JR (2000) Membrane estrogen receptor engagement activates endothelial nitric oxide synthase via the PI3-kinase-Akt pathway in human endothelial cells. Circ Res 87:677–682
12. Kumar V, Green S, Stack G, Berry M, Jin JR, Chambon P (1987) Functional domains of the human estrogen receptor. Cell 51:941–951
13. Lin CL, Shih HC, Dumont AS, Kassell NF, Lieu AS, Su YF, Hwong SL, Hsu C (2006) The effect of 17beta-estradiol in attenuating experimental subarachnoid hemorrhage-induced cerebral vasospasm. J Neurosurg 104:298–304
14. MacArthur PH, Shiva S, Gladwin MT (2007) Measurement of circulating nitrite and S-nitrosothiols by reductive chemiluminescence. J Chromatogr B Analyt Technol Biomed Life Sci 851:93–105
15. Macdonald RL, Weir BK (1991) A review of hemoglobin and the pathogenesis of cerebral vasospasm. Stroke 22:971–982
16. McNeill AM, Zhang C, Stanczyk FZ, Duckles SP, Krause DN (2002) Estrogen increases endothelial nitric oxide synthase via estrogen receptors in rat cerebral blood vessels: effect preserved after concurrent treatment with medroxyprogesterone acetate or progesterone. Stroke 33:1685–1691
17. Murphy S, Simmons ML, Agullo L, Garcia A, Feinstein DL, Galea E, Reis DJ, Minc-Golomb D, Schwartz JP (1993) Synthesis of nitric oxide in CNS glial cells. Trends Neurosci 16:323–328
18. Odenlund M, Ekblad E, Nilsson BO (2008) Stimulation of oestrogen receptor-expressing endothelial cells with oestrogen reduces proliferation of cocultured vascular smooth muscle cells. Clin Exp Pharmacol Physiol 35:245–248
19. Pelligrino DA, Galea E (2001) Estrogen and cerebrovascular physiology and pathophysiology. Jpn J Pharmacol 86:137–158
20. Pluta RM (2006) Dysfunction of nitric oxide synthases as a cause and therapeutic target in delayed cerebral vasospasm after SAH. Neurol Res 28:730–737
21. Rachman IM, Unnerstall JR, Pfaff DW, Cohen RS (1998) Regulation of neuronal nitric oxide synthase mRNA in lordosis-relevant neurons of the ventromedial hypothalamus following short-term estrogen treatment. Brain Res Mol Brain Res 59:105–108
22. Schreihofer DA, Ma Y (2013) Estrogen receptors and ischemic neuroprotection: who, what, where, and when? Brain Res 1514:107–122
23. Scordalakes EM, Shetty SJ, Rissman EF (2002) Roles of estrogen receptor alpha and androgen receptor in the regulation of neuronal nitric oxide synthase. J Comp Neurol 453:336–344
24. Simoncini T, Hafezi-Moghadam A, Brazil DP, Ley K, Chin WW, Liao JK (2000) Interaction of oestrogen receptor with the regulatory subunit of phosphatidylinositol-3-OH kinase. Nature 407:538–541
25. Thompson LP, Pinkas G, Weiner CP (2000) Chronic 17beta-estradiol replacement increases nitric oxide-mediated vasodilation of guinea pig coronary microcirculation. Circulation 102:445–451
26. Weiner CP, Lizasoain I, Baylis SA, Knowles RG, Charles IG, Moncada S (1994) Induction of calcium-dependent nitric oxide synthases by sex hormones. Proc Natl Acad Sci U S A 91:5212–5216
27. Yang SH, He Z, Wu SS, He YJ, Cutright J, Millard WJ, Day AL, Simpkins JW (2001) 17-beta estradiol can reduce secondary ischemic damage and mortality of subarachnoid hemorrhage. J Cereb Blood Flow Metab 21:174–181

Cilostazol Administration with Combination Enteral and Parenteral Nutrition Therapy Remarkably Improves Outcome After Subarachnoid Hemorrhage

Hidehito Kimura, Yusuke Okamura, Yosiyuki Chiba, Miyake Shigeru, Taiji Ishii, Tatsuo Hori, Ryoji Shiomi, Yuusuke Yamamoto, Yousuke Fujimoto, Masahiro Maeyama, and Eiji Kohmura

Abstract *Objective*: In order to prevent cerebral vasospasm (VS) following aneurysmal subarachnoid hemorrhage (SAH), we introduced combined enteral nutrition (EN) and parenteral nutrition (PN) with oral cilostazol administration to the postoperative patient after SAH and investigated the effect on VS.

Methods: After aneurysmal SAH, 130 postoperative patients were enrolled in this study between April 2008 and March 2012. The patients enrolled before April 2010 were treated by conventional therapy (control group). The patients enrolled after April 2010 were administrated cilostazol 200 mg/day and received EN and PN simultaneously (combined group).

Results: The combined group consisted of 62 patients and the control group of 68 patients. Angiographic VS occurred in 33.9 % ($n=21$) of the combined group and in 51.5 % ($n=35$) of the control group ($p=0.051$, Fisher exact test). The incidence of symptomatic VS was significantly lower in the combined group ($p=0.001$). The incidence of new cerebral infarctions was also significantly lower in the combined group ($p=0.0006$). Clinical outcome at discharge was also significantly better in the combined group than in control group ($p=0.031$).

Conclusions: Cilostazol administration with combination EN and PN is remarkably effective in preventing cerebral VS after aneurysmal SAH.

Keywords SAH • Vasospasm • Cilostazol • Combined nutrition • Enteral nutrition • Parenteral nutrition

Introduction

Cerebral vasospasm (VS) is a main cause of morbidity and mortality following aneurysmal subarachnoid hemorrhage (SAH). Cilostazol, a selective inhibitor of phosphodiesterase 3, is recently known to attenuate cerebral VS owing to its antiplatelet and vasodilatory effects [32, 36, 40]. On the other hand, malnutrition has been reported to occur in critically ill patients as well as in acute stroke patients [7, 11, 34, 39]. Current recommendations suggest the initiation of enteral nutrition (EN) feeding as soon as possible whenever the gastrointestinal tract is functioning in critically ill patients [2, 21, 31] because negative energy balance is associated with increased morbidity and mortality [9–11, 39]. However, it is reported to be difficult to achieve targeted nutritional goals with EN alone, at least during the early phase after intensive care unit (ICU) admission [1, 17, 18].

Therefore, several studies recommend combined EN and parenteral nutrition (PN) support, especially when EN alone failed to achieve the caloric goal [14–16]. The European Society for Parenteral and Enteral Nutrition (ESPEN) guideline also recommends that supplementary PN be initiated if the nutritional goals cannot be achieved using EN alone [21]. In April 2010, we introduced combined EN and PN for postoperative patients with aneurysmal SAH. The objective of the current study is to investigate whether combined EN and PN in addition to cilostazol administration improves the outcomes of the patients with aneurysmal SAH.

H. Kimura, MD, PhD (✉) • Y. Okamura • T. Ishii • T. Hori • Y. Yamamoto • M. Maeyama • E. Kohmura
Department of Neurosurgery, Kobe University Graduate School of Medicine, 7-5-1, Kusuniki-cho, Chuo-ku, Kobe 650-0017, Japan
e-mail: hkimura@med.kobe-u.ac.jp

Y. Chiba
Department of Neurosurgery, Toyooka Public Hospital, Chuo-ku, Kobe, Japan

M. Shigeru • R. Shiomi • Y. Fujimoto
Department of Neurosurgery, Toyooka Public Hospital, 1094 Tobera, Toyooka 668-8501, Japan

J. Fandino et al. (eds.), *Neurovascular Events After Subarachnoid Hemorrhage*, Acta Neurochirurgica Supplement, Vol. 120,
DOI 10.1007/978-3-319-04981-6_25, © Springer International Publishing Switzerland 2015

Materials and Methods

Patients

Between April 2008 and March 2012, patients with SAH who were transferred to Kobe University Hospital and an affiliated hospital, Toyooka Hospital, were enrolled in this study. We first considered surgical clipping rather than endovascular coiling for the treatment of ruptured cerebral aneurysms. Generally, patients with Hunk and Kosnik Grades of I–IV were enrolled in this study. However, even if a patient suffered a severe SAH (Hunt and Kosnik Grade V), we sometimes performed surgical slipping as long as the patient were thought to be treatable and were wished for further life. Therefore, this study included patients admitted to our hospitals with SAH caused by a ruptured cerebral aneurysm with Hunt and Kosnik Grades I–V who were treated by clipping within 72 h after the onset of SAH. Subarachnoid hemorrhage was diagnosed by computed tomography (CT) scanning. Thereafter, CT angiography (CTA) or digital subtraction angiography (DSA) was usually performed 7–9 days postoperatively to evaluate radiological cerebral VS. Exclusion criteria were nonaneurysmal SAH, untreatable severe SAH in Hunt and Kosnik Grade V, endovascular treatment, allergy to cilostazol, and hemorrhagic complications such as gastrointestinal bleeding.

Treatment Protocol

We introduced combined EN and PN with oral cilostazol administration to postoperative patients with SAH from April 2010. On the next day of surgery, they had a CT scan. After it was confirmed that there were no major hemorrhagic events on the scan, the patients started to receive cilostazol (Otsuka Pharmaceutical Co.) orally or through a nasogastic tube, 100 mg twice daily for 14 days. Patients also began to be fed orally or receive enteral feeding as EN on the same day, and a central venous catheter was inserted within a few days with total PN beginning as soon as possible. If the patient was likely amenable to oral feeding considering their neurological status, the first attempt at feeding was oral. However, at the time the total amount of oral intake was judged less than 50 % of the served volume, enteral feeding was started in place of oral intake. This treatment continued by 14 days from the onset. By means of this treatment, patients were expected to receive at least approximately 2,800 kcal/day. These patients were categorized into the combined group. In addition to these treatments, conventional treatment for VS was also performed, which included maintaining a normal circulating blood volume, avoid hypovolemia, administering 30 mg fasudil hydrochloride (Asahi Kasei Pharma Corp.) three times per day for 14 days, and intravenous low molecular weight dextran continuously at 20 ml/h for 14 days. Fasudil hydrochloride is a vasodilator that causes Rho-kinase inhibition and is recommended for use under the Japanese guidelines for the management of aneurysmal SAH. Patients treated before March 2010 were categorized into the control group. On the day after surgery, they also had a CT scan. After it was confirmed that they had no major hemorrhagic complication on the scan, they began to be fed orally or began enteral feeding if they were not amenable to oral feeding, and did not have oral cilostazol administration. PN was administered only when both oral feeding and enteral feeding were not suitable because of their clinical status, such as pneumonia, gastrointestinal dysfunction, and so on. With this nutrition protocol, they received approximately 1,600 kcal/day. They also received the conventional VS treatment described above. In addition, the patients in control group were administered low-dose intravenous nicardipine 2 mg/h continuously for 14 days.

Radiological and Clinical Evaluations

Subarachnoid hemorrhage was diagnosed using CT scanning, and the severity was assessed by Hunt and Kosnik grade. A ruptured aneurysm was confirmed by CTA or DSA. Either DSA or CTA was performed between 7 and 9 days after the onset of SAH to assess angiographic VS. Angiographic VS was defined as greater than 50 % decrease in vessel diameter from the initial images. All patients were closely observed and clinical symptoms of cerebral VS were evaluated for 14 days. Symptomatic VS was defined as the development of a new focal or global neurological deficit or deterioration that was not explained by initial hemorrhage, rebleeding, hydrocephalus, surgical complications, fever, infections, electrolytes, or metabolic disturbances.

Clinical outcomes were evaluated using the modified Rankin Scale (mRS) at discharge with outcomes divided into mRS scores of 0–2, 3–5, and 6. New cerebral infarctions related to VS were defined as the presence of new low-density areas on follow-up CT scanning, not related to procedure-related infarctions or brain damage. These findings were assessed by more than two neurosurgeons.

Statistical Analysis

Data are presented as means and standard deviation, and categorical variables as percentages. Student's *t* test and Fisher's exact test were used to compare continuous variables and proportions. Clinical factors affecting angiographic and symptomatic VS were assessed using multiple logistic regression analysis. All statistical analyses were performed with R-Commander 2.0-0, a basic statistics graphical user interface for R 3.0.1 (R Foundation for Statistical Computing, Vienna, Austria). A p value <0.05 was considered statistically significant.

Results

Patient Characteristics

Between April 2008 and March 2012, 200 patients with SAH were transferred to our hospital. Among them, 31 patients had untreatable severe SAH in Hunt and Kosnik Grade V, 18 patients received coil embolization, and 8 patients were diagnosed as having nonaneurysmal SAH. Excluding these 57 patients, 143 patients with SAH in Hunt and Kosnik Grades I to V were treated by clipping within 48 h from the SAH onset. Among the 143 patients, 130 patients received either DSA or CTA between 7 and 9 days after the onset to assess angiographic VS and were enrolled in this study. The control group consisted of 68 patients and the combined group of 62 patients. No significant difference in the background data of the patients, including age, sex, severity of SAH, and location of aneurysm, was found between the groups (Table 1).

Table 1 Clinical and radiological characteristics of patients in the combined and control groups

	Value[a]		
Characteristic	Combined group	Control group	p value[b]
No. of patients	62	68	
Mean age (years)	65.6 ± 14.0	65 ± 13.52	0.921
Female	44 (71.0)	54/68 (79.4)	0.539
H&K Grade			0.984
I	4 (6.5)	5 (7.4)	
II	24 (38.7)	25 (36.8)	
III	14 (22.6)	16 (23.5)	
IV	15 (24.2)	18 (26.4)	
V	5 (8.1)	4 (5.9)	
Hemorrhage location			0.045
AcomAN	17 (27.4)	29 (42.6)	
Distal ACA	6 (9.7)	0 (0)	
IC	16 (25.8)	14 (20.6)	
MCA	16 (25.8)	19 (27.5)	
VABA	5 (8.1)	6 (8.8)	
Other	2 (3.2)	0 (0)	

H&K Hunt and Kosnik, *AcomAN* anterior communicating artery aneurysm, *ACA* anterior communicating artery, *IC* internal carotid, *MCA* middle cerebral artery, *VABA* vertebrobasilar artery

[a]Mean values are presented as the mean ± SD. All other values are the number of patients (%)

[b]Calculated using Student's t-test, the Fisher exact probability test

Study Evaluations

Angiographic VS occurred in 33.9 % (n=21) of the combined group and in 51.5 % (n=35) of the control group (odds ratio 0.48 [95 % CI, 0.24–0.98], p=0.051) (Table 2). The incidence of symptomatic VS was significantly lower in the combined group than in the control group (11.3 % vs 36.8 %; odds ratio 0.22 [95 % CI, 0.09–0.55], p=0.001) (Table 2). The incidence of new cerebral infarctions was also significantly lower in the combined group than in the control group (6.4 % vs 30.9 %; odds ratio 0.15 [95 % CI, 0.05–0.48], p=0.0006) (Table 2). Clinical outcomes at discharge were also significantly better in the combined group than in the control group (mRS ≦2: 48.4 % vs 29.4 %, odds ratio 2.25 [95 % CI, 1.09–4.63], p=0.031). The mortality rate was also lower in the combined group than in the control group, although the difference was not statistically significant (1.7 % vs 10.3 %, odds ratio 0.14 [95 % CI, 0.02–1.20], p=0.064) (Table 2). Multiple logistic analyses demonstrated that introduction of cilostazol administration and EN plus PN was the only factor affecting angiographic VS as well as symptomatic VS (Table 3). No major adverse effects were related to cilostazol use. By performing both enteral feeding and PN, hyperglycemia and elevated serum levels of transaminase were detected, which were treated safely by continuous infusion of human insulin and glycyrrhizin, respectively. No major adverse events were related to EN and PN.

Table 2 Stratified analysis of angiographic vasospasm (VS), symptomatic VS, cerebral infarction, and mRS in the combined and control groups

	No. of patients (%)		
Parameter	Combined group	Control group	p value[a]
Angiographic VS	21 (33.9)	35 (51.5)	0.051
Symptomatic VS	7 (11.3)	25 (36.8)	0.001
Cerebral infarction	7 (11.3)	25 (36.8)	0.0006
mRS			0.022
0–2	30 (48.4)	20 (29.4)	
3–5	31 (50)	41 (60.3)	
6	1 (1.7)	7 (10.3)	

mRS modified Rankin Scale

[a]Calculated using the Fisher exact probability test

Table 3 Factors affecting angiographic vasospasm (VS) and symptomatic VS based on the results of multiple logistic analyses

Factor	Odds ratio	95 % CI	*p* value
H&K Grade I or II			
Angiographic VS	1.510	0.739–3.090	0.258
Symptomatic VS	0.818	0.3490–1.92	0.644
Cilostazol & EN+PN			
Angiographic VS+	0.418	0.196–0.894	0.0245
Symptomatic VS	0.189	0.0713–0.50	0.000795
CSF drainage			
Angiographic VS	1.540	0.706–3.370	0.278
Symptomatic VS	1.630	0.6630–4.02	0.286

H&K Hunt and Kosnik, *EN* enteral nutrition, *PN* parenteral nutrition, *CSF* cerebrospinal fluid

Discussion

Recent some reports recommended endovascular coil embolization as the first treatment option rather than surgical clipping [24–26, 35]. However, we decided to consider surgical clipping as a first line of treatment because long-term follow-up data demonstrated that the risk of rebleeding was lower in patients treated by surgical clipping than by endovascular coiling even the patients with ruptured posterior circulation aneurysms were treated by surgical clipping when the aneurysm was assessed as being relative easy to access by craniotomy.

In this study, our combined EN and PN with cilostazol administration significantly reduced the frequency of symptomatic VS and the incidence of cerebral infarction related to VS, which significantly improved the clinical outcomes. Based on the multiple logistic analyses, introduction of combined EN and PN with cilostazol administration reduced angiographic VS to 42 % and symptomatic VS to 19 %. Combined EN and PN with cilostazol administration was the only factor that reduced angiographic VS and symptomatic VS.

The effects of cilostazol are basically mediated by inhibition of phosphodiesterase 3 in smooth muscle cells and platelets, leading to relaxation of intact smooth muscle cells and inhibition of platelet aggregation. Previous studies reported the effectiveness of cilostazol administration for cerebral VS [32, 36, 40]. Yoshimoto et al. reported the efficacy of cilostazol for cerebral VS in their series of patients who were treated by cilostazol administration in the same way as in our study. In their series, symptomatic VS occurred in 5 of the 26 (19.2 %) patients in the cilostazol group and 9 of the 24 (37.5 %) patients in the control group, showing a reduction in symptomatic VS by cilostazol, but not significantly. They also reported that new lesions caused by VS on CT or MR scans were detected in 3 of the 26 patients in the cilostazol group and 7 of the 24 patients in the control group, showing no significant difference [40]. In 2011, Suzuki et al. reported on a series of patients treated in the same way, in which the frequency of symptomatic VS was occurred in 11 of 49 patients (22.4 %) in the cilostazol group and 19 of 51 patients in the control group (37.3 %) in the control group, with findings of new cerebral infarction caused by VS detected in 5 of the 49 patients (10.2 %) in the cilostazol group and 14 of the 51 patients (27.5 %) in the control group, showing no significant difference. However, they showed an improvement in clinical outcomes [36]. In 2013, Senbokuya et al. performed a multicenter prospective, randomized, open-label, blinded endpoint trial under the same treatment protocol as used in our study. In their series, the frequency of symptomatic VS was 7 of 54 patients (13.0 %) in the cilostazol group, 22 of 55 patients (40 %) in the control group; and cerebral infarction was detected in 6 of 54 patients (11.1 %) and 16 of 55 patients (29.1 %), respectively. There were significant differences between two groups. However, they failed to prove significant improvement of clinical outcomes. Comparing with these data, the occurrence of symptomatic VS was 19.2, 22.4, 13.0 % in the cilostazol groups previously reported and 12.0 % in our series and the findings of cerebral infarction was detected in 11.5, 10.2, 11.1 % in the cilostazol group, and no more than 6.9 % in our series. Comparing our data with the previous studies, the incidence of symptomatic VS may be slightly lower and the incidence of cerebral infarction may be slightly suppressed with the aid of the combined nutrition.

In general, the medical treatment for cerebral VS after SAH consists of calcium antagonist [5], Rho kinase inhibitor [33], and triple-H therapy [28]. Endovascular treatments, including angioplasty [12] and intraarterial drug administration [27, 30, 37] have also been reported to be effective for cerebral VS. As attending neurosurgeons caring for the postoperative patient after SAH, nutrition may often tend to be a secondary priority. Critically ill patients are reported to be frequently hypermetabolic and catabolic. And it is reported that there was a risk of underfeeding in critically ill patients [11, 34, 39] including acute stroke patients [7, 13]. Badjatia et al. investigated the relationship between energy balance and complications after SAH and reported that these patients tend to be underfed because of either inadequate caloric intake or increased energy expenditure, and that this led to increases in infectious complications. They suggested that adjunctive use of PN to EN may by effective even for short periods to reach nutrition goals [3]. Kasuya et al. reported that postoperative patients after SAH experienced a profound increase in metabolic rate that may be attributed to cerebral VS [19]. Furthermore, they stated that a favorable outcome after SAH might be expected with early PN because the most important management of patients with SAH is to avoid hypovolemia to prevent VS, and that diarrhea and vomiting, as complications of enteral feedings, make it difficult to maintain an adequate water balance [19]. However, supplemental PN to EN has not been reported as a management for the patients with SAH in any previous studies. Our current study showed the possibility of improving patient outcomes with SAH by supplemental PN to EN leading to reduced frequency of VS.

Limitations

There are several limitations to our study. First, we did not evaluate nitrogen balance and serum turnover proteins. Therefore, it is still unclear whether combined EN and PN actually improve patient nutrition and outcomes. Improved visceral proteins were observed in patients receiving EN and PN compared with those receiving EN alone in two studies [4, 8]. Second, as described above, some authors reported that even cilostazol administration alone is effective in reducing incidence of VS. In our study, the occurrence of symptomatic VS and cerebral infarction were much lower, compared with the those previously reported treated by cilostaozol alone. However, it is unclear how much the combined EN and PN play a role in avoiding cerebral VS. Third, we could not clarify the optimal energy volume to feed patients after SAH because we did not investigate actual calories given to the patients in this study. Although malnutrition tends to occur in critically ill patients as well as in acute stroke patients [7, 11, 34, 39], overfeeding is reported to be avoided as well as underfeeding [22, 29]. Various complications of overfeeding have been reported in several studies: hyperglycemia, hyperlipidemia, hepatic dysfunction, and ventilation-weaning difficulties [6, 20, 23, 38]. In general, to estimate energy needs in critically ill patients, the Harris-Benedict Equation is used. A "stress factor," one of the variables in the equation, for the patient with SAH does not exist. By assuming the value, we can estimate energy need and setup caloric goal [3, 7]. Because achieving targeted nutritional goals with EN alone is known to be often difficult, at least during the early phase after ICU admission [1, 17, 18], combined EN and PN support may be recommended, especially when EN alone failed to achieve the caloric goal as previously reported [14–16]. In executing this, total calorie intake ought to be set just 100 % of their estimated nutritional requirements, avoiding underfeeding or overfeeding, which may lead to better outcomes in patients with SAH. Last, our current study is a retrospective study, and a prospective randomized study is needed to confirm the results of the current study. We have launched into prospective randomized study in which evaluation of nitrogen balance and serum turnover proteins, estimation of individual energy requirements, and inspection of actual given energy to resolve the problems described above.

Conclusions

In conclusion, the results of the current retrospective study suggested that combined EN and PN could improve the outcome of the postoperative patients with SAH. Future prospective studies will confirm the effectiveness of this combined therapy.

Conflict of Interest Statement We declare that we have no conflict of interest.

References

1. Adam S, Batson S (1997) A study of problems associated with the delivery of enteral feed in critically ill patients in five ICUs in the UK. Intensive Care Med 23(3):261–266
2. Artinian V, Krayem H, DiGiovine B (2006) Effects of early enteral feeding on the outcome of critically ill mechanically ventilated medical patients. Chest 129(4):960–967
3. Badjatia N, Fernandez L, Schlossberg MJ, Schmidt JM, Claassen J, Lee K, Connolly ES, Mayer SA, Rosenbaum M (2010) Relationship between energy balance and complications after subarachnoid hemorrhage. JPEN J Parenter Enteral Nutr 34(1):64–69
4. Bauer P, Charpentier C, Bouchet C, Nace L, Raffy F, Gaconnet N (2000) Parenteral with enteral nutrition in the critically ill. Intensive Care Med 26(7):893–900
5. Bederson JB, Connolly ES, Batjer HH, Dacey RG, Dion JE, Diringer MN, Duldner JE, Harbaugh RE, Patel AB, Rosenwasser RH (2009) Guidelines for the management of aneurysmal subarachnoid hemorrhage: a statement for healthcare professionals from a special writing group of the Stroke Council, American Heart Association. Stroke 40(3):994–1025
6. Van den Berg B, Stam H (1988) Metabolic and respiratory effects of enteral nutrition in patients during mechanical ventilation. Intensive Care Med 14(3):206–211
7. Chalela JA, Haymore J, Schellinger PD, Kang D-W, Warach S (2004) Acute stroke patients are being underfed: a nitrogen balance study. Neurocrit Care 1(3):331–334
8. Chiarelli AG, Ferrarello S, Piccioli A, Abate A, Chini G, Berioli MB, Peris A, Lippi R (1996) Total enteral nutrition versus mixed enteral and parenteral nutrition in patients at an intensive care unit. Minerva Anestesiol 62(1–2):1–7
9. Correia MITD, Waitzberg DL (2003) The impact of malnutrition on morbidity, mortality, length of hospital stay and costs evaluated through a multivariate model analysis. Clin Nutr 22(3):235–239
10. da Cunha HFR, da Rocha EEM, Hissa M (2013) Protein requirements, morbidity and mortality in critically ill patients: fundamentals and applications. Rev Bras Ter Intensiva 25(1):49–55
11. Dvir D, Cohen J, Singer P (2006) Computerized energy balance and complications in critically ill patients: an observational study. Clin Nutr 25(1):37–44
12. Eskridge JM, McAuliffe W, Song JK, Deliganis AV, Newell DW, Lewis DH, Mayberg MR, Winn HR (1998) Balloon angioplasty for the treatment of vasospasm: results of first 50 cases. Neurosurgery 42(3):510–516; discussion 516–517
13. Esper DH, Coplin WM, Carhuapoma JR (2006) Energy expenditure in patients with nontraumatic intracranial hemorrhage. JPEN J Parenter Enteral Nutr 30(2):71–75
14. Heidegger CP, Berger MM, Thibault R, Zingg W, Pichard C (2013) Supplemental parenteral nutrition in critically ill patients – authors' reply. Lancet 381(9879):1716–1717

15. Heidegger C-P, Darmon P, Pichard C (2008) Enteral vs. parenteral nutrition for the critically ill patient: a combined support should be preferred. Curr Opin Crit Care 14(4):408–414
16. Heidegger C-P, Romand J-A, Treggiari MM, Pichard C (2007) Is it now time to promote mixed enteral and parenteral nutrition for the critically ill patient? Intensive Care Med 33(6):963–969
17. Heyland D, Cook DJ, Winder B, Brylowski L, Van deMark H, Guyatt G (1995) Enteral nutrition in the critically ill patient: a prospective survey. Crit Care Med 23(6):1055–1060
18. De Jonghe B, Appere-De-Vechi C, Fournier M, Tran B, Merrer J, Melchior JC, Outin H (2001) A prospective survey of nutritional support practices in intensive care unit patients: what is prescribed? What is delivered? Crit Care Med 29(1):8–12
19. Kasuya H, Kawashima A, Namiki K, Shimizu T, Takakura K (1998) Metabolic profiles of patients with subarachnoid hemorrhage treated by early surgery. Neurosurgery 42(6):1268–1274; discussion 1274–1275
20. Klein CJ, Stanek GS, Wiles CE (1998) Overfeeding macronutrients to critically ill adults: metabolic complications. J Am Diet Assoc 98(7):795–806
21. Kreymann KG, Berger MM, Deutz NEP et al (2006) ESPEN guidelines on enteral nutrition: intensive care. Clin Nutr 25(2):210–223
22. Krishnan JA, Parce PB, Martinez A, Diette GB, Brower RG (2003) Caloric intake in medical ICU patients: consistency of care with guidelines and relationship to clinical outcomes. Chest 124(1): 297–305
23. Lo H-C, Lin C-H, Tsai L-J (2005) Effects of hypercaloric feeding on nutrition status and carbon dioxide production in patients with long-term mechanical ventilation. JPEN J Parenter Enteral Nutr 29(5):380–387
24. McDougall CG, Spetzler RF, Zabramski JM, Partovi S, Hills NK, Nakaji P, Albuquerque FC (2012) The barrow ruptured aneurysm trial. J Neurosurg 116(1):135–144
25. Molyneux A, Kerr R, Stratton I, Sandercock P, Clarke M, Shrimpton J, Holman R (2002) International subarachnoid aneurysm trial (ISAT) of neurosurgical clipping versus endovascular coiling in 2143 patients with ruptured intracranial aneurysms: a randomised trial. Lancet 360(9342):1267–1274
26. Molyneux AJ, Kerr RSC, Yu L-M, Clarke M, Sneade M, Yarnold JA, Sandercock P (2005) International subarachnoid aneurysm trial (ISAT) of neurosurgical clipping versus endovascular coiling in 2143 patients with ruptured intracranial aneurysms: a randomised comparison of effects on survival, dependency, seizures, rebleeding, subgroups, and aneurysm occlusion. Lancet 366(9488):809–817
27. Musahl C, Henkes H, Vajda Z, Coburger J, Hopf N (2011) Continuous local intra-arterial nimodipine administration in severe symptomatic vasospasm after subarachnoid hemorrhage. Neurosurgery 68(6): 1541–1547; discussion 1547
28. Origitano TC, Wascher TM, Reichman OH, Anderson DE (1990) Sustained increased cerebral blood flow with prophylactic hypertensive hypervolemic hemodilution ("triple-H" therapy) after subarachnoid hemorrhage. Neurosurgery 27(5):729–739; discussion 739–740
29. Radrizzani D, Iapichino G (1998) Nutrition and lung function in the critically ill patient. Clin Nutr 17(1):7–10
30. Sawada M, Hashimoto N, Tsukahara T, Nishi S, Kaku Y, Yoshimura S (1997) Effectiveness of intra-arterially infused papaverine solutions of various concentrations for the treatment of cerebral vasospasm. Acta Neurochir 139(8):706–711
31. Scurlock C, Mechanick JI (2008) Early nutrition support in the intensive care unit: a US perspective. Curr Opin Clin Nutr Metab Care 11(2):152–155
32. Senbokuya N, Kinouchi H, Kanemaru K et al (2012) Effects of cilostazol on cerebral vasospasm after aneurysmal subarachnoid hemorrhage: a multicenter prospective, randomized, open-label blinded end point trial. J Neurosurg 118(1):121–130
33. Shibuya M, Suzuki Y, Sugita K, Saito I, Sasaki T, Takakura K, Nagata I, Kikuchi H, Takemae T, Hidaka H (1992) Effect of AT877 on cerebral vasospasm after aneurysmal subarachnoid hemorrhage. Results of a prospective placebo-controlled double-blind trial. J Neurosurg 76(4):571–577
34. Singh H, Watt K, Veitch R, Cantor M, Duerksen DR (2006) Malnutrition is prevalent in hospitalized medical patients: are housestaff identifying the malnourished patient? Nutrition 22(4): 350–354
35. Spetzler RF, McDougall CG, Albuquerque FC, Zabramski JM, Hills NK, Partovi S, Nakaji P, Wallace RC (2013) The barrow ruptured aneurysm trial: 3-year results. J Neurosurg 119(1):146–157
36. Suzuki S, Sayama T, Nakamura T, Nishimura H, Ohta M, Inoue T, Mannoji H, Takeshita I (2011) Cilostazol improves outcome after subarachnoid hemorrhage: a preliminary report. Cerebrovasc Dis 32(1):89–93
37. Tachibana E, Harada T, Shibuya M, Saito K, Takayasu M, Suzuki Y, Yoshida J (1999) Intra-arterial infusion of fasudil hydrochloride for treating vasospasm following subarachnoid haemorrhage. Acta Neurochir 141(1):13–19
38. Takiguchi SA (1990) Report of a hidden case of overfeeding. Heart Lung 19(6):639–640
39. Villet S, Chiolero RL, Bollmann MD, Revelly J-P, Cayeux RNM-C, Delarue J, Berger MM (2005) Negative impact of hypocaloric feeding and energy balance on clinical outcome in ICU patients. Clin Nutr 24(4):502–509
40. Yoshimoto T, Shirasaka T, Fujimoto S, Yoshidumi T, Yamauchi T, Tokuda K, Kaneko S, Kashiwaba T (2009) Cilostazol may prevent cerebral vasospasm following subarachnoid hemorrhage. Neurol Med Chir 49(6):235–240; discussion 240–241

Pharmacological Modulation of Spreading Depolarizations

Renán Sánchez-Porras, Zelong Zheng, and Oliver W. Sakowitz

Abstract Spreading depolarization (SD) is a wave of almost complete depolarization of the neuronal and glial cells. Nowadays there is sufficient evidence demonstrating its pathophysiological effect in migraine with aura, transient global amnesia, stroke, subarachnoid hemorrhage, intracerebral hemorrhage, and traumatic brain injury. In these cases, occurrence of SD has been associated with functional neuronal damage, neuronal necrosis, neurological degeneration, and poor clinical outcome. Animal models show that SD can be modulated by drugs that interfere with its initiation and propagation. There are many pharmacological targets that may help to suppress SD occurrence, such as Na^+, K^+, Cl^-, and Ca^{2+}channels; Na^+/K^+-ATPase; gap junctions; and ligand-based receptors, for example, adrenergic, serotonin, sigma-1, calcitonin gene-related peptide, $GABA_A$, and glutamate receptors. In this regard, *N*-methyl-d-aspartate (NMDA) receptor blockers, in particular, ketamine, have shown promising results. Therefore, theoretically pharmacologic modulation of SD could help diminish its pathological effects.

Keywords Spreading depolarization • Ketamine • NMDA receptor • Therapy

Introduction

Spreading depolarization (SD) is a wave of neuronal and glial depolarization that propagates across the cortex; it is characterized by neuronal swelling, distortion of dendritic spines, and depression of neuronal activity [9]. Underlying this phenomenon is a dramatic failure of brain ion homeostasis, acidification, efflux of excitatory amino acids, and increase of energy metabolism [29]. Experimentally, SD can be elicited through chemical, mechanical, or electrical stimulations. However, this depolarization also occurs spontaneously after mechanical damage, hypoxia, ischemia, or hypoglycemia [45]. SD is associated with important hemodynamic changes. The physiological hemodynamic response during SD development is arteriolar vasodilation. As a result, increments of more than 100 % of cerebral blood flow (spreading hyperemia) occur, followed by a mild but prolonged hypoperfusion (spreading oligemia). In tissue at risk, such as areas adjacent to subarachnoid hemorrhage (SAH), an inverse hemodynamic response with hypoperfusion (spreading ischemia) can be observed. It has been shown that, under pathologic circumstances, SD can produce oxidative stress, worsen hypoxia, and induce neuronal death [9, 10].

Since its original description by the Brazilian physiologist Aristides Leão in 1944, SD has been extensively characterized in animal models [31]. Not until the past decade has an electrophysiological confirmation of SD in human brain been found and its role in the pathophysiological basis of several neurological conditions addressed [20, 29]. Today there is sufficient evidence showing that SD plays an important role in migraine with aura (MA), transient global amnesia, stroke, SAH, intracerebral hemorrhage, and traumatic brain injury (TBI), where SD occurrence has been associated with functional neuronal damage, neuronal necrosis, neurological degeneration, and poor clinical outcome [20, 29]. Therefore, therapeutic modulation of SD has raised high expectations.

In the human brain, pharmaceutical targeting of SD is still in its infancy. Nonetheless, a large body of experimental study shows that SD can be presumably modulated by drugs that interfere with its initiation and propagation. The range of targets is wide and includes ion trafficking such as Ca^{2+}, K^+, and voltage-gated Na^+ and Cl^- channels, along with Na^+/

R. Sánchez-Porras, MD (✉) • Z. Zheng • O.W. Sakowitz
Department of Neurosurgery, Heidelberg University Hospital, Im Neuenheimer Feld 400, 69120 Heidelberg, Germany
e-mail: renan.sanchez-porras@med.uni-heidelberg.de

J. Fandino et al. (eds.), *Neurovascular Events After Subarachnoid Hemorrhage*, Acta Neurochirurgica Supplement, Vol. 120,
DOI 10.1007/978-3-319-04981-6_26,

K^+-ATPase and gap junctions, and many ligand-based receptors, for example, adrenergic, serotonin, sigma-1, and glutamate receptors [2, 16, 45]. In addition, many analgesics and sedatives seem to exert an impact on the susceptibility and occurrence of SD [27]. In particular, *N*-methyl-d-aspartate (NMDA) receptor antagonists have been shown to inhibit SD initiation and/or propagation and they seem to be, at the moment, the most effective drugs for SD suppression [48]. Based on these observations, pharmacological modulation of SD in humans as a neuroprotective therapy could be feasible. Here, we briefly review some important aspects of pharmacological modulation of SD.

Clinical Implications of Spreading Depolarization

SD has been observed in patients suffering from SAH using subdural electrocorticographic strip electrodes. It has been shown that SD has a high incidence in this type of cerebrovascular disease, reported to be between 66 and 100 %; there is also a relationship between delayed cerebral ischemia (DCI) and SD occurrence in approximately 44–88 % of the cases [40]. Repeated SDs with prolonged depression periods have been found as an early indicator of DCI after SAH [15]. This finding called into question the role of angiographic cerebral vasospasm as the main cause of DCI, suggesting that SD has a potential pathophysiological mechanism in its development [52]. It is expected that pathological conditions that occur after SAH, such as hypoxia, low glucose, high extracellular concentrations of K^+, and nitric oxide depletion by free hemoglobin products, are capable of triggering SD [11, 12]. Then, SD is initiated under conditions when (1) metabolic demands are not met per se and (2) the hemodynamic response is turned from hyperemia to spreading ischemia. This could lead into a self-perpetuating cycle with consecutive cortical necrosis and DCI formation [9]. Therefore, treatments targeting SD should decrease DCI and improve clinical outcome. In this regard, there is indirect evidence that the L-type Ca^+ inhibitors, nimodipine [14, 49] and nicardipine [50], or the NMDA receptor blocker ketamine [25] could improve outcome by SD suppression in patients.

In other cerebrovascular diseases, spontaneous SDs have also been observed with high incidence. In stroke, for example, SDs are present in 86–100 % of patients and their presence is associated with infarct growth. It is hypothesized that prevention and treatment of SD may also help to avoid secondary ischemia and fatal brain edema [8]. SDs have been found in 50–60 % of TBI patients and their presence is related to unfavorable outcome [22, 23].

SD is now widely recognized to be the neurophysiological substrate of MA and a potential trigger of the headache [29]. Genetic factors that favor hyperexcitability of the visual cortex may enhance susceptibility to SD, such is the case for familial hemiplegic migraine (FHM), a genetic form of migraine that involves mutations in genes that encode for voltage-gated P/Q-type Ca^{2+} channel subunits (FHM1), Na^+/K^+-ATPase subunits (FHM2) [19], or Na^+ channel subunits (FHM3) [38]. Transgenic mice carrying FHM mutations show increased susceptibility to SD, with a vastly reduced triggering threshold, an increased propagation velocity, and frequently multiple SDs after a single stimulus [33]. Another example is the K^+ channel, TRESK, which is regulated by Ca^{2+} concentrations, where it has been shown that a dominant-negative mutation is linked to MA and SD [17]. Over the past years, several antimigraine drugs have been tested on SD. Tonabersat, a benzoylaminobenzopyran anticonvulsant, suppresses SDs in animal models after intraperitoneal administration; however, the clinical trials show conflicting results [2, 16]. Many other antimigraine drugs have been tested or are under investigation, e.g., valproate, propranolol, methysergide, amitriptyline, topiramate, gabapentin, lamotrigine, flunarizine, and olcegepant, although the results are contradictory. These drugs have an inhibitory effect on ion channels, receptors, and neurotransmitters such as Na^+, L-type Ca^{2+}, P/Q- and N-type Ca^{2+} channels, gap junctions, $GABA_A$, and calcitonin gene-related peptide receptors, thus, supporting the role of multiple targets [6]. Research into SD inhibitory antimigraine drugs could, therefore, have a collateral impact on cerebrovascular diseases and brain trauma.

Pharmacological Targets and SD Modulation

When SD develops, a surge of $[K^+]_e$ occurs, which leads to depolarization of adjacent neurons and glial cells. At the same time, $[Na^+]_e$ decreases as it enters the cells accompanied by water. This process is followed by neuronal swelling and shrinkage of the extracellular space. At the same time, influx of Ca^{2+} also occurs, leading to release of glutamate and other neurotransmitters. Glutamate induces NMDA receptor activation, which may contribute to SD initiation, propagation, and, if released in excess, can generate excitotoxicity. Moreover, gap junctions are thought to play an important role in SD expansion by promoting intercellular Ca^{2+} and K^+ waves. After SD, $[K^+]_e$ is restored by Na^+/K^+-ATPase and astrocytes [44]. This suggests Na^+, K^+, Ca^{2+} channels, Na^+/K^+-ATPase, gap junctions, and NMDA receptors as the main targets for SD modulation.

Voltage-Gated Na^+ Channels

The role of Na^+ channels in SD generation or propagation is under debate. Tetrodotoxin (TTX), one inhibitor of voltage-gated Na^+ channels, is sufficient to diminish the SD phenomenon or reduce the propagation velocity, but it does not prevent SD. Actually, TTX has a stronger effect on hypoxic spreading depolarization than on SD [45]. Conversely, other studies demonstrated there is no sign of any attenuation of SD in the presence of TTX [46]. However, dysfunction of Na^+ channels has been confirmed in FHM3, which provides further support for the potential role of these channels in generation of SD [7].

K^+ Channels

Voltage-gated K^+ channels control neuronal excitability and inhibit hyperexcitability. Generally, the increase of membrane K^+ conductance will lower neuronal excitability by hyperpolarization. Concurrent with this, several studies have shown that blockages of K^+ channels (e.g., Ba^{2+}, Rb^+, Cs^+ , tetraethylammonium chloride (TEA), and 4-aminopyridine) lower the threshold of SD, and some of these substances can even induce spontaneous SDs [18]. K^+ channel opening can reduce SD incidence and propagation velocity [51]. However, it is unclear whether these effects are specific for special channel types or a nonspecific outcome from hyperpolarization.

Ca^{2+} Channels

Ca^{2+} channels have a potential role in SD generation or propagation [33]. Important Ca^{2+} channels subtypes seem to be P/Q-type (Cav2.1) and N-type (Cav2.2), which have been related to special types of migraine [28]. After the blockage of P/Q-type Ca^{2+} channels by ωAgaIVA, SD cannot be induced in mouse cortical slices, whereas blockage of N- or R-type Ca^{2+} channels by ωCgtxVIA and SNX-482 has only a small inhibitory effect on SD threshold and propagation velocity [47]. Many of the medications blocking this channel currently tested on animal models are primarily antimigraine drugs such as gabapentin, flunarizine, topiramate, and valproate. They seem to elevate the electrical threshold, and decrease the frequency, duration, and propagation of SD. However, the results remain inconclusive [2, 3]. In general, L-type Ca^{2+} channels have no direct effect on SD generation and propagation. Nonetheless, blockers of this subtype channel, such as nimodipine and nicardipine, can suppress the vasoconstriction effect of high $[K^+]_e$. Thus, they can correct the inverse hemodynamic response induced by SD under pathological conditions [30, 50].

Na^+/K^+-ATPase

Na^+/K^+-ATPase is important for restoring $[K^+]_e$ after SD, so it is critical for SD occurrence. Consistent with this, inhibitors (e.g., ouabain) of Na^+/K^+-ATPase are capable to enhance SD susceptibility [21]. Additionally, a ketogenic diet related to augmentation of Na^+/K^+-ATPase activity can suppress SD [4].

Gap Junctions

Gap junctions are the basis of a functional synchronization between neighboring cells. Some studies have shown that gap junction blockers (e.g., heptane, octane, quinine, quinidine, mefloquine, halothane, isoflurane, and tonabersat) inhibit SD propagation or duration [34, 35]. However, it is difficult to ascertain the role of neural or glial gap junctions in SD because of the lack of specificity of gap junction blockers. Moreover, the specific gap junction blocker, carbenoxolone, seems to have no effect on SD [37]. More evidence is needed to support the role of gap junctions in SD.

NMDA Receptors

N-methyl-d-aspartate (NMDA) receptors have a critical role in excitatory synaptic transmission, excitotoxicity, and plasticity in the central neuronal system. Both competitive and noncompetitive NMDA receptors blockers are able to modulate SDs. Some of the drugs already tested are AP5, AP7, CPP, CP-101,606, PCP, MK-801, ketamine, Mg^{2+}, Zn^{2+}, and N_2O, which have shown the capacity to elevate SD electrical threshold, block or slow SD propagation, and reduce SD duration and speed [2, 24, 25]. However, the use of most of them is limited because of their harmful side effects.

Many other receptors could be pharmacological targets for SD modulation, such as sigma-1, serotonin, adrenergic, and $GABA_A$ receptors. Studies have shown that drugs acting on these receptors can inhibit SD. However, mechanisms of SD suppression by these receptors are not clear and there are inconsistent results with different dosages and animal models.

Ketamine as a Therapeutic Agent Against Spreading Depolarization

Ketamine, a noncompetitive NDMA receptor blocker, is a phencyclidine derivate used as an anesthetic drug in emergency medicine and intensive care. The active enantiomer is S(+)-ketamine [36]. Ketamine has a number of properties that make it useful for neurointensive care patients, such as improved hemodynamic stability [43], decreased cerebral infarct volume, ameliorated neurological dysfunction after head trauma [41, 42], protection against excitotoxicity [5] and against status epilepticus [32], and, as mentioned above, the capacity of suppressing SD in animal models [24].

There is preliminary evidence of the inhibitory effect of ketamine on SD in patients with neurological disorders. A number of clinical studies explored the use of ketamine on MA and FHM, reporting that an application of 25 mg intranasal ketamine can reduce aura symptoms and severity [1, 26]. A report on two patients suffering from intracranial hemorrhage showed that ketamine perfused at 2–3 mg/kg/h was able to suppress SD development [39]. However, there is conflicting data in a clinical study reporting a case of a patient with SAH where clustered SDs were not suppressed by 2 mg/kg/h of ketamine [13]. This contradictory result can probably be attributed to ketamine's dose-dependent effect on SD. Recently Hertle et al. [25], studying 115 patients with acute brain injury and the effect of different analgesics on SD occurrence, found that ketamine is associated with a reduction of SD and SD in clusters. However, additional prospective clinical trials are needed to explore ketamine's effects and benefits in patients with acute brain injury.

Conclusions

SD is accompanied by significant ionic, metabolic, and hemodynamic changes, which, under pathological conditions, can damage the brain. Even though SD has been known for 69 years, it is only in the past decade that a relationship with migraine aura, traumatic brain injury, and cerebrovascular diseases has been confirmed, and as negatively impacting clinical outcome. Pharmacological modulation of SD could help in diminishing its pathological effects. Many pharmacological targets may help to suppress SD. NMDA receptor blockers, in particular, ketamine, are promising drugs. We expect more testing and development of drugs that modulate SD in the years to come.

Conflict of Interest Statement We declare that we have no conflict of interest.

References

1. Afridi SK, Giffin NJ, Kaube H, Goadsby PJ (2013) A randomized controlled trial of intranasal ketamine in migraine with prolonged aura. Neurology 80(7):642–647
2. Ayata C (2009) Spreading depression: from serendipity to targeted therapy in migraine prophylaxis. Cephalalgia 29(10):1095–1114
3. Ayata C, Jin H, Kudo C, Dalkara T, Moskowitz MA (2006) Suppression of cortical spreading depression in migraine prophylaxis. Ann Neurol 59(4):652–661
4. Bough KJ, Schwartzkroin PA, Rho JM (2003) Calorie restriction and ketogenic diet diminish neuronal excitability in rat dentate gyrus in vivo. Epilepsia 44(6):752–760
5. Brunson KL, Khanna A, Cromwell HC, Cohen RW (2001) Effect of the noncompetitive NMDA antagonists MK-801 and ketamine on the spastic Han-Wistar mutant: a rat model of excitotoxicity. Dev Neurosci 23(1):31–40
6. Costa C, Tozzi A, Rainero I, Cupini LM, Calabresi P, Ayata C, Sarchielli P (2013) Cortical spreading depression as a target for anti-migraine agents. J Headache Pain 14(1):62
7. Dichgans M, Freilinger T, Eckstein G et al (2005) Mutation in the neuronal voltage-gated sodium channel SCN1A in familial hemiplegic migraine. Lancet 366(9483):371–377
8. Dohmen C, Sakowitz OW, Fabricius M et al (2008) Spreading depolarizations occur in human ischemic stroke with high incidence. Ann Neurol 63(6):720–728
9. Dreier JP (2011) The role of spreading depression, spreading depolarization and spreading ischemia in neurological disease. Nat Med 17(4):439–447
10. Dreier JP, Drenckhahn C, Woitzik J et al (2013) Spreading ischemia after aneurysmal subarachnoid hemorrhage. Acta Neurochir Suppl 115:125–129
11. Dreier JP, Ebert N, Priller J et al (2000) Products of hemolysis in the subarachnoid space inducing spreading ischemia in the cortex and focal necrosis in rats: a model for delayed ischemic neurological deficits after subarachnoid hemorrhage? J Neurosurg 93(4):658–666
12. Dreier JP, Körner K, Ebert N et al (1998) Nitric oxide scavenging by hemoglobin or nitric oxide synthase inhibition by N-nitro-L-arginine induces cortical spreading ischemia when K+ is increased in the subarachnoid space. J Cereb Blood Flow Metab 18(9):978–990
13. Dreier JP, Major S, Manning A et al (2009) Cortical spreading ischaemia is a novel process involved in ischaemic damage in patients with aneurysmal subarachnoid haemorrhage. Brain 132(Pt 7):1866–1881
14. Dreier JP, Windmüller O, Petzold G, Lindauer U, Einhäupl KM, Dirnagl U (2002) Ischemia triggered by red blood cell products in the subarachnoid space is inhibited by nimodipine administration or moderate volume expansion/hemodilution in rats. Neurosurgery 51(6):1457–1465; discussion 1465–1467
15. Dreier JP, Woitzik J, Fabricius M et al (2006) Delayed ischaemic neurological deficits after subarachnoid haemorrhage are associated with clusters of spreading depolarizations. Brain 129(Pt 12): 3224–3237
16. Eikermann-Haerter K, Can A, Ayata C (2012) Pharmacological targeting of spreading depression in migraine. Expert Rev Neurother 12(3):297–306
17. Enyedi P, Braun G, Czirják G (2012) TRESK: the lone ranger of two-pore domain potassium channels. Mol Cell Endocrinol 353(1–2): 75–81
18. Fujimoto M, Yanase H (1991) The effect of K(+)-conductance-blocking substances on the occurrence of retinal spreading depression. Exp Eye Res 53(3):333–336
19. De Fusco M, Marconi R, Silvestri L, Atorino L, Rampoldi L, Morgante L, Ballabio A, Aridon P, Casari G (2003) Haploinsufficiency

of ATP1A2 encoding the Na+/K+ pump alpha2 subunit associated with familial hemiplegic migraine type 2. Nat Genet 33(2): 192–196
20. Gorji A (2001) Spreading depression: a review of the clinical relevance. Brain Res Brain Res Rev 38(1–2):33–60
21. Haglund MM, Schwartzkroin PA (1990) Role of Na-K pump potassium regulation and IPSPs in seizures and spreading depression in immature rabbit hippocampal slices. J Neurophysiol 63(2): 225–239
22. Hartings JA, Bullock MR, Okonkwo DO et al (2011) Spreading depolarisations and outcome after traumatic brain injury: a prospective observational study. Lancet Neurol 10(12):1058–1064
23. Hartings JA, Watanabe T, Bullock MR et al (2011) Spreading depolarizations have prolonged direct current shifts and are associated with poor outcome in brain trauma. Brain 134(Pt 5):1529–1540
24. Hernándéz-Cáceres J, Macias-González R, Brozek G, Bures J (1987) Systemic ketamine blocks cortical spreading depression but does not delay the onset of terminal anoxic depolarization in rats. Brain Res 437(2):360–364
25. Hertle DN, Dreier JP, Woitzik J et al (2012) Effect of analgesics and sedatives on the occurrence of spreading depolarizations accompanying acute brain injury. Brain 135(Pt 8):2390–2398
26. Kaube H, Herzog J, Käufer T, Dichgans M, Diener HC (2000) Aura in some patients with familial hemiplegic migraine can be stopped by intranasal ketamine. Neurology 55(1):139–141
27. Kudo C, Toyama M, Boku A, Hanamoto H, Morimoto Y, Sugimura M, Niwa H (2013) Anesthetic effects on susceptibility to cortical spreading depression. Neuropharmacology 67:32–36
28. Kunkler PE, Kraig RP (2004) P/Q Ca2+ channel blockade stops spreading depression and related pyramidal neuronal Ca2+ rise in hippocampal organ culture. Hippocampus 14(3):356–367
29. Lauritzen M, Dreier JP, Fabricius M, Hartings JA, Graf R, Strong AJ (2011) Clinical relevance of cortical spreading depression in neurological disorders: migraine, malignant stroke, subarachnoid and intracranial hemorrhage, and traumatic brain injury. J Cereb Blood Flow Metab 31(1):17–35
30. Leng LZ, Fink ME, Iadecola C (2011) Spreading depolarization: a possible new culprit in the delayed cerebral ischemia of subarachnoid hemorrhage. Arch Neurol 68(1):31–36
31. Leo AAP (1944) Spreading depression of activity in the cerebral cortex. J Neurophysiol 7(6):359–390
32. Loss CM, Córdova SD, de Oliveira DL (2012) Ketamine reduces neuronal degeneration and anxiety levels when administered during early life-induced status epilepticus in rats. Brain Res 1474:110–117
33. Van den Maagdenberg AMJM, Pizzorusso T, Kaja S et al (2010) High cortical spreading depression susceptibility and migraine-associated symptoms in Ca(v)2.1 S218L mice. Ann Neurol 67(1): 85–98
34. Margineanu DG, Klitgaard H (2006) The connexin 36 blockers quinine, quinidine and mefloquine inhibit cortical spreading depression in a rat neocortical slice model in vitro. Brain Res Bull 71(1–3):23–28
35. Martins-Ferreira H, Ribeiro LJ (1995) Biphasic effects of gap junctional uncoupling agents on the propagation of retinal spreading depression. Braz J Med Biol Res 28(9):991–994
36. Mion G, Villevieille T (2013) Ketamine pharmacology: an update (pharmacodynamics and molecular aspects, recent findings). CNS Neurosci Ther 19(6):370–380
37. Peters O, Schipke CG, Hashimoto Y, Kettenmann H (2003) Different mechanisms promote astrocyte Ca2+ waves and spreading depression in the mouse neocortex. J Neurosci 23(30):9888–9896
38. Russell MB, Ducros A (2011) Sporadic and familial hemiplegic migraine: pathophysiological mechanisms, clinical characteristics, diagnosis, and management. Lancet Neurol 10(5):457–470
39. Sakowitz OW, Kiening KL, Krajewski KL, Sarrafzadeh AS, Fabricius M, Strong AJ, Unterberg AW, Dreier JP (2009) Preliminary evidence that ketamine inhibits spreading depolarizations in acute human brain injury. Stroke 40(8):e519–e522
40. Sánchez-Porras R, Zheng Z, Santos E, Schöll M, Unterberg AW, Sakowitz OW (2013) The role of spreading depolarization in subarachnoid hemorrhage. Eur J Neurol 20(8):1121–1127
41. Shapira Y, Artru AA, Lam AM (1992) Ketamine decreases cerebral infarct volume and improves neurological outcome following experimental head trauma in rats. J Neurosurg Anesthesiol 4(4): 231–240
42. Shapira Y, Lam AM, Eng CC, Laohaprasit V, Michel M (1994) Therapeutic time window and dose response of the beneficial effects of ketamine in experimental head injury. Stroke 25(8): 1637–1643
43. Smischney NJ, Beach ML, Loftus RW, Dodds TM, Koff MD (2012) Ketamine/propofol admixture (ketofol) is associated with improved hemodynamics as an induction agent: a randomized, controlled trial. J Trauma Acute Care Surg 73(1):94–101
44. Smith JM, Bradley DP, James MF, Huang CL-H (2006) Physiological studies of cortical spreading depression. Biol Rev Camb Philos Soc 81(4):457–481
45. Somjen GG (2001) Mechanisms of spreading depression and hypoxic spreading depression-like depolarization. Physiol Rev 81(3):1065–1096
46. Tobiasz C, Nicholson C (1982) Tetrodotoxin resistant propagation and extracellular sodium changes during spreading depression in rat cerebellum. Brain Res 241(2):329–333
47. Tottene A, Urbani A, Pietrobon D (2011) Role of different voltage-gated Ca2+ channels in cortical spreading depression: specific requirement of P/Q-type Ca2+ channels. Channels (Austin) 5(2):110–114
48. Wang M, Chazot PL, Ali S, Duckett SF, Obrenovitch TP (2012) Effects of NMDA receptor antagonists with different subtype selectivities on retinal spreading depression. Br J Pharmacol 165(1): 235–244
49. Windmüller O, Lindauer U, Foddis M, Einhäupl KM, Dirnagl U, Heinemann U, Dreier JP (2005) Ion changes in spreading ischaemia induce rat middle cerebral artery constriction in the absence of NO. Brain 128(Pt 9):2042–2051
50. Woitzik J, Dreier JP, Hecht N et al (2012) Delayed cerebral ischemia and spreading depolarization in absence of angiographic vasospasm after subarachnoid hemorrhage. J Cereb Blood Flow Metab 32(2):203–212
51. Wu Y-J, Boissard CG, Greco C et al (2003) (S)-N-[1-(3-morpholin-4-ylphenyl)ethyl]- 3-phenylacrylamide: an orally bioavailable KCNQ2 opener with significant activity in a cortical spreading depression model of migraine. J Med Chem 46(15):3197–3200
52. Zheng Z, Sanchez-Porras R, Santos E, Unterberg AW, Sakowitz OW (2012) Delayed cerebral ischemia after subarachnoid hemorrhage: from vascular spasm to cortical spreading depolarizations. Curr Neurovasc Res 9(4):310–319

Imaging and Endovascular Management

Relationship Between Angiographic Vasospasm, Cerebral Blood Flow, and Cerebral Infarction After Subarachnoid Hemorrhage

Rajat Dhar and Michael N. Diringer

Abstract Delayed cerebral ischemia (DCI) and cerebral infarction are major contributors to poor functional recovery after subarachnoid hemorrhage (SAH). Cerebral vasospasm, the narrowing of proximal intracranial arteries after SAH, has long been assumed to be the primary cause of DCI, and has therefore been the primary therapeutic target in attempts to diminish disability after SAH. However, emerging evidence has questioned the strength and causality of the relationship between vasospasm and DCI. To address this fundamental question, we performed two parallel studies assessing the relationship between the presence of vasospasm in a vascular territory and both regional reductions in cerebral blood flow (CBF) and development of cerebral infarction.

In a cohort of SAH patients at high-risk for DCI, we identified regions of hypoperfusion using positron emission tomography (PET) and compared their distribution with territories exhibiting vasospasm on concurrent angiography. We found that regional hypoperfusion was common in the absence of proximal vasospasm and that some patients without any significant vasospasm still could have hypoperfused brain regions. Similarly, our parallel study demonstrated that both patients and brain territories without vasospasm could develop delayed cerebral infarction, and that such vasospasm-independent infarcts account for more than a quarter of the infarct burden from DCI. These findings suggest that other processes, perhaps at a microvascular level, contribute at least part of the burden of DCI and future interventions should also address these other pathophysiologic processes.

Michael N. Diringer, MD • R. Dhar, MD (✉)
Department of Neurology (Neurocritical Care Section),
Washington University in St. Louis School of Medicine,
Campus Box 8111 660S Euclid Avenue,
St. Louis, MO 63110, USA
e-mail: dharr@neuro.wustl.edu

Keywords Subarachnoid hemorrhage • Cerebral vasospasm • Cerebral blood flow • Cerebral infarction

Introduction

Delayed cerebral ischemia (DCI) is a major threat to recovery in those surviving the ictus of aneurysmal rupture and early period after subarachnoid hemorrhage (SAH). This pathologic process encompasses the development of ischemic neurological deficits and can lead to cerebral infarction and persistent disability. In fact, cerebral infarction is the complication most strongly associated with poor outcome after SAH [15]. Shortly after the recognition that infarcts could occur with SAH, a pathologic narrowing of intracranial arteries was also noted to occur in the days after aneurysmal rupture, an observation made possible by the advent of cerebral angiography [5]. This phenomenon, termed cerebral vasospasm (CVS) is found in as many of 70 % of patients after SAH and thereafter became implicated as the primary factor in the pathogenesis of DCI and infarction. DCI is presumed to result from critical reductions in cerebral blood flow (CBF) that impair energy metabolism, leading to ischemic deficits and, if not corrected, infarction. CVS may reduce distal perfusion, when severe, and was associated with reductions in regional CBF following the development of blood flow measurement techniques such as 15-oxygen PET [7]. Furthermore, patients with CVS appeared to be at high risk for developing delayed neurological deficits [6].

The strength of this relationship between CVS and DCI has promoted confusing nomenclature, such as the term, "symptomatic vasospasm," based on the assumption that the anatomic/angiographic abnormality underlies all or most cases of delayed ischemia after SAH. The presumed causality of this association also formed the basis for numerous trials over the past few decades that have focused on

DOI 10.1007/978-3-319-04981-6_27, © Springer International Publishing Switzerland 2015

preventing or treating CVS, with the ultimate goal of ameliorating the impact of DCI on functional recovery after SAH.

However, the causal and linear relationship between subarachnoid bleeding, proximal artery vascular constriction, reductions in CBF (i.e., hypoperfusion), and delayed ischemia has been challenged by a number of recent observations [11]. First, the majority of patients who develop CVS do not become symptomatic and most do not develop infarcts [2]. Other factors clearly modulate tissue perfusion along with proximal vasospasm, including degree of collaterals, capacity for distal arteriolar vasodilation, systemic blood pressure, and volume status. Notably, there has been discordance between treatments that can significantly reduce vasospasm and the ability of these interventions to improve clinical endpoints such as infarction or functional recovery after SAH [8, 9]. In addition, nimodipine, the only intervention shown to improve outcomes after SAH, did not reliably reduce CVS in most studies [12]. Finally, infarction and not CVS has emerged as the principal intermediate outcome measure that best relates to functional recovery [15, 16]. These inconsistencies, coupled with an increasing appreciation that SAH and DCI involve a complex and multifactorial cascade of processes, has led to a reevaluation of the assumed linear path between CVS and DCI/infarction [17]. To further explore the degree of such discordances between vascular anatomy, physiology, and tissue outcome, we undertook two parallel studies; specifically evaluating the relationship between both cerebral regional hypoperfusion (using quantitative CBF measured by PET) and cerebral infarction with angiographic CVS in vascular territories supplying the same brain regions.

Table 1 Characteristics of two study cohorts

	Cohort 1	Cohort 2
	Hypoperfusion	Cerebral Infarction
Population	Aneurysmal SAH	Aneurysmal SAH
Inclusion criteria	^{15}O-PET performed within 1 day of angiogram	Both postprocedure and predischarge CT (at least 7 days after SAH) performed
Assessment of angiography	Quantitative measurement of proximal stenosis, qualitative assessment of distal vessels	Qualitative assessment by neuroradiologist (retrospective)
Vasospasm defined as	Stenosis ≥50 % or moderate-severe distal narrowing	Moderate-severe in proximal and/or distal vessels
Radiographic measurement	Cerebral blood flow measured in 28 brain regions by PET Hypoperfusion: CBF<25 ml/100 g/min	Cerebral infarct seen on final CT after exclusion of early/ postprocedural infarcts
Number of patients	25	134
Poor Grade (WFNS IV-V)	10 (40 %)	42 (31 %)
Modified Fisher Grade 3-4	23 (92 %)	119 (89 %)
Clip/Coil	15/10	67/67
Angiographic vasospasm in	14 (56 %)	54 (34 %)
Death or discharge to LTC	3 (12 %)	18 (13 %)

Methods

The first study analyzed 25 patients with aneurysmal SAH who underwent ^{15}O-PET imaging within 24 h of cerebral angiography, both performed 4–14 days after SAH when CVS and DCI are at their peak risk [3]. Each delayed angiogram was compared with the patient's baseline study to quantitatively assess the degree of CVS in each proximal intracranial artery, as well as qualitatively assess distal CVS in second- and third-order branches. CVS was judged significant if proximal narrowing was ≥50 % or if distal vasospasm was adjudicated to be moderate-severe in the same territory. For patients who underwent endovascular treatment of CVS and had PET after angiography ($n=4$), we used postintervention measurements of stenosis. PET was processed as previous described, with alignment performed to Talairach atlas space to allow regional measurement of CBF in 28 stereotactically defined brain regions of 10-mm diameter, 3 in each anterior cerebral artery (ACA) and posterior cerebral artery (PCA) territory, and 8 in each middle cerebral artery (MCA) territory [4]. Regions were classified as hypoperfused if CBF was <25 ml/100 g/min; hypoperfusion was then related to presence or absence of significant vasospasm in arteries supplying that region.

In a parallel study, we analyzed the incidence of delayed cerebral infarction and its relationship to CVS in a second cohort of 134 SAH patients [1]. This broader sample included all patients with aneurysmal SAH admitted to our neuro intensive care unit (ICU) within 48 h of rupture, over a 4-year period, who had undergone the necessary sequential brain imaging to adequately delineate and classify infarcts as early vs. delayed (Table 1). To exclude early (including periprocedural infarcts), we only included patients who had imaging at 24–48 h after aneurysm-securing procedures. Presence of eventual infarction was determined from imaging performed 7 or more days after SAH. Patients were excluded if they died within 7 days of SAH or if either CT scans (or routine cerebral angiography) were not available. All final CT scans were analyzed for the presence of well-defined hypodensities, excluding lesions related to hematoma, ventriculostomy, or surgical intervention. Infarcts seen on postprocedure CT (even as evolving low-density regions) were excluded as early infarcts and thus not related to DCI. The volume of all infarcts was calculated by a perimeter tracing method, and each infarct was classified as cortical, deep, or both. Infarct location was also classified into specific vascular territories (ACA, MCA, or PCA), or watershed location. All delayed infarcts were then adjudicated to be related or unrelated to CVS based on whether moderate or severe CVS was reported on any angiograms in the corresponding vascular territory. Watershed infarcts were attributed to CVS if there was moderate-severe CVS in either of the vessels supplying that watershed. Infarcts occurring in the absence of any corresponding CVS were categorized as vasospasm independent.

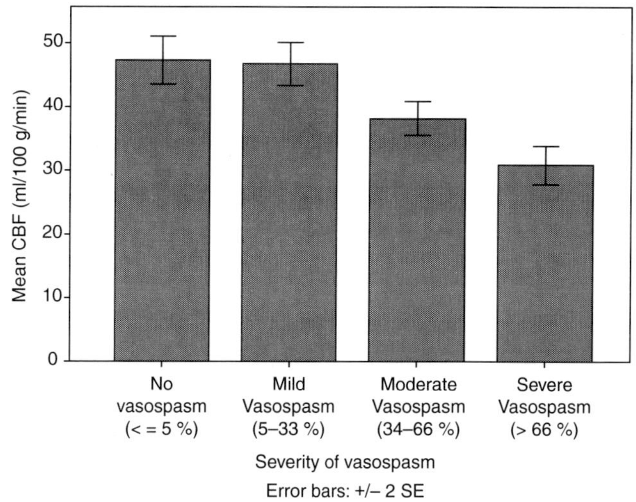

Fig. 1 Mean regional CBF in territories with varying severities of cerebral vasospasm (excluding three patients on vasopressors)

Results

Relationship of Vasospasm and CBF

PET was performed a median of 6 h from time of angiography in this cohort of 25 patients. Fourteen patients had moderate-severe CVS in at least one vascular territory. Although 12 of the patients had symptomatic DCI at some point in their course, only 3 patients were being actively treated with hypertensive therapy at time of PET. Excluding these patients, mean arterial blood pressure was not different between those with and those without CVS. Twenty-four percent of all brain regions were affected by significant (proximal and/or distal) CVS, involving 34 vascular territories across the 14 affected patients. Global mean CBF tended to be lower in patients with CVS (38.4 ± 9.7 vs. 44.3 ± 14.5 ml/100 g/min in those without CVS, $p = 0.07$). Regional CBF was also lower (mean 38.6 ± 11.7) in regions affected by CVS compared with 48.7 ± 16.5 ml/100 g/min in brain regions without CVS ($p < 0.001$). A graded reduction in CBF was seen between mild, moderate, and severe degrees of CVS (Fig. 1). This reduction in perfusion was present whether there was only proximal, only distal, or both proximal and distal CVS present.

More relevant to the question at hand, however, regional hypoperfusion (rCBF < 25 ml/100 g/min) was not confined or even preferentially located within territories affected by CVS. We found regions with low CBF in 10 of 25 patients, including 7 of 14 patients with CVS but also 3 of 11 patients without significant CVS. Nine of these ten patients with hypoperfusion had neurological symptoms during their course, but none were on vasopressors at the time of PET. Interestingly, two of the three patients with hypoperfusion but no CVS still had neurological deficits. A total of 46 brain regions exhibited hypoperfusion (CBF < 25 ml/100 g/min) across ten patients. Regional hypoperfusion did not occur more frequently in territories with significant CVS (15 of 157 affected regions, 10 %) vs. 20 of 217 (9 %) of unaffected regions, even when restricting analysis to only patients with CVS (i.e., comparing territories with and without vasospasm in the same group of patients). Therefore, the majority of regions with hypoperfusion were found outside territories with CVS. In fact, 54 % of hypoperfused regions were located in vascular territories with no CVS anywhere in the ipsilateral carotid (or, if appropriate, vertebrobasilar) circulation. When the 11 patients without CVS were also included, a total of 31 of the 46 (67 %) hypoperfused regions were not in the territory of any affected vessels (Fig. 2). This relationship persisted even after excluding the three patients on vasopressors, in whom treatment could have masked an association between vasospasm and hypoperfusion.

Relationship of Vasospasm to Delayed Cerebral Infarction

Delayed cerebral infarcts were seen in 20 of the 134 patients (15 %) after exclusion of early/procedural infarcts (which accounted for an equivalent proportion of the total infarcts); moderate-severe angiographic CVS was present in 34 % of this cohort. The rate of delayed infarction was higher in those with CVS compared with those without CVS (31 % vs. 4 %, $p < 0.001$), although in one of these patients with CVS and infarction, the infarct actually occurred in a vascular territory without CVS. Fifteen of the 20 patients with delayed infarcts had infarcts in territories with CVS, 4 had infarcts unrelated to CVS, and 1 patient had both infarcts related and

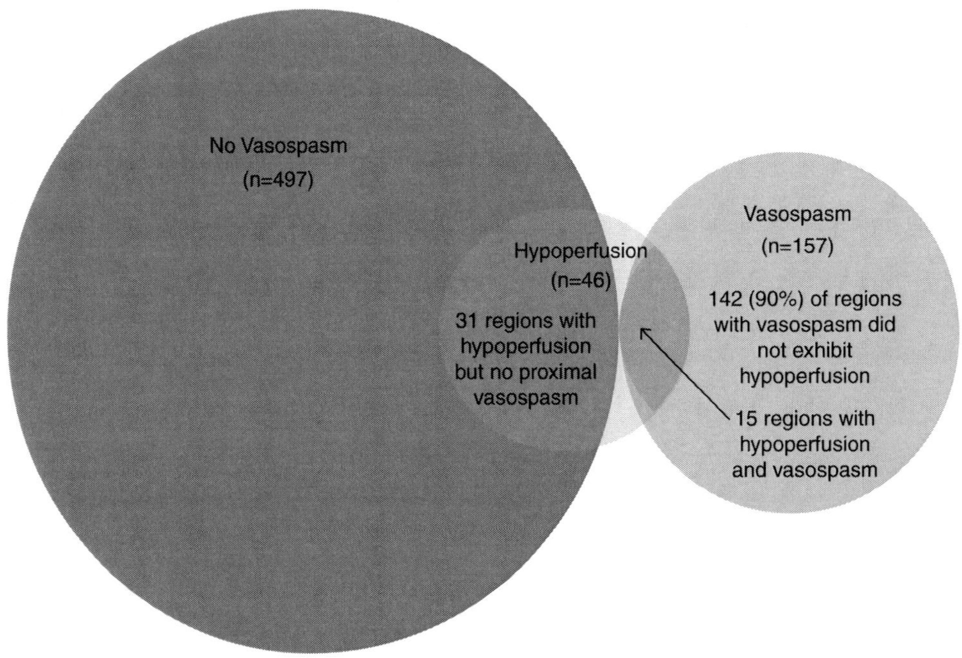

Fig. 2 Venn diagram of brain regions within territories affected and unaffected by cerebral vasospasm, overlapping with regions exhibiting hypoperfusion (CBF < 25 ml/100 g/min)

unrelated to vasospasm. There were no patient characteristics that differentiated these groups, although the number of patients in each group was admittedly low. There were a total of 29 delayed cerebral infarcts, of which 21 were associated with corresponding angiographic CVS, whereas 8 (28 %) occurred in the absence of any proximal CVS. Half of the vasospasm-related infarcts were in the ACA territory whereas no infarcts unrelated to CVS were in the ACA region. Rather, half the vasospasm-unrelated infarcts occurred in watershed territories, compared with 10 % of infarcts seen with CVS ($p=0.03$). There was no difference in volume of these two infarct types and they were evenly divided between cortical and subcortical regions.

Discussion

Vasospasm and Hypoperfusion

We demonstrated that CVS is associated with lower global CBF in affected patients as well as lower regional CBF within affected territories. Still, this association does not confirm a causal or pathophysiologic link between radiographic narrowing and hypoperfusion. It may be that other processes coexist in those with CVS, and it may be these that are primarily responsible or contribute concurrently to reductions in CBF. For example, those at high risk for angiographic CVS are also more likely to develop microcirculatory dysfunction, and the latter could also contribute to tissue hypoperfusion. Our main finding that cerebral hypoperfusion occurs as commonly in the absence of proximal CVS as in its presence further questions the direct relationship between CVS and CBF. Even for patients who had some territories with CVS, hypoperfusion was equally likely to be found in brain regions located outside territories with angiographic abnormality. A similar discordance was found in a study that compared transcranial Doppler (TCD)-defined CVS with PET measurements of hemispheric CBF [10]. Such findings suggest that hypoperfusion (and therefore likely ischemia/DCI) are mediated in significant part by processes other than angiographic CVS alone. These may include distal microcirculatory abnormalities that reduce tissue perfusion, such as impaired vasodilation, microvascular thrombosis, capillary endothelial dysfunction, and cortical spreading depolarizations [13].

Vasospasm and Cerebral Infarction

Our analysis of infarcts after SAH uncovered two major findings. First, delayed infarcts (those typically attributed to DCI and CVS) only account for half of the infarct burden after SAH. This highlights the importance of also addressing early contributors to brain injury such as inflammation, edema, and minimizing procedural complications that could lead to infarcts. Second, a significant minority of even delayed infarcts occurred in territories (and some patients) without angiographic CVS. Although we corroborated that CVS remains a strong risk factor for infarction, fully more than a quarter of delayed infarcts occurred in the absence of corresponding CVS. Such vasospasm-independent infarcts have been previously described [14], but here we captured the size and location of such infarcts in detail. Although they did not appear to differ appreciably from typical vasospasm-related infarcts, they were more likely to be located in a watershed territory. Similar infarct types have been noted in association with cortical spreading depolarization, a phenomenon tied closely to DCI and recently noted to persist even when CVS has been successfully treated [18, 19].

Implications

Although CVS may be associated with and implicated in reductions in cerebral perfusion and the development of cerebral infarcts after SAH, it is becomingly increasingly apparent that this radiographically defined large-vessel process is only the tip of the iceberg of what is going on in the brain of patients after SAH and is only one factor in a complex cascade that cumulatively culminates in ischemia, neuronal injury, and infarction. Such findings remind us that CVS should not continue to be the primary surrogate marker for DCI in clinical trials or be used as the sole target for therapeutic interventions. Instead, minimizing cerebral infarction (and perhaps maintain or restoring cerebral perfusion) appear to the most important targets for future studies [16]. To provide durable benefit to the clinical outcome of patients with SAH, it appears increasingly likely that we must address these other processes that contribute to hypoperfusion and not focus entirely on CVS or its treatment. More research is being undertaken to explore aspects of SAH such as neuroinflammation, cortical depolarizations, and microcirculatory abnormalities. Only with this more holistic viewpoint can we hope to fully understand and mitigate the burden of DCI.

Conflict of Interest This work was supported by grants from the American Heart Association (10SDG3440008) and the National Institutes of Health (NINDS 5P50NS35966-10 and P50NS55977-04).

References

1. Brown RJ, Kumar A, Dhar R, Sampson TR, Diringer MN (2013) The relationship between delayed infarcts and angiographic vasospasm after aneurysmal subarachnoid hemorrhage. Neurosurgery 72(5):702–708
2. Dankbaar JW, Rijsdijk M, Van der Schaaf IC, Velthuis BK, Wermer MJH, Rinkel GJE (2009) Relationship between vasospasm, cerebral perfusion, and delayed cerebral ischemia after aneurysmal subarachnoid hemorrhage. Neuroradiology 51(12):813–819
3. Dhar R, Scalfani MT, Blackburn S, Zazulia AR, Videen T, Diringer M (2012) Relationship between angiographic vasospasm and regional hypoperfusion in aneurysmal subarachnoid hemorrhage. Stroke 43(7): 1788–1794
4. Dhar R, Zazulia AR, Videen TO, Zipfel GJ, Derdeyn CP, Diringer MN (2009) Red blood cell transfusion increases cerebral oxygen delivery in anemic patients with subarachnoid hemorrhage. Stroke 40(9):3039–3044
5. Ecker A, Riemenschneider P (1951) Arteriographic demonstration of spasm of the intracranial arteries, with special reference to saccular arterial aneurysms. J Neurosurg 8(6):660–667
6. Fisher CM, Roberson GH, Ojemann RG (1977) Cerebral vasospasm with ruptured saccular aneurysm – the clinical manifestations. Neurosurgery 1(3):245–248
7. Grubb RL Jr, Raichle ME, Eichling JO, Gado MH, Grubb RL (1977) Effects of subarachnoid hemorrhage on cerebral blood volume, blood flow, and oxygen utilization in humans. J Neurosurg 46(4):446–453
8. Haley EC, Kassell NF, Torner JC (1993) A randomized controlled trial of high-dose intravenous nicardipine in aneurysmal subarachnoid hemorrhage. A report of the Cooperative Aneurysm Study. J Neurosurg 78(4):537–547
9. Macdonald RL, Higashida RT, Keller E et al (2011) Clazosentan, an endothelin receptor antagonist, in patients with aneurysmal subarachnoid haemorrhage undergoing surgical clipping: a randomised, double-blind, placebo-controlled phase 3 trial (CONSCIOUS-2). Lancet Neurol 10(7):618–625
10. Minhas PS, Menon DK, Smielewski P, Czosnyka M, Kirkpatrick PJ, Clark JC, Pickard JD (2003) Positron emission tomographic cerebral perfusion disturbances and transcranial Doppler findings among patients with neurological deterioration after subarachnoid hemorrhage. Neurosurgery 52(5):1017–1024
11. Nolan CP, Macdonald RL (2006) Can angiographic vasospasm be used as a surrogate marker in evaluating therapeutic interventions for cerebral vasospasm? Neurosurg Focus 21(3):E1
12. Petruk KC, West M, Mohr G, Weir BK, Benoit BG, Gentili F, Disney LB, Khan MI, Grace M, Holness RO (1988) Nimodipine treatment in poor-grade aneurysm patients. Results of a multicenter double-blind placebo-controlled trial. J Neurosurg 68(4):505–517
13. Pluta RM, Hansen-Schwartz J, Dreier J et al (2009) Cerebral vasospasm following subarachnoid hemorrhage: time for a new world of thought. Neurol Res 31(2):151–158
14. Rabinstein AA, Friedman JA, Weigand SD, Robyn L, Fulgham JR, Manno EM, Atkinson JLD, Wijdicks EF, McClelland RL (2004) Predictors of cerebral infarction in aneurysmal subarachnoid hemorrhage. Stroke 35(8):1862–1866
15. Rosengart AJ, Schultheiss KE, Tolentino J, Macdonald RL (2007) Prognostic factors for outcome in patients with aneurysmal subarachnoid hemorrhage. Stroke 38(8):2315–2321
16. Vergouwen MDI, Etminan N, Ilodigwe D, Macdonald RL (2011) Lower incidence of cerebral infarction correlates with improved functional outcome after aneurysmal subarachnoid hemorrhage. J Cereb Blood Flow Metab 31(7):1545–1553
17. Vergouwen MDI, Vermeulen M, Van Gijn J et al (2010) Definition of delayed cerebral ischemia after aneurysmal subarachnoid hemorrhage as an outcome event in clinical trials and observational studies: proposal of a multidisciplinary research group. Stroke 41(10):2391–2395
18. Weidauer S, Lanfermann H, Raabe A, Zanella F, Seifert V (2007) Impairment of cerebral perfusion and infarct patterns attributable to vasospasm after aneurysmal subarachnoid hemorrhage. Stroke 38:1831–1836
19. Woitzik J, Dreier JP, Hecht N et al (2011) Delayed cerebral ischemia and spreading depolarization in absence of angiographic vasospasm after subarachnoid hemorrhage. J Cereb Blood Flow Metab 32(2):203–211

Prophylactic Intra-arterial Administration of Fasudil Hydrochloride for Vasospasm Following Subarachnoid Haemorrhage

Satoshi Iwabuchi, M. Hayashi, T. Yokouchi, K. Sato, H. Nakayama, J. Harashina, J. Iwama, M. Ishii, Y. Hiramoto, N. Hirai, Y. Hirata, N. Saito, K. Ito, H. Kimura, and K. Aoki

Abstract *Purpose*: We evaluated patients treated with prophylactic intra-arterial administration of fasudil hydrochloride (IAF) after subarachnoid haemorrhage (SAH).

Materials and Methods: Between August 1998 and December 2012, 92 patients with aneurysmal SAH were treated with IAF for angiographic vasospasm without ischemic symptoms after their follow-up angiography. Patients comprised 50 women and 42 men, aged 24–83 (mean 56.6) years. IAF consisted of 15 mg of fasudil hydrochloride dissolved in 20 ml physiological saline and injected through a catheter during approximately 15 min, after diagnostic angiography. The clinical outcome was evaluated using the Glasgow Outcome Scale (GOS) at discharge and ischemic lesions resulting from vasospasm were assessed on computed tomography (CT) scan at discharge.

Results: Forty-eight patients underwent surgical clipping and 44 patients underwent endovascular coiling. Angiographic improvement was observed in all patients (100 %). At discharge, 76 (83.0 %) of 92 patients showed good recovery on GOS. Nine patients developed progression of delayed ischemic neurological deficits (DIND) and three of these patients had ischemic lesions on CT scans. No patient had any significant changes in vital signs or any other adverse effects resulting from IAF.

Conclusion: IAF therapy was safe and effective for patients with vasospasm following SAH. Prophylactic IAF therapy may prevent symptomatic vasospasm.

Keywords Vasospasm • Fasudil hydrochloride • Intra-arterial administration

Introduction

Fasudil hydrochloride is an inhibitor of myosin light chain kinase [1], which is essential in smooth muscle contraction. Fasudil hydrochloride also inhibits Rho-associated protein kinase, which affects vascular smooth muscle contraction by inactivating myosin light chain phosphatase [2, 8, 10]. Fasudil hydrochloride is effective in preventing vasospasm after subarachnoid haemorrhage [6, 7, 9] and is widely administered intravenously in Japan. In the present study, we evaluated patients treated with prophylactic intra-arterial administration of fasudil hydrochloride (IAF).

Materials and Methods

Between August 1998 and December 2012, 92 patients with aneurysmal subarachnoid haemorrhage (SAH) were treated with IAF for angiographic vasospasm without ischemic symptoms at initial follow-up angiography. Patients comprised 50 women and 42 men, aged 24–83 (mean 56.6) years. A 4-French catheter was inserted via the femoral artery into the cervical portion of the internal carotid artery. IAF consisted of 15 mg of fasudil hydrochloride dissolved in 20 ml physiological saline and injected through a catheter during approximately 15 min, after diagnostic angiography. The procedure was performed once or twice. Overall outcome was assessed at discharge using the Glasgow Outcome Scale (GOS), consisting of five levels [5]: good recovery

S. Iwabuchi (✉) • M. Hayashi • T. Yokouchi • K. Sato
H. Nakayama • J. Harashina • J. Iwama • M. Ishii • Y. Hiramoto
N. Hirai • Y. Hirata • N. Saito • K. Ito • H. Kimura, MD, PhD
K. Aoki
Department of Neurosurgery,
Toho University Ohashi Medical Center, 2-17-6 Ohashi,
Meguro-ku, Tokyo 153-8515, Japan
e-mail: iwabuchi@med.toho-u.ac.jp; hkimura@med.kobe-u.ac.jp

J. Fandino et al. (eds.), *Neurovascular Events After Subarachnoid Hemorrhage*, Acta Neurochirurgica Supplement, Vol. 120,
DOI 10.1007/978-3-319-04981-6_28,

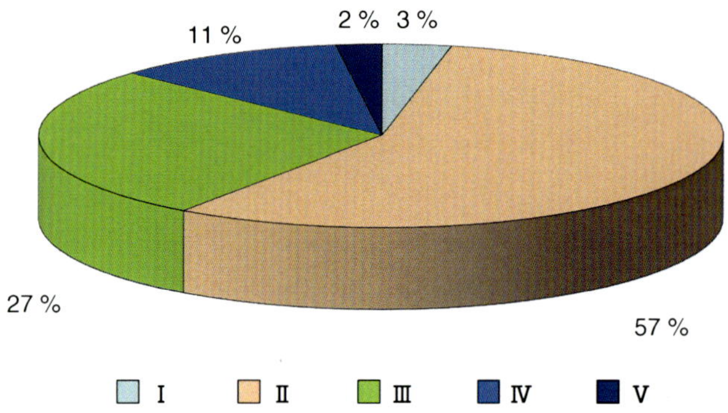

Fig. 1 Hunt and Kosnik grade

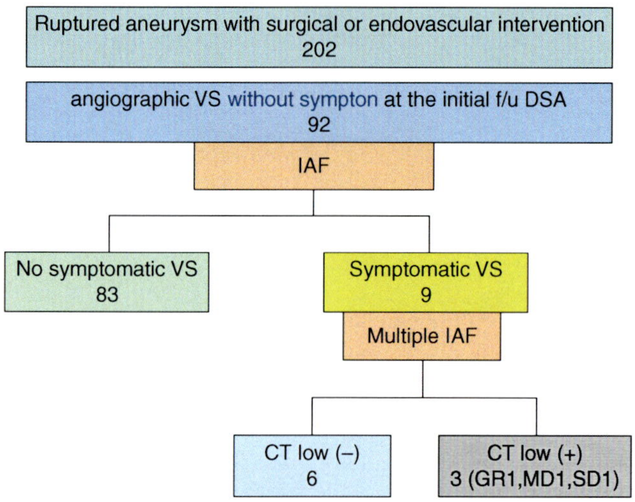

Fig. 2 GOS at discharge

(GR), moderate disability (MD), severe disability (SD), vegetative state (VS) and death (D). This study was approved by the Ethics Committee of Toho University Ohashi Medical Center (approval number 13–31).

Results

Forty-eight patients underwent surgical clipping, and 44 patients underwent endovascular coiling. Hunt and Kosnik grading revealed that 3 % were in Grade I, 57 % in Grade II, 27 % in Grade III, 11 % in Grade IV, and 2 % in Grade V (Fig. 1). Of 202 patients with ruptured aneurysms treated with surgical or endovascular intervention between August 1998 and December 2012, 92 patients presented with angiographic vasospasm without ischemic symptoms at the initial follow-up angiography. Despite IAF treatment for angiographic vasospasm, nine patients developed delayed ischemic neurological deficits (DIND). The interval between prophylactic IAF and presenting DIND was 2–7 (mean 3.8) days. These patients underwent multiple IAF treatment and three had ischemic lesions caused by vasospasm on CT scan at discharge (Fig. 2). GOS at discharge showed that 83 % were in GR, 9 % in MD, 4 % in SD, 3 % in VS, and 1 % in D (Fig. 3). Angiographic improvement was observed on all occasions (100 %). No patient showed any significant changes in vital signs, such as lower blood pressure or symptomatic autonomic responses, or any other adverse effects resulting from IAF.

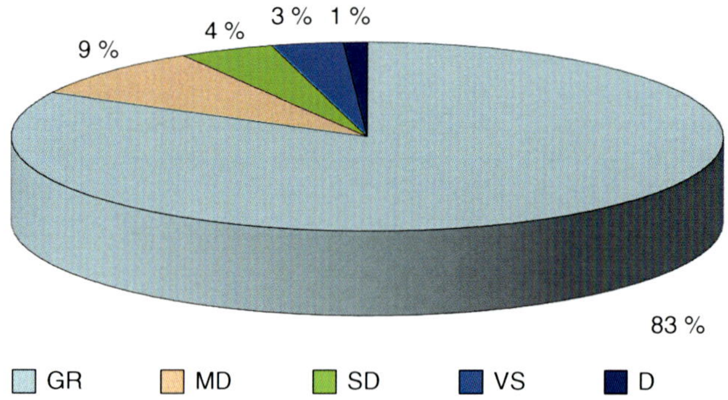

Fig. 3 Number of patients

Discussion

We previously reported the effectiveness of IAF by measuring cerebral circulatory dynamics, as determined by cerebral angiography performed before and after IAF [3]. We found that that the time to peak opacification and the time to half-peak opacification were significantly reduced in the proximal portion of the middle cerebral artery in the early arterial phase after intra-arterial administration of fasudil hydrochloride, and that the time to peak opacification was significantly reduced both in the distal portion of the middle cerebral artery in the late arterial phase and in the transverse sinus in the venous phase. IAF induced dilation of the proximal arteries and improved cerebral microcirculation in patients with vasospasm. We also reported that IAF was clinically safe and effective treatment for patients with vasospasm following SAH [4]. In this study, only three patients (3.2 %) of 92 patients treated with IAF for angiographic vasospasm without ischemic symptom had evidence of ischemic lesion caused by vasospasm on CT at discharge. IAF performed before presentation of symptomatic vasospasm could improve outcome in patients with SAH. IAF for patients with angiographic vasospasm may prevent further progression of vasospasm.

Conclusion

IAF therapy was safe and effective for patients with vasospasm following SAH. Prophylactic IAF therapy may prevent symptomatic vasospasm.

Conflict of Interest Statement The authors have no personal financial or institutional interest in any of the drugs, materials, or devices in the article. All authors have registered online Self-reported Conflict of Disclosure Statement Forms through the website for the Japan Neurosurgical Society members.

References

1. Asano T, Suzuki T, Tsuchiya M, Satoh S, Ikegaki I, Shibuya M, Suzuki Y, Hidaka H (1989) Vasodilator actions of HA1077 in vitro and in vivo putatively mediated by the inhibition of protein kinase. Br J Pharmacol 98:1091–1100
2. Ito K, Shimomura E, Iwanaga T, Shiraishi M, Shindo K, Nakamura J, Nagumo H, Seto M, Sasaki Y, Takuwa Y (2003) Essential role of rho kinase in the Ca^{2+} sensitization of prostaglandin $F_2\alpha$-induced contraction of rabbit aortae. J Physiol 546:823–836
3. Iwabuchi S, Yokouchi T, Hayashi M, Uehara H, Ueda M, Samejima H (2006) Intra-arterial administration of fasudil hydrochloride for vasospasm following subarachnoid hemorrhage: analysis of time-density curve with digital subtraction angiography. Neurol Med Chir (Tokyo) 46:535–540
4. Iwabuchi S, Yokouchi T, Hayashi M, Sato K, Saito N, Hirata Y, Harashina J, Nakayama H, Akahata M, Ito K, Aoki K (2011) Intra-arterial administration of fasudil hydrochloride for vasospasm following subarachnoid haemorrhage. Experience of 90 cases. Acta Neurochir Suppl 110:179–181
5. Jannett B, Bond M (1975) Assessment of outcome after severe brain damage. A practical scale. Lancet 1:480–484
6. Masaoka H, Takasato Y, Nojiri T, Hayakawa T, Akimoto H, Yatsushige H, Toumori H, Miyazaki Y, Honma M (2001) Clinical effect of Fasudil hydrochloride for cerebral vasospasm following subarachnoid hemorrhage. Acta Neurochir Suppl (Wien) 77:209–211
7. Satoh S, Yamamoto Y, Toshima Y, Ikegaki I, Asano T, Suzuki Y, Shibuya M (1999) Fasudil, a protein kinase inhibitor, prevents the development of endothelial injury and neutrophil infiltration in a two-haemorrhage canine subarachnoid model. J Clin Neurosci 6:394–399
8. Seto M, Takuwa Y, Sasaki Y (1992) The molecular mechanism of vasospasm and the attenuation by fasudil. Nippon Yakurigaku Zasshi 114:66–70
9. Shibuya M, Suzuki Y, Sugita K, Saito I, Sasaki T, Takakura K, Nagata I, Kikuchi H, Takemae T, Hidaka H et al (1992) Effect of AT877 on cerebral vasospasm after aneurysmal subarachnoid hemorrhage. J Neurosurg 76:571–577
10. Shimokawa H, Seto M, Katsumata N, Amano M, Kozai T, Yamawaki T, Kuwata K, Kandabashi T, Egashira K, Ikegaki I, Asano T, Kaibuchi K, Takeshita A (1999) Rho-kinase-mediated pathway induces enhanced myosin light chain phosphorylations in a swine model of coronary artery spasm. Cardiovasc Res 43:1029–1039

Proximal Arterial Diameters on CT Angiography and Digital Subtraction Angiography Correlate Both at Admission and in the Vasospasm Period After Aneurysmal Subarachnoid Hemorrhage

Hassen Kerkeni, Bawarjan Schatlo, Hiroki Dan-Ura, Luca Remonda, Carl Muroi, Michael Diepers, Javier Fandino, and Ali-Reza Fathi

Abstract *Background*: Comparison of artery diameters between CT angiography (CTA) and subtraction arteriography (DSA) has the limitation that measurements on DSA are provided as relative units, making a quantitative comparison difficult. On CTA, artery diameters may depend on windowing settings and may lead to false measurements. This study assesses the correlation between CTA and DSA based on measurements in a basic imaging viewer using normalized DSA values, and assesses whether the validity is time dependent.

Methods: Patients with aneurysmal subarachnoid hemorrhage (aSAH) were included if they underwent both CTA and DSA within 24 h. The analysis was performed using the basic imaging application Centricity Enterprise PACS viewer (GE Healthcare). A total of 15 arterial locations were assessed on CTA and DSA and a specific measurement protocol with normalization of all artery diameters to the cavernous segment of the internal carotid artery was used. Pearson correlation analysis was calculated to access the correlation of normalized arterial diameters measured with both methods at admission and at clinical onset of CVS.

Results: A total of 627 arteries in 38 patients were analyzed in both CTA and DSA. There was a significant correlation coefficient ($R=0.706$) of artery diameters between CTA and DSA measures ($p<0.0001$). This correlation remained high when comparing CTA and DSA at admission (correlation coefficient: 0.641; $p<0.0001$) vs. in the vasospasm period (0.835; $p<0.0001$). The correlation was good in all proximal artery segments and lost significance only when distal vessel segments were considered.

Conclusion: Using basic imaging viewers, mostly accessible for clinicians, CTA is a noninvasive and reliable method to assess proximal arterial diameters of the brain in the management of cerebral vasospasm in the acute phase after aSAH. Significance is reached, independent of whether CTA is obtained in the acute phase or during the period of vasospasm, by normalization of basal cerebral artery diameters to a nonvariable anatomic landmark, i.e., the petrous or cavernous internal carotid artery diameter.

Keywords Cerebral angiography • Subarachnoid hemorrhage • CT angiography • Intracranial aneurysm • Vasospasm

H. Kerkeni • B. Schatlo, MD • H. Dan-Ura, MD
J. Fandino, MD • A.-R. Fathi, MD (✉)
Department of Neurosurgery, Kantonsspital Aarau, Aarau, Switzerland
e-mail: javier.fandino@ksa.ch; ali-reza.fathi@ksa.ch

C. Muroi, MD
Department of Neurosurgery, Kantonsspital Aarau, Tellstrasse 1, Aarau 5001, Switzerland

Department of Intensive Care Medicine, University and University Hospital Bern, Bern, Switzerland

Department of Neuropharmacology, Faculty of Pharmaceutical Sciences, Fukuoka University, Fukuoka, Japan

Neurocritical Care Unit, Department of Neurosurgery, University Hospital Zurich, Zurich, Switzerland
e-mail: carl.muroi@ksa.ch

L. Remonda, MD • M. Diepers
Department of Neuroradiology, Kantonsspital Aarau, Tellstrasse, Aarau 5001, Switzerland

Division of Neuroradiology, Department of Radiology, Kantonsspital Aarau, Aarau, Switzerland

J. Fandino et al. (eds.), *Neurovascular Events After Subarachnoid Hemorrhage*, Acta Neurochirurgica Supplement, Vol. 120,
DOI 10.1007/978-3-319-04981-6_29, © Springer International Publishing Switzerland 2015

Introduction

Delayed cerebral vasospasm remains a severe complication following aneurysmal subarachnoid hemorrhage (aSAH). Its timely detection is one of the goals of intensive care monitoring in these patients. CT angiography (CTA) is established as a routine screening tool and provides noninvasive information on cerebral artery diameters [1, 2]. However, it is unclear whether this information is potentially equivalent to the gold standard imaging modality, digital subtraction arteriography (DSA) resolution images. Measurements of vessel diameter on DSA depend on various factors, including magnification, source of image to detector distance, and viewing angle. Moreover, when images are evaluated using basic imaging viewers, measurements are often only available in relative units. Therefore, there is a need for a standardized assessment without the use of an absolute scale. The goals of our study were (1) to develop and evaluate a standardized measurement paradigm to compare CTA and DSA arterial diameters and (2) to assess whether the correlation depends on whether a scan is obtained early after admission or in the vasospasm phase.

Methods

Patients from an institutional database at the Kantonsspital Aarau with aSAH were included if they underwent both CTA and DSA within 24 h. The time points of CTA and DSA were assigned to the early (<4 days after SAH) and vasospasm period (>4 days) group. Analyses were performed by neurosurgeons using the basic imaging application, Centricity Enterprise PACS viewer (GE Healthcare). A total of 15 arterial locations (7 arteries on each side plus the basilar artery (BA)) were examined: the suprasellar internal carotid artery (ICA), the M1 and M2 segments of the middle cerebral artery, the A1 and A2 segments of the anterior cerebral artery, the P1 and P2 segments of the posterior cerebral artery, and the basilar artery. Measures in DSA were taken in anterior–posterior views for the following arteries: the proximal and distal segments of the anterior cerebral artery (A1 and A2), the proximal and distal segments of the middle cerebral artery (M1 and M2), and the petrous or cavernous and communicating segments of the internal carotid artery. Additionally, measures of the basilar artery and of the proximal and distal segments of the posterior cerebral arteries (P1 and P2) were taken in anterior–posterior DSA views. In CTA, measures of the petrous or cavernous segment of the internal carotid artery and those of the basilar artery were taken in sagittal views. Measures of the proximal and distal segments of anterior cerebral artery (A1 and A2) and those of the middle cerebral artery (M1and M2) were obtained in coronal views. Measures of the proximal and the distal segments of the posterior cerebral artery (P1 and P2) were obtained with transverse views.

On DSA, arterial diameters were recorded as relative values by normalizing them to the diameter of the petrous or cavernous segment of the internal carotid artery (Fig. 1). The relative values for vessel diameter are obtained using the formula (diameter of measured vessel/diameter of petrous or cavernous ICA) × 100. CTA arterial diameters were measured in millimeters. Contrast was adjusted manually. Diameters were arbitrarily normalized to the petrous or cavernous segment of the internal carotid artery in the sagittal plane (Fig. 1). Pearson correlation analysis was calculated to access the correlation of normalized arterial diameters measured with both methods.

Results

Between 2009 and 2012, we retrospectively studied 128 cases of aneurysmal subarachnoid hemorrhage. Of these, a total of 91 patients underwent CTA due to clinically suspected vasospasm (the appearance of a new neurological deficit or increased Doppler velocity values). Of these, 38 patients had DSA within 24 h of CTA and were available for the final analysis. Fifteen of these were men and 23 women with ages ranging from 42 to 64 years (mean, 53 years). The mean time difference between the CTA and DSA was 10 h and 18 min. A total of 627 arteries were studied in both CTA and DSA. We assessed the correlation between CTA and DSA at admission and at clinical onset of CVS. The correlation between CTA and DSA at admission was 0.641 ($p<0.0001$; Fig. 2). The correlation between CTA and DSA in the vasospasm period was 0.835, with a significant p value ($p<0.0001$; Fig. 2). The overall correlation regardless of the timing of the imaging between CTA and DSA was 0.706, with a significant p value ($p<0.0001$; Fig. 2). The correlations for the different measured arterial segments are displayed in detail in Table 1. All proximal arterial segments (BA, A1, M1, P1) revealed significant correlations between CTA and DSA ($p<0.05$). However, distal arterial segments appeared to not be reliable enough for the assessment of the arterial diameter on CTA, with a low correlation ($p>0.05$). The correlation for the proximal middle cerebral artery (M1) is displayed in Fig. 2.

Discussion

The main finding of this study is that CTA is a reliable, fast, and noninvasive tool to assess proximal cerebral artery diameters during the management of cerebral vasospasm

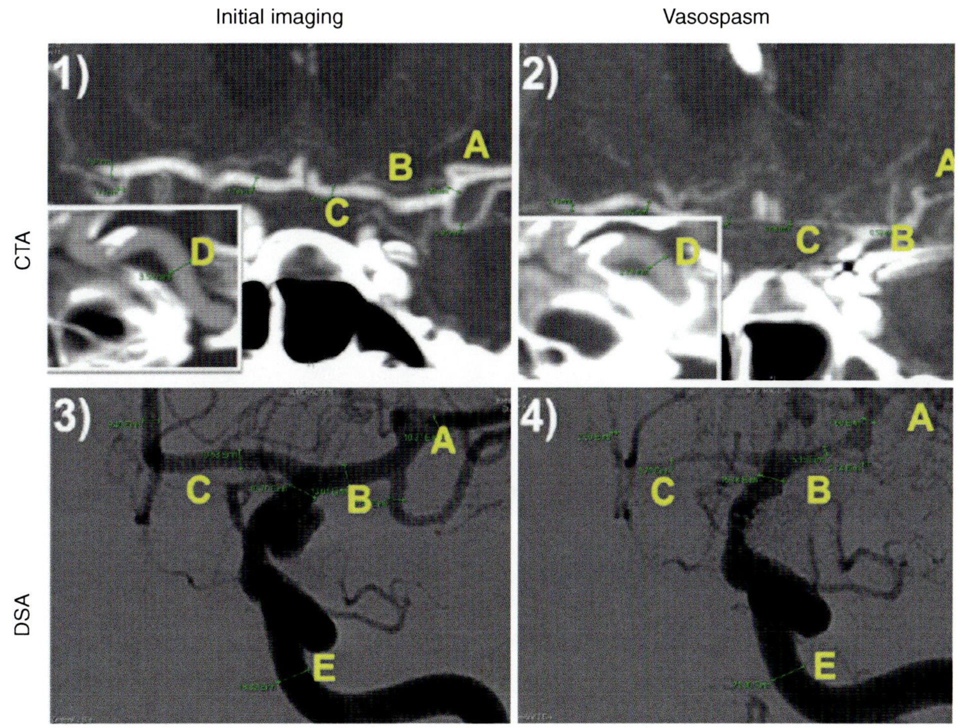

Fig. 1 Illustration of a selection of measured parameters. *Above*: CTA, *below*: DSA. *Left*: Initial imaging at admission. *Right*: imaging during the vasospasm period. The petrous or cavernous segments (depending on visibility) were taken as reference for normalization in the AP view. *A* Middle cerebral artery, M2 segment; *B* M1 segment of the middle cerebral artery; *C* anterior cerebral artery, A1 segment; *D* and *E* internal carotid artery, cavernous and petrous segments, respectively

after aSAH. CTA has emerged as an alternative noninvasive modality for imaging of the cerebral arteries. Its usefulness was demonstrated for imaging and therapeutic decision making for cerebral aneurysms [3–5]. In this study, we assessed the reliability of CTA as a noninvasive, alternative imaging tool for the diagnosis of cerebral arterial vasospasm. Angiographic vasospasm is seen up to 40–70 % of patients and leads to ischemic deficits in 15–36 % of patients [6–9]. It usually occurs in a delayed fashion from 48 h to 14 days after hemorrhage [10, 11]. CTA has been compared with DSA for assessment of vasospasm in several prospective [12, 13] and retrospective [1, 14–16] studies. These studies showed high accuracy of CTA for the diagnosis of severe and proximal vasospasm. However, there is little mention of how vessel diameters were measured, and inaccuracies induced by using maximum intensity projections on CTA or by the lack of a millimeter scale in DSA have not been addressed to date. By normalizing all arterial diameters to the diameter of the extradural segment of the internal carotid artery, we tried to develop an objective and easy tool for clinicians to evaluate vasospasm in patients after aneurysmal SAH. This method succeeded in all proximal artery segments independently of the time point of measurements. Moreover, our study yielded lower correlation between CTA and DSA for the diagnosis of peripheral vasospasm as compared with proximal vasospasm. This finding confirms the notion that in vasospasm, the evaluation of post-bifurcation segments A1, M2, and P2 is beyond the resolution of CTA. Another limitation is poor image quality of CTA caused by movement artifact or the presence of streak artifacts from metal devices that obscure adjacent arteries.

The strength of the present analysis is that CTA and DSA were performed within 24 h, which is a relatively short succession in clinical terms. This is explained by the fact that, after documentation of vasospasm on CTA, a trial of hyperdynamic therapy was performed which, in case of failure, was rapidly complemented with DSA. Nonetheless, the concern of potential time-dependent vascular caliber fluctuations remains. Future investigations should include the correlation between vasospasm severity in both CTA and DSA and the likelihood of perfusion abnormality in perfusion imaging.

Conclusions

Even when measuring vessels on a basic imaging viewer, CTA is a reliable noninvasive screening tool for assessing diameters of proximal cerebral artery segments. Significant correlations between CTA and DSA can be obtained using basic viewers for the assessment of delayed cerebral vasospasm by normalization of basal cerebral artery diameters to a nonvariable anatomical landmark, i.e., the petrous or cavernous internal carotid artery diameter. Further investigation toward an optimized and standardized comparison protocol is warranted.

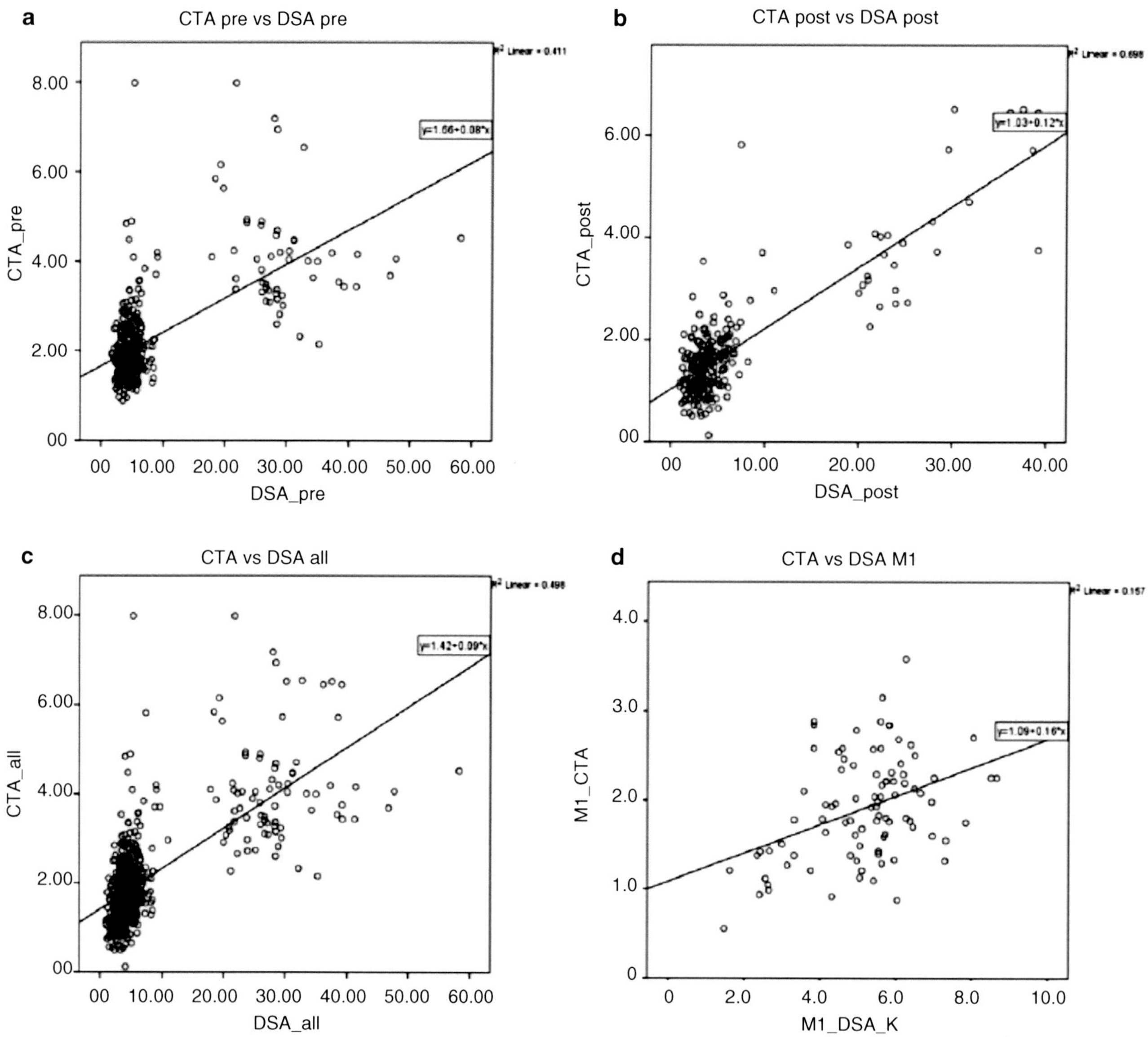

Fig. 2 The x-axis represents diameters obtained from DSA after normalization. The y-axis represents diameters obtained from CTA. (**a**) CTA and DSA by admission before the vasospasm period showed a significant correlation of 0.641 ($p<0.0001$); (**b**) CTA and DSA also correlated in the vasospasm period (Pearson coefficient of 0.835 ($p<0.0001$)); (**c**) the overall correlation of CTA and normalized DSA values was good, at 0.706 ($p<0.0001$); (**d**) example of correlation between CTA and DSA of M1 segment caliber showing a correlation of 0.396 ($p<0.0001$)

Table 1 Pearson's Correlation Coefficient and significance levels were calculated for CTA and DSA in the following artery segments: M1 (proximal middle cerebral artery), M2 (post bifurcation branches of middle cerebral artery), A1 (anterior cerebral artery), A2 (pericallosal artery), P1 (pre-communicating posterior cerebral artery), P2 (post-communicating posterior cerebral artery), and basilar artery trunk

Segment	Correlation	*P*-value
A1	0.488	<0.0001
A2	0.149	0.152
M1	0.396	<0.0001
M2	0.093	0.385
P1	0.344	0.003
P2	0.201	0.078
Basilar	0.450	0.005

Conflict of Interest Statement We declare that we have no conflict of interest

References

1. Anderson GB et al (2000) CT angiography for the detection of cerebral vasospasm in patients with acute subarachnoid hemorrhage. AJNR Am J Neuroradiol 21:1011–1015
2. Shankar JJS, Tan IYL, Krings T, Terbrugge K, Agid R (2012) CT angiography for evaluation of cerebral vasospasm following acute subarachnoid haemorrhage. Neuroradiology 54: 197–203
3. Agid R, Lee SK, Willinsky RA, Farb RI, terBrugge KG (2006) Acute subarachnoid hemorrhage: using 64-slice multidetector CT angiography to "triage" patients' treatment. Neuroradiology 48:787–794
4. Westerlaan HE, Gravendeel J, Fiore D, Metzemaekers JD, Groen RJ, Mooij JJ, Oudkerk M (2007) Multislice CT angiography in the selection of patients with ruptured intracranial aneurysms suitable for clipping or coiling. Neuroradiology 49:997–1007
5. Schuknecht B (2007) High-concentration contrast media (HCCM) in CT angiography of the carotid system: impact on therapeutic decision making. Neuroradiology 49(Suppl 1):S15–S26
6. van Gijn J, Kerr RS, Rinkel GJ (2007) Subarachnoid haemorrhage. Lancet 369:306–318
7. Kidwell CS, Saver JL, Mattiello J et al (2001) Diffusion-perfusion MRI characterization of post-recanalization hyperperfusion in humans. Neurology 57:2015–2021
8. Cenic A, Nabavi DG, Craen RA et al (2000) A CT method to measure hemodynamics in brain tumors: validation and application of cerebral blood flow maps. AJNR Am J Neuroradiol 21:462–470
9. ICRP (1990) Recommendation of the international commission on radiological protection, ICRP publication no. 60. Pergamon, Oxford
10. Deitrich HH, Dacey RG (2000) Molecular keys to the problems of cerebral vasospasm. Neurosurgery 46:517–530
11. Sehba FA, Ding WH, Chereshnev I, Bederson JB (1999) Effects of S-nitrosoglutathione on acute vasoconstriction and glutamate release after subarachnoid hemorrhage. Stroke 30:1955–1961
12. Chaudhary SR, Ko N, Dillon WP, Yu MB, Liu S, Criqui GI, Higashida RT, Smith WS, Wintermark M (2008) Prospective evaluation of multidetector-row CT angiography for the diagnosis of vasospasm following subarachnoid hemorrhage: a comparison with digital subtraction angiography. Cerebrovasc Dis 25:144–150
13. Goldsher D, Shreiber R, Shik V, Tavor Y, Soustiel JF (2004) Role of multisection CT angiography in the evaluation of vertebrobasilar vasospasm in patients with subarachnoid hemorrhage. AJNR Am J Neuroradiol 25:1493–1498
14. Takagi R, Hayashi H, Kobayashi H, Kumazaki T, Isayama K, Ikeda Y, Teramoto A (1998) Three-dimensional CT angiography of intracranial vasospasm following subarachnoid haemorrhage. Neuroradiology 40:631–635
15. Otawara Y, Ogasawara K, Ogawa A, Sasaki M, Takahashi K (2002) Evaluation of vasospasm after subarachnoid hemorrhage by use of multislice computed tomographic angiography. Neurosurgery 51:939–942; discussion 942–943
16. Yoon DY, Choi CS, Kim KH, Cho BM (2006) Multidetector-row CT angiography of cerebral vasospasm after aneurysmal subarachnoid hemorrhage: comparison of volume-rendered images and digital subtraction angiography. AJNR Am J Neuroradiol 27:370–377

Invasive Intracranial Arterial Pressure Monitoring During Endovascular Cerebral Aneurysms Embolization for Cerebral Perfusion Evaluation

Andriy M. Netlyukh, Volodymyr M. Shevaga, Leonid M. Yakovenko, Angelika V. Payenok, Victor M. Salo, and Oleg Ja. Kobyletskiy

Abstract The purpose of the study was to define a method of estimation of cerebral blood flow by a determination of parameters of the hemodynamics during neuroendovascular procedures.

Materials and Methods. Extracranial and intracranial mean arterial pressure (MAP) was invasively monitored with the help of a transducing system during an endovascular coiling procedure in 19 patients. The measurements were performed at the tip of the guiding catheter and microcatheter placed into internal carotid artery (ICA) C1 segments and of the microcatheter placed into C4 ICA segments, at different stages of the aneurysm repair.

Results. As measured, the diameter of the ICA in the C1 and C4 segments did not differ substantially. MAP in the ICA was determined to be 91.2 ± 9.6 mmHg in the skull cavity, and 102.4 ± 6.3 mmHg outside of the skull cavity, with an average difference of 9.2 ± 3.0 mmHg.

Conclusion. The difference in MAP, as measured in the ICA outside and inside the skull cavity, was ascribed to the influence of intracranial pressure. Further investigation is required to check the accuracy of invasive intra-arterial pressure recording for an objective and direct measurement of the cerebral perfusion in reference to the intracranial pressure level.

Keywords Cerebral arterial aneurysm • Endovascular treatment • Cerebral perfusion pressure • Intracranial pressure • Invasive arterial pressure monitoring

A.M. Netlyukh, MD (✉) • V.M. Shevaga
A.V. Payenok • O.J. Kobyletskiy
Lviv National Medical University named after Danylo Halitsky, Pekarska str. 69, Lvov 79010, Ukraine
e-mail: romaivanova-mail@rambler.ru

L.M. Yakovenko
The State Institution "Institute of Neurosurgery named after acad. A.P. Romodanov of NAMS of Ukraine",
Mayborody str. 32, Kyiv 04050, Ukraine

V.M. Salo
Lviv Municipal Emergency Hospital,
Mykolaichuka str. 9, Lvov 79059, Ukraine

Introduction

Invasive intra-arterial pressure monitoring is commonly used in intensive care departments [1] and is also often used during surgical operations. The purpose of intra-arterial measurement of the blood pressure is to record the arterial pressure during every heartbeat [3]. Factors such as vasospasm and intracranial hypertension (ICH) result in worsening of postoperative results after operations on arterial aneurysms of brain vessels and are well documented. ICH and vasospasm occurring separately do not always result in ischemic damage to the brain during a subarachnoid hemorrhage (SAH). However, the combined action of both factors can promote cerebral ischemia. If vasospasm occurs together with ICH, it causes an increase of the cerebral blood flow resistance, which can result in the development of a secondary ischemic brain damage, followed by a neurological deficit, increase of intracranial pressure (ICP), and brain distortion and herniation [6]. In accordance with the generally accepted standards of intensive therapy, the correction of ICH must be conducted with the ICP under control. Intraparenchymal sensors are the most modern devices for ICP control, in which a transducer is located on the distal end of a catheter inserted into the brain parenchyma (the fiber optic transducer "Camino" and the microsensor "Codman" are commonly used). Sensors of this type are characterized by high precision and minimal injury to the brain tissue and do not require repeated calibration. This method of monitoring has not been widely adopted because of a lack of specialized equipment and the high cost of the sensors [1].

Diagnosing brain ischemia is also possible on the basis of a continuous registration of the cerebral perfusion pressure (CPP). CPP is the difference between the mean arterial pressure (MAP) and the ICP. Estimation of CPP requires both implantation of an ICP sensor and an invasive placement of an arterial catheter for measurement of the arterial pressure (AP). Adequate CPP under normal conditions is 70–100 mmHg. Cerebral blood circulation fails to meet

J. Fandino et al. (eds.), *Neurovascular Events After Subarachnoid Hemorrhage*, Acta Neurochirurgica Supplement, Vol. 120,
DOI 10.1007/978-3-319-04981-6_30,

the metabolic requirements of the brain tissue, resulting in hypoxia and cerebral ischemia, if CPP falls below 50 mmHg [9]. Decline of CPP below this threshold caused by arterial hypotension is especially dangerous for the damaged brain, because it strengthens ischemia, which, in turn, amplifies the syndrome of ICH. Based on data by Russian authors [6], CPP below 70 mmHg is a factor that provokes neuronal ischemia and a secondary neurological deficit [6]. The disadvantages of this method are that it relies on a calculation, in that CPP is the difference between the MAP and the ICP, and on the use of invasive procedures, a puncture and cannulation of an artery (for MAP) and an implantation of intracranial sensor (for ICP). Thus, an error in one of the measurements results in a calculation error for CPP.

Grinenko et al. [8] conducted an evaluation of cerebral blood flow by transcranial dopplerography measuring systolic linear flow velocity (LFVsyst) and a continuous registration of ICP simultaneously. This allowed the authors to adequately estimate the severity of both complications of acute SAH, namely, of vasospasm and ICH, in their interdependence. The combined study of ICP and blood flow showed that LFVsyst itself is not an indicator for severity and dynamics of vasospasm under ICH. Early diagnosis of ICH allows for a timely application of dehydration therapy, amelioration of the venous blood outflow from the skull cavity, an improvement of the arterial blood flow by decreasing the peripheral vascular resistance, and an adequate delivery of oxygen to the brain tissues. Absence of an adequate response to the therapy as evidenced by the persistent syndrome of ICH (ICP ≥ 30 mmHg) at LFVsyst even ≤200 cm/s was accompanied by ischemic damage to the brain tissue, which resulted in worsening of the neurological deficit and in unfavorable treatment results [8].

For patients in critical condition, intra-arterial pressure monitoring provides access for frequent arterial blood specimens and also helps in the differential diagnosis of certain malicious conditions. It is an additional instrument that can be used by an experienced clinician for improving a patient's treatment [2]. Below, we list the general principles of invasive AP monitoring during endovascular cerebral aneurysm embolization and also describe equipment that can provide high accuracy for invasive AP measurement [3]. In general, (1) the catheter in the artery must be as short as possible, with a maximal diameter; (2) the length of the liquid line must be as short as possible; (3) the catheter and tubes must have rigid walls; and (4) the diaphragm of the transducer must be as rigid as possible.

According to information by other authors [4, 7], although intravascular catheters of small diameter reduce the natural frequency of vibrations, they allow for improved functionalities of the system with a low dumping coefficient and for diminishment of the risk of complications. Figure 1 shows a typical curve observed during invasive measurement of AP in an aorta.

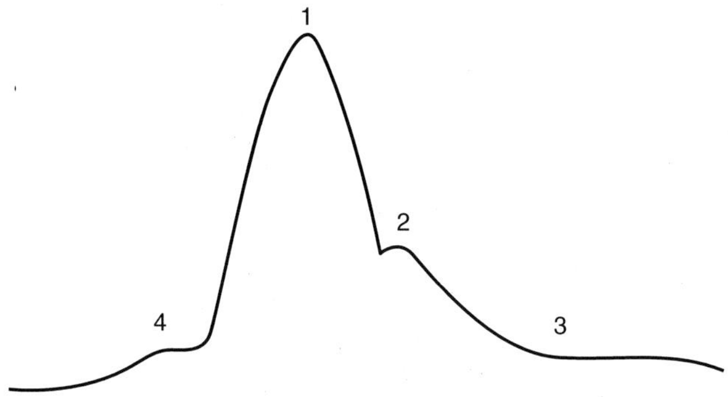

Fig. 1 Typical pattern of AP dynamics measured invasively in aorta: (*1*) peak systolic pressure; (*2*) dicrotic notch; (*3*) diastolic pressure; (*4*) anacrotic notch [5]

Dicrotic notch occurs at the instant of the closing of the aortic valve, when the pressure in aorta becomes higher than in the left ventricle. This moment signifies the end of systole and the beginning of diastole. An anacrotic notch occurs at the beginning of systole, before the instant of the opening of the aortic valve, and is only observed during monitoring of the pressure in the aorta, or during certain pathologic conditions [5]. To summarize, existing methods to study cerebral perfusion exhibit a series of limitations: invasiveness, insufficient accuracy, and high probability of diagnostic errors. Thus, improvement is needed.

Materials and Methods

This study of the procedure for invasive measurement of AP was conducted during endovascular operations on 19 patients. Operations were performed on patients with ruptures of anterior circulation arterial aneurysms. Real-time comparative recordings of AP were performed in the internal carotid artery (ICA) inside and outside of the skull cavity, and also inside the aneurysm lumen; AP was also measured noninvasively on the humeral artery with a blood pressure cuff.

The invasive monitoring of AP was executed under fluoroscopic control during different stages of operation; in the magisterial artery, with standard guiding catheters (length, 100 cm; internal diameter, 1.63 mm) and, in the cavity of the aneurysm, with a standard microcatheter (length, 150 cm; internal diameter, 0.4 mm). Measurements of AP in the magisterial artery both inside and outside of the skull cavity were conducted through a standard microcatheter. Invasive measurement of AP inside the skull cavity was conducted in the proximal (vertical) part of the C4 segment of the ICA. Outside the skull cavity, the measurement was carried out in the distal part of the C1 segment of the ICA (Fig. 2). Results were recorded by the monitor "Utas" UM 300 with the help of a transducer that was calibrated, then attached through a liquid line to the cannula of the catheter. Before

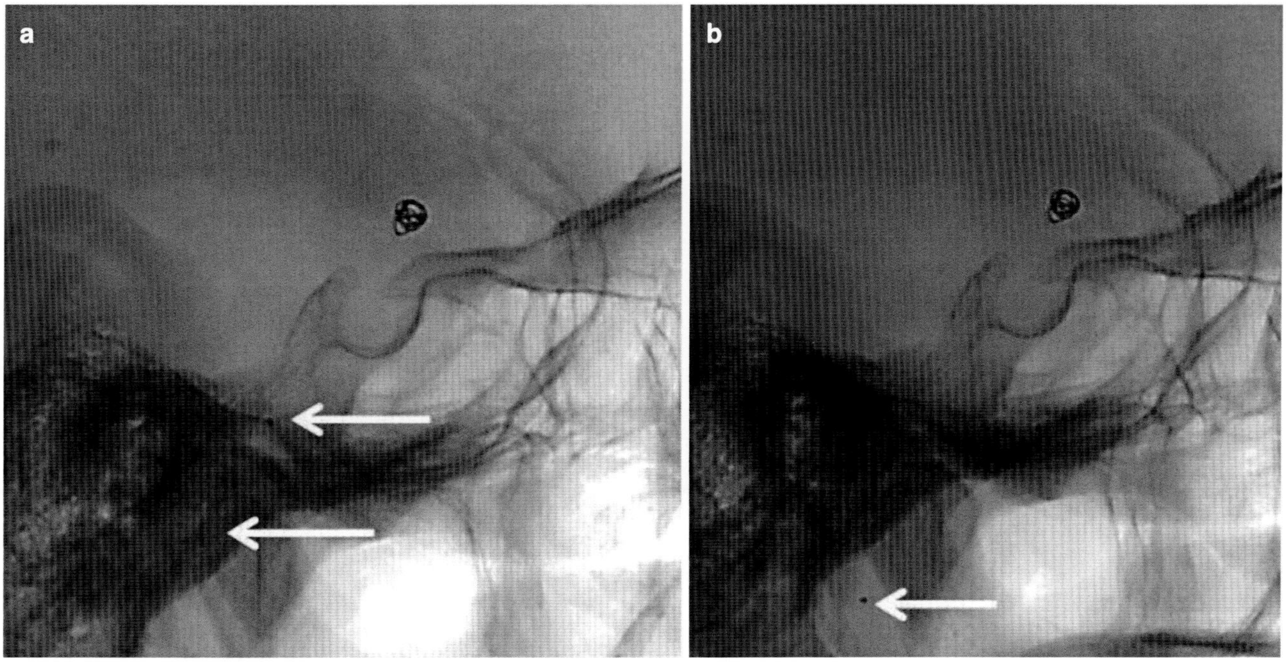

Fig. 2 Position of marks of microcatheter (*arrows*) during measurement of pressure in the segment C4 of ICA (**a**) and in the distal part of C1 segment of ICA (**b**)

every measurement, the sensor was calibrated. Data was processed for statistics on a personal computer with the program "Statistic 6.0".

Results and Discussion

Principles of Invasive AP Monitoring During Endovascular Neurointerventional Procedures

We conducted a series of simultaneous measurements of AP through catheters of different diameters (a guiding catheter and microcatheter) in the extracranial section of the ICA (segment C1). We observed that the amplitudes of fluctuations during measurements through the microcatheter were decreased, which was reflected in smaller values of systolic and pulse pressures and also in the growth of the diastolic pressure. These differences can be explained by the peculiarities of the functioning of the system with a high dumping coefficient, where elastic and very long tubes (the microcatheters) were used. The length of the catheter should not exceed 3–4 ft (91–122 cm) [2], and the length of the microcatheter, 150 cm. The patterns are shown on a curve recorded from the monitor (Fig. 3).

According to our data, measured values of MAP (a basic characteristic of the perfusion pressure) are practically independent of the catheter diameters. They are 98.3 ± 5.6 mmHg on average, if measured through a guiding catheter; and 102.4 ± 6.3 mmHg, if measured through a microcatheter; $p > 0.5$. When measured by a noninvasive method on the humeral artery, MAP was recorded to be 103.8 ± 4.9 mmHg. Thus, MAP appears a precise parameter independent of the method of AP measurement (see Table 1). This explains why we will use this index for establishing the main characteristics of cerebral hemodynamics and brain perfusion in the future.

Intraoperative Parameters of Cerebral Perfusion

Certain differences were observed between the AP measurements in the ICA inside the cranial cavity (C4 segment), and outside the cranial cavity (distal part of C1 segment). The AP in the ICA was recorded to be 91.2 ± 9.6 mmHg in the skull cavity and 102.4 ± 6.3 mmHg outside the skull cavity. The difference fluctuated from 1.7 to 25.0 mmHg, and was 9.2 ± 3.0 mmHg on average (see Table 2).

To estimate the possible influence of the smaller artery diameter in the distal direction on the level of pressure inside the artery, during angiography, we conducted a measurement of the ICA diameter at the points of the invasive measurements of AP in the C1 and C4 segments. The obtained data are listed in Table 3. The diameter of the ICA in the C1 and C4 segments did not differ substantially, with an average difference of 0.19 ± 0.08 mm, $p > 0.5$. Thus, we ascribe the difference of MAP, as measured in the ICA outside and inside the skull cavity, to the influence of the ICP (see Table 2). Therefore, we suggest that a direct

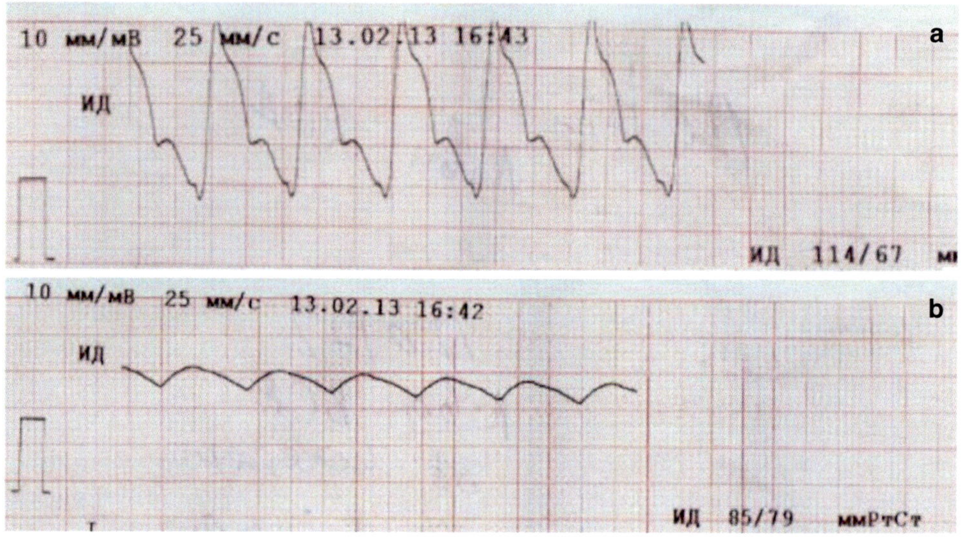

Fig. 3 A record of the direct measurements of AP in ICA: (**a**) through a guiding catheter; (**b**) through a microcatheter

Table 1 AP parameters measured by cuff and directly, through catheters of various inner diameter

N = 14	Systolic AP	Diastolic AP	MAP	Pulse AP
Non-invasive AP measurement	143.5 ± 7.1	84.8 ± 3.9	103.8 ± 4.9	58.8 ± 4.2
Invasive, microcatheter AP measurement Ø 0.4 mm	108.0 ± 7.0	99.3 ± 5.6	102.4 ± 6.3	8.7 ± 1.8
Invasive, guiding catheter AP measurement Ø 1.63 mm	141.8 ± 10.9	77.7 ± 3.6	98.3 ± 5.6	65.3 ± 8.0

Table 2 Distribution of MAP in ICA, if measured inside and outside the skull cavity (mmHg)

	Mean AP
Outside cranial cavity, ICA C1 segment	102.4 ± 6.3
Inside cranial cavity, ICA C4 segment	91.2 ± 9.6
C1-C4 = intracranial pressure (ICP)	9.3 ± 3.0

Table 3 Mean diameter of ICA in C1 and in C4 segments, and their mean difference

	Ø of ICA in C1 segment, mm	Ø of ICA in C4 segment, mm	Difference, mm
M	4.11	4.17	0.19
±m	0.16	0.23	0.08

recording of intra-arterial pressure can yield objective real-time information regarding cerebral perfusion during endovascular procedures in reference to the ICP level.

Conclusions

The procedure of an invasive AP measurement does not substantially influence the duration of an operation and does not cause additional trauma to the patient. During endovascular neuroradiologic aneurysm coiling, the invasive AP measurement and estimate of parameters of hemodynamics in different parts of intracranial and extracranial arteries can provide additional important information regarding the level of ICP and cerebral perfusion. Further investigations are required to check the accuracy of invasive extracranial and intracranial intra-arterial pressure recording for an objective and direct measurement of the cerebral perfusion in reference to the ICP level.

Conflict of Interest Statement We declare that we have no conflict of interest.

References

1. Aliya A (2007) Anaesthesia for interventional neuroradiology. J Ayub Med Coll Abbottabad 19(3):80–84
2. Orlando Health (2011) Fundamentals of hemodynamic monitoring self-learning packet. Orlando Health, Education & Development, Orlando, p 52
3. Gupta B (2012) Invasive blood pressure monitoring. Intensive Care Med Spec Ed 28:36–42
4. Hackman JL, Johnson MD, Ma OJ (2010) Spontaneous subarachnoid and intracerebral hemorrhage. In: Tintinalli JE, Stapczynski JS, Ma OJ (eds) Tintinalli's emergency medicine: a comprehensive study guide, 7th edn. McGraw-Hill, New York

5. Headley JM (2002) Invasive hemodynamic monitoring: physiological principles and clinical applications. Irvine, Edwards Lifesciences LLC
6. Krylov VV, Tsarenko SV (2005) Diagnostics and management of secondary brain damages. Neirochirurgia 1: 4–8. Russian (Крылов В.В., Царенко С.В. Диагностика и принципы лечения вторичных повреждений головного мозга. Нейрохирургия, 2005. № 1. С.4–8)
7. Malyshev VD (2000) Intensive care. Reanimation. First aid. Medicine. Moscow. Russian (Интенсивная терапия. Реанимация. Первая помощь: учебное пособие/под ред. В.Д. Малышева. М.: Медицина. 2000.- 464 с.: іл.- ISBN 5-225-04560-X)
8. Pub. No.: RU 2353297 A61B8/06 Appl. No.: 2007145238/14 Appl. Date Dec. 7, 2007 Pub. Date Apr. 27, 2009. Assignee: Research institute of neurosurgery named after acad. N.N.Burdenko RAMS. Inventors: Grinenko EA, Parfenov AL Method for prognostication of ischemic brain damage after acute subarachnoid hemorrhage produced by arterial aneurysm rupture at intracranial hypertension and arterial vasospasm occurence. Russian Federation
9. Teasdale GM, Rowan JO et al (1990) Relationship between cardiac output and CBF in patients with intact and improper autoregulation. J Neurosurg 73:268–274

Real-Time Changes in Brain Tissue Oxygen During Endovascular Treatment of Cerebral Vasospasm

Rune Rasmussen, Søren Bache, Trine Stavngaard, Jane Skjøth-Rasmussen, and Bertil Romner

Abstract The use of endovascular intervention to treat cerebral vasospasm after subarachnoid hemorrhage has increased. Although the effect on angiographic vasospasm can be easily demonstrated, the effect on cerebral blood flow and clinical outcome is still controversial. In this report, we investigate minute-by-minute changes in brain tissue oxygen during balloon angioplasty and intraarterial administration of vasodilators in three patients.

Our results confirm that endovascular intervention is capable of not only resolving angiographic vasospasm, but also of normalizing values of brain tissue oxygen pressure ($PtiO_2$) in target parenchyma. However, during the intervention, dangerously low levels of brain tissue oxygen, leading to cerebral infarction, may occur. Thus, no clinical improvement was seen in two of the patients and a dramatic worsening was observed in the third patient. Because the decrease in brain tissue oxygen was seen after administration of vasopressor agents, this may be a contributing factor.

Keywords Subarachnoid hemorrhage • Cerebral vasospasm • Endovascular intervention • Brain tissue oxygen monitoring

R. Rasmussen (✉) • J. Skjøth-Rasmussen • B. Romner
Department of Neurosurgery,
Copenhagen University Hospital,
9 Blegdamsvej, Copenhagen, Denmark
e-mail: rune.rasmussen@rh.regionh.dk

S. Bache
Department of Neuroanesthesiology,
Copenhagen University Hospital,
Blegdamsvej 9, Copenhagen, Denmark

T. Stavngaard
Department of Radiology, Copenhagen University Hospital,
9 Blegdamsvej, Copenhagen, Denmark

Introduction

Delayed cerebral ischemia (DCI) is the leading cause of poor outcome in the weeks after subarachnoid hemorrhage (SAH) [3]. The presumed cause of DCI is cerebral vasospasm, although this causality has been challenged lately [1]. No fully effective treatment of DCI exists, but, during the last decade, the use of endovascular intervention has increased. Mechanical dilation (percutaneous transluminal angioplasty (PTA)) and/or intraarterial administration of vasodilating drugs has been used to resolve cerebral vasospasm to prevent or treat DCI. The effect of endovascular intervention is, however, still controversial [6].

To evaluate the effect of endovascular intervention, neuroradiologic imaging has traditionally been performed. However, because the causality between angiographic vasospasm and DCI is complex, other measurements are needed to guide and evaluate treatment. Brain tissue oxygen pressure ($PtiO_2$) offers a continuous measurement of cerebral oxygenation and can be used as a surrogate measure of cerebral blood flow [5]. In this way, measurement of $PtiO_2$ offers a unique way of monitoring the response in target brain parenchyma during manipulation of the feeding arteries. Although some reports describe changes in $PtiO_2$ before and after endovascular intervention [2, 4, 7], none so far has described the minute-by-minute changes during the intervention.

The aim of this study was to investigate changes in $PtiO_2$ during PTA and intraarterial administration of vasodilators. In this report, we describe three cases of responses in $PtiO_2$ during endovascular intervention.

Materials and Methods

During 2012, 12 patients with aneurysmal SAH were monitored with brain tissue oxygen pressure ($PtiO_2$) (Licox, Integra) for clinical reasons at our institution. Three of these

J. Fandino et al. (eds.), *Neurovascular Events After Subarachnoid Hemorrhage*, Acta Neurochirurgica Supplement, Vol. 120,
DOI 10.1007/978-3-319-04981-6_31, © Springer International Publishing Switzerland 2015

patients developed symptoms of DCI and underwent endovascular intervention. During the intervention, changes in $PtiO_2$ and the exact time of balloon inflation and intraarterial administration of a vasodilator were prospectively collected. Later, the data were retrospectively analyzed. In all three cases, the $PtiO_2$ probe was placed in the white matter of the left frontal lobe. Indications for endovascular intervention were DCI (as defined by Vergouwen et al. [8]) and no response to triple-H (hypertension, hypervolemia, and hemodilution) treatment.

Results

Case 1

Figure 1 shows changes in $PtiO_2$ in the left frontal lobe during endovascular intervention in a 47-year-old woman 5 days after ictus. The clinical symptoms consisted of right-sided hemiparesis and decreased level of consciousness; and bilateral vasospasm was demonstrated on computed tomography (CT) angiography. PTA was performed in the internal carotid artery (ICA), middle cerebral artery (MCA), and anterior cerebral artery (ACA) on both sides, and 2 mg of nimodipin was injected during 20 min into the ICA bilaterally. As can be seen, PTA leads to a rapid response in the level of $PtiO_2$. Initially, a drop in $PtiO_2$ is observed corresponding to the inflation of the balloon in ICA. After 20 min, during which PTA on the MCA and ACA is performed and nimodipin is administrated, values rise above the levels before the intervention. Interestingly, inflation in the right ICA also initially causes a significant drop in $PtiO_2$. At the end of the intervention, $PtiO_2$ values rise to normal levels. Angiography demonstrated resolution of the vasospasm. $PtiO_2$ values in the next 4 days after the intervention was between 20 and 40 mmHg, as compared with below 10 mmHg before intervention; thus, showing a lasting improvement. However, no clinical improvement was observed.

Case 2

A 54-year-old man developed a mild right-sided hemiparesis and confusion 6 days after SAH, and CT angiography revealed vasospasm bilaterally. Figure 2 shows the development of $PtiO_2$ in the left frontal lobe during anesthesia, verapamil infusion, and bilateral PTA. A decrease in MAP after anesthesia made the use of vasopressor agents (ephedrine and phenylephrine) necessary. After initiation of continuous phenylephrine infusion, $PtiO_2$ values decreased to near zero. No immediate effect of intraarterial verapamil was observed; the $PtiO_2$ rose to normal levels and even to

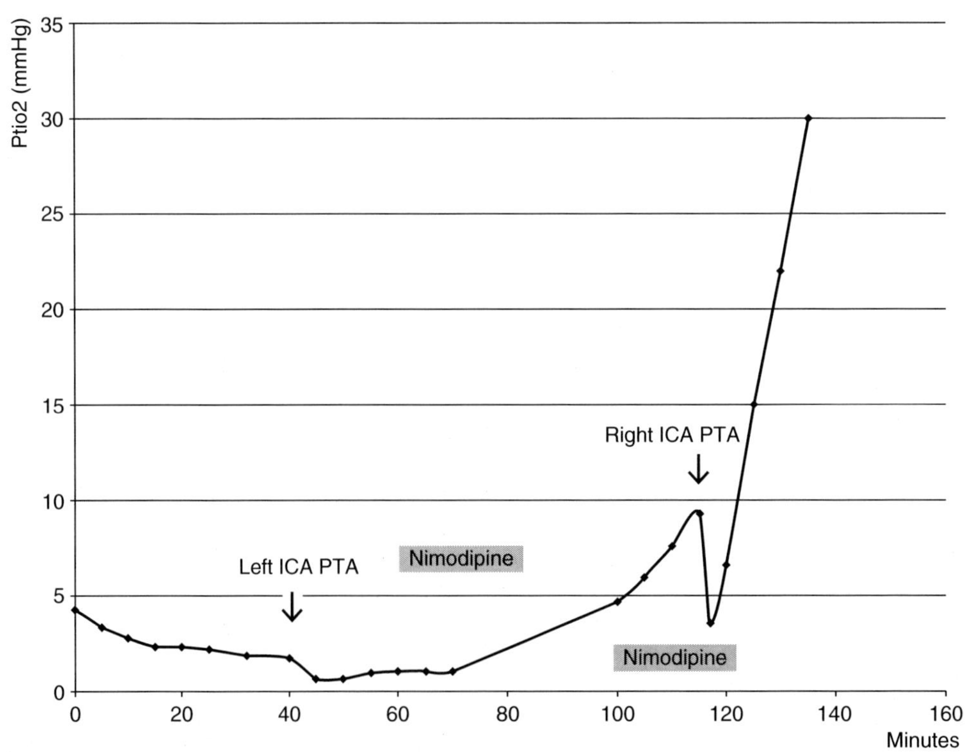

Fig. 1 Development of $PtiO_2$ in the left frontal lobe during endovascular intervention. Times for PTA in the left and right internal carotid artery and period of nimodipin administration are indicated

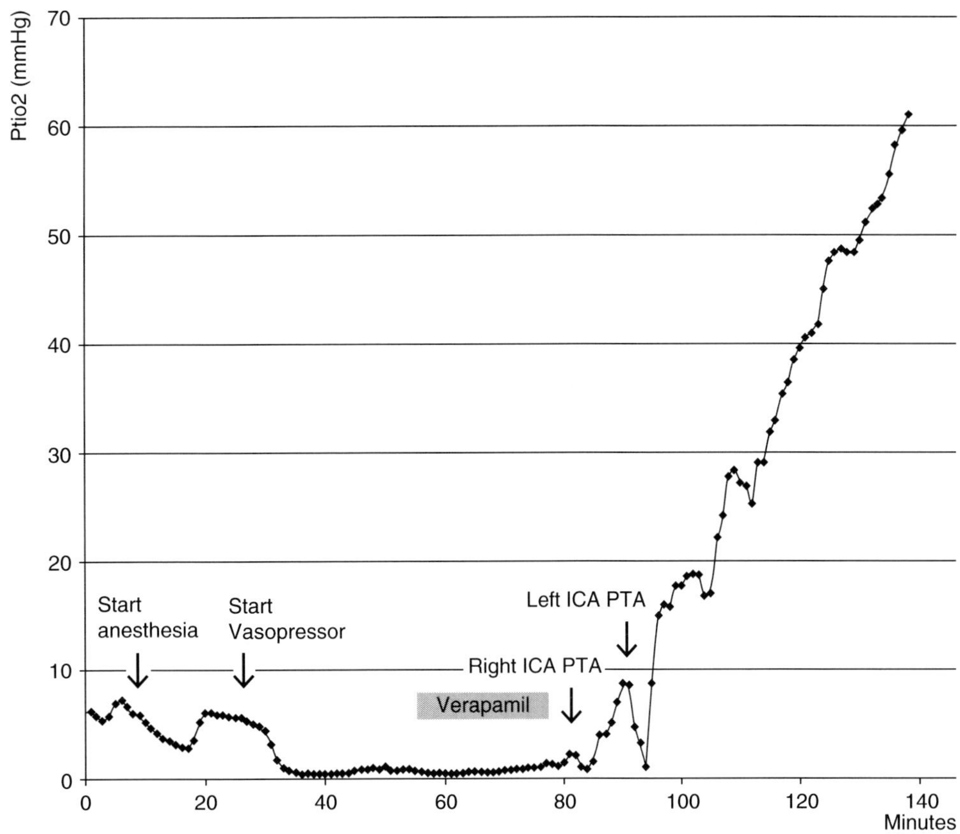

Fig. 2 $PtiO_2$ values in the left frontal lobe during endovascular intervention. Times for anesthesia, vasopressor administration, intraarterial verapamil administration, and PTA are indicated

values suggesting hyperperfusion (>80 mmHg) only after PTA. Angiography after the intervention showed resolution of the vasospasm.

The increased $PtiO_2$ values obtained during intervention were not lasting. Within 24 h after intervention, $PtiO_2$ decreased to the level observed before the intervention and even below. Clinically, a dramatic worsening was observed after the intervention in this case. The mild paresis worsened to paralysis and the Glasgow Coma Scale (GCS) dropped from 14 to 6. CT scan revealed infarction in the left frontal lobe.

Case 3

Figure 3 shows $PtiO_2$ values during administration of vasopressor agents and intraarterial administration of nimopidin (2 mg in the ICA, bilaterally). A significant drop in $PtiO_2$ is observed after administration of vasopressor agents. After nimodipine administration, the $PtiO_2$ level rose to the preintervention level, but not above. No clinical improvement was seen after the intervention.

Discussion

The above cases show that decreases in $PtiO_2$ values can be dramatically improved by mechanic/pharmacological dilation of the main cerebral arteries. However, no clinical improvement was seen in any of the cases. Several reasons can account for this. In Figs. 1 and 3, very low levels of $PtiO_2$ are seen during the intervention. In Fig. 1, the $PtiO_2$ level dropped to values below 2 mmHg for several minutes as the feeding artery was manipulated during PTA. No vasopressors were used in this case. In Fig. 3, a dramatic drop in $PtiO_2$ to near 0 mmHg was seen after initiation of vasopressor agents. The curves suggest that both manipulation of the arteries and the use of vasopressors in patients with cerebral vasospasm can cause ischemia, potentially leading to poorer outcome than without any intervention.

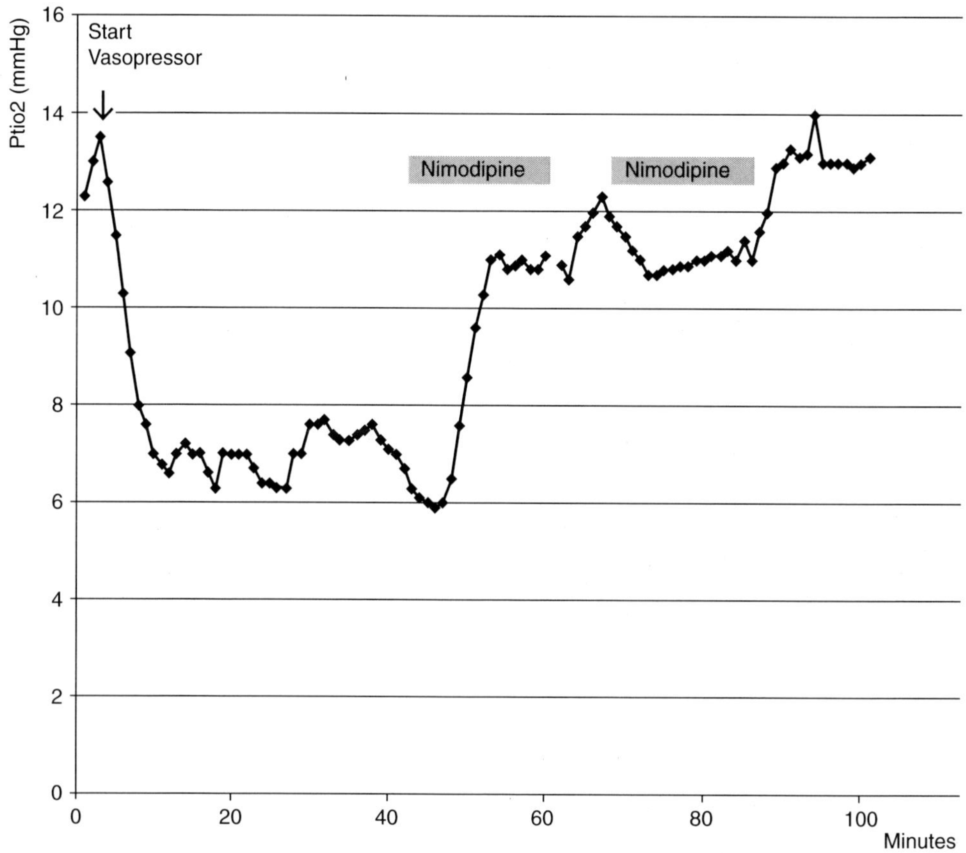

Fig. 3 $PtiO_2$ values in the left frontal lobe during endovascular intervention. Times for vasopressor administration and intraarterial nimodipin administration are indicated

Conclusion

Endovascular intervention is capable of not only resolving angiographic vasospasm, but also normalizing values of $PtiO_2$ in the target parenchyma. However, dangerously low levels of $PtiO_2$ leading to cerebral infarction can be seen during interventions. One reason for this may be the use of vasopressor agents during the anesthesia, but manipulation within the arteries may also be a cause. Further studies are needed for clarification.

Conflict of Interest Statement We declare that we have no conflict of interest.

References

1. Al-Tamimi YZ, Orsi NM, Quinn AC, Homer-Vanniasinkam S, Ross SA (2010) A review of delayed ischemic neurologic deficit following aneurysmal subarachnoid hemorrhage: historical overview, current treatment, and pathophysiology. World Neurosurg 73:654–667
2. Deshaies EM, Jacobsen W, Singla A, Li F, Gorji R (2012) Brain tissue oxygen monitoring to assess reperfusion after intra-arterial treatment of aneurysmal subarachnoid hemorrhage-induced cerebral vasospasm: a retrospective study. AJNR Am J Neuroradiol 33:1411–1415
3. Dorsch NW (1995) Cerebral arterial spasm – a clinical review. Br J Neurosurg 9:403–412
4. Hoelper BM, Hofmann E, Sporleder R, Soldner F, Behr R (2003) Transluminal balloon angioplasty improves brain tissue oxygenation and metabolism in severe vasospasm after aneurysmal subarachnoid hemorrhage: case report. Neurosurgery 52:970–974
5. Jaeger M, Soehle M, Schuhmann MU, Winkler D, Meixensberger J (2005) Correlation of continuously monitored regional cerebral blood flow and brain tissue oxygen. Acta Neurochir (Wien) 147:51–56
6. Keyrouz SG, Diringer MN (2007) Clinical review: prevention and therapy of vasospasm in subarachnoid hemorrhage. Crit Care 11:220
7. Stiefel MF, Spiotta AM, Udoetuk JD, Maloney-Wilensky E, Weigele JB, Hurst RW, LeRoux PD (2006) Intra-arterial papaverine used to treat cerebral vasospasm reduces brain oxygen. Neurocrit Care 4:113–118
8. Vergouwen MD, Vermeulen M, van Gijn J, Rinkel GJ, Wijdicks EF, Muizelaar JP, Mendelow AD, Juvela S, Yonas H, Terbrugge KG, Macdonald RL, Diringer MN, Broderick JP, Dreier JP, Roos YB (2010) Definition of delayed cerebral ischemia after aneurysmal subarachnoid hemorrhage as an outcome event in clinical trials and observational studies: proposal of a multidisciplinary research group. Stroke 41:2391–2395

Acute Angiographic Vasospasm and the Incidence of Delayed Cerebral Vasospasm: Preliminary Results

Hiroki Danura, Bawarjan Schatlo, Serge Marbacher, Hassen Kerkeni, Michael Diepers, Luca Remonda, Ali-Reza Fathi, and Javier Fandino

Abstract *Background:* More than half of subarachnoid hemorrhage (SAH) patients develop angiographically detectable delayed cerebral vasospasm (dCVS). It mostly occurs between days 4 and 15 after ictus and can be associated with neurological deficits that contribute to increased morbidity and mortality after SAH. Although dCVS is well studied, there are only a handful of reports on the acute phase of vasospasm (APV) occurring after treatment of intracranial aneurysms, whether ruptured or not. The aim of the current study is to elucidate the association of intraoperative cerebral vasospasm (iCVS) with the incidence of dCVS.

Method: We retrospectively reviewed consecutive patients who were treated for aneurysmal SAH or incidental aneurysms during the study period. Angiograms of patients undergoing aneurysm treatment were reviewed. Spasm severity was classified with respect to reduction in the transverse diameter. Mild vasospasm was defined as a reduction in vessel diameter of 10–30 %; moderate, 30–50 %; and severe vasospasm, >50 %. Statistical significance was tested using the X^2 test with $p<0.05$. Correlations between iCVS and other factors were investigated.

Results: Of 109 patients, 77 patients (33 men and 44 women) presented with acute SAH and 32 patients (9 men and 23 women) were treated for incidental aneurysms. Seventeen (22 %) of 77 patients presenting with acute SAH had evidence of acute (within 72 h after SAH ictus) CVS. In 16 of 17 (94.1 %) patients, this vasospasm was observed immediately after treatment and was therefore termed iCVS. Eleven (30 %) of 36 patients undergoing clipping and 5 (14 %) of 36 patients with endovascular aneurysm occlusion had iCVS ($p=0.07$). Patients presenting with acute SAH had a higher incidence of iCVS than patients undergoing elective aneurysm treatment ($p=0.02$). Only one patient (3 %) had iCVS in the elective treatment group whereas 16 (20 %) had iCVS after SAH. The incidence of dCVS, delayed ischemic neurological deficits (DNDs), and poor outcome in patients presenting with iCVS during surgical treatment of ruptured aneurysms was 56 % ($p=0.001$), 63 % ($p=0.02$), and 38 % ($p=0.14$), respectively.

Conclusion: APV exists and is a common finding in patients with SAH. Further studies are warranted to correlate the presence of APV with postoperative ischemia, dCVS, and outcome.

Keywords Subarachnoid Hemorrhage • Intraoperative • Cerebral Vasospasm • Clipping • Coiling • Hybride OR

H. Danura, MD • B. Schatlo, MD • H. Kerkeni
S. Marbacher, MD, MSc • A.-R. Fathi, MD
J. Fandino, MD (✉)
Department of Neurosurgery, Kantonsspital Aarau, Aarau, Switzerland
e-mail: neurosurgery@ksa.ch

M. Diepers, MD • L. Remonda, MD
Division of Neuroradiology, Department of Radiology, Kantonsspital Aarau, Aarau, Switzerland

Introduction

Delayed cerebral vasospasm (dCVS) after subarachnoid hemorrhage (SAH) is major contributor to poor outcome after aneurysmal SAH. It occurs between days 4 and 15 after hemorrhage and is associated with delayed ischemic neurological deficits (DNDs). The amount of blood in the subarachnoid space is a predictive factor for the occurrence of dCVS [5].

As early as 1975, Weir et al. described that the presence of vasospasm before surgery was predictive of poor outcome and therefore advocated against operating in such cases [11].

DOI 10.1007/978-3-319-04981-6_32,

However, it remains unclear whether these patients were admitted later in the vasospasm period or whether the described phenomenon was indeed an ultra-early spasm as reported by Taneda et al. [8]. Studies that are more recent found vasospasm at admission in 10 % [1] and 13 % [6] of patients with SAH. In both studies, the presence of early vasospasm was predictive of delayed cerebral ischemia. Whether the early phase spasm itself can be treated and how it may affect aneurysm treatment nowadays is unknown. Surgical manipulation of vessels may induce "mechanical vasospasm" and catheter manipulation may also lead to vasospasm [10]. Therefore, in addition to early and delayed vasospasm, there is also a "treatment-induced" or iatrogenic vasospasm. The recent advance of intraoperative angiography in hybrid operating rooms (ORs) [4] opened the possibility of assessing the success of aneurysm occlusion as well as the presence of vessel narrowing. Our aim was to assess the incidence of intraoperative cerebral vasospasm (iCVS) during aneurysm treatment. Moreover, we assessed whether the presence of iCVS was associated with dCVS, ischemia, and/or outcome.

Materials and Methods

All neurovascular surgeries were performed in a hybrid OR at our institution (Philips, Allura XT). The hybrid OR is equipped with a C-arm capable of 3D rotational angiography. All patients underwent diagnostic angiography before aneurysm treatment. After surgical clipping of an aneurysm, we routinely obtained an intraoperative angiogram to exclude vessel occlusion. This offered us the unique opportunity to evaluate the presence of acute spasm related to aneurysm treatment.

We retrospectively reviewed intraoperative angiograms of 130 consecutive patients who underwent surgical or interventional aneurysm occlusion during a 4-year period at our institution (January 2009 to January 2013). Patients admitted or operated after 72 h after ictus were excluded from the study.

Angiographic vasospasm was defined as a decrease in diameter of greater than 30 % compared with the adjacent contiguous vessel segment. Particular attention was paid to possible differences in preoperative to postoperative vessel diameter. Patients with SAH undergo regular neurological exams and transcranial Doppler ultrasonography. If patients show a decline in neurological performance or mean middle cerebral artery (MCA) flow velocity above 200 cm/s, we perform CT angiography with perfusion imaging to detect vasospasm or hypoperfusion. In cases of dCVS with no improvement of symptoms despite maximal hyperdynamic therapy, the need for angiography and subsequent angioplasty are evaluated.

Poor outcome at discharge was defined as a modified Rankin scale (mRS) >3. The degree of iCVS was defined as % stenosis $= [1-(D_{stenosis}/D_{normal})] \times 100$, where $D_{stenosis}$ is the diameter of the artery at the site of the most severe stenosis, and D_{normal} is the diameter of the same artery before treatment. Vasospasm severity was classified with respect to reduction in transverse diameter (mild 10–30 %, moderate 30–50 %, and severe >50 %).

We recorded age, sex, the location and size (the maximum diameter) of aneurysm, Fisher grade at admission, the presence of vasospasm on angiography intraoperatively and postoperatively (iCVS and dCVS), the degree of vasospasm (mild, moderate, severe) based on our vasospasm criteria [7], the presence of DND, and the patients' status at discharge based on mRS.

Statistical significance was determined as $p<0.05$ using the X^2 test. The presence of iCVS and its association with Fisher grade at admission, dCVS, DND, and outcome at discharge with mRS were investigated. The Mann Whitney U test was used for comparison of severity of vasospasm among groups.

Results

Candidates in this study were 130 patients who underwent microsurgical or endovascular aneurysmal occlusions during a 4-year period in our institution (January 2009 to January 2013). The final analysis included 109 patients: 77 patients (33 men and 44 women) who presented with acute SAH and 32 patients (9 men and 23 women) who were treated for incidental aneurysms.

Overall, 17 (22 %) of 77 patients presenting with acute SAH had evidence of acute (within 72 h after SAH ictus) cerebral vasospasm (CVS). In 16 (94.1 %) of 17 patients, this vasospasm was observed immediately after treatment and was therefore termed iCVS. The majority of these patients underwent microsurgical occlusion of the aneurysm (n = 11, 68.8 %). Vasospasm at admission after acute SAH was present in only 1 of 77 patients (1.3 %) and did not lead to neurological symptoms, delayed vasospasm, or poor outcome. The degree of vasospasm was not different in the surgical or endovascular groups ($p=0.529$). Mild iCVS was observed in 9 (52.9 %) of the 17 patients, moderate in 5 (29.4 %), and severe in 3 (17.7 %). Fisher grade at admission was documented as follows: grade 1 (n = 0), grade 2 (n = 2; 11.8 %), grade 3 (n = 4; 23.5 %), and grade 4 (n = 11; 64.7 %). Of the patients with iCVS, 9 (56.3 %) developed dCVS, 10 (62.5 %) developed DND. Six (37.5 %) had a poor outcome. Eleven of 36 patients undergoing clipping and 5 of 36 patients with endovascular aneurysm occlusion had iCVS. Of the 60 patients presenting with acute SAH

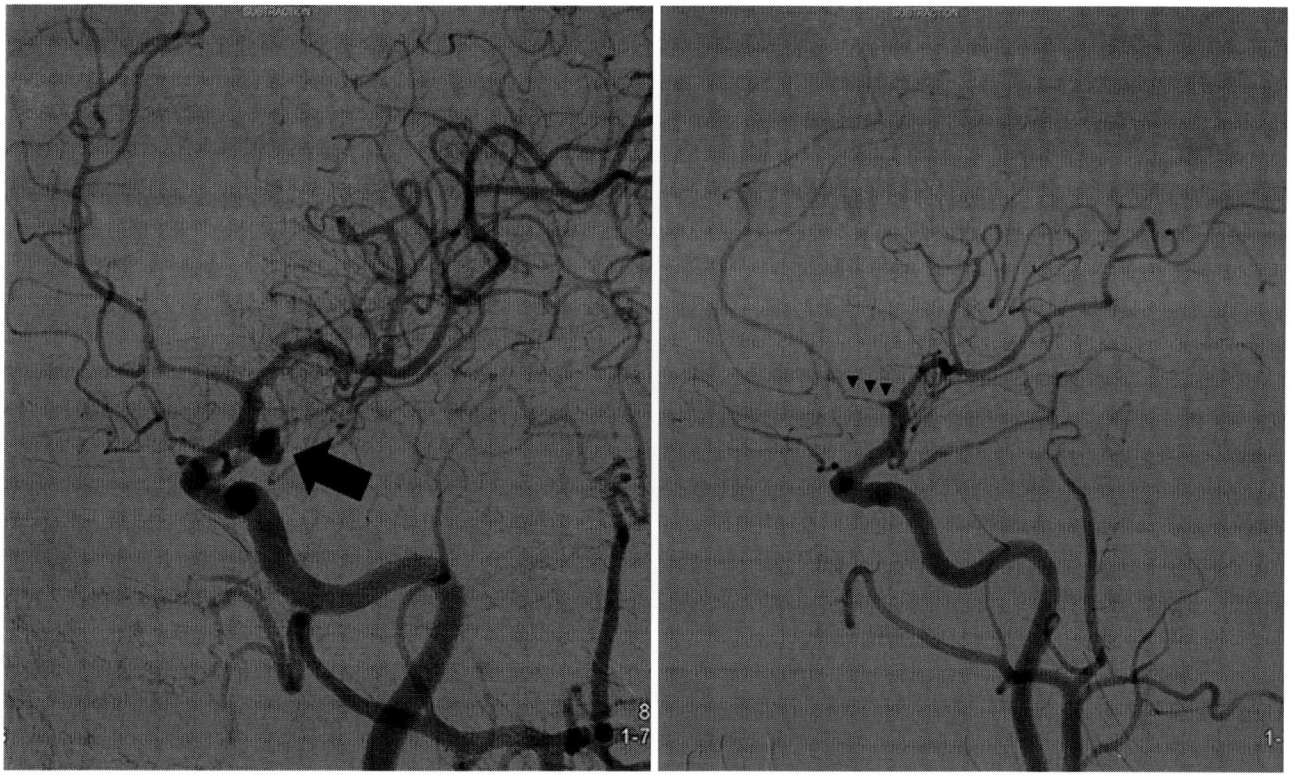

Fig. 1 *Case 1*: 68-year-old man with acute SAH caused by ruptured left posterior communicating artery aneurysm (*arrow*) with Hunt & Hess grade II, World Federation of Neurosurgical Societies (WFNS) grade I, and Fisher grade 4. On the same day, the patient underwent microsurgical occlusion of the aneurysm. The intraoperative angiogram illustrated severe iCVS (53.2 % stenosis) in the left A1 segment (*arrow heads*)

and no evidence of iCVS or acute vasospasm, 13 (21.7 %) patients developed dCVS, 19 (31.7 %) developed DND, and 12 (20.0 %) had poor outcome. Patients presenting with acute SAH had a higher incidence of iCVS than patients undergoing elective aneurysm treatment ($p=0.02$). Only one patient (3 %) had iCVS in the elective treatment group whereas 16 (20 %) had iCVS after SAH. The incidence of dCVS, DND, and poor outcome in patients presenting with iCVS during surgical treatment of ruptured aneurysms was 56 % ($p=0.001$), 63 % ($p=0.02$), and 38 % ($p=0.14$), respectively (Figs. 1 and 2).

Discussion

The incidence of iCVS in patients undergoing treatment for ruptured intracranial aneurysms has been underestimated, especially during surgical occlusion of ruptured aneurysms. In the present series, we found a rate of iCVS of 30 % in clipped patients and 14 % in coiled patients with SAH. Although this finding fell short of statistical significance ($p=0.07$), there was a trend toward a higher rate of iCVS in the surgery group. One of the possible explanations is that surgical manipulation of the larger arterial vessels may lead to vasospasm of the microvasculature [9]. These results are analogous to the data showing that coiling is associated with a lower rate of vasospasm and delayed cerebral ischemia [3]. Moreover, patients who had iCVS also had a higher risk of suffering from delayed cerebral ischemia, suggesting that iCVS reflects vulnerable vasculature that is also prone to delayed vasospasm. Hypothetically, manipulation of vessels may lead to decreased vasoreactivity and, therefore, favor ischemia later on [2]. The causes of iCVS remain controversial, but surgically induced iCVS has to be considered as an important factor. This preliminary series suggests an association between iCVS and CVS or DND. Further studies are warranted to investigate the pathogenesis of iCVS, namely acute CVS, and its influence on the outcome after acute treatment of SAH.

Conclusion

APV exists and is a common finding in patients with SAH. Further studies are warranted to correlate the presence of APV with postoperative ischemia, dCVS, and outcome.

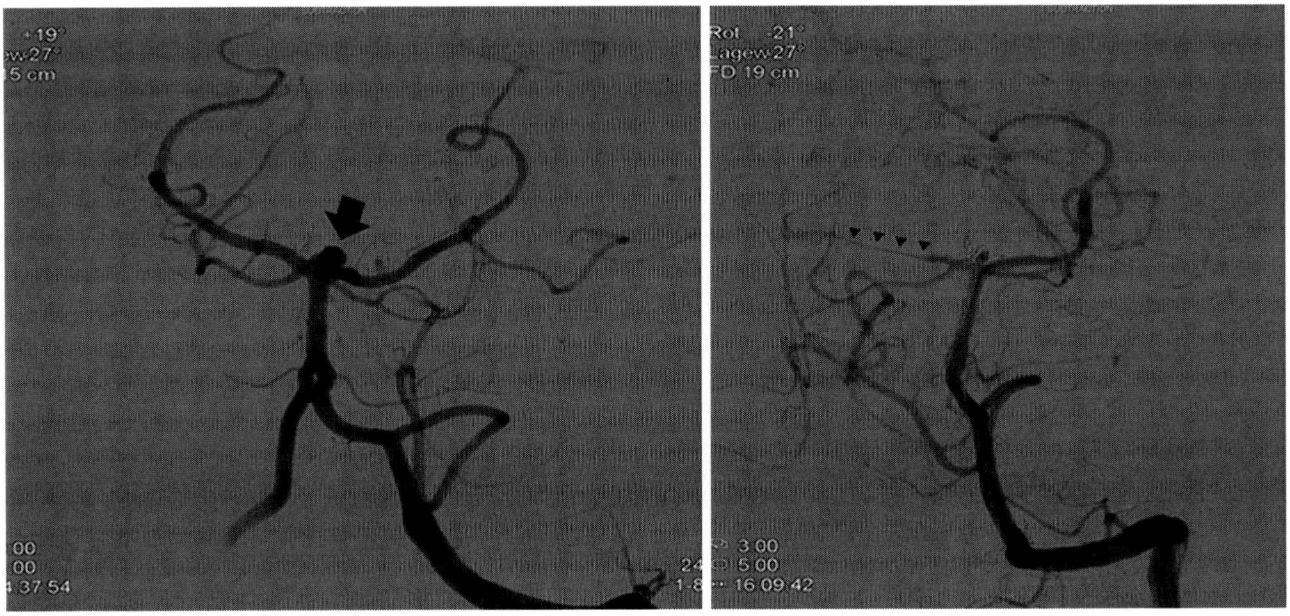

Fig. 2 *Case 2*: 51-year-old woman with acute SAH caused by a ruptured basilar tip aneurysm (*arrow*) with Hunt & Hess grade IIb, WFNS grade II, and Fisher grade 4. On the same day, she underwent coiling of the ruptured aneurysm. The angiogram demonstrated severe iCVS (62.9 % stenosis) of the right posterior cerebral artery (*arrow heads*)

Conflict of Interest Statement We declare that we have no conflict of interest.

References

1. Baldwin ME, Macdonald RL, Huo D, Novakovic RL, Goldenberg FD, Frank JI, Rosengart AJ (2004) Early vasospasm on admission angiography in patients with aneurysmal subarachnoid hemorrhage is a predictor for in-hospital complications and poor outcome. Stroke 35:2506–2511
2. Budohoski KP, Czosnyka M, Kirkpatrick PJ, Smielewski P, Steiner LA, Pickard JD (2013) Clinical relevance of cerebral autoregulation following subarachnoid haemorrhage. Nat Rev Neurol 9:152–163
3. Dumont AS, Crowley RW, Monteith SJ, Ilodigwe D, Kassell NF, Mayer S, Ruefenacht D, Weidauer S, Pasqualin A, Macdonald RL (2010) Endovascular treatment or neurosurgical clipping of ruptured intracranial aneurysms: effect on angiographic vasospasm, delayed ischemic neurological deficit, cerebral infarction, and clinical outcome. Stroke 41:2519–2524
4. Fandino J, Taussky P, Marbacher S, Muroi C, Diepers M, Fathi AR, Remonda L (2013) The concept of a hybrid operating room: applications in cerebrovascular surgery. Acta Neurochir Suppl 115:113–117
5. Fergusen S, Macdonald RL (2007) Predictors of cerebral infarction in patients with aneurysmal subarachnoid hemorrhage. Neurosurgery 60:658–667; discussion 667
6. Qureshi AI, Sung GY, Suri MA, Straw RN, Guterman LR, Hopkins LN (1999) Prognostic value and determinants of ultraearly angiographic vasospasm after aneurysmal subarachnoid hemorrhage. Neurosurgery 44:967–973; discussion 973–974
7. Samuels OB, Joseph GJ, Lynn MJ, Smith HA, Chimowitz MI (2000) A standardized method for measuring intracranial arterial stenosis. AJNR Am J Neuroradiol 21:643–646
8. Taneda M, Otsuki H, Kumura E, Sakaguchi T (1990) Angiographic demonstration of acute phase of intracranial arterial spasm following aneurysm rupture. Case report. J Neurosurg 73:958–961
9. Uhl E, Lehmberg J, Steiger HJ, Messmer K (2003) Intraoperative detection of early microvasospasm in patients with subarachnoid hemorrhage by using orthogonal polarization spectral imaging. Neurosurgery 52:1307–1315; discussion 1315–1317
10. Wanke I, Dorfler A, Dietrich U, Aalders T, Forsting M (2000) Combined endovascular therapy of ruptured aneurysms and cerebral vasospasm. Neuroradiology 42:926–929
11. Weir B, Rothberg C, Grace M, Davis F (1975) Relative prognostic significance of vasospasm following subarachnoid hemorrhage. Can J Neurol Sci 2:109–114

The Penumbra Coil 400 System for Treatment of Wide-Necked Intracranial Aneurysms: Initial Single-Center Experience

Mark R. Villwock, Amit Singla, David J. Padalino, and Eric M. Deshaies

Abstract Endovascular treatment of wide-necked intracranial aneurysms frequently requires stent- or balloon-assisted coiling to prevent coil herniation into the parent artery. Provided that coils can be securely deployed within the aneurysm sac, these adjunctive devices and their associated risk can be avoided. The Penumbra 400 Coil (PC-400) has a larger diameter than conventional coils and is constructed completely of metal, a feature that increases the coil stability and may improve its ability to respect the aneurysm neck. The purpose of this study was to examine the frequency of adjunctive stent usage when coiling wide-necked intracranial aneurysms with the PC-400 in comparison with conventional coils. We examined consecutive patients with unruptured wide-necked aneurysms treated at our institution with endovascular coils. Aneurysm characteristics and procedural outcomes were compared between patients treated with PC-400 compared with a control group treated with conventional coils. Thirty-eight patients met criteria for this study. Stent-assisted coiling was required in 34 % fewer cases using PC-400 compared with conventional coils ($P = .049$). Fewer coils and less length were required with the PC-400 to obtain the same packing densities, occlusion types, and short-term stability. This may reduce treatment cost and prove to be valuable in patients with contraindications to dual antiplatelet therapy.

M.R. Villwock, MS • A. Singla, MD • D.J. Padalino, MD
Department of Neurosurgery, SUNY Upstate Medical University, Syracuse, NY 13210, USA

E.M. Deshaies, MD (✉)
Department of Neurosurgery,
SUNY Upstate Medical University,
Syracuse, NY, USA
e-mail: eric.m.deshaies@gmail.com

Keywords Intracranial aneurysm • Embolization • Penumbra Coil 400 • Stent-assisted coiling • Wide necked

Introduction

Coil embolization has become the leading treatment modality for intracranial aneurysms. However, this technique can be particularly challenging for wide-necked aneurysms, often requiring neck remodeling to provide a mechanical scaffold that prevents coil herniation into the parent artery [5]. Adjunctive balloon assistance or stent placement can accomplish this feat, but not without increased risk of procedural complications and long-term morbidity [1, 3, 10, 12].

Balloon-assisted coiling is one adjunctive technique used to maintain arterial lumen patency during coil placement in wide-necked aneurysms and provides the benefits of avoiding a stent and the need for long-term antiplatelet agents. Disadvantages of balloon assistance include the possibility of aneurysm or parent artery rupture and repeated episodes of cerebral ischemia during balloon inflation, thromboembolic events, and coil migration into the parent artery after deflation. There are mixed reports regarding the safety of balloon remodeling for wide-necked aneurysms; some reveal no increased adverse events whereas others demonstrate a high complication rate and advise against its use when possible [7, 8, 12, 13].

Stent-assisted coil embolization of wide-necked aneurysms increases the risk of procedural complications as well, specifically, of thromboembolic occlusions, stent migration, vessel wall injury, delayed thromboembolic events, and in-stent stenosis [1, 3]. Dual antiplatelet therapy is recommended for at least 6 weeks to minimize the delayed complications, but their use introduces the higher risk of a new set of potential bleeding problems [14, 15].

J. Fandino et al. (eds.), *Neurovascular Events After Subarachnoid Hemorrhage*, Acta Neurochirurgica Supplement, Vol. 120,
DOI 10.1007/978-3-319-04981-6_33, © Springer International Publishing Switzerland 2015

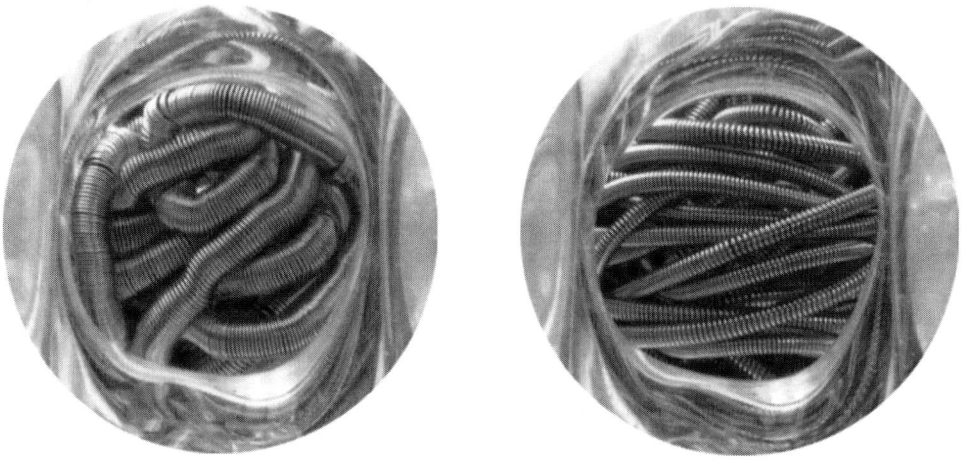

Fig. 1 The image on the *left* depicts the Penumbra Coil 400 System and its 0.020″ diameter loops. The image on the *right* is of a conventional coil with 0.010″ coil loops (Image reprinted with permission from Penumbra Inc.)

Provided that a coil can be securely deployed into the sac while respecting the aneurysm neck–parent artery interface, the additional risk from adjunctive remodeling can be eliminated from the treatment of wide-necked aneurysms. Presumably, a coil construct that is more stable, such as that seen with the Penumbra Coil 400 System (PC-400) (Penumbra, Inc., Alameda CA, USA), may be better able to respect the aneurysm neck than conventional coils.

PC-400 coils are designed with a larger outer diameter (0.020″) than most conventional coils (e.g., 0.010″ for GDC 10) (Fig. 1). Conventional coils are constructed with a nonmetallic polymer, whereas the PC-400 is designed with three layers of metal providing a more robust and sturdier construct (Fig. 2). The innermost layers of the PC-400 coils are composed of Nitinol wire, a memory-shape material designed to resist the stress of hemodynamic forces encountered within the aneurysm sac. This added resistance to mechanical stressors purportedly prevents coil compaction after placement and promotes coil loop stability within the aneurysm sac. This latter coil characteristic may provide the additional advantage of stabilizing the coils securely on the shoulders of the aneurysm neck to prevent herniation into the parent artery, thus avoiding the need for adjunctive remodeling and stent placement. Despite the physical properties of these completely metallic coils, we hypothesized that there would be no difference in adjunctive stent usage for wide-neck aneurysms between those treated with the PC-400 system and those occluded with conventional coils.

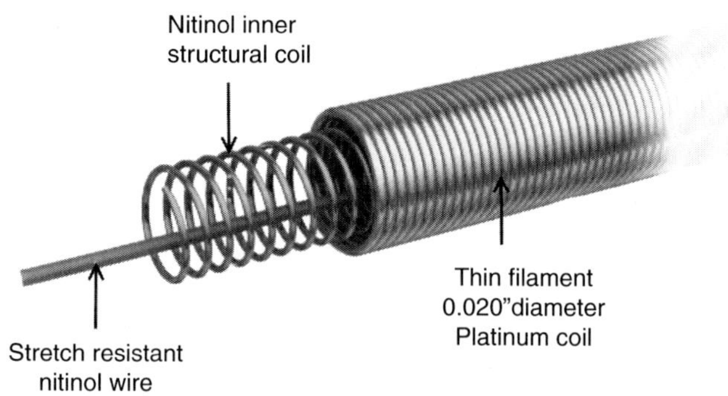

Fig. 2 The design of the Penumbra Coil 400 System is composed of three metal layers (Image reprinted with permission from Penumbra Inc.)

Methods

Approval was obtained from the Institutional Review Board of our university for this study. We retrospectively collected data from consecutive patients with unruptured intracranial aneurysms with a wide-neck (≥4-mm neck or dome:neck ratio <2:1) treated by the senior author (EMD) between October 2008 and December 2012. Patients were divided into two groups based on the choice of endovascular coils: (1) PC-400 and (2) conventional coils (Cashmere, Micrusphere, DeltaWind, and Ultipaq: Codman & Shurtleff, Inc., Raynham MA, USA; Hydrogel, Cosmos, Complex, and HyperSoft: MicroVention, Inc., Tustin CA, USA). All patients had planned adjunctive stenting with either an Enterprise (Codman & Shurtleff, Inc., Raynham MA, USA) or Neuroform (Stryker Corporation, Kalamazoo MI, USA) intracranial stent. Only unruptured aneurysms were considered in the present analysis because adjunctive stent placement is a rarity after aneurysm subarachnoid hemorrhage where antiplatelet therapy is a relative contraindication.

In our series, the first framing coil was placed into the aneurysm sac and its ability to respect the ostium of the neck was tested to confirm that it would not herniate into the parent vessel before detachment. In the PC-400 group, the stiffer standard coils were typically inserted first to frame the aneurysm so that they would maintain their position within the sac better and minimize the chance of coil loop herniation into the parent vessel. Subsequently, the coils were rapidly downsized and soft or extra-soft PC-400 coils were used to finish the packing to avoid pushing the previous coils out of the aneurysm sac. The initial PC-400 framing coil typically was chosen based on the maximum aneurysm sac diameter, downsizing to the closest loop size that matched the dome because of their more robust nature. Similar techniques were used with the conventional coils, except that the first framing coil was upsized to the closest loop length to secure them against the sac wall; our initial experience demonstrated that when the PC-400 system was chosen in the same manner, the coils were too large and would push out of the aneurysm. In both cases, if the first framing coil herniated into the parent vessel, it was removed and the process was repeated with a larger-sized framing coil and when stent assistance was required, a Neuroform or Enterprise stent was placed across the neck to act as a scaffold for the coil mass according to our standard treatment preferences.

The goal of every coiling was total occlusion of the aneurysm, aneurysm embolization grade (AEG) = A, with stent assistance only when framing coils would not respect the aneurysm neck. The AEG system was used because of its unique angiographic filling characteristics, which have been demonstrated to have predictive value for determining aneurysm sac thrombosis [2, 11]. The filling characteristics include persistent contrast in the aneurysm neck (AEG = B) or dome (AEG = C) in the capillary or venous phase of the angiogram, and emptying of contrast from the aneurysm neck (AEG = D) or dome (AEG = E) during the arterial phase in sync with the parent artery.

Coil insertion was stopped when total occlusion of the aneurysm was achieved or the microcatheter dislodged from the aneurysm neck and could not be accessed again, thus preventing additional coils from being inserted into the sac. An AEG was assigned by the interventionalist based on the flow of contrast material into the aneurysm neck and dome immediately after embolization. The packing density was calculated using AngioCalc (www.angiocalc.com) for all treated aneurysms. The length of coils and aneurysm volume were also used to calculate the total coil length per unit aneurysm volume (cm/mm^3). Short-term radiographic occlusion was noted at follow-up imaging typically scheduled 6 months postprocedure. The long-term occlusion durability of the PC-400 is being examined on a larger scale in the Aneurysm Coiling Efficiency Clinical Trial (NCT01465841).

Data were analyzed using SPSS Version 17 (IBM Corporation, Armonk NY, USA). Nominal variables were compared between the PC-400 and conventional coil groups using Fisher's Exact test. Continuous variables were compared between groups using independent samples t-tests. Two-sided probability values less than .05 were considered statistically significant for all analyses.

Table 1 Elective wide-necked intracranial aneurysm patient population characteristics and treatment details

	Penumbra Coil 400 System (N = 15)	Conventional coils (N = 23)	P value
Age, years; mean (SD)	58 (14)	59 (14)	.799
Aneurysm Embolization Grade (AEG)			
A; n (%)	6 (40 %)	9 (39 %)	.269
B; n (%)	3 (20 %)	9 (39 %)	
C; n (%)	4 (27 %)	5 (22 %)	
D; n (%)	2 (13 %)	0 (0 %)	
E; n (%)	0 (0 %)	0 (0 %)	
Stent assistance; n (%)	6 (40 %)	17 (74 %)	.049
Neck size, mm; mean (SD)	5.2 (1.8)	5.7 (1.5)	.425
Maximum aneurysm dimension, mm; mean (SD)	10.5 (4.2)	10.1 (3.5)	.760
Coil length, cm; mean (SD)	47 (31)	137 (117)	.002
Coil length per aneurysm volume (cm/mm^3); mean (SD)	0.20 (0.12)	0.43 (0.24)	.000
Number of coils; mean (SD)	6 (4)	10 (6)	.021
Packing density[a], %; mean (SD)	38 (22)	32 (18)	.379

[a]Calculated using AngioCalc

Results

Thirty-eight patients (59 ± 14 years) were identified who underwent coil embolization for wide-necked intracranial aneurysms. Fifteen patients were treated with the PC-400 system and the remaining 23 with conventional coils (Table 1). There were no significant differences in neck size or the maximum aneurysm dimension between groups (P = .760 and P = .425, respectively).

Adjunctive Stent

In patients treated with conventional coils, adjunctive stent placement was required in 74 % of the cases (17 of 23). The PC-400 resulted in a significantly reduced need for stent assistance, with only 40 % of the cases (6 of 15) requiring adjunctive stent placement (P = .049).

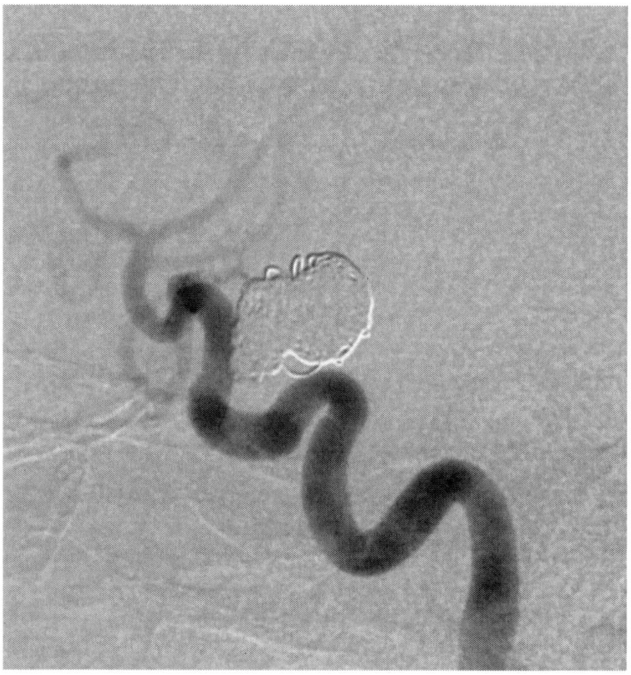

Fig. 3 Left paraophthalmic artery aneurysm after embolization with the Penumbra Coil 400 System without adjunctive intracranial stent (Aneurysm Embolization Grade = A)

Initial Occlusion

Total occlusion of the aneurysm neck and dome (AEG = A) was noted in 40 % of the PC-400 cases (Fig. 3) and 39 % of the conventional coil cases. Minimal residual dome filling with contrast stasis (AEG = C), suggesting a high likelihood of autothrombosis, was observed in 27 % of PC-400 cases and 22 % of the conventional coil cases. The packing density was not significantly different between PC-400 and conventional coils ($P = .379$). The number of coils necessary to occlude the aneurysm, total coil length, and length per unit sac volume were all significantly lower for cases treated with PC-400 compared with conventional coils (Table 1). No procedural complications occurred in either group.

Short-Term Follow-Up Occlusion

The mean time at follow-up was 5.3 ± 2.4 months. Stable or improved aneurysm occlusion was noted in 11 (85 %) of 13 patients treated with PC-400 (2 patients were excluded because of lack of imaging). One aneurysm exhibited a significant recurrence with recommended retreatment. Another aneurysm worsened from complete obliteration to a small residual neck with recommended observation rather than treatment. Neither worsened aneurysm was treated with adjunctive stent.

Patients treated with conventional coils exhibited stable or improved aneurysm occlusion in 20 (87 %) of 23 cases. Three aneurysms exhibited significant recurrence with recommended retreatment, two of which were initially treated with adjunctive stent placement. There was no significant difference in occlusion stability between PC-400 versus conventional coils ($P = 1.000$). Additionally, 2 of 23 patients treated with stent assistance in the conventional coil group demonstrated asymptomatic in-stent stenosis at follow-up.

Discussion

Stenosis and thromboembolic complications associated with the use of neck-remodeling devices increase the risk of treating wide-necked intracranial aneurysms [9]. A retrospective review of 161 patients treated with stent–coil embolization of an intracranial aneurysm documented a procedural morbidity rate of 14.9 %, along with stenosis and thromboembolic complications in 6.8 % of patients [6]. Delayed in-stent stenosis is not a rare occurrence. A review of 156 cerebral aneurysms treated with a Neuroform stent demonstrated stenosis in 5.8 % of patients at follow-up [4]. The stenosis can be symptomatic and may require endovascular treatment or surgical bypass. In addition to delayed complications, Piotin et al. recently reported a large series of 216 patients in which the periprocedural mortality rate in patients treated with adjunctive stent placement was 6.0 %, considerably higher than the 1.2 % in their procedures without stents [10].

For these reasons, avoidance of adjunctive stent usage and balloon assistance is a goal during endovascular treatment of aneurysms at our university. A coil that can respect the geometry of a wide-necked aneurysm without the need for a mechanical scaffold is highly desirable. In this study, the PC-400 was noted to rely less on adjunctive stent placement to secure the coil mass within the aneurysm sac than conventional coils. This may be because of its larger 0.020″ loops and inner Nitinol design, providing more stability of the coil mass within the aneurysm sac.

Techniques that minimize device dependence should be fully explored to minimize the risk and cost of these procedures to patients and health care insurers. Balloon-assisted coil embolization is one such technique that avoids the long-term complications associated with endovascular placement of a permanent metallic device. However, the potential for repeated episodes of cerebral ischemia and arterial wall injury may be increased with this technique and its use is not without controversy [12, 13]. Balloon assistance was not compared in this study because it is not the preferred adjunctive coiling technique at our university and is rarely used for aneurysm treatment.

The Penumbra-Slim microcatheter (0.025″ ID; 2.95Fr Proximal OD; 2.6Fr Distal OD) is recommended for placement of the PC-400 coils and requires a 6F (0.070″ ID) guide catheter. One of the main disadvantages of using the Penumbra-Slim microcatheter through a 6F guide is that the simultaneous use of a balloon catheter or a second microcatheter for stent deployment using the jailing technique is essentially prohibitive with the 0.070″ ID. A larger guide catheter is needed for dual microcatheter use in conjunction with the Penumbra-Slim. Additionally, the larger microcatheter size needed for this coil system may be prohibitive in patients with tortuous cervicocranial vasculature and very narrow-necked aneurysms, increasing the difficulty in accessing the aneurysm. The microcatheter size can also be an impediment when trying to access individual lobes of a multilobulated aneurysm or when trying to cross a stent wall for aneurysm access.

An additional finding in this study was that there was no significant difference between immediate postembolization packing densities and filling characteristics between the PC-400 and conventional coil systems. Despite the packing densities being similar, the total coil length and number of coils was significantly lower with the larger diameter PC-400 coil system. Short-term follow-up was included in the present study and demonstrated no significant difference in occlusion stability between PC-400 versus conventional coils. Long-term occlusion durability is being examined in the Aneurysm Coiling Efficiency Clinical Trial (NCT01465841) and will ultimately be important when evaluating the performance of the PC-400 system.

The limitations of this study include the small sample size, single interventionalist, and retrospective examination. However, limiting the results to a single interventionalist reduces technique variation and results in consistent procedural decisions across all cases.

Conclusion

Embolization of wide-necked aneurysms with the PC-400 system required significantly less stent assistance, fewer coils, and shorter coil length than conventional coils, resulting in similar short-term angiographic outcomes. This may reduce treatment cost and prove to be valuable in patients with contraindications to dual antiplatelet therapy.

Conflict of Interest Statement Dr. Eric Deshaies consults for MicroVention Inc., Covidien Neurovascular, Integra LifeSciences Corporation, and McKesson Health Solutions.

References

1. Akpek S, Arat A, Morsi H, Klucznick RP, Strother CM, Mawad ME (2005) Self-expandable stent-assisted coiling of wide-necked intracranial aneurysms: a single-center experience. AJNR Am J Neuroradiol 26(5):1223–1231
2. Deshaies EM, Adamo MA, Boulos AS (2007) A prospective single-center analysis of the safety and efficacy of the hydrocoil embolization system for the treatment of intracranial aneurysms. J Neurosurg 106(2):226–233
3. Fiorella D, Albuquerque FC, Han P, McDougall CG (2004) Preliminary experience using the Neuroform stent for the treatment of cerebral aneurysms. Neurosurgery 54(1):6–16; discussion 16–17
4. Fiorella D, Albuquerque FC, Woo H, Rasmussen PA, Masaryk TJ, McDougall CG (2006) Neuroform in-stent stenosis: incidence, natural history, and treatment strategies. Neurosurgery 59(1):34–42; discussion 34–42
5. Jabbour P, Koebbe C, Veznedaroglu E, Benitez RP, Rosenwasser R (2004) Stent-assisted coil placement for unruptured cerebral aneurysms. Neurosurg Focus 17(5):E10
6. Kanaan H, Jankowitz B, Aleu A et al (2010) In-stent thrombosis and stenosis after neck-remodeling device-assisted coil embolization of intracranial aneurysms. Neurosurgery 67(6):1523–1532; discussion 1532–1533
7. Layton KF, Cloft HJ, Gray LA, Lewis DA, Kallmes DF (2007) Balloon-assisted coiling of intracranial aneurysms: evaluation of local thrombus formation and symptomatic thromboembolic complications. AJNR Am J Neuroradiol 28(6):1172–1175
8. Lefkowitz MA, Gobin YP, Akiba Y, Duckwiler GR, Murayama Y, Guglielmi G, Martin NA, Viñuela F (1999) Balloon-assisted Guglielmi detachable coiling of wide-necked aneurysms: Part II – Clinical results. Neurosurgery 45(3):531–537; discussion 537–538
9. McDonald JS, Norgan AP, McDonald RJ, Lanzino G, Kallmes DF, Cloft HJ (2012) In-hospital outcomes associated with stent-assisted endovascular treatment of unruptured cerebral aneurysms in the USA. J Neurointerv Surg. doi:10.1136/neurintsurg-2012-010349
10. Piotin M, Blanc R, Spelle L, Mounayer C, Piantino R, Schmidt PJ, Moret J (2010) Stent-assisted coiling of intracranial aneurysms: clinical and angiographic results in 216 consecutive aneurysms. Stroke 41(1):110–115
11. Singla A, Villwock MR, Jacobsen W, Deshaies EM (2012) Aneurysm embolization grade: a predictive tool for aneurysm recurrence after coil embolization. Acta Neurochir (Wien). doi:10.1007/s00701-012-1554-3
12. Sluzewski M, van Rooij WJ, Beute GN, Nijssen PC (2006) Balloon-assisted coil embolization of intracranial aneurysms: incidence, complications, and angiography results. J Neurosurg 105(3):396–399
13. Soeda A, Sakai N, Sakai H, Iihara K, Yamada N, Imakita S, Nagata I (2003) Thromboembolic events associated with Guglielmi detachable coil embolization of asymptomatic cerebral aneurysms: evaluation of 66 consecutive cases with use of diffusion-weighted MR imaging. AJNR Am J Neuroradiol 24(1):127–132
14. Toyoda K, Yasaka M, Iwade K et al (2008) Dual antithrombotic therapy increases severe bleeding events in patients with stroke and cardiovascular disease: a prospective, multicenter, observational study. Stroke 39(6):1740–1745
15. Tumialán LM, Zhang YJ, Cawley CM, Dion JE, Tong FC, Barrow DL (2008) Intracranial hemorrhage associated with stent-assisted coil embolization of cerebral aneurysms: a cautionary report. J Neurosurg 108(6):1122–1129

Quality of Life and Outcome After Treatment of Ruptured Cerebral Aneurysms: Results of a Single Center in Switzerland

Lucia Schwyzer, Evelin Soleman, Rolf Ensner, Angel Mironov, Hans Landolt, and Javier Fandino

Abstract *Object:* To evaluate the subjective outcome and quality of life (QoL) of patients who suffered from aneurysmal subarachnoid hemorrhage and underwent endovascular coiling or microsurgical clipping in a single center.

Methods: For this retrospective single-center study, we included patients who underwent aneurysm occlusion at the Cantonal Hospital of Aarau between January 2000 and December 2006. The QoL, the functional status, and the level of independence were assessed by means of the Short Form (SF)-12 Health Survey, the modified Rankin Scale (mRS), and the Barthel Index. The questionnaires were sent to and completed by the patients. A total of 104 patients with a mean age of 53.14 years (range, 18–80 years) were included in the study. In 63 (60.6 %) of the cases, the aneurysm was clipped; in 41 (39.4 %) of the cases, endovascular coiling was performed.

Results: The SF-12 scores for the PCS (Physical Component Summary) and MCS (Mental Component Summary) were similar for both clipped (PCS 45.35; MCS 46.55) and coiled (PCS 46.31; MCS 47.87) patients. The mean values were, on average, 4.17 points lower for the PCS and 2.79 points lower for the MCS when compared with the mean of the US population, with a mean of 50 (standard deviation (SD) 10). The mean Barthel Index for the entire group was 92.26 (SD 16.8) and was almost identical for both the clipped (92.54; SD 16.21) and coiled (91.83; SD 17.9) patients ($p=0.56$). The mean mRS did not differ between the coiled and clipped patients (coiled 1.63; clipped 1.56; $p=0.97$)

Conclusions: There were no significant differences in the functional and mental health scores between the two groups of clipped and coiled patients who were treated at our center, but both groups were lower than population-based scores. Although the neurologic condition and the imaging results on admission were worse in the coiled group, the long-term results did not differ significantly.

Keywords Subarachnoid hemorrhage • Ruptured aneurysm Quality of life • Outcome • Clipping • Coiling

L. Schwyzer, MD • E. Soleman, MD • J. Fandino, MD (✉)
Department of Neurosurgery, Kantonsspital Aarau,
Aarau, Switzerland
e-mail: neurosurgery@ksa.ch

H. Landolt, MD
Department of Neurosurgery, Kantonsspital Aarau,
Tellstrasse, Aarau, 5001, Switzerland

R. Ensner, MD
Department of Intensive Care Medicine, Kantonsspital Aarau,
Aarau, Switzerland

A. Mironov, MD
Division of Neuroradiology, Department of Radiology,
Kantonsspital Aarau, Aarau, Switzerland

Introduction

Although the mortality and morbidity in patients after subarachnoid hemorrhage (SAH) caused by rupture of an aneurysm has greatly decreased within the last decades with advancements in microsurgical techniques and the development of the endovascular coiling technique [11], for many patients, the impact on quality of life (QoL), independence, and cognitive function remains enormous. Although many patients may have objectively a good or even excellent neurological outcome, they may have to deal with emotional and neuropsychological disturbances that complicate their social reintegration [5, 19].8

To evaluate the overall well-being of the patients, subjective physical and mental health has to be taken into account along with objective measurements. Previous studies have shown that the QoL of patients who suffered an aneurysmal SAH is very often substantially affected and diminished [8]. A number of self-administered instruments to measure the subjective functional and mental health status exist [3, 13]. The Short Form (SF)-12 Health Survey is a shorter version

J. Fandino et al. (eds.), *Neurovascular Events After Subarachnoid Hemorrhage*, Acta Neurochirurgica Supplement, Vol. 120,
DOI 10.1007/978-3-319-04981-6_34, © Springer International Publishing Switzerland 2015

Table 1 Patient characteristcs and clinical grading on admission distributed by treatment modality

	All patients (%)	Clipped patients (%)	Coiled patients (%)
Men	33 (31.7)	20 (31.7)	13 (31.7)
Women	71 (68.3)	43 (68.3)	28 (68.3)
Mean age in years; range	53.14 years; 18–80 years	53.89 years; 18–80 years	51.86 years; 20–76 years
Glasgow Coma Scale (GCS)			
GCS 3 – 6	26 (25)	10 (15.9)	16 (39)
GCS 7 – 12	10 (9.6)	5 (8)	5 (12)
GCS 13 – 14	30 (28.9)	21 (33.3)	9 (22)
GCS 15	35 (33.7)	26 (41.3)	9 (22)
Hunt & Hess Scale (HH)			
HH 0	1 (1)	1 (1.6)	
HH 1	2 (1.9)	2 (3.2)	
HH 2	59 (56.7)	40 (63.5)	19 (46.3)
HH 3	16 (15.4)	11 (17.5)	5 (12.2)
HH 4	19 (18.3)	7 (11.1)	12 (29.3)
HH 5	7 (6.7)	2 (3.2)	5 (12.2)
Fisher Scale (on admission CT scan)			
1	2 (1.9)	1 (1.6)	1 (2.4)
2	11 (10.6)	8 (12.7)	3 (7.3)
3	40 (38.5)	30 (47.6)	10 (24.4)
4	50 (48.1)	23 (36.5)	27 (65.9)
Treatment			
Clipping	63 (60.6)		
Coiling	41 (39.4)		

of the SF-36 [4]. It covers the same eight health domains as the SF-36, but has only 12 questions and, therefore, can be completed in a much shorter time. This questionnaire has been shown to be a reliable and valid tool that measures the same health domains as the SF-36 (physical, mental, and social functioning; bodily pain; vitality; and handicaps) [9].

In addition to the SF-12 score, we assessed the Barthel Index and the modified Rankin scale (mRS) to evaluate the level of independence and disability, respectively. The purpose of our study was to evaluate the QoL and subjective functional outcome of patients who underwent treatment for a ruptured aneurysm at our center between 2000 and 2006.

Materials and Methods

Patient Population and Characteristics

A total of 174 patients presenting with aneurysmal SAH were admitted and treated in our institution between January 2000 and December 2006. Among those patients, 33 died during the follow-up period and 37 patients were lost to follow-up or could not be included in the study because of incomplete questionnaires. The final analysis included 71 women (68.3 %) and 33 men (31.7 %), with a mean age of 53.1 years (range 18–80 years). Sixty-three patients (60.6 %) underwent microsurgical clipping of their ruptured aneurysm and 41 patients (39.4 %) underwent endovascular coiling.

On admission, the neurologic condition was assessed by the Glasgow Coma Scale (GCS), the Hunt & Hess Scale (HH), and the Fisher Scale on computed tomography (CT) scan [14]. The patient characteristics and imaging grading on admission CT scan are shown in Table 1.

Measurement of Outcome and Quality of Life

Quality of life was assessed using the QoL questionnaire SF-12 Health Survey for self-administration, which is a shorter version of the SF-36 Health Survey (QualiMetric Inc., Lincoln, RI, USA) [18]. The results of the SF-12 questionnaire are composed of a Physical Component Summary (PCS) score and a Mental Component Summary (MCS) score and are obtained by standard algorithms. The SF-12 PCS and MCS scores of the US population have a mean of 50, with a standard deviation (SD) of 10. Lower scores mean a worse health status, higher scores a better health status. The written German version of the SF-12 was mailed to the patients and standard scoring algorithms were used to score their responses to the 12 multiple choice questions.

To evaluate the functional health status, the mRS score and the Barthel Index [6, 17] were assessed. The mRS ranges from 0 to 6 and the scores are defined as: (0) no symptoms at all; (1) no significant disability despite symptoms, able to carry out all usual duties and activities; (2) slight disability, unable to carry out all previous activities, but able to look after own affairs without assistance; (3) moderate disability, requiring some help, but able to walk without assistance; (4) moderately severe disability, unable to walk without assistance and unable to attend to own bodily needs without assistance; (5) severe disability, bedridden, incontinent, and requiring constant nursing care and attention; and (6) dead.

Additionally, the Self Evaluation of Health State test, which is a visual analog scale (VAS), was used to evaluate the present subjective health state. In the VAS, 100 points is defined as the best and 0 as the worst imaginable state.

The questionnaires were filled out by the patients themselves or by the help of a close relative.

Results

Study Population

The mean age for all of the patients was 53.14 years (range 18–80 years) and was 53.89 years (range 18–80 years) for the clipped group versus 51.86 years (range 20–76 years) for the coiled group. The median Glasgow Coma Scale (GCS) score (± SD) on presentation was 11 (±5) for all patients; and GCS 12 (±4) for the clipped and GCS 9 (±5) for the coiled patients. The median Hunt and Hess Score was 3 (±1) for all patients; in the coiled patients was 2 (±1) and in the clipped patients was 3 (±1).

The location and thickness of the subarachnoid blood clot was scaled by the Fisher Grading Scale (± SD) on CT scan. The mean grade was 3 (±1) for the whole group and was, on average, 1 point higher in the coiled (mean, 4 ±1) than in the clipped (mean, 3 ±1) patients.

SF-12 Results

The results of the SF-12 Health survey, which are split into a PCS score and a MCS score, were as follows (Figs. 1 and 2). The mean overall PCS was 45.73 (range, 23.32–60.04) and the mean overall MCS was 47.07 (range, 17.76–67.99). For the clipped patients, the mean SF-12 score for PCS was 45.35 (range, 23.32–60.04) and for MCS was 46.55 (range, 17.76–67.14) and did not differ significantly from those of the coiled patients, where the PCS was 46.31 (range, 26.22–57.9) and the MCS was 47.87 (range, 23.32–67.99). The mean values were, on average, 4.17 points lower for the PCS and 2.79 points lower for the MCS when compared with the mean of the US population, with a mean of 50 (standard deviation (SD) 10).

Barthel Index Results

The mean Barthel Index for the whole group was 92.26 (SD 16.8), with a range between 10 and 100 (Fig. 3). The indexes were practically identical for both clipped (mean, 92.54; SD 16.21) and coiled (mean, 91.83; SD 17.9) patients ($p=0.56$).

Modified Rankin Scale Results

Fifty-six (53.9 %) of all study patients had mRS scores of 0 or 1, meaning that they had no significant disability and were fully independent (Fig. 4). A moderate to severe disability was observed in 16 patients (15.4 %) of the whole group. The mRS scores did not differ between the coiled and clipped patients (mean coiled, 1.63; mean clipped, 1.56; $p=0.97$).

Self-Evaluation of Health State (VAS) Results

The mean VAS score for the whole group was 71.57 (SD 23.20), and ranged from 5 to 100 % (Fig. 5). The mean VAS scores were similar for both clipped (mean, 70.97; SD 24.03) and coiled (mean, 72.49; SD 22.14) patients ($p=0.000$).

Discussion

This single-center study provides the outcome and QoL from the patient's perspective after either endovascular or microsurgical treatment of a ruptured aneurysm. Within recent years, reliable tools to measure outcome and QoL have become more widespread, related to the increasing demand of evaluation of cost-effectiveness and evidence-based medicine. With skyrocketing health care costs, the public interest and need for measuring long-term effectiveness of different therapeutic interventions, such as for aneurysmal SAH, has increased [10, 20]. In Switzerland, there is a lack of studies addressing treatment outcome after a ruptured aneurysm [2].

To measure the outcome and different QoL domains, standardized scores are most valuable to compare patients series and treatments. Both the SF-36 and the SF-12 health survey are valid and reliable instruments to measure QoL [4, 9,

15, 18]. The advantages of the SF-12 questionnaire are that it is an easy to understand and short multiple choice survey that can be completed by the patient within minutes and that it incorporates the physical as well as the mental health status.

The results of previous studies addressing outcome after aneurysmal SAH have demonstrated the importance of measurements that address not only the neurologic condition but also subjective well-being and functional status [9, 15]. It has been shown that the subjective outcome can differ significantly from the objective impression and that many patients with a good neurological outcome suffer from neuropsychological long-term problems [1, 2, 7, 15, 16]. So far, only few studies exist that used the SF-12 score to measure the QoL after treatment for a ruptured cerebral aneurysm [9].

The aim of our study was to evaluate and document the outcome of those patients who were treated for a ruptured intracranial aneurysm at our institution. The comparison of the two therapeutical modalities was not a major objective in our study, although we analyzed the two groups separately to detect differences regarding the outcome. We did not observe differences in the QoL between clipped and coiled patients. Other studies assessing the long-term outcome domains after treatment for a ruptured intracranial aneurysm also showed no major differences between clipping and coiling, although neuropsychological assessments after SAH have suggested that the treatment modality affects the outcome specifically in regard to the location of the aneurysm [1, 12].

Among the weak points of our study are the facts that it is a single-center study with a relatively small patients series and that the length of the follow-up time after treatment varies from 1 to 6 years. In addition, we did not obtain any response from a number of patients. Further, it has to be taken into consideration that the response to such QoL questionnaires may be higher for patients with good outcomes and high levels of independence.

Although the conclusions that can be drawn from our data might be limited, this study emphasizes the importance of QoL evaluations to document the treatment outcome in combination with objective outcome assessments. To detect specific and slight differences between the treatment modalities, multicenter studies with patient matching and a clear standardized study design of QoL measurements, neuropsychological tests, and follow-up time points would be crucial. Such studies would help to better predict the long-term outcome and to define guidelines that are more precise for therapeutic management.

Conclusion

We present the outcome and QoL of patients who were treated either by clipping or coiling for a ruptured aneurysm between January 2000 and December 2006 in our single-center study. Our results do not show any major long-term difference regarding the functional and mental health after either treatment, coiling or clipping, but demonstrate a diminished overall QoL when compared with the norm.

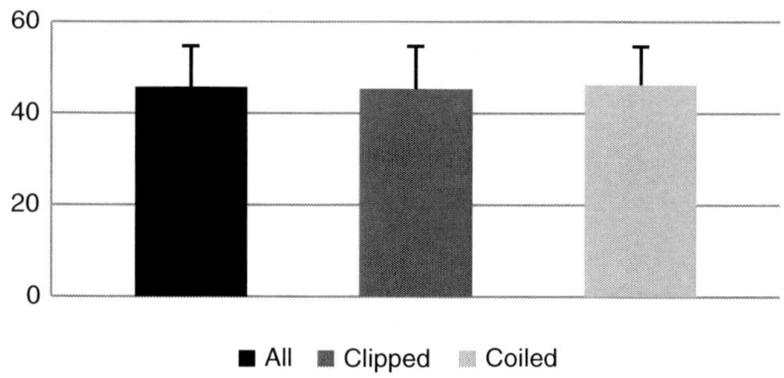

Fig. 1 SF-12 PCS (Physical Component Summary)

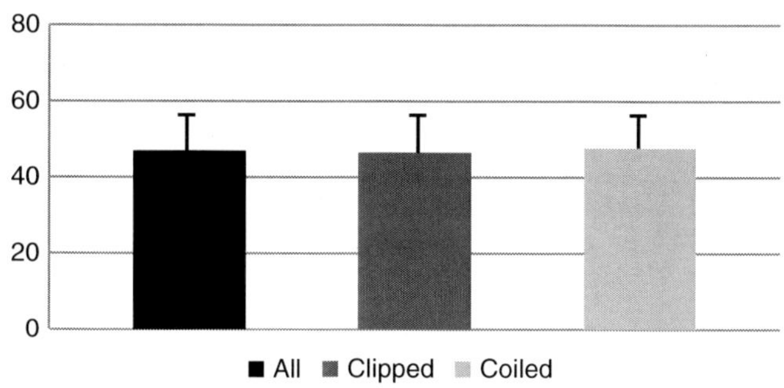

Fig. 2 SF-12 MCS (Mental Component Summary)

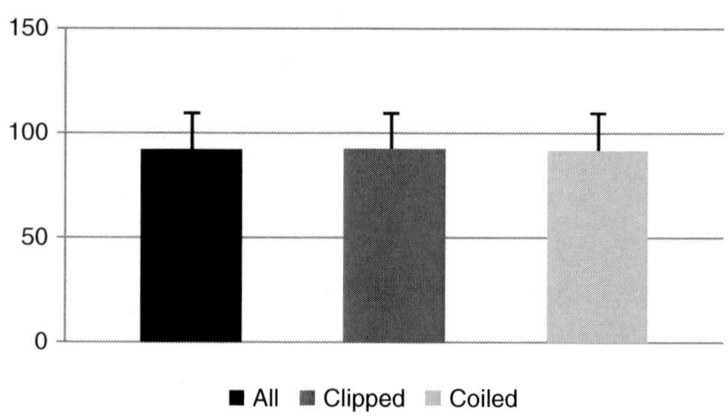

Fig. 3 Barthel Index

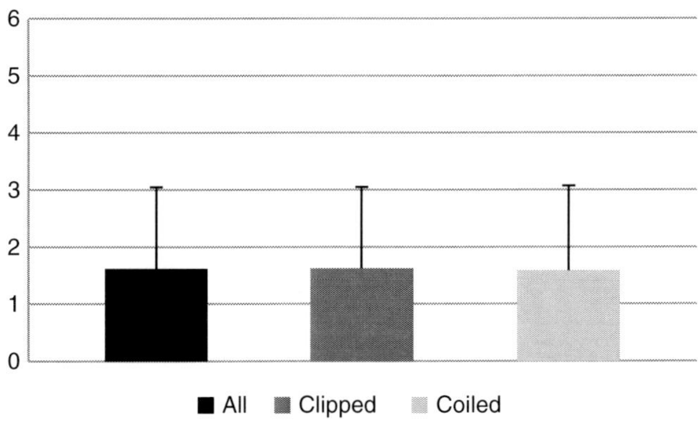

Fig. 4 mRS (modified Rankin Scale)

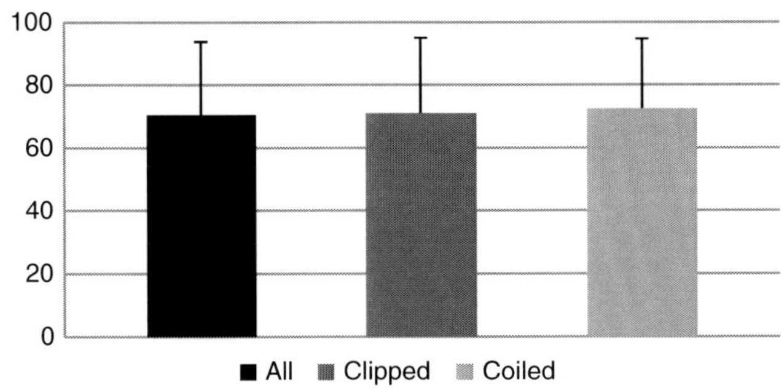

Fig. 5 VAS (visual analog scale)

Conflict of Interest Statement We declare that we have no conflict of interest.

References

1. Bellebaum C, Schafers L, Schoch B, Wanke I, Stolke D, Forsting M, Daum I (2004) Clipping versus coiling: neuropsychological follow up after aneurysmal subarachnoid haemorrhage (SAH). J Clin Exp Neuropsychol 26:1081–1092
2. Bjeljac M, Keller E, Regard M, Yonekawa Y (2002) Neurological and neuropsychological outcome after SAH. Acta Neurochir Suppl 82:83–85
3. Brazier J, Roberts J, Deverill M (2002) The estimation of a preference-based measure of health from the SF-36. J Health Econ 21:271–292
4. Brazier JE, Roberts J (2004) The estimation of a preference-based measure of health from the SF-12. Med Care 42:851–859
5. Carter BS, Buckley D, Ferraro R, Rordorf G, Ogilvy CS (2000) Factors associated with reintegration to normal living after subarachnoid hemorrhage. Neurosurgery 46:1326–1333; discussion 1333–1334
6. Collin C, Wade DT, Davies S, Horne V (1988) The Barthel ADL Index: a reliability study. Int Disabil Stud 10:61–63
7. Hackett ML, Anderson CS (2000) Health outcomes 1 year after subarachnoid hemorrhage: an international population-based study. The Australian Cooperative Research on Subarachnoid Hemorrhage Study Group. Neurology 55:658–662
8. Katati MJ, Santiago-Ramajo S, Perez-Garcia M, Meersmans-Sanchez Jofre M, Vilar-Lopez R, Coin-Mejias MA, Caracuel-Romero A, Arjona-Moron V (2007) Description of quality of life and its predictors in patients with aneurysmal subarachnoid hemorrhage. Cerebrovasc Dis 24:66–73
9. King JT Jr, Horowitz MB, Kassam AB, Yonas H, Roberts MS (2005) The short form-12 and the measurement of health status in patients with cerebral aneurysms: performance, validity, and reliability. J Neurosurg 102:489–494
10. Maud A, Lakshminarayan K, Suri MF, Vazquez G, Lanzino G, Qureshi AI (2009) Cost-effectiveness analysis of endovascular versus neurosurgical treatment for ruptured intracranial aneurysms in the United States. J Neurosurg 110:880–886
11. Prestigiacomo CJ (2006) Historical perspectives: the microsurgical and endovascular treatment of aneurysms. Neurosurgery 59:S39–S47; discussion S3–S13
12. Proust F, Martinaud O, Gerardin E, Derrey S, Leveque S, Bioux S, Tollard E, Clavier E, Langlois O, Godefroy O, Hannequin D, Freger P (2009) Quality of life and brain damage after microsurgical clip occlusion or endovascular coil embolization for ruptured anterior communicating artery aneurysms: neuropsychological assessment. J Neurosurg 110:19–29
13. Rabin R, de Charro F (2001) EQ-5D: a measure of health status from the EuroQol Group. Ann Med 33:337–343
14. Rosen DS, Macdonald RL (2005) Subarachnoid hemorrhage grading scales: a systematic review. Neurocrit Care 2:110–118
15. Scharbrodt W, Stein M, Schreiber V, Boker DK, Oertel MF (2009) The prediction of long-term outcome after subarachnoid hemorrhage as measured by the Short Form-36 Health Survey. J Clin Neurosci 16(11):1409–1413
16. Scott RB, Farmer E, Smiton A, Tovey C, Clarke M, Carpenter K (2004) Methodology of neuropsychological research in multicentre randomized clinical trials: a model derived from the International Subarachnoid Aneurysm Trial. Clin Trials 1:31–39
17. Wade DT, Collin C (1988) The Barthel ADL Index: a standard measure of physical disability? Int Disabil Stud 10:64–67
18. Ware J Jr, Kosinski M, Keller SD (1996) A 12-Item Short-Form Health Survey: construction of scales and preliminary tests of reliability and validity. Med Care 34:220–233
19. Wermer MJ, Kool H, Albrecht KW, Rinkel GJ (2007) Subarachnoid hemorrhage treated with clipping: long-term effects on employment, relationships, personality, and mood. Neurosurgery 60:91–97; discussion 97–98
20. Zubair Tahir M, Enam SA, Pervez Ali R, Bhatti A, ul Haq T (2009) Cost-effectiveness of clipping vs coiling of intracranial aneurysms after subarachnoid hemorrhage in a developing country–a prospective study. Surg Neurol 72:355–360; discussion 360–361

Repeated Combined Endovascular Therapy with Milrinone and Nimodipine for the Treatment of Severe Vasospasm: Preliminary Results

Camillo Sherif, Bernhard Wambacher, Michel Loyoddin, Radenko Karaic, Peter Krafft, Andreas Valentin, Dimiter Tscholakoff, and Guenther Kleinpeter

Abstract *Background*: Delayed vasospasm (VSP) following aneurysmal subarachnoid hemorrhage (aSAH) remains a major source of morbidity. Milrinone was recently suggested as an invasive VSP treatment option. It is a phosphodiesterase III inhibitor with vasodilating and additional positive inotrope and anti-inflammatory effects.

Methods: In this preliminary series, we included patients with severe VSP and unsuccessful maximum conservative therapy. Inclusion criteria were (1) transcranial Doppler (TCD) mean >180 cm/s; (2) increase of >50 % of TCD mean values within 6 h to values >150 cm/s; and/or (3) neurological deterioration (after exclusion of hemorrhage, hydrocephalus, and other systemic reasons). Patients received endovascular therapy with nimodipine 2 mg followed by milrinone 4–8 mg. Reinterventions were indicated aggressively in cases of persistent neurological deficits or persistent high mean TCD >180 cm/s.

Results: Of 121 consecutive aSAH patients, 16 (13.2 %) received endovascular VSP therapy. Of these, 11 patients (68.5 %) received ≥3 interventions (median 4; maximum 9); 14 (87.5 %) showed postinterventional angiographic improvement of vessel diameters; and 11 (68.5 %) showed improvement of their neurological deficits after a mean follow-up time of 4.5 months. No cardiovascular adverse events attributed to milrinone were observed.

Conclusions: Milrinone may be a useful supplementary substance for endovascular VSP therapy. Aggressive reintervention indications did not cause additional adverse events.

Keywords Cerebral • Vasospasm • Milrinone • Endovascular • Intervention • Treatment

Introduction

A main cause of mortality and poor neurological outcome after aneurysmal subarachnoid hemorrhage (aSAH), in addition to the direct effects of the initial hemorrhage and rebleed, are cerebral infarctions associated with delayed ischemic neurological deficits (DINDs) secondary to cerebral vasospasm (VSP). Between 15 and 20 % of patients die or develop a stroke, leading to increased morbidity and mortality [7]. If the standard recommended conservative therapy consisting of prophylactic nimodipine and induced hypertension and hemodilution [16] fails, several invasive treatment options remain. The present guidelines of the American Heart Association [7] recommend a class 2a invasive endovascular treatment, without differentiating between the multiple endovascular approaches. In addition to mechanical techniques using balloon dilation [2], many different substances, such as papaverine, nimodipine, verapamil, fasudil, and many others have been proposed [1, 12].

C. Sherif, MD (✉)
Department of Neurosurgery, Krankenanstalt Rudolfstiftung, Juchgasse 25, A-1030 Vienna, Austria

Department of Neurosurgery, Cerebrovascular Research Group, Krankenanstalt Rudolfstiftung, Juchgasse 25, A-1030 Vienna, Austria

Department of Neurosurgery, Ludwig Boltzmann Cluster for Cardiovascular Research, Vienna, Austria
e-mail: camillo.sherif@cerebrovascular.at

B. Wambacher • G. Kleinpeter, MD
Department of Neurosurgery, Krankenanstalt Rudolfstiftung, Juchgasse 25, A-1030 Vienna, Austria

Cerebrovascular Research Group, Krankenanstalt Rudolfstiftung, Juchgasse 25, A-1030 Vienna, Austria

M. Loyoddin, MD
Department of Neurosurgery, Krankenanstalt Rudolfstiftung, Juchgasse 25, A-1030 Vienna, Austria

R. Karaic, MD • D. Tscholakoff, MD
Department of Radiology, Krankenanstalt Rudolfstiftung, Vienna, Austria

P. Krafft, MD
Department of Anesthesiology and Intensive Care Medicine, Krankenanstalt Rudolfstiftung, Vienna, Austria

A. Valentin, MD
Intensive Care Unit, Department of Cardiology, Krankenanstalt Rudolfstiftung, Vienna, Austria

J. Fandino et al. (eds.), *Neurovascular Events After Subarachnoid Hemorrhage*, Acta Neurochirurgica Supplement, Vol. 120,
DOI 10.1007/978-3-319-04981-6_35,

Milrinone, widely used in cardiology for heart failure, is a phosphodiesterase III inhibitor with vasodilating but also positive inotrope and anti-inflammatory effects [15]. In the present series, we present our preliminary results of endovascular milrinone application supplementary to nimodipine. To minimize the effects of postinterventional VSP recurrence, we used a policy of aggressive reinterventions.

Patients and Methods

Inclusion Criteria

Beginning on January 1, 2012, all aSAH patients with severe VSP refractory to maximum conservative treatment were included in the study. In detail, the inclusion criteria were (1) transcranial Doppler (TCD) mean >180 cm/s; (2) increase of >50 % of TCD mean values within 6 h to values >150 cm/s; and/or (3) neurological deterioration (after exclusion of hemorrhage, hydrocephalus, and other systemic reasons). Patients received endovascular therapy with nimodipine 2 mg followed by milrinone 4–8 mg. Reinterventions were indicated aggressively in cases with persistent neurological deficits or persistent high mean TCD >180 cm/s values.

Data Collection

In our department, all data of aSAH patients are prospectively collected in a database. The following parameters were extracted retrospectively from this database for the present evaluations: demographic data (age, gender); aneurysm locations; Fisher grades; Hunt and Hess grades; treatment modality (clipping, endovascular); time to first intervention; reason for intervention; number of interventions; clinical follow up of preinterventional and postinterventional neurological symptoms, including modified Rankin Scale (independently evaluated by anesthesiologist/intensive care specialists); time of last follow-up; TCD values preinterventional and postinterventional at the level of the MCA (independently evaluated by three subspecialized anesthesiologists/intensive care specialists). The degree of VSP (as compared with the vessel diameter on the initial digital subtraction angiography (DSA)/CT angiography, with severe VSP defined as ≤70 % and moderate VSP as 50–70 %) and the success of the endovascular intervention was evaluated retrospectively by an independent blinded neurosurgeon.

Statistical Evaluation

For all statistical comparisons, we used the software program SAS 8.01 (SAS Institute Inc., Cary, NC). A P value <0.05 was considered statistically significant. All data are given as mean value ± standard deviation. The Wilcoxon matched-pairs test was used for intraindividual comparisons (before vs. after).

Results

Of 121 consecutive aSAH patients, 16 patients (13.2 %) received endovascular VSP therapy. In our series of 121 aSAH patients, 103 patients were clipped (85.1 %) and 18 patients coiled (14.8 %). Among the 16 patients receiving endovascular VSP therapy, we had 13 clipped (81.25 %) and 3 coiled patients (18.75 %).

In the anterior circulation (87.5 %), aneurysms were located at the anterior cerebral artery in six patients (37.5 %), at the internal carotid artery in six patients (37.5 %), and at the medial cerebral artery in two patients (12.5 %). In the posterior circulation (12.5 %), aneurysms were found at the basilar bifurcation in one patient (6.25 %) and at the posterior inferior cerebellar artery in one patient (6.25 %). Eleven patients (68.75 %) had severe VSP and five patients (31.25 %) had moderate VSP.

One patient (6.25 %) had Fisher grade 2, nine patients (56.25 %) had Fisher grade 3, and six patients (37.5 %) had Fisher grade 4. Four patients (25 %) had Hunt and Hess grade (HH) 1; six patients had HH2 (37.5 %); one patient (6.25 %) had HH3; and five patients (31.25 %) had HH4.

The mean time to the first intervention was 8d ± 3.16d. Indications were clinical neurological deterioration (hemiparesis, aphasia, impaired consciousness) ± TCD elevation in 11 patients (68.75 %); in 5 sedated patients (31.25 %), indications were based on TCD worsening alone. A total of 11 patients (68.5 %) received ≥3 interventions (median, 4; maximum, 9). Fourteen patients (87.5 %) showed DSA improvement after each intervention. We observed an additional effect on vasodilation of milrinone over nimodipine in all patients (see Fig. 1). The mean preinterventional TCD before the first intervention reached 200.9 ± 57.8 cm/s and was reduced to 95 ± 23.7 cm/s ($p = 0.001$) after intervention. For repetitive interventions, the preinterventional mean TCD value was 193.6 ± 66.2 cm/s versus 88.2 ± 11.3 cm/s after intervention ($p = 0.0156$). In 15 (93.8 %) of 16 patients, we found TCD improvement after each intervention.

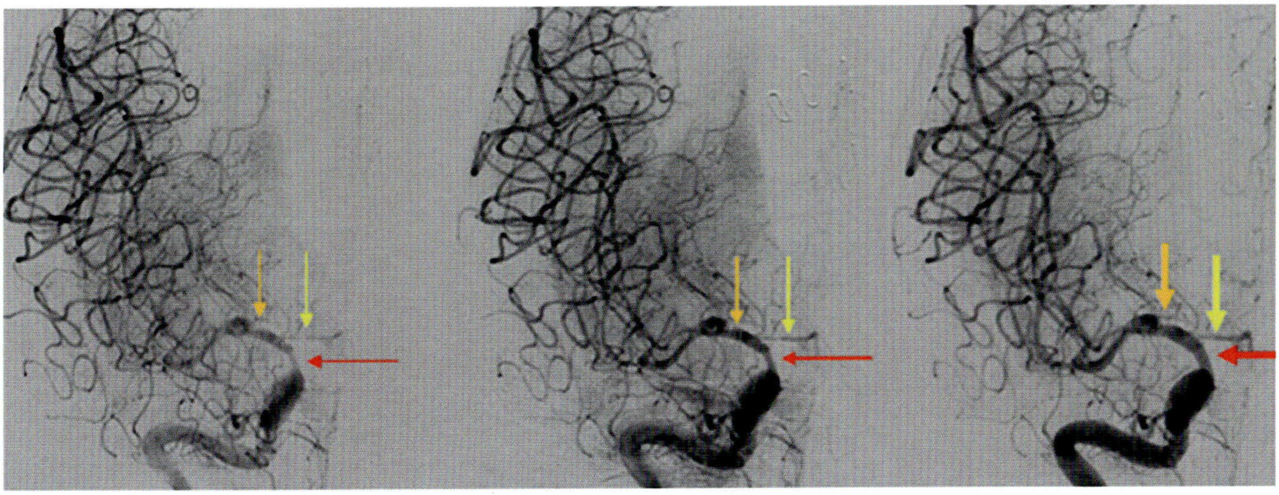

Fig. 1 Third intervention for patient No. 5; DSA anterior/posterior projection. Note the typical additional effect on vasodilation of milrinone supplementary to nimpodipine (*orange arrow* M1 segment, *yellow arrow* A1 segment, *red arrow* ICA)

Outcome Parameter

After a mean follow-up time of 4.5 months, 68.5 % of the patients (11 of 16) showed a good clinical outcome, with mRS ≤ 2. Preinterventional neurological deficits improved in 68.5 % of the patients. Mortality was low, at 6.25 % (one patient).

Poor initial clinical condition was correlated with therapy failure and bad outcome. We had five patients without postinterventional recovery and a bad clinical outcome of mRS ≥ 3. Of those, four patients had initial HH4 and Fisher grade 4, and one patient had HH3 and Fisher grade 3. We did not observe severe cardiovascular adverse events attributed to milrinone despite increased use of vasopressors and multiple treatments.

Discussion

The recommended and widely accepted standard conservative treatment for VSP includes prophylactic administration of nimodipine, triple-H therapy (hypertension, hypervolemia, and hemodilution; without hypervolemia [16]) and cerebrospinal fluid drainage [7]. If these standard treatments fail, intraarterial injection of vasodilators such as verapamil [14], papavarine [11], nimodipine [6], nicardipine [5], or balloon angioplasty with or without additional intraarterial vasodilators [8] have been proposed as rescue therapies. Several alternative substances such as fasudil [20], mainly used in Japan, and colforsin daropate [21] for local endovascular as well as systemic intraarterial or intravenous administration have also been tried. A main problem with all the interventional techniques remains the reversibility of the vasodilation and, thus, clinical treatment effects. Using balloon angioplasty, there is even a potential for serious life-threatening complications, including vessel rupture, branch occlusion, displacement of surgical clips, and rupture of untreated aneurysms despite improved techniques and catheters [22]. The first randomized controlled trial, the IMCVS trial (ClinicalTrials.gov Identifier: NCT01400360), using mainly balloon angioplasty with or without intraarterial application of vasodilators, was interrupted because of statistical significant higher mortality in the interventional group as compared with the conservative treatment group [23].

Therefore, researchers are seeking approaches that are new and more effective. Milrinone, widely used in cardiology for heart failure, has vasodilating effects in addition to positive inotrope and antiinflammatory effects. As described by Lannes et al. [13] in detail, milrinone is a potent selective phosphodiesterase III (PDE III) inhibitor that affects cyclic adenosine monophosphate (cAMP) pathways with both inotropic and vasodilatory effects [24]. Milrinone has also antiinflammatory effects through the inhibition of interleukin 1B and interleukin 6 [10]. Thus, several authors have used milrinone in smaller cohorts, but without aggressive reintervention indications [4, 9, 13, 17–19].

In this preliminary series, we used milrinone supplementary to the more commonly used nimodipine. To minimize the effects of postinterventional VSP recurrence, we indicated reinterventions aggressively in cases with persistent neurological deficits or persistent high mean TCD > 180 cm/s. The baseline data show a representative patient cohort with typical age, gender, aneurysm location, and clinical severity distribution. Only the high rate of clipped patients may be atypical. With the present algorithm, we could reach a very low mortality of 6.25 % as compared with the up to 15 % mortality in the literature for conservative treatment alone and contradictory to the negative results of the IMCVS trial [7]. Clinical improvement at a mean of 4.5 months was observed in 68.5 % of patients. Very good and good clinical outcomes with mRS ≤ 2 were reached in 68.5 % of patients. This is in the higher range when compared with the literature, with mRS ≤ 2 rates between 57 % [3] and 75 % [13]. Interestingly, milrinone showed a clear supplementary vasodilating effect over nimodipine in all interventions, leading to 87.5 % DSA improvement. We did not observe any negative side effects of multiple interventions, nor did we find severe cardiovascular adverse events of milrinone, because we used relatively low doses.

Limitations

The present study had a retrospective design and did not have a control group. Comparability may be reduced because of the high rate (81.25 %) of clipped patients. We did not perform perfusion imaging.

Conclusions

Milrinone may be a useful supplementary substance for endovascular VSP therapy. Aggressive reintervention indications did not cause additional adverse events in the present series.

Conflict of Interest Sherif is shareholder of NVTec. Ltd., Vienna, Austria.

References

1. Abruzzo T, Moran C, Blackham K, Eskey C, Lev R, Meyers P, Narayanan S, Prestigiacomo CJ (2012) Invasive interventional management of post-hemorrhagic cerebral vasospasm in patients with aneurysmal subarachnoid hemorrhage. J NeuroInterv Surg 4:169–177
2. Appelboom G, Strozyk D, Hwang B, Prowda J, Badjatia N, Helbok R, Meyers P (2010) Bedside use of a dual aortic balloon occlusion for the treatment of cerebral vasospasm. Neurocrit Care 13:385–388
3. Arakawa Y, Kikuta K, Hojo M, Goto Y, Ishii A, Yamagata S (2001) Milrinone for the treatment of cerebral vasospasm after subarachnoid hemorrhage: report of seven cases. Neurosurgery 48:723–730
4. Arakawa Y, Kikuta K, Hojo M, Goto Y, Yamagata S, Nozaki K, Hashimoto N (2004) Milrinone reduces cerebral vasospasm after subarachnoid hemorrhage of WFNS grade 4 or 5. Neurol Med Chir (Tokyo) 44:393–401
5. Badjatia N, Topcuoglu M, Pryor J, Rabinov J, Ogilvy C, Carter B, Rordorf G (2004) Preliminary experience with intra-arterial nicardipine as a treatment for cerebral vasospasm. AJNR Am J Neuroradiol 25:819–826
6. Biondi A, Ricciardi G, Puybasset L, Abdennour L, Longo M, Chiras J, Van Effenterre R (2004) Intra-arterial nimodipine for the treatment of symptomatic cerebral vasospasm after aneurysmal subarachnoid hemorrhage: preliminary results. AJNR Am J Neuroradiol 25:1067–1076
7. Connolly E, Rabinstein A, Carhuapoma J, Derdeyn C, Dion J, Higashida R, Hoh B, Kirkness C, Naidech A, Ogilvy C, Patel A, Thompson B, Vespa P (2012) Guidelines for the management of aneurysmal subarachnoid hemorrhage: a guideline for healthcare professionals from the American Heart Association/American Stroke Association. Stroke 43:1711–1737
8. Delgado A, Jahromi B, Müller N (2008) Endovascular therapy of cerebral vasospasm: two year experience with angioplasty and/or intra-arterial administration of nicardipine and verapamil. Acta Neurochir Suppl 1004:347–351
9. Fraticelli A, Cholley B, Losser M, Saint Maurice J, Payen D (2008) Milrinone for the treatment of cerebral vasospasm after aneurysmal subarachnoid hemorrhage. Stroke 39:893–898
10. Hayashida N, Tomoeda H, Oda T, Tayama E, Chihara S, Kawara T, Aoyagi S (1999) Inhibitory effect of milrinone on cytokine production after cardiopulmonary bypass. Ann Thorac Surg 68:1661–1667
11. Kaku Y, Yonekawa Y, Tsukahara T, Kazekawa K (1992) Superselective intra-arterial infusion of papaverine for the treatment of cerebral vasospasm after subarachnoid hemorrhage. J Neurosurg 77:842–847
12. Khajavi K, Ayzman I, Shearer D, Jones S, Levy J, Prayson R, Skibinski C, Hahn J, Chyatte D (1997) Prevention of chronic cerebral vasospasm in dogs with milrinone. Neurosurgery 40:354–362
13. Lannes M, Teitelbaum J, del Pilar Cortés M, Cardoso M, Angle M (2012) Milrinone and homeostasis to treat cerebral vasospasm associated with subarachnoid hemorrhage: the Montreal Neurological Hospital protocol. Neurocrit Care 16:354–362
14. Lavine S, Wang M, Etu J, Meyers P, Joshi S (2007) Augmentation of cerebral blood flow and reversal of endothelin-1-induced vasospasm: a comparison of intracarotid nicardipine and verapamil. Neurosurgery 60:742–748
15. Nishiguchi M, Ono S, Iseda K, Manabe H, Hishikawa T, Date I (2010) Effect of vasodilation by milrinone, a phosphodiesterase III inhibitor, on vasospastic arteries after a subarachnoid hemorrhage in vitro and in vivo: effectiveness of cisternal injection of milrinone. Neurosurgery 66:158–164
16. Rinkel G, Feigin V, Algra A, van Gijn J (2004) Circulatory volume expansion therapy for aneurysmal subarachnoid haemorrhage. Cochrane Database Syst Rev (4):CD000483
17. Romero CM, Morales E, Reccius A, Mena F, Prieto J, Bustos P, Larrondo J, Castro J (2009) Milrinone as a rescue therapy for symptomatic refractory cerebral vasospasm in aneurysmal subarachnoid hemorrhage. Neurocrit Care 11:165–171
18. Schmidt U, Bittner E, Pivi S, Marota J (2010) Hemodynamic management and outcome of patients treated for cerebral vasospasm with intraarterial nicardipine and/or milrinone. Anesth Analg 110:895–902
19. Shankar J, dos Santos M, Deus-Silva L, Lum C (2011) Angiographic evaluation of the effect of intra-arterial milrinone therapy in patients with vasospasm from aneurysmal subarachnoid hemorrhage. Neuroradiology 53:123–128
20. Shibuya M, Suzuki Y, Sugita K, Saito I, Sasaki T, Takakura K, Nagata I, Kikuchi H, Takemae T, Hidaka H (1992) Effect of AT877

on cerebral vasospasm after aneurysmal subarachnoid hemorrhage. Results of a prospective placebo-controlled double-blind trial. J Neurosurg 77:424–431

21. Suzuki S, Ito O, Sayama T, Goto K (2010) Intra-arterial colforsin daropate for the treatment of cerebral vasospasm after aneurysmal subarachnoid hemorrhage. Neuroradiology 52:837–845
22. Terry A, Zipfel G, Milner E, Cross D, Moran C, Diringer M, Dacey R, Derdeyn C (2006) Safety and technical efficacy of over-the-wire balloons for the treatment of subarachnoid hemorrhage-induced cerebral vasospasm. Neurosurg Focus 15:E14
23. Vatter H (Lucerne, July 10-12) The IMCVS trial and current recommendations. Vasospasm 2013 Lucerne
24. Vroom M, Pfaffendorf M, van Wezel H, van Zwieten P (1996) Effect of phosphodiesterase inhibitors on human arteries in vitro. Br J Anaesth 76:122–129

Techniques and Surgical Innovations

Perioperative Measures to Improve Outcome After Subarachnoid Hemorrhage—Revisiting the Concept of Secondary Brain Injury

Hans-Jakob Steiger, Thomas Beez, Kerim Beseoglu, Daniel Hänggi, and Marcel A. Kamp

Abstract Progress in the management of aneurysmal subarachnoid hemorrhage (SAH) is reflected most clearly in a continuously decreasing case fatality rate over the last decades. The purpose of the present review is to identify the relevant factors responsible for this progress and to outline future possibilities of improvement. Although data on intracerebral hemorrhage and ischemic stroke are less homogeneous, the respective data suggest that reduction of case fatalities could also be achieved with these types of stroke. Therefore, advances of general neurocritical care may be the common denominator responsible for the decreasing case fatality rates. Additionally, a change in practice with regard to treatment of elderly patients that is more active may also be a factor. Regarding SAH, the majority of unfavorable outcomes is still related to early or delayed cerebral injury. Therefore, efforts to pharmacologically prevent secondary neuronal damage are likely to play a certain role in achieving improvement in overall outcome. However, the data from previous randomized clinical trials conducted during the last three decades does not strongly support this. A clear benefit has only been proven for oral nimodipine, whereas other calcium antagonists and the rho-kinase inhibitors were not conclusively shown to have a significant effect on functional outcome, and all other tested substances disappointed in clinical trials. Regarding ischemic stroke and traumatic brain injury, intensive clinical research has also been conducted during the last 30 years to improve outcome and to minimize secondary neuronal injury. For ischemic stroke, treatment focusing on reversal of the primary pathomechanism, such as thrombolysis, proved effective, but none of the pharmacological neuroprotective concepts resulted in any benefit. To date, decompressive hemicraniectomy has been the only effective effort focused at reducing secondary damage that resulted in a clear reduction of mortality. In the case of traumatic brain injury, none of the pharmacological or other efforts to limit secondary damage met our hopes. In summary, although limited, pharmacotherapy to limit delayed neuronal injury is more effective for SAH than for ischemic stroke and traumatic brain injury. The disappointing results of most trials addressing secondary damage force one to question the general concept of mechanisms of secondary damage that do not also have a positive side in the natural course of the disease. For example, in the case of SAH, the data from the Cooperative Study from the 1960s showed that vasospasm to some degree protects against rerupture of unsecured aneurysms. Thus, one could argue from an evolutionary standpoint that the purpose of vasospasm was not exclusively a detrimental or suicide pathomechanism, but an attempt to protect against life-threating aneurysm rerupture. Because of the above-discussed arguments, SAH may indeed differ from ischemic stroke and traumatic brain injury with regard to the usefulness of blocking secondary mechanisms pharmacologically. Further efforts to limit vasospasm should therefore be made, and the most promising drugs, calcium antagonists, deserve further development. Because, with various drugs, systemic side effects counteracted the local beneficial effect, future efforts should focus on topical administration of drugs instead of systemic administration. Furthermore, efforts for a better understanding of the variations of the calcium channels and the interplay between the different types of calcium channels should be made.

Keywords Aneurysmal subarachnoid hemorrhage • Cerebral vasospasm • Secondary brain injury • Delayed neurological deficit • Secondary brain injury • Neuroprotection • Calcium channel vasospasm

H.-J. Steiger, MD (✉) • T. Beez • K. Beseoglu, MD • D. Hänggi, MD
M.A. Kamp
Department of Neurosurgery, Medical Faculty,
Heinrich-Heine-University, Moorenstraße 5, Geb. 13.71,
D-40225, Düsseldorf, Germany
e-mail: steiger@uni-duesseldorf.de;
beseoglu@med.uni-duesseldorf.de

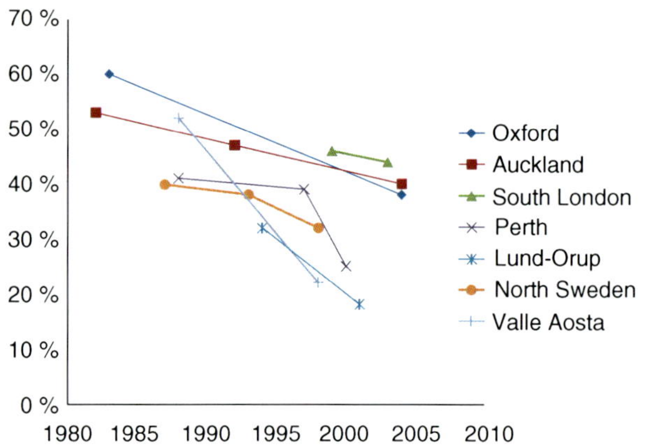

Fig. 1 Decreasing case fatality rates with aneurysmal SAH over the last 3 decades (according to Lovelock et. al. [18]). Over the last 3 decades, case fatality rates continuously decreased in these population-based studies

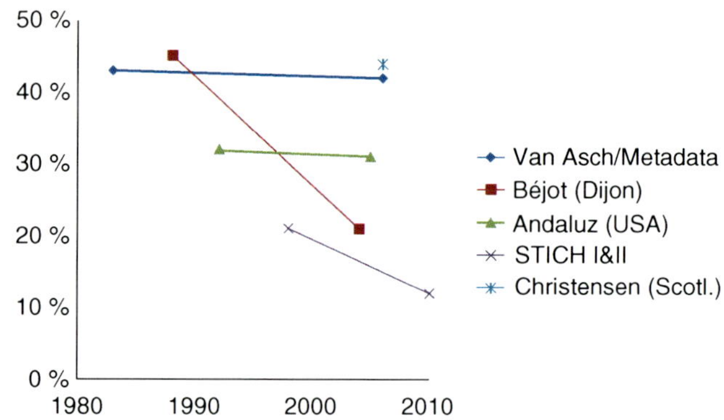

Fig. 2 Inhomogeneously decreasing case fatality rates for spontaneous intracerebral hemorrhage. Overall, a similar trend is seen as with SAH, i.e., a decreasing case fatality rate. The trends at the different locations vary considerably. The low fatality rate in the STICH trials compared with population-based data is noteworthy

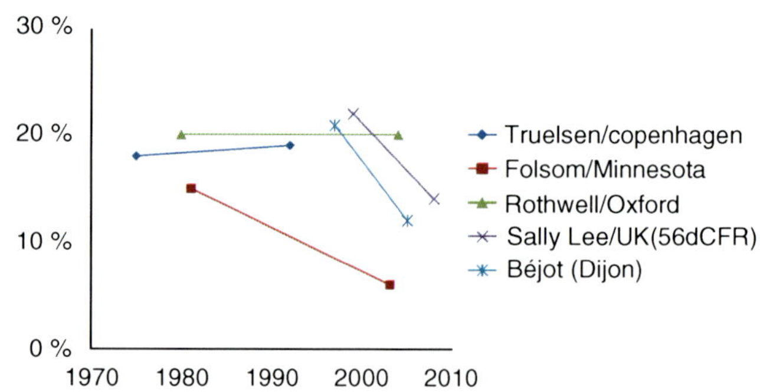

Fig. 3 Inhomogeneously decreasing case fatality rates for ischemic stroke. Population-based evaluations also show a general trend toward decreasing cases fatality rates after ischemic stroke

What Has Perioperative "Management" of Subarachnoid Hemorrhage Achieved?

The most apparent progress in the treatment of aneurysmal subarachnoid hemorrhage (SAH) is reflected in the distinct reduction of the mortality [18]. Although data from 1980 indicated an overall case fatality rate of around 55 %, extrapolation suggests that it decreased to approximately 30 % around 2010 (Fig. 1). The reasons for this improvement are not obvious. Is the progress caused by better management of the specific complications of SAH or by better general intensive care unit (ICU) care? A recent analysis of our own cases treated during the last decade showed that at least 50 % of the case fatality rate with SAH is related to early or delayed brain injury [3]. Therefore, we concluded that changing fatality rates reflect, to a substantial degree, but not entirely, improved quality in the management of specific cerebral complications of SAH.

Comparison with Other Stroke Entities

To gain a better feeling for the significance of prevention and correction of vasospasm for improved prognosis, it appears reasonable to look at other stroke entities with regard to the evolution of case fatality rates [4]. Here, we looked at the major population-based surveys on intracerebral hemorrhage and ischemic stroke (Figs. 2 and 3). In the case of intracerebral hemorrhage, the situation is confounded by massively changing demographics of this patient group [1, 2, 5, 17, 19, 20, 32]. The proportion of younger patients decreased in the Western countries clearly during the last three decades, probably mainly because of better control of arterial hypertension. Simultaneously, the proportion of older patients increased. The data found in the different surveys appear somewhat inhomogeneous. While, for example, in Dijon, a decrease of case fatalities of around 50 % was observed, no significant improvement was found in the United States or in Scotland [1, 2, 5]. For illustrative purposes, we also included the STICH data in the analysis, although the STICH cohort does not represent the population of a specific region [19, 20]. The STICH case fatality rates were substantially lower than those of the population-based surveys from the same time frame. Interestingly, the case fatality rates decreased by almost 50 % between the first and the second STICH trial, regardless of the different inclusion criteria in both trials (deep vs. lobar intracerebral hemorrhage, respectively). The relatively low case fatalities in the STICH trials, compared with other patient cohorts, confirm the assumption of a substantial selection bias in the STICH cohorts.

For ischemic stroke, there is also some heterogeneity with respect to geographical or demographical data [2, 27, 30, 31]. In general, as with cerebral hemorrhage, a trend toward decreasing case fatality rates is apparent. Persistent high case fatality rates were reported from Copenhagen and from Oxford, whereas overall data from the UK, Dijon, and Minnesota show steeply decreasing mortality rates.

Study or subgroup	Experimental Events	Experimental Total	Control Events	Control Total	Weight	Risk ratio M - H, Fixed, 95 % CI
Allen 1983	3	56	5	26	1.0 %	0.28 [0.07, 1.08]
Assano 1996	8	80	16	82	2.2 %	0.51 [0.23, 1.13]
Chou 2008	0	19	3	20	0.5 %	0.15 [0.01, 2.72]
Findlay 1995	8	51	11	49	1.6 %	0.70 [0.31, 1.59]
Haley 1993	81	438	83	448	11.5 %	1.00 [0.76, 1.32]
Haley 1995	24	184	8	61	1.7 %	0.99 [0.47, 2.10]
Haley 1997	86	597	48	300	8.9 %	0.90 [0.65, 1.25]
Hop 2000	1	24	2	26	0.3 %	0.54 [0.05, 5.60]
Kassel 1996	143	762	52	253	10.9 %	0.91 [0.69, 1.21]
Lanzino 1999a	72	398	74	409	10.9 %	1.00 [0.75, 1.34]
Lanzino 1999b	52	399	62	398	8.7 %	0.84 [0.59, 1.18]
Lynch 2005	0	19	3	20	0.5 %	0.15 [0.01, 2.72]
Macdonald 2008	20	313	4	96	0.9 %	1.53 [0.54, 4.38]
Mendelow 1982	5	27	5	26	0.7 %	0.96 [0.32, 2.94]
Mell-Dwyer 1987	4	38	10	37	1.4 %	0.39 [0.13, 1.13]
Ohta 1986	24	102	16	106	2.2 %	1.56 [0.88, 2.76]
Ono 1984	3	65	9	68	1.2 %	0.35 [0.10, 1.23]
Petruk 1988	34	72	32	82	4.2 %	1.21 [0.84, 1.74]
Pickard 1989	43	278	60	276	8.4 %	0.71 [0.50, 1.01]
Saito 1998	12	145	15	141	2.1 %	0.78 [0.38, 1.60]
Shaw 2000	32	207	33	213	4.6 %	1.00 [0.64, 1.56]
Shibuya 1992	7	131	9	136	1.2 %	0.81 [0.31, 2.10]
Siironen 2003	7	85	4	85	0.6 %	1.75 [0.53, 5.76]
Springborg 2007	4	24	2	30	0.2 %	2.50 [0.50, 12.51]
Suzuki 1989	21	170	8	86	1.5 %	1.33 [0.61, 2.87]
Tseng 2005	2	40	8	40	1.1 %	0.25 [0.06, 1.11]
Tseng 2009	6	40	7	40	1.0 %	0.86 [0.32, 2.33]
Vajkoczy 2005	3	15	3	17	0.4 %	1.13 [0.27, 4.79]
Vam den bergh 2006	9	87	7	74	1.1 %	1.09 [0.43, 2.79]
Van den bergh 2005	27	139	31	144	4.3 %	0.90 [0.57, 1.43]
Vergeuwen 2009	2	16	2	16	0.3 %	1.00 [0.16, 6.25]
Wong 2010	17	169	19	159	2.7 %	0.84 [0.45, 1.56]
Ohman 1988	10	104	15	109	2.0 %	0.74 [0.33, 1.48]
Total (95 % CI)		5294		4073	100.0 %	0.90 [0.82, 0.99]
Total events	770		666			

Heterogeneity; chi^2 = 30.63, df = 32 (P = 0.54): I^2 = 0 %
Test for overall effect: Z = 2.08 (P = 0.04)

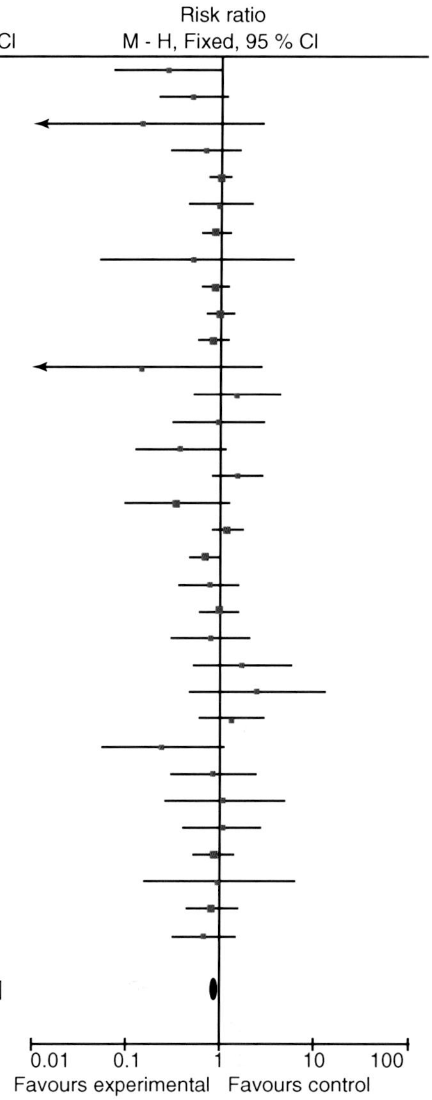

Fig. 4 Summary of prospective randomized trials with aim to limit secondary damage after SAH (work in progress). In this analysis, all prospective, randomized, placebo-controlled trials addressing secondary mechanisms after SAH were included. The analysis was restricted to case fatality rate. Overall, a number of drugs proved to provide a favorable trend or clear-cut benefit, e.g., oral nimodipine and fasudil

Although the overall trends cannot be simplified and local factors may play a certain role, it is clear that progress with SAH may be comparable with other types of stroke. Here, improvement of neurocritical care may be the common denominator. On the other hand, it appears likely that changing attitudes accompanying aging populations are also a significant factor, e.g., treatment that is more invasive in patients older than 70–80 years or acceptance of functional deficits in elderly patients.

The Benefit of Neuroprotective Intervention in General

As highlighted, at least 50 % of the case fatality rate with SAH is related to early or delayed brain injury. Thus, a focus on the respective improvements of prevention and therapy should also result in beneficial effects on outcome. A review of the various prospective and randomized clinical trials of the last 30 years illustrates that only oral nimodipine has been definitely proven to improve outcome (Fig. 4). For other pharmacological interventions, a distinct but nonsignificant trend is seen, e.g., the rho kinase inhibitor, fasudil. However, the current smaller trials on statins seem to be promising in this respect, but larger trials are required to explore the potential of this drug type.

Intensive preclinical and clinical research has been conducted during the last 30 years in the field of neuroprotection following ischemic stroke. Although efforts to reverse the initial injury, e.g., by thrombolysis, proved to be very effective, none of the pharmacologic concepts or other interventional concepts, such as hypothermia, for neuroprotection resulted in any beneficial effect on functional outcome. To date, decompressive craniotomy remains the only intervention

Study or subgroup	Dexamethasone Events	Total	Placebo Events	Total	Weight	Risk ratio M - H, Fixed, 95 % CI
De Gans 2002	11	157	21	144	8.4 %	0.48 [0.24, 0.96]
Molyneux 2002	96	307	91	295	35.7 %	1.01 [0.80, 1.29]
Nguyen 2007	22	217	26	218	10.0 %	0.85 [0.50, 1.45]
Odio 1991	1	52	1	49	0.4 %	0.94 [0.06, 14.65]
Quazi 1996	12	48	5	41	2.1 %	2.05 [0.79, 5.33]
Thwaites 2004	87	274	112	271	43.4 %	0.77 [0.61, 0.96]
Total (95 % CI)		1055		1018	100.0 %	0.87 [0.75, 1.01]
Total events	229		256			

Heterogeneity; $Chi^2 = 8.68$, df = 5 ($P = 0.12$): $I^2 = 42$ %

Test for overall effect: $Z = 1.86$ ($P = 0.06$)

Risk ratio M - H, Fixed, 95 % CI

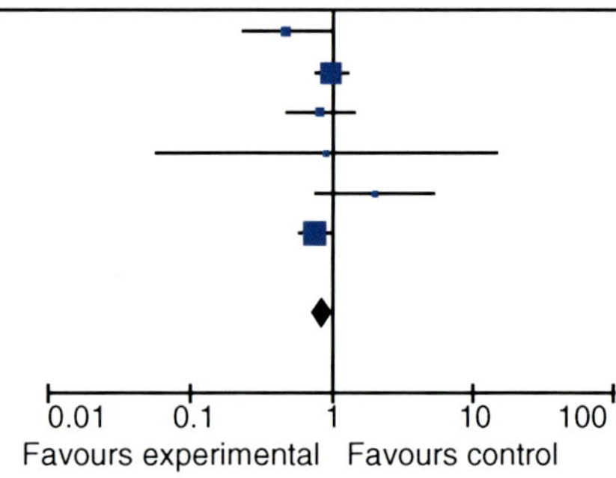

Fig. 5 Summary of prospective randomized trials on corticosteroids for meningitis (work in progress). Case fatality rate was used as the outcome parameter. In general, adding dexamethasone to antibiotic treatment reduces secondary complications. It is important to stress the point that dexamethasone is only beneficial under the protection of antibiotics. Therefore, experimental treatment does not compare with the "natural" course

focusing on limiting secondary brain damage that resulted in a clear reduction of mortality [11, 15].

Regarding traumatic brain injury, the data on the effect of neuroprotective strategies to limit secondary brain damage remain disappointing. To date, none of the larger clinical trials on pharmacological or interventional (hypothermia or decompressive craniectomy) treatments were able to demonstrate a beneficial effect on neurological outcome [6–8].

Common Denominators and Explanation

Looking at the clinical trials on corticosteroid therapy for meningitis may provide an explanation for the differences in benefit of neuroprotective measures (Fig. 5). Most of the few trials evaluating corticosteroids in addition to antibiotics for bacterial meningitis demonstrated a reduction of poor outcome and mortality [9, 10, 16, 21–26, 28]. It appears clear that steroids are only beneficial under concomitant treatment with antibiotics. Therefore, experimental treatment does not compare with the "natural" course for this entity, because corticosteroid treatment without antibiotic treatment would inevitably result in poor outcome or death in patients with bacterial meningitis.

There is a similar scenario in the case of SAH. Blocking secondary negative reactions by nimodipine has only been proven beneficial in the case of secured aneurysms, which means that the control group was not exposed to the true natural course of the disease. If we assume that evolution or nature has not developed "suicide pathomechanisms," why would patients develop vasospasm during the course of this disease? For obvious reasons, there is no recent data on the natural course after aneurysmal SAH to underline this assumption, but the data from the Cooperative Study from the 1960s might provide some insight in this respect [14]. The registry dates back to the time before the introduction of early aneurysm surgery and can therefore provide information on the natural course after SAH. Although the data show a clear association between the occurrence of vasospasm and poor outcome, the data also show a clear negative association between the occurrence of vasospasm and aneurysm rerupture during the unsecured phase. Therefore, it appears that, in the natural course after SAH, macrovascular spasm might have been evolutionarily meant to protect patients against aneurysm rerupture. The protective effect of vasospasm was not readily evident in clinical practice, because risk factors to develop macrovascular spasm parallel those for rehemorrhage, i.e., severe SAH [29]. The protective effect of vasospasm against rerupture could only be distilled by multifactorial statistical correlation analysis. Thus, one could argue from an evolutionary standpoint that the purpose of macrovascular spasm was not exclusively a detrimental or suicide pathomechanism, but an attempt to protect against life-threating aneurysm rerupture.

The models of meningitis and SAH suggest that the concepts of secondary brain damage must be revised. For the natural course, nature does not appear to have developed suicide mechanisms that need to be fought, i.e., blocked pharmacologically. In contrast, nature has to limit resources for repair, and therefore also mechanisms of compensation following brain injury. Insufficient potential for repair and compensation need to be supported by medical intervention. On the other hand, current data do not indicate that blocking biochemical reactions after brain injury and stroke makes much sense. The pharmaceutical industry has realized that there is not much to gain and has largely withdrawn from drug development and clinical studies. Because of the above-discussed arguments, the situation may be different with SAH, and the most effective drugs, calcium antagonists, deserve further development.

Conclusions and Consequences

Nimodipine was introduced into clinical practice in the 1980s. Although we have a much more detailed understanding of the various types of calcium channels compared with 30 years ago, many open questions remain regarding calcium channels and their function following SAH. In particular, a variable response is seen after local application of nimodipine or intraarterial delivery. In a monocentric prospective trial at our department on intraarterial application of nimodipine for severe vasospasm, no response was seen in one of three patients [12]. The question of these nonresponders to calcium antagonists needs to be addressed. Are there substantial genetic variations of the calcium channels? How important is the balance between different types of calcium channels and how are they upregulated or downregulated?

Furthermore, in some clinical and experimental settings, the antispastic effect of nimodipine appears to decrease with increasing dose. We observed this effect in a study on the dose-related efficacy of continuous intracisternal nimodipine treatment for cerebral vasospasm in the rat double-SAH model [13]. The question of decreasing effect with increasing dose remains enigmatic and further research is needed to elucidate the underlying cause of the decreasing nimodipine effect at higher dosage. Differential effects on the individual types of calcium channels might play a role.

Last but not least, the concepts of systems theory defining the general principles governing the hierarchy and interactions between genes, cells, organs, the organism, and society should be considered more seriously by physicians and neuroscientists. A better understanding of systems theory would have made it clear that the assumption of suicide mechanisms in the brain rests on shaky grounds [8].

Conflict of Interest Statement We declare that we have no conflict of interest

References

1. Andaluz N, Zuccarello M (2009) Recent trends in the treatment of spontaneous intracerebral hemorrhage: analysis of a nationwide inpatient database. J Neurosurg 110(3):403–410
2. Bejot Y, Rouaud O, Durier J, Caillier M, Marie C, Freysz M, Yeguiayan JM, Chantegret A, Osseby G, Moreau T, Giroud M (2007) Decrease in the stroke case fatality rates in a French population-based twenty-year study. A comparison between men and women. Cerebrovasc Dis 24:439–444
3. Beseoglu K, Holtkamp K, Steiger HJ, Hänggi D (2013) Fatal aneurysmal subarachnoid haemorrhage: causes of 30-day in-hospital case fatalities in a large single-centre historical patient cohort. Clin Neurol Neurosurg 115(1):77–81
4. Biotti D, Jacquin A, Boutarbouch M, Bousquet O, Durier J, Ben Salem D, Ricolfi F, Beaurain J, Osseby GV, Moreau T, Giroud M, Béjot Y (2010) Trends in case-fatality rates in hospitalized nontraumatic subarachnoid hemorrhage: results of a population-based study in Dijon, France, from 1985 to 2006. Neurosurgery 66(6):1039–1043
5. Christensen MC, Munro V (2008) Ischemic stroke and intracerebral hemorrhage: the latest evidence on mortality, readmissions and hospital costs from Scotland. Neuroepidemiology 30(4):239–246
6. Clifton GL, Miller ER, Choi SC, Levin HS, McCauley S, Smith KR Jr, Muizelaar JP, Wagner FC Jr, Marion DW, Luerssen TG, Chesnut RM, Schwartz M (2001) Lack of effect of induction of hypothermia after acute brain injury. N Engl J Med 344(8):556–563
7. Cooper DJ, Rosenfeld JV, Murray L, Arabi YM, Davies AR, D'Urso P, Kossmann T, Ponsford J, Seppelt I, Reilly P, Wolfe R, DECRA Trial Investigators; Australian and New Zealand Intensive Care Society Clinical Trials Group (2011) Decompressive craniectomy in diffuse traumatic brain injury. N Engl J Med 364(16):1493–1502
8. Drack M, Apfalter W, Pouvreau D (2007) On the making of a system theory of life: Paul A Weiss and Ludwig von Bertalanffy's conceptual connection. Q Rev Biol 82(4):349–373
9. Escobar JA, Belsey MA, Dueñas A, Medina P (1975) Mortality from tuberculous meningitis reduced by steroid therapy. Pediatrics 56(6):1050–1055
10. Geiman BJ, Smith AL (1992) Dexamethasone and bacterial meningitis. A meta-analysis of randomized controlled trials. West J Med 157(1):27–31
11. Geurts M, van der Worp HB, Kappelle LJ, Amelink GJ, Algra A, Hofmeijer J, on behalf of the HAMLET Steering Committee (2013) Surgical decompression for space-occupying cerebral infarction: outcomes at 3 years in the randomized HAMLET trial. Stroke 44:2506–8
12. Hänggi D, Turowski B, Beseoglu K, Yong M, Steiger HJ (2008) Intra-arterial nimodipine for severe cerebral vasospasm after aneurysmal subarachnoid hemorrhage: influence on clinical course and cerebral perfusion. AJNR Am J Neuroradiol 29(6):1053–1060
13. Hänggi D, Eicker S, Beseoglu K, Rapp M, Perrin J, Nawatny J, Turowski B, Sommer C, Steiger HJ (2009) Dose-related efficacy of a continuous intracisternal nimodipine treatment on cerebral vasospasm in the rat double subarachnoid hemorrhage model. Neurosurgery 64(6):1155–1159
14. Henderson WG, Torner JC, Nibbelink DW, Henderson WG, Torner JC, Nibbelink DW (1977) Intracranial aneurysms and subarachnoid hemorrhage—report on a randomized treatment study. IV—B. Regulated bed rest— statistical evaluation. Stroke 8:579–589
15. Jüttler E, Schwab S, Schmiedek P, Unterberg A, Hennerici M, Woitzik J, Witte S, Jenetzky E, Hacke W, DESTINY Study Group (2007) Decompressive surgery for the treatment of malignant infarction of the middle cerebral artery (DESTINY): a randomized, controlled trial. Stroke 38(9):2518–2525
16. Lebel MH, Freij BJ, Syrogiannopoulos GA, Chrane DF, Hoyt MJ, Stewart SM, Kennard BD, Olsen KD, McCracken GH Jr (1988) Dexamethasone therapy for bacterial meningitis. Results of two double-blind, placebo-controlled trials. N Engl J Med 319(15):964–971
17. Lee S, Shafe ACE, Cowie MR (2011) UK stroke incidence, mortality and cardiovascular risk management 1999–2008: time-trend analysis from the General Practice Research Database. BMJ Open 1:e000269. doi:10.1136/bmjopen-2011-000269
18. Lovelock CE, Rinkel GJ, Rothwell PM (2010) Time trends in outcome of subarachnoid hemorrhage: population-based study and systematic review. Neurology 74(19):1494–1501
19. Mendelow AD, Gregson BA, Fernandes HM, Murray GD, Teasdale GM, Hope DT, Karimi A, Shaw MD, Barer DH, STICH investigators (2005) Early surgery versus initial conservative treatment in patients with spontaneous supratentorial intracerebral haematomas in the international surgical trial in intracerebral haemorrhage (STICH): a randomised trial. Lancet 365(9457):387–397

20. Mendelow AD, Gregson BA, Rowan EN, Murray GD, Gholkar A, Mitchell PM, for the STICH II Investigators (2013) Early surgery versus initial conservative treatment in patients with spontaneous supratentorial lobar intracerebral haematomas (STICH II): a randomised trial. Lancet 382:397–408. doi:10.1016/S0140-6736(13)60986-1, pii: S0140-6736(13)60986-1
21. Molyneux EM, Walsh AL, Forsyth H, Tembo M, Mwenechanya J, Kayira K, Bwanaisa L, Njobvu A, Rogerson S, Malenga G (2002) Dexamethasone treatment in childhood bacterial meningitis in Malawi: a randomised controlled trial. Lancet 360(9328): 211–218
22. Mongelluzzo J, Mohamad Z, Ten Have TR, Shah SS (2008) Corticosteroids and mortality in children with bacterial meningitis. JAMA 299(17):2048–2055, PubMed [citation] PMID: 18460665
23. Nguyen TH, Tran TH, Thwaites G, Ly VC, Dinh XS, Ho Dang TN, Dang QT, Nguyen DP, Nguyen HP, To SD, Nguyen VC, Nguyen MD, Campbell J, Schultsz C, Parry C, Torok ME, White N, Nguyen TC, Tran TH, Stepniewska K, Farrar JJ (2007) Dexamethasone in Vietnamese adolescents and adults with bacterial meningitis. N Engl J Med 357(24):2431–2440
24. Odio CM, Faingezicht I, Paris M, Nassar M, Baltodano A, Rogers J, Sáez-Llorens X, Olsen KD, McCracken GH Jr (1991) The beneficial effects of early Dexamethasone administration in infants and children with bacterial meningitis. N Engl J Med 324(22):1525–1531, PubMed [citation] PMID: 2027357
25. Pécoul B, Varaine F, Keita M, Soga G, Djibo A, Soula G, Abdou A, Etienne J, Rey M (1991) Long-acting chloramphenicol versus intravenous ampicillin for treatment of bacterial meningitis. Lancet 338(8771):862–866
26. Qazi SA, Khan MA, Mughal N, Ahmad M, Joomro B, Sakata Y, Kuriya N, Matsuishi T, Abbas KA, Yamashita F (1996) Dexamethasone and bacterial meningitis in Pakistan. Arch Dis Child 75(6):482–488
27. Rothwell PM, Coull AJ, Giles MF, Howard SC, Silver LE, Bull LM, Gutnikov SA, Edwards P, Mant D, Sackley CM, Farmer A, Sandercock PA, Dennis MS, Warlow CP, Bamford JM, Anslow P, Oxford Vascular Study (2004) Change in stroke incidence, mortality, case-fatality, severity, and risk factors in Oxfordshire, UK from 1981 to 2004 (Oxford Vascular Study). Lancet 363(9425):1925–33
28. Scarborough M, Gordon SB, Whitty CJ, French N, Njalale Y, Chitani A, Peto TE, Lalloo DG, Zijlstra EE (2007) Corticosteroids for bacterial meningitis in adults in sub-Saharan Africa. N Engl J Med 357(24):2441–2450
29. Steiger HJ, Fritschi J, Seiler RW (1994) Current pattern of in-hospital aneurysmal rebleeds. Analysis of a series treated with individually timed surgery and intravenous nimodipine. Acta Neurochir (Wien) 127(1–2):21–26
30. Sturgeon JD, Folsom AR (2007) Trends in hospitalization rate, hospital case fatality, and mortality rate of stroke by subtype in Minneapolis-St. Paul, 1980–2002. Neuroepidemiology 28(1):39–45
31. Truelsen T, Grønbaek M, Schnohr P, Boysen G (2002) Stroke case fatality in Denmark from 1977 to 1992: the Copenhagen City Heart Study. Neuroepidemiology 21(1):22–27
32. van Asch CJ, Luitse MJ, Rinkel GJ, van der Tweel I, Algra A, Klijn CJ (2010) Incidence, case fatality, and functional outcome of intracerebral haemorrhage over time, according to age, sex, and ethnic origin: a systematic review and meta-analysis. Lancet Neurol 9(2):167–176

Craniotomy Without Flap Replacement for Ruptured Intracranial Aneurysms to Reduce Ischemic Brain Injury: A Preliminary Safety and Feasibility Analysis

Jehuda Soleman, Bawarjan Schatlo, Hiroki Dan-Ura, Luca Remonda, Javier Fandino, and Ali-Reza Fathi

Abstract *Background:* Cortical and subcortical brain ischemia following aneurysmal subarachnoid hemorrhage (aSAH) remains a central challenge in improving patient outcome. Generally the bone flap is replaced after surgical clipping and no decompression is practiced in endovascularly treated patients. The aim of this preliminary safety and feasibility study is to clarify whether a first-line decompression would improve brain perfusion and salvage more tissue at risk in patients who developed delayed vasospasm. In addition, we assessed whether the risks involved with a second surgery to replace the bone flap would affect patient outcome.

Methods: We retrospectively analyzed patients with aSAH who underwent surgical clipping and developed cerebral vasospasm from 2009 to 2012 at our institution. We selected cases where the bone flap was not replaced at initial surgery and needed a second procedure for bone flap replacement. Primary end points were new delayed ischemic neurological deficits (DINDs), the extent of brain infarctions, and patient functional outcome. Secondary end points were hazards of the second procedure for bone replacement.

Results: We identified six patients in whom the surgeon chose not to replace the bone flap. In four patients, this was a pterional bone flap (standard), and in two patients it was a larger frontotemporoparietal flap. Despite the limited extent of the craniotomy, only one patient (16 %) required additional decompression. Two patients (33%) developed DINDs and five patients (83 %) showed delayed cerebral infarctions on computed tomography. Of those, three patients showed good outcome (Glasgow Outcome Scale score >4 and modified Rankin Scale score <3). No complications or new neurological deficits occurred during the second surgery for bone replacement.

Conclusions: To date, no standardized criteria exist to decide whether the bone flap should be removed or replaced at initial surgery. Our single-center experience in a limited number of patients reveals a pattern with respect to initial clinical parameters and imaging findings that might be a first step in developing standardized decision parameters. This may prevent secondary surgery for decompression in deleterious conditions during the vasospasm phase. Based on these findings, we have developed a protocol for a prospective study that will further investigate the benefits of this management.

Keywords Subarachnoid hemorrhage • Cerebral aneurysm • Craniectomy • Ischemic deficit

Introduction

The incidence of subarachnoid hemorrhage caused by ruptured intracranial aneurysm (aSAH) varies from 3 to 23 per 100,000 persons per year [6, 14]. Clinically, presentation with a poor neurological grade after aSAH correlates with worse outcome [2, 4, 9, 11, 13]. One reason for this is delayed brain swelling with elevation of intracranial pressure (ICP) [4, 13]. Thus far, several studies have shown good outcomes after performing decompressive hemicraniectomy (DHC) in a selected group of aSAH patients [1, 4, 5, 7, 12, 13], whereas others have shown no benefit [10]. In aSAH patients, the most common indication for DHC adjunct to clipping is a concomitant intraparenchymal hemorrhage or hemispheric infarction caused by vasospasm. We postulate that removing the bone flap at the conclusion of surgical clipping in cases where the probability of delayed diffuse brain tissue swelling is high (e.g., patients at risk for delayed cerebral vasospasm)

J. Soleman, MD • B. Schatlo, MD • H. Dan-Ura, MD
L. Remonda, MD • J. Fandino, MD • A.-R. Fathi, MD (✉)
Department of Neurosurgery, Kantonsspital Aarau,
Aarau, Switzerland
e-mail: ali-reza.fathi@ksa.ch

J. Fandino et al. (eds.), *Neurovascular Events After Subarachnoid Hemorrhage*, Acta Neurochirurgica Supplement, Vol. 120,
DOI 10.1007/978-3-319-04981-6_37, © Springer International Publishing Switzerland 2015

could help preserve the existing penumbra, improve brain perfusion, and therefore save vital brain tissue. The effects of a second surgery to replace the bone flap and benefits of this approach have not been systematically studied thus far. Furthermore, no standardized criteria exist that would justify the decision of removing the bone flap at the initial surgery. The purpose of this preliminary study is to analyze the safety and feasibility of treating aSAH by neurosurgical clipping without bone flap replacement and to assess the clinical and radiological ramifications of this approach.

Methods

We retrospectively analyzed 44 consecutive patients who underwent emergency neurosurgical aneurysm clipping following aSAH at our institute from 2009 to 2012. Inclusion criteria were patients who had no bone flap replacement at initial surgical clipping and who also developed delayed cerebral vasospasm. We recorded patient demographic parameters retrieved from our SAH database. Data related to Glasgow Coma Scale (GCS), Hunt and Hess and World Federation of Neurosurgical Societies (WFNS) grading, modified Rankin scale (mRS), neurologic deficits at hospital admission, discharge and follow-up (after 4–18 months; mean 6.5 months), and duration of hospitalization were collected. Radiological data included aneurysm location and size, Fisher grade, midline shift (MLS), and volume of intraparenchymal hemorrhage (IHV; using Broderick's Method $(a \times b \times c)/2$) [3].

Aneurysm clipping was performed within 48 h of presentation after angiographically proven aSAH according to standard microsurgical techniques. In all cases except one (case 2), an intraoperative angiogram was performed to ensure complete aneurysm occlusion [8]. According to the surgeons' assessment of potential delayed swelling of the brain and risk for delayed vasospasm, the bone flap was frozen for deferred replacement or reimplanted at the end of surgery. In the case of obvious brain edema or hematoma, the surgeon chose to enlarge the initial pterional craniotomy and perform a duroplasty to achieve a frontotemporoparietal decompressive craniectomy flap.

Postoperatively, all patients were managed in the surgical intensive care unit (ICU) with continuous neurological examination. Twenty-four hours postoperatively, we routinely performed a computed tomography scan (CT) with angiography and perfusion sequences to exclude early postoperative complications (e.g., intracranial hemorrhage, cerebral ischemia, and early vasospasm). Transcranial Doppler (TCD) was performed daily in all cases during the ICU stay. In case the patient developed signs or symptoms of DIND, CT-angiography with evaluation of brain perfusion was performed. If conservative ICU treatment failed to improve the new deficits and vasospasm was radiologically confirmed, cerebral angiography and treatment with percutaneous angioplasty and/or papaverine or nimodipine infusion into the vasospastic vessels was performed. Ventriculostomies were converted to ventriculoperitoneal shunts within 7–14 days if weaning was not possible. Patients were discharged to a rehabilitation center after completion of acute neurosurgical treatment and were followed up with in our outpatient clinic. Bone flap replacement was performed between 3 weeks and 7 months after surgical clipping. New adverse events at the second surgery were recorded.

Radiographic films were analyzed retrospectively by an investigator who was not involved in patient surgical treatment.

The study was approved by the Institutional Review Board of the Kantonsspital Aarau, Switzerland. Written informed consent was obtained preoperatively from all patients or family members.

Results

Six patients met the inclusion criteria with decompressive craniectomy at initial surgery for clipping of a ruptured aneurysm and by developing delayed vasospasm. The mean age of this group was 46 years (±12.4 years) with two male and four female (66.7 %) patients. Three patients (50 %) presented with a communicans anterior artery aneurysm (A-com), and three had an aneurysm of the middle cerebral artery (MCA). Two patients (33.3 %) had a Fisher grade 3 hemorrhage and four had a Fisher grade 4. One patient (16.7 %) had a second unruptured aneurysm (MCA aneurysm on the right), and one patient showed four additional aneurysms (MCA aneurysm on the left and three aneurysms along the internal carotid artery on the right). These unruptured aneurysms were not treated during the first acute management.

The bone flap was a pterional flap (standard flap; Fig. 1) in four patients (66 %) and a large frontotemporoparietal flap (Fig. 2) in two patients (33 %). The mean MLS (1.25 mm ± 2.5 mm vs. 14.5 mm ± 3.54 mm) and IHV (14.25 cm^3 ± 17.86 cm^3 vs. 79.2 cm^3 ± 22.91 cm^3) was lower in the group with a standard flap compared with the group with a large flap. The mean admission GCS was 12 (±2.9); in the standard flap group, the mean admission GCS was 13.75 ± 1.26 compared with 8.5 ± 0.7 in the large flap group. Three patients showed a Hunt and Hess score of 3, two a score of 2, and one patient showed a score of 4. A WFNS score of IV was seen in three patients, a score of III in two patients, and a score of II in one patient.

One patient (16.7 %) presented with aphasia at admission, three patients (50 %) with focal neurologic deficits, and three patients (50 %) with cranial nerve palsy. In one case (16.7 %), a ventriculitis occurred, which was treated with intrathecal and i.v. antibiotics. Two of six patients showed a progression

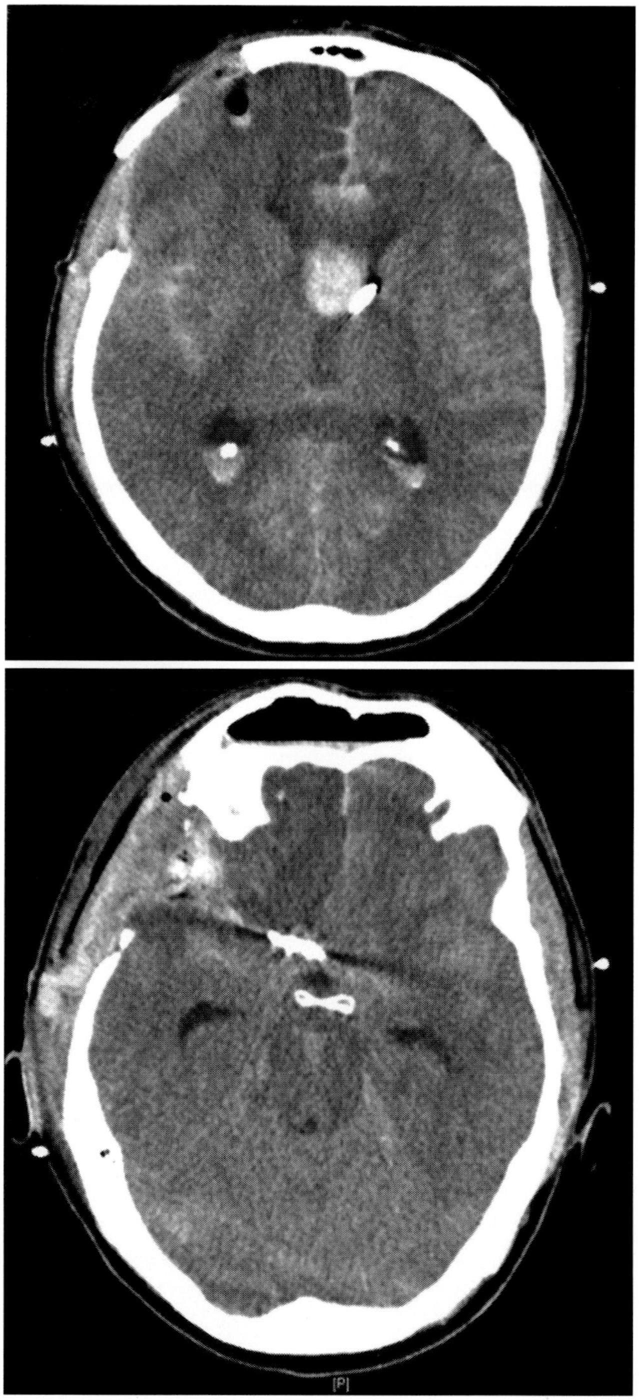

Fig. 1 Axial computed tomography scans without contrast agent showing the dimension of a pterional flap (standard flap)

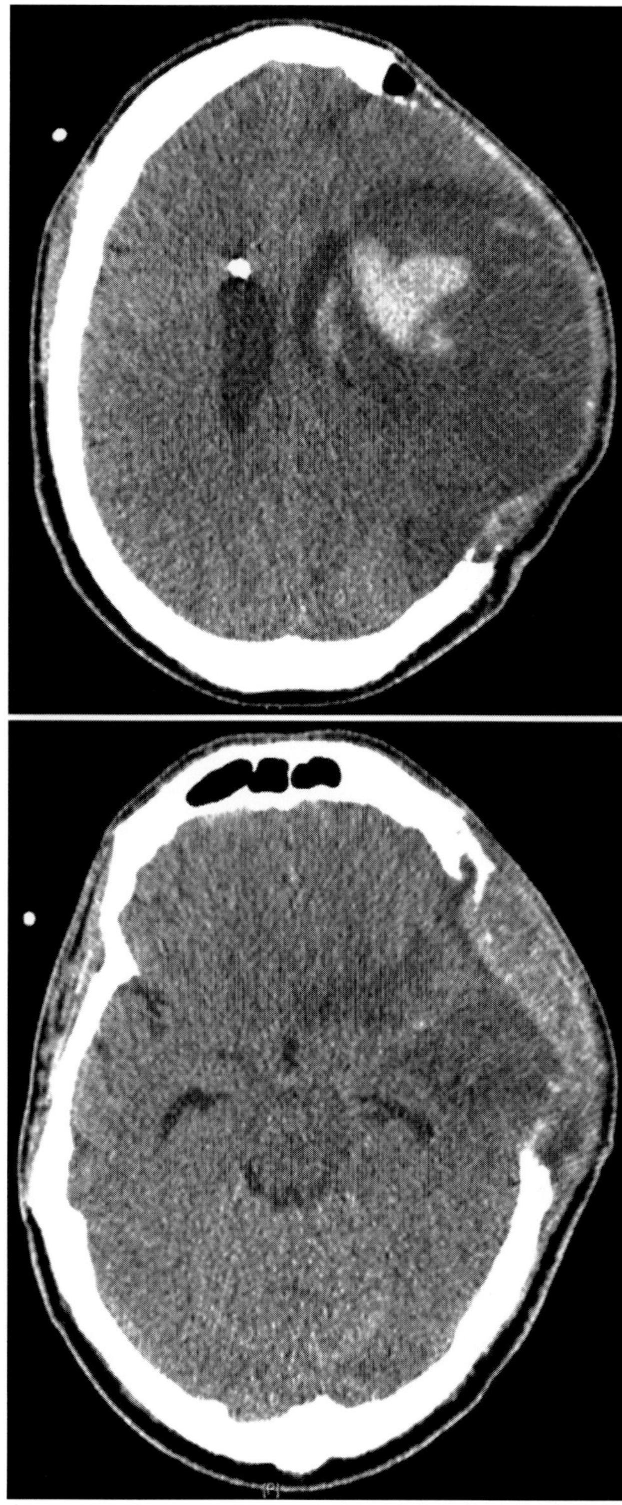

Fig. 2 Axial computed tomography scans without contrast agent showing the dimension of a large frontotemporoparietal flap (large flap)

of neurologic deficits or postoperative complication, leading to a morbidity of 33 %. Mortality was 16.7 % ($n=1$; case 2), caused by rebleeding of the aneurysm and vasospasm with hemispheric infarction.

All patients ($n=6$) developed vasospasm and in all cases a hypertensive therapy was instaurated. In two cases (33 %), intra-arterial transfemoral angioplasty and/or papaverine infusion was indicated. In two cases (33 %), delayed cerebral ischemia led to DIND, and, in three cases (50 %), a perfusion deficit was seen on CT with angiographic and perfusion sequences. In five cases (83 %), cerebral infarction was seen on radiologic examinations. One patient with a pterional bone flap (case 6) required additional surgical decompression because of diffuse brain swelling.

Table 1 Results of decompressive hemicraniectomy group vs. pterional flap group

	Pterional flap (n=4)	Decompressive flap (n=2)
Admission GCS	13.75 (±1.26)	8.5 (±0.7)
Admission mRS	1.75 (±1.5)	4.5 (±0.7)
Discharge GCS	9.75 (±5.31)	7.0 (±0)
Discharge mRS	3.75 (±2.06)	4.5 (±0.7)
Midline shift	1.25 (±2.5)	14.25 (±17.86)
Hematoma volume	14.50 (±3.56)	79.20 (±22.91)

At discharge, the mean GCS was 8.8 (±4.4). The mean GCS of the standard flap group (9.75±5.31) was better than in the large flap group (7±0). Mini Mental Scores (MMS) were not assessable in two patients because of aphasia. Two patients had a MMS of 29 and two patients a MMS of 27 and 15. The mRS was 1 in three patients, and 3, 5, and 6 in one patient each (mean 4±1.7). The Glasgow Outcome scale (GOS) was 3 in three patients and 1, 2, and 5 in the other three (mean 2.8±1.3), while a Barthel Index (BI) of 100 was seen in two patients and a BI of 0 in three patients (mean 33.3±51.6). Five patients (83.3 %) showed focal neurological deficits at discharge, four patients (66.7 %) showed cranial nerve palsy, and one patient (16.7 %) had aphasia.

In one case (case 3), bone flap reimplantation was not concluded because the patient deceased because of rebleeding and diffuse brain swelling. Three patients recovered to a sufficient clinical state to justify bone flap reimplantation after 2–7 months, and, in two cases, reimplantation was carried out earlier, after 3–4 weeks, because of hydrocephalus needing ventriculoperitoneal shunt placement. No complications or new neurologic deficits occurred after bone flap reimplantation.

At follow-up (n=5, range 4–18 months, mean 6.5 months), four patients showed a GCS of 15, while one patient had a GCS of 10 (mean 14±2.2). The mRS was in three patients 1, 3, and 5 in one patient each (mean 2.2±1.8). The GOS was 5 in three patients, and 2 and 3 in one patient each (mean 4±1.4), and a BI of 100 was seen in two patients and a BI of 50, 30, and 5 in one patient each (mean 57±42.4). MMS was not assessable in two patients because of aphasia. Two patients had a MMS of 27 and one patient a MMS of 29 (mean 16.6±15.8). All patients displayed improvement of neurologic deficits at follow up compared with discharge. Tables 1 and 2 summarize the patient characteristics and results.

Discussion

This preliminary single-center study investigated the clinical and radiological features of patients with aSAH in which the surgeon decided to remove the bone flap on the basis of preoperative clinical and intraoperative parameters. In this small six-patient cohort, a pattern was revealed that might guide cases in which the bone flap should be removed and what size craniotomy should be applied.

In patients with a GCS <10, a MLS >5 mm, and a hematoma volume >40 cm^3, a moderate frontotemporoparietal decompressive craniectomy should be performed. In patients with a GCS of ≥10, MLS ≤5 mm, and hematoma volume ≤40 cm^3, a standard pterional flap may suffice. However, once intraoperative brain swelling is observed, removal of the pterional bone flap may be a viable alternative to a larger decompression.

Although all patients developed vasospasm with resulting ischemia in five cases, this led to permanent DIND in only two patients. Moreover, an enlargement of the previous craniectomy was necessary in one case only, leading to improved clinical results. We think that avoiding a second surgical decompression during the phase of cerebral vasospasm may contribute more harm to patients than performing it. We were reluctant to reoperate on one case because of the seriousness of the condition resulting in death caused by diffuse rebleeding combined with severe vasospasm and ischemia. New complications or neurological deficits following the second procedure for bone replacement did not occur.

It has been shown that DHC leads to normalization of ICP values [10, 12, 13]. This normalization of ICP is associated with an immediate, significant improvement in tissue perfusion and oxygenation [4, 10, 13]. Therefore, studies were conducted to evaluate the indications and outcomes of DHC during or after clipping of aneurysms. Smith et al. concluded that prophylactic DHC in a subcategory of patients with aSAH and large sylvian fissure hematomas is safe, is associated with rapid and sustained control of ICP, and leads to good outcomes [13]. Arikan et al. postulated that primary DHC after surgical or endovascular treatment of aSAH may be beneficial in a select subgroup of patients [1]. Schirmer et al. concluded that DHC can be useful in the management of refractory intracranial hypertension in patients with high grade (Hunt and Hess grade ≥4) aSAH, even in absence of large hemorrhage [12]. According to Buschmann et al., patients with progressive brain edema lacking radiological signs of infarctions and those with hematoma and consecutive ICP elevations might benefit most from decompressive craniectomy, while patients manifesting severe infarctions on CT scans should be excluded from this treatment option [4]. Jaeger et al. showed, in a small study with three patients, that while DHC has a beneficial effect on ICP and brain tissue oxygenation, it does not improve clinical outcome [10]. These conducted studies are all too small to have statistical impact and to offer guidelines concerning indications and timing of DHC. It seems that, in patients with high-grade aSAH (Hunt and Hess grade ≥4) in addition to large hematomas or diffuse ischemia, DHC might lead to a better clinical outcome. Yet whether it should be performed primarily or

Table 2 Patient characteristics

	Characteristics		Radiology				Operation
Patient no.	Gender	Location	Fisher grade	MLS	Hematoma volume (cm^3)	Age (years)	Flap
1	m	MCA	3	17	95.4	46	Large
2	f	MCA	4	12	63	61	Large
3	f	A-com	4	0	None	25	Standard
4	f	A-com	4	0	None	53	Standard
5	m	A-com	3	0	37	48	Standard
6	f	MCA	4	5	20	50	Standard

	Admission				Discharge						Follow-up					
Patient no.	H&H grade	WFNS grade	GCS	Neurologic deficits	GCS	mRS	GOS	BI	MMS	Neurologic deficits	GCS	mRS	GOS	BI	MMS	Neurologic deficits
1	3	4	8	Yes	7	5	2	0	0	Unchanged	10	5	2	5	0	Unchanged
2	4	4	9	Yes	7	4	3	0	0	Unchanged	15	1	5	50	27	Improved
3	2	2	15	No	3	6	1	–	–	Exitus	–	–			–	Exitus
4	2	3	14	Yes	14	1	5	100	27	Unchanged	15	1	5	100	27	No
5	2	4	12	No	8	4	3	0	15	New	15	3	3	30	0	Improved
6	3	3	14	Yes	14	4	3	100	29	Unchanged	15	1	5	100	29	Improved

in a secondary manner remains unclear. To our knowledge, no study exists that evaluates the indication, effect, or outcome of a standard-sized pterional craniectomy in patients with aSAH.

We postulated that, in a selected group of patients with aSAH, a pterional craniectomy would be sufficient for the brain to be decompressed, with potential beneficial effects on the perihematoma penumbra. We hypothesize an improved recovery and outcome and a decreased incidence of infarcts. In our study, of the four patients with pterional craniectomy (standard bone flap), two patients (50 %) showed perfusion deficits on CT angiography, yet only one patient needed an extension of the existing craniectomy. Of the two patients with DHC (decompressive flap), one patient showed perfusion deficits. Because of the size of the patient cohort, no conclusions or guidelines can be derived, but this preliminary data suggests that, in a carefully selected subgroup of patients, a pterional craniectomy would be sufficient.

Our study has several limitations. Above all this is a preliminary study and consists of a very small number of patients, making it difficult to draw statistical conclusions. However, the MLS, ICH, and GCS at admission were clearly different (standard flap vs. decompressive flap), despite the small sample size. This is a retrospective study and subject to the limitations of data collection inherent in such studies. The follow-up time was short, particularly in patients with aSAH, where rehabilitation takes months and outcome measures and conclusions are limited.

Conclusion

This preliminary study suggests that in patients who are at risk for cerebral infarction or delayed vasospasm, a first line decompression could improve brain perfusion and save brain tissue at risk. In addition, primary bone flap removal after aneurysm clipping might lead to reduced re-operation rates. To date no standardized criteria exist to determine whether the bone flap should be removed at initial surgery. Our single center experience in a limited number of patients suggests a pattern which might be helpful in this decision making process. In patients with intraoperative brain swelling, presentation of GCS >10, midline shift ≤5mm, and hematoma volume ≤40 cm3, a standard pterional craniotomy with flap removal (standard flap) should be conducted, while in all other cases DHC (large flap) is recommended. Based on this preliminary analysis a standard protocol was developed which will be prospectively studied at our institution.

Conflict of Interest Statement We declare that we have no conflict of interest.

References

1. Arikan F, Vilalta J, Romero FJ, Porta I, Martinez-Ricarte FR, Sahuquillo J (2010) Primary decompressive craniectomy in patients with aneurysmatic subarachnoid hemorrhage. Results of a pilot study in 11 cases. Neurocirugia (Astur) 21:452–460
2. Bailes JE, Spetzler RF, Hadley MN, Baldwin HZ (1990) Management morbidity and mortality of poor-grade aneurysm patients. J Neurosurg 72:559–566
3. Broderick JP, Brott TG, Tomsick T, Barsan W, Spilker J (1990) Ultra-early evaluation of intracerebral hemorrhage. J Neurosurg 72:195–199
4. Buschmann U, Yonekawa Y, Fortunati M, Cesnulis E, Keller E (2007) Decompressive hemicraniectomy in patients with subarachnoid hemorrhage and intractable intracranial hypertension. Acta Neurochir (Wien) 149:59–65
5. D'Ambrosio AL, Sughrue ME, Yorgason JG, Mocco JD, Kreiter KT, Mayer SA, McKhann GM II, Connolly ES Jr (2005) Decompressive hemicraniectomy for poor-grade aneurysmal subarachnoid hemorrhage patients with associated intracerebral hemorrhage: clinical outcome and quality of life assessment. Neurosurgery 56:12–19; discussion 19–20
6. de Rooij NK, Linn FH, van der Plas JA, Algra A, Rinkel GJ (2007) Incidence of subarachnoid haemorrhage: a systematic review with emphasis on region, age, gender and time trends. J Neurol Neurosurg Psychiatry 78:1365–1372
7. Dorfer C, Frick A, Knosp E, Gruber A (2010) Decompressive hemicraniectomy after aneurysmal subarachnoid hemorrhage. World Neurosurg 74:465–471
8. Fandino J, Taussky P, Marbacher S, Muroi C, Diepers M, Fathi AR, Remonda L (2013) The concept of a hybrid operating room: applications in cerebrovascular surgery. Acta Neurochir Suppl 115:113–117
9. Haley EC Jr, Kassell NF, Torner JC (1992) The International Cooperative Study on the timing of aneurysm surgery. The North American experience. Stroke 23:205–214
10. Jaeger M, Soehle M, Meixensberger J (2003) Effects of decompressive craniectomy on brain tissue oxygen in patients with intracranial hypertension. J Neurol Neurosurg Psychiatry 74: 513–515
11. Kassell NF, Torner JC, Jane JA, Haley EC Jr, Adams HP (1990) The International Cooperative Study on the timing of aneurysm surgery. Part 2: Surgical results. J Neurosurg 73:37–47
12. Schirmer CM, Hoit DA, Malek AM (2007) Decompressive hemicraniectomy for the treatment of intractable intracranial hypertension after aneurysmal subarachnoid hemorrhage. Stroke 38:987–992
13. Smith ER, Carter BS, Ogilvy CS (2002) Proposed use of prophylactic decompressive craniectomy in poor-grade aneurysmal subarachnoid hemorrhage patients presenting with associated large sylvian hematomas. Neurosurgery 51:117–124; discussion 124
14. TISoUIA I (1998) Unruptured intracranial aneurysms – risk of rupture and risks of surgical intervention. International Study of Unruptured Intracranial Aneurysms Investigators. N Engl J Med 339:1725–1733

Endovascular Treatment of Vasospasm Related to Acute Subarachnoid Hemorrhage from Ruptured Aneurysms

Dmitry V. Scheglov, Mykola E. Polischuk, Viktor I. Scheglov, Maryna Y. Mamonova, and Lee H. Monsein

Abstract In the first 2 weeks after subarachnoid hemorrhage caused by a ruptured aneurysm, 30–35 % of surviving patients treated with conservative nonoperative therapy experience rebleeding. This is fatal in 60–90 % of cases and leads to significant disability in 17–20 % of cases. A major factor for this poor outcome is thought to be the vasospasm that occurs in up to 38.7 % by the third day, 46.3 % by the ninth day, and eventually in up to 70 % of patients. Endovascular treatment of aneurysms associated with acute subarachnoid hemorrhage has the potential to decrease the occurrence of rebleeding and therefore decrease the high mortality and morbidity associated with this disease. Treatment of vasospasm, if it does occur, has the potential to further improve patient outcomes. We describe the outcomes of 174 of our patients with acute subarachnoid hemorrhage caused by a ruptured aneurysm who were treated with endovascular techniques. Overall, the majority of our patients experienced a good or excellent outcome.

Keywords Aneurysm • Subarachnoid • Hemorrhage • Endovascular • Vasospasm

D.V. Scheglov, MD, PhD (✉) • V.I. Scheglov
Department of Vascular Pathology of the Brain Spinal Cord, Scientific -Practical Center of Endovascular Neuroradiology, National Academy of Medical Sciences of Ukraine, Kyiv, Ukraine
e-mail: info@neuroradiology.org.ua

M.E. Polischuk
Chair of Neurosurgery, National Medical Academy of Postgraduate Education Named After P.L. Shupyk, Kyiv, Ukraine

M.Y. Mamonova, MD, PhD
Chair of Anesthesiology and Critical Care, National Medical University Named After O.O. Bogomolec, Kyiv, Ukraine

L.H. Monsein, MD, MPH
Medstar Washington Hospital Center, Washington, DC, USA

Introduction

Cerebrovascular disease or stroke is a significant global health problem. It is the second leading cause of death worldwide after cardiovascular disease. Approximately 1–7 % of strokes are caused by subarachnoid hemorrhage (SAH) [1]. In 85 % of cases, the SAH is caused by a ruptured cerebral aneurysm. Even though it is an infrequent cause of stroke, the impact of SAH on global health is comparable to ischemia, the most common type of stroke, because of the relatively younger patient ages and poorer outcomes.

The incidence of cerebral aneurysms has been estimated at approximately 4 % [2]. The frequency of an aneurysm rupturing is dependent on its size and location; however, it may be up to 1–2 % per year. The peak age for aneurysm rupture is between 40 and 70 years of age. When rupture occurs, the mortality rate is 25–50 %. Of those that survive, approximately 50 % will have permanent disability. Disability is primarily caused by vasospasm, which occurs in the majority of these patients and is maximal between days 6 and 14 after SAH. If vasospasm can be minimized or reversed, patient outcomes can be improved.

The conservative and endovascular management of vasospasm is well described [3]. Conservative therapy, which is often used prophylactically, consists of cerebral protective agents such as nimodipine and "triple-H therapy" (hypertension, hypervolemia, and hemodilution). Mainstream endovascular treatments have included intraarterial infusions, most commonly papaverine [4, 5] and angioplasty [6, 7]. The degree of vasospasm is thought to be caused by the amount of SAH, which can significantly increase if there is rebleeding. This occurs with greatest frequency between days 14 and 20 and days 20 and 25. Therefore, successful aneurysm ablation, which prevents rebleeding, will improve patient outcomes.

DOI 10.1007/978-3-319-04981-6_38,

Materials and Methods

We retrospectively reviewed the records of 174 consecutive patients from 2003 to 2009 in our institution with a ruptured cerebral aneurysm that was treated within 21 days of SAH with endovascular coiling. All patients had diagnostic cerebral angiography (CA) and computed tomography (CT) scans. The degree of vasospasm was determined from the CA results using the method of Krylov [8].

For aneurysm or vasospasm treatment, the tip of a 5-F or 6-F guiding catheter was placed in the internal carotid artery (ICA). For aneurysm treatment, a microcatheter (Balt, Stryker, Codman, Microvention) was then used with compatible coils. Preservation of the parent vessel was attempted in all cases. If this was not possible, then the parent vessel was sacrificed. For vasospasm treatment via intraarterial infusion, the same microcatheters were used, through which a bolus of 2–4 ml of 2 % papaverine was infused followed by continuous infusion of up to 16 ml (320 mg). The infusion was performed directly into the vessel in spasm unless this was not possible, in which case, the infusion was performed in the ICA. For vasospasm treatment with angioplasty, a wire-guided angioplasty balloon (Balt, EV3, various manufacturers of coronary angioplasty balloons) was used. In some cases, repeat aneurysm or vasospasm treatments were performed if the patient's condition warranted.

The Fisher grade [9], World Federation of Neurosurgical Societies (WFNS) scale [10], and modified Rankin outcome (MRO; [11, 12]) was determined for each patient. Records were reviewed by a clinical trial professional. Cerebral angiography and CT images were independently assessed by two senior endovascular neurosurgeons. If there was a discrepancy between interpretations, a third endovascular neurosurgeon was used for consensus.

Table 1 Presentation

	N	%
Subarachnoid hemorrhage		
SAH	83	47
SAH and IVH	38	21.8
SAH and IPH	29	16.7
SAH and IVH and IPH	24	13.8
Location of aneurysms		
ACOM	79	45.4
ICA (non PICOM)	50	28.7
MCA	23	13.2
PICOM	22	12.7
Fisher grade		
1 (No hemorrhage evident)	2	1.2
2 (SAH <1-mm thick)	27	15.5
3 (SAH >1-mm thick)	51	29.3
4 (SAH with IVH and/or IPH)	94	54
WFNS scale (Glasgow Coma Scale, GCS)		
I (GCS = 15 without motor deficit)	31	17.8
II (GCS = 14–13 without motor deficit)	48	27.6
III (GCS = 14–13 with motor deficit)	58	33.3
IV (GCS = 12–7)	36	20.7
V (GCS = 6–3)	1	0.6
Vasospasm (Krylov)		
0 (none)	31	17.8
I (<50 % narrowing in 1–2 segments)	53	30.5
II (>50 % narrowing in 1–2 segments)	28	16.1
III (<50 % narrowing in >2 segments)	42	24.1
IV (>50 % narrowing in >2 segments)	20	11.5

Results

Presentation *(Table 1)*

We treated a total of 174 patients with a ruptured cerebral aneurysm. The majority had isolated SAH ($N=83$; 47 %). Thirty-eight (21.8 %) also had intraventricular hemorrhage (IVH), 29 (16.7 %) also had intraparenchymal hemorrhage (IPH), and 24 (13.8 %) also had both IVH and IPH. The most frequent location of a ruptured aneurysm in our population was in proximity to the anterior communicating artery (ACOM; $N=79$; 45.4 %). This was followed by the internal carotid artery (ICA; $N=50$; 28.7 %), the middle cerebral artery (MCA; $N=23$; 13.2 %), and the posterior communicating artery (PICOM; $N=22$; 12.7 %).

The majority of our patients, 54 %, presented with Fisher grade 4 (SAH with IVH and/or IPH). The least number, 1.2 %, had no visible hemorrhage on CT but had SAH determined by lumbar puncture. As many of our patients presented with a good WFNS scale [I ($N=31$; 17.8 %) or II ($N=48$; 27.6 %] as presented with a poor WFNS clinical scale [III ($N=58$; 33.3 %), IV ($N=42$; 24.1 %) and V ($N=1$; 0.6 %)]. Most of our patients presented with angiographically detectable vasospasm ($N=143$; 82 %). Approximately one-third had extensive vasospasm (Krykov III and IV; $N=62$; 35.6 %). A small number of our patients did not demonstrate vasospasm ($N=31$; 17.8 %).

We analyzed the relationship between the location of a patient's ruptured aneurysm and their Fisher grade (Fig. 1). We found that, for all locations, a Fisher grade of 4 was most common. We found this most prominently with MCA and PICOM aneurysms. We examined the relationship between

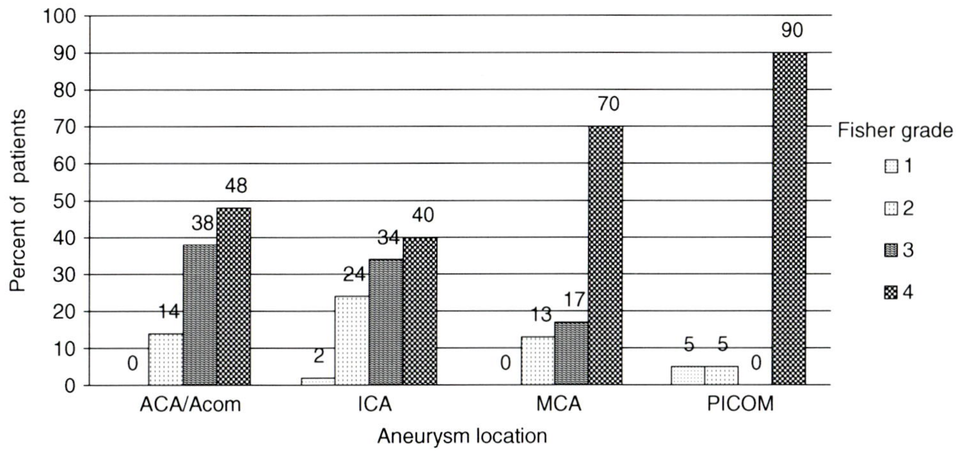

Fig. 1 Relationship between aneurysm location and Fisher grade

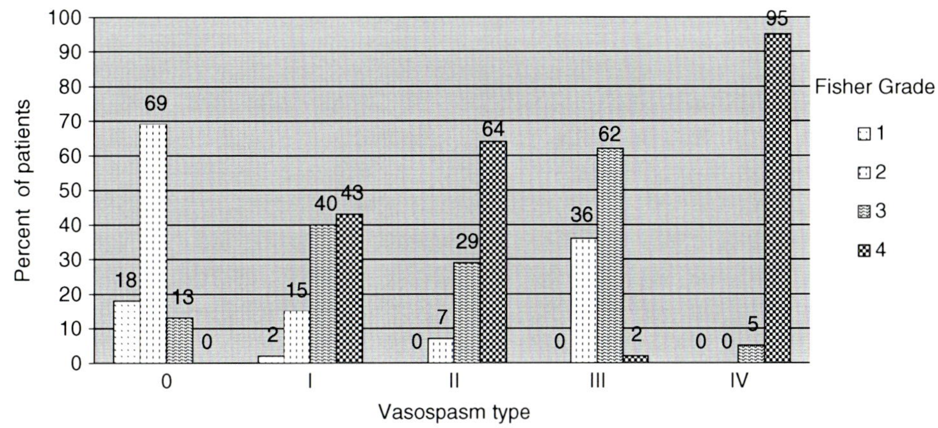

Fig. 2 Relationship between vasospasm severity and Fisher grade

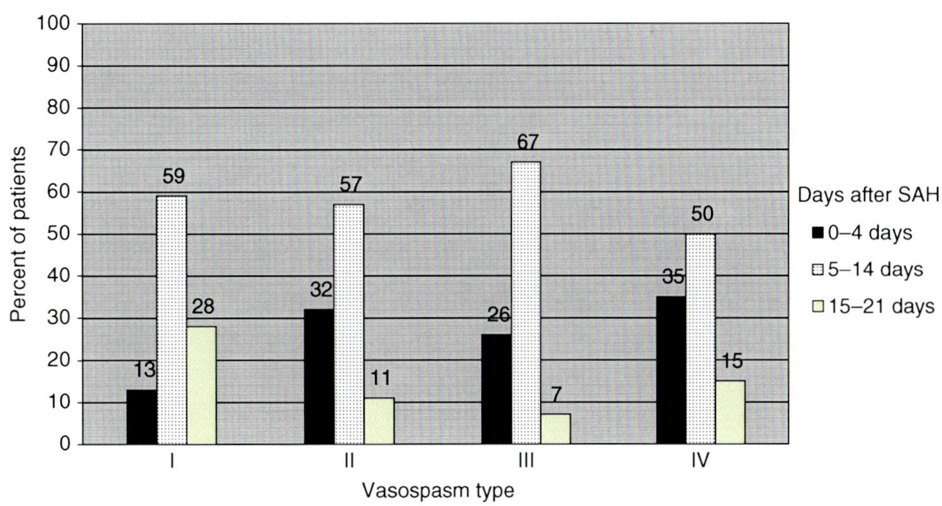

Fig. 3 Relationship between severity of vasospasm and days after SAH

a patient's Fisher grade and their development of vasospasm (Fig. 2). Not unexpectedly, the patients with the most significant vasospasm (Krylov IV) had the highest Fisher grades. We studied the relationship between the severity of vasospasm and the days after SAH (Fig. 3). All severities of vasospasm were most commonly found in the 5- to 14-day period after SAH.

Management and Outcomes *(Table 2)*

All 174 patients had a ruptured aneurysm that was treated with endovascular techniques. In 131 patients (75.3 %), there was complete ablation. In 12 of these, the parent vessel was sacrificed. In the remaining patients, the aneurysm was subtotally (N=29; 16.7 %), partially (N=10; 5.8 %), or not occluded

Table 2 Management and outcomes

	N	%
Aneurysm treatment		
Complete occlusion	131	75.3
Complete occlusion with preservation of parent vessel	119	
Complete occlusion without preservation of parent vessel	12	
Subtotal occlusion	29	16.7
Partial occlusion	10	5.8
No occlusion	4	2.2
Vasospasm		
Initial	124	71.3
Delayed	29	16.7
None	21	12.0
Treatment of vasospasm		
Medical treatment	174	100
Endovascular treatment	153	87.9
Infusion	42	27.5
Angioplasty	38	24.8
Infusion and angioplasty	73	47.7
No endovascular treatment	21	12.0
Adverse outcomes		
Any adverse outcomes	37	21.3
No adverse outcome	137	78.7
Hemorrhagic	14 (3 caused by procedure)	8.1
Ischemic	20	11.5
Other	3	1.7
Death	13 (3 caused by procedure)	7.5
Modified Rankin outcome		
0 no disability	61	35.1
1	48	27.6
2	35	20.1
3	13	7.5
4	3	1.7
5	1	0.5
6 death	13	7.5

(*N*=4; 2.2 %). In 33 patients (19 %), there was reoccurrence of at least part of the aneurysm. Twenty-seven patients (15.5 %) had one or more additional endovascular aneurysm ablations. Further details of treatment will be reported elsewhere.

Vasospasm was found at initial CA and coil treatment in most of our patients (*N*=124; 71.3 %). Delayed vasospasm, after initial angiography and coil treatment, occurred in fewer patients (*N*=29; 16.7 %). Twenty-one patients (12 %) had no angiographically detectable vasospasm. All of our patients received optimal medical therapy for vasospasm (hypertension, hypervolemia, and hemodilution). Those who demonstrated angiographic vasospasm (*N*=153; 87.9 %) received endovascular therapy, which consisted of angioplasty with a nondetachable balloon in 38 (24.8 %), intraarterial infusion in 42 (27.5 %), or both in 73 (47.7 %) patients.

The majority of our patients had a good outcome. Fourteen patients (8.1 %) had hemorrhagic events after initial presentation. Three of these were related to aneurysm treatment and the patients died. Another 20 (11.5 %) patients experienced infarcts or had other adverse events (*N*=3; 7.5 %). Using the MRO Scale, 61 (35.1 %) patients had no residual sequelae from their disease (MRO=0). Another almost 50 % (*N*=83) had a MRO of 1–2 (slight or no significant disability). A minority had an MRO of 3–5 (*N*=17; 9.7 %) or died (MRO=6; *N*=13, 7.5 %). Examples of vasospasm treatment are shown in Figs. 4, 5, and 6).

Discussion

Ruptured cerebral aneurysms usually result in isolated SAH but are often associated with IVH and IPH, which we also observed. Approximately half of our patients had associated IVH, IPH, or both (i.e., Fisher grade 4). Not unexpectedly, with a higher Fisher grade, we saw a greater severity of vasospasm (Fig. 2). Similar to the literature, approximately half of our patients presented with a poor WFNS scale (III, IV, or V).

Approximately 80 % of cerebral aneurysms arise from the Circle of Willis. They are most often found in the region of the ACOM (30–35 %), ICA (includes PICOM; 30–35 %), and MCA (20 %), and infrequently occur in other locations (10 %) [13]. In our experience, ACOM aneurysms were also the most frequent (45.4 %). In contrast, we found PICOM aneurysms in only 12.7 % of cases. Although the PICOM aneurysms were the least frequent, we found the highest frequency of Fisher grades (i.e., associated IPH and IVH) with these lesions (Fig. 1).

An estimated 50 % of patients die from their ruptured aneurysm before reaching the hospital. Of the remaining 50 %, an estimated 50 % develop angiographic vasospasm, which is clinically significant in approximately half (i.e., 25 % of the surviving patients). We demonstrated angiographic vasospasm in almost 90 % of our patients. We hypothesize that this higher frequency in our patients is caused by referral patterns in our community resulting in more critically ill patients in our institution than reported elsewhere. Similar to the literature, we found the highest percentage of each vasospasm severity (i.e., Krylov) in the 5- to 14-day period after SAH (Fig. 3).

The first cerebral aneurysm treated surgically was by Dandy in 1938 [14]. In 1974, Sebinenko described the first

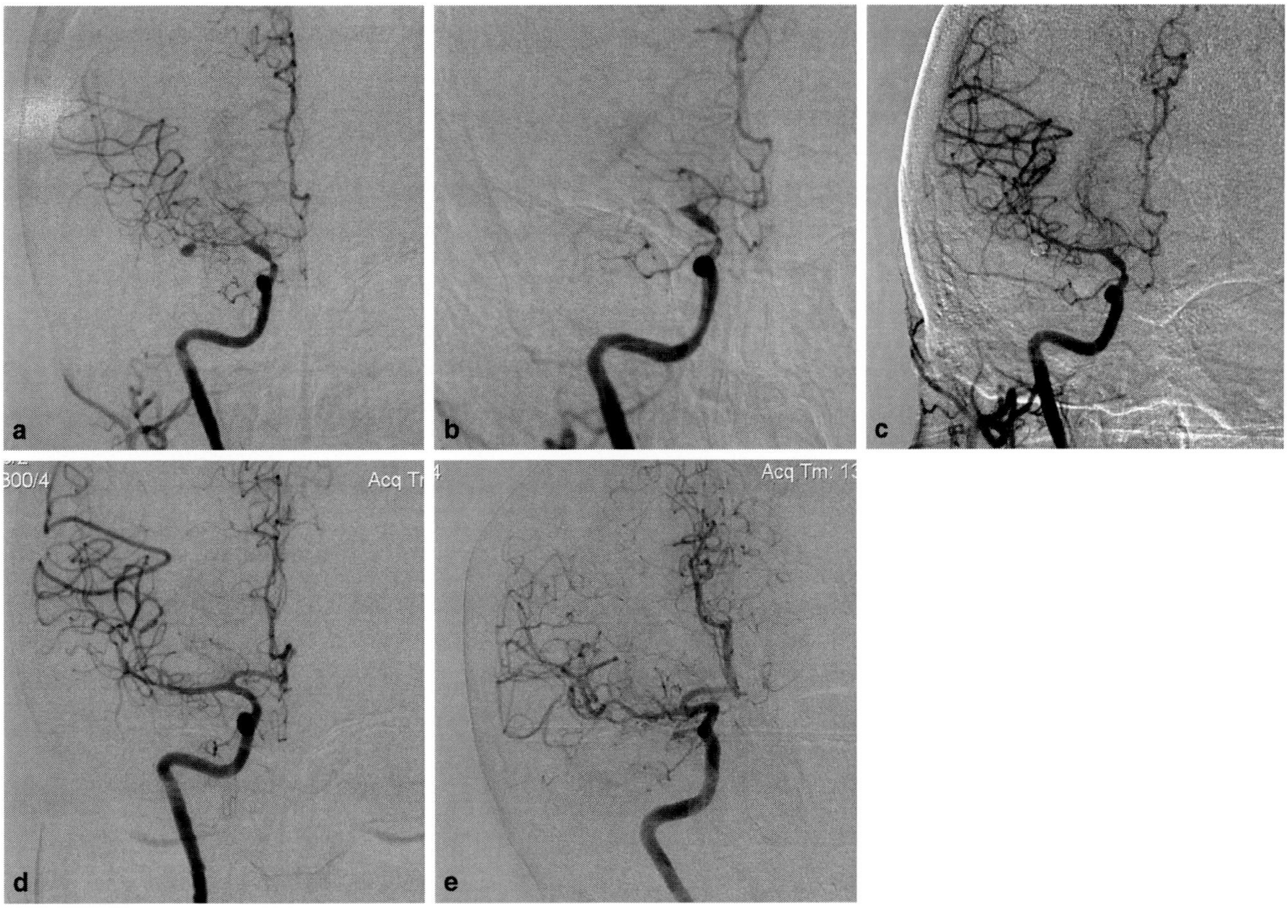

Fig. 4 (**a**) Eighth day after SAH in a 50-year-old woman with an aneurysm of the right MCA, common multisegmental angiospasm. (**b**) Intraoperative occlusion of MCA against vasospasm with subsequent catheterization. (**c**) MCA lumen restoring by super-selective infusion of papaverine in low titer (240 mg) and total reconstructive occlusion. (**d**) Early angiographic control in 1 month. (**e**) Remote angiographic control in 4 months (MRO scale 0)

successful treatment of an intracranial aneurysm without resorting to a craniotomy [15]. Initially, detachable balloon [16] and pushable coils [17] were used; however, detachable coils have been used since they were introduced in 1991 [18, 19]. Occasional balloons, stents, and liquid agents are used to supplement, or instead of, the detachable coils. High success rates of complete aneurysm ablation with low complication rates are now routine. We were successful in fully ablating the aneurysms in 131 patients (75.3 %) with preservation of the parent vessel in 119 patients. We had a serious complication in three cases caused by procedural rupture of the aneurysm and subsequent hemorrhage and death.

All of our patients received conservative therapy similar to previously described. We also used a combination of intraarterial infusion and angioplasty in the patients who demonstrated angiographic vasospasm. In all cases, there was improved angiographic vasospasm. There were no procedural complications related to vasospasm treatment. Other investigators have demonstrated intraarterial infusion, angioplasty, or both to be successful in treating vasospasm [4, 5, 7]. Although there have been reports of intraarterial infusion of a number of medications for vasospasm, papaverine has been the most widely used.

The overall outcome of our patients was quite good compared with the natural history of patients with SAH caused by ruptured cerebral aneurysms described in the literature. Approximately 85 % of our patients suffered no significant disability. Thirty-five percent had no sequelae. Less than 10 % died, including three patients in whom the deaths were procedure related. Our complication and fatality rate of less than 2 % was acceptable but unfortunate.

Conclusion

Endovascular methodology allows not only occlude the aneurysms but also helps to treat vasospasm, as a main complication of acute aneurysmal hemorrhage and thus can significantly improve outcomes.

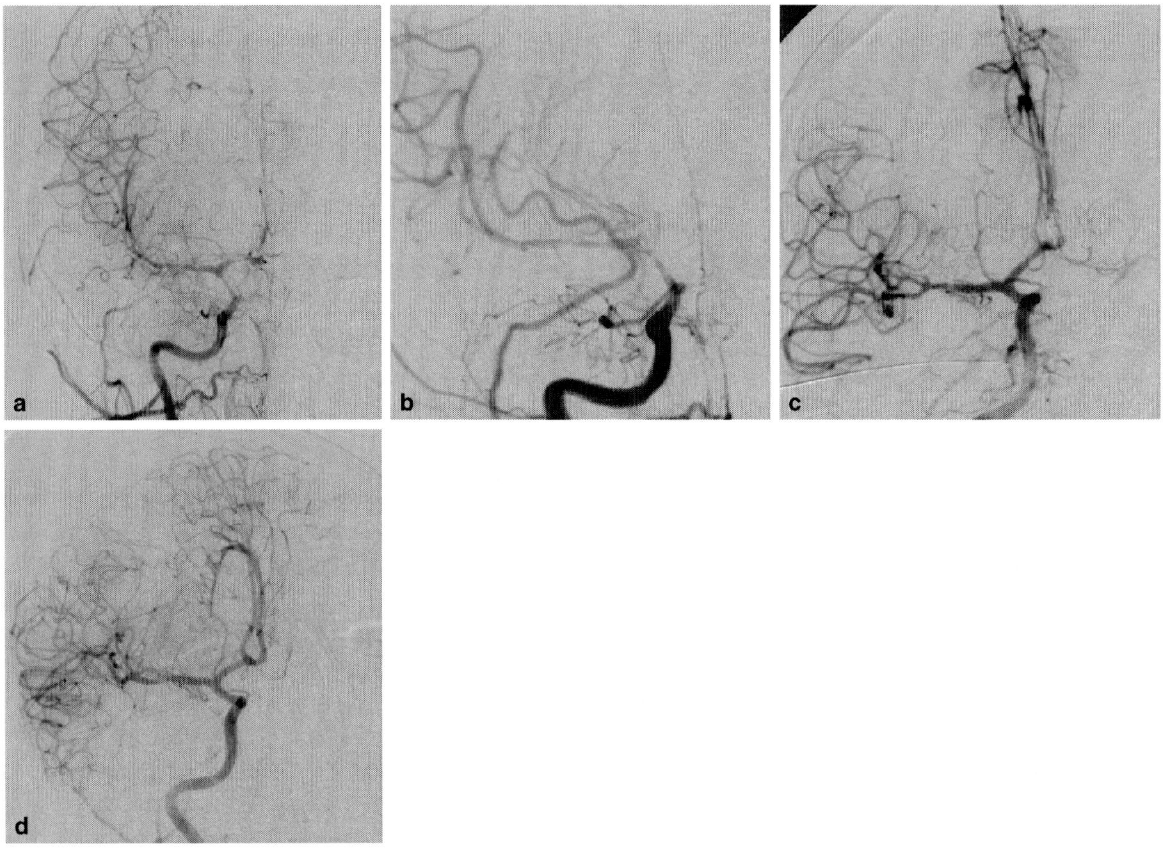

Fig. 5 (**a**) Sixth day after SAH in a 32-year-old woman with an aneurysm of the right ACA/ACOM, common multisegmental angiospasm. (**b**) Vasospasm increasing, critical stenosis of ICA and MCA; ACA/ACOM are not visualized. (**c**) The reconstructive precervical occlusion of the aneurysm performed simultaneously with balloon angioplasty of the ICA and MCA and pharmacological dilation of the ACA. (**d**) Remote angiographic control in 4 months (MRO scale 1)

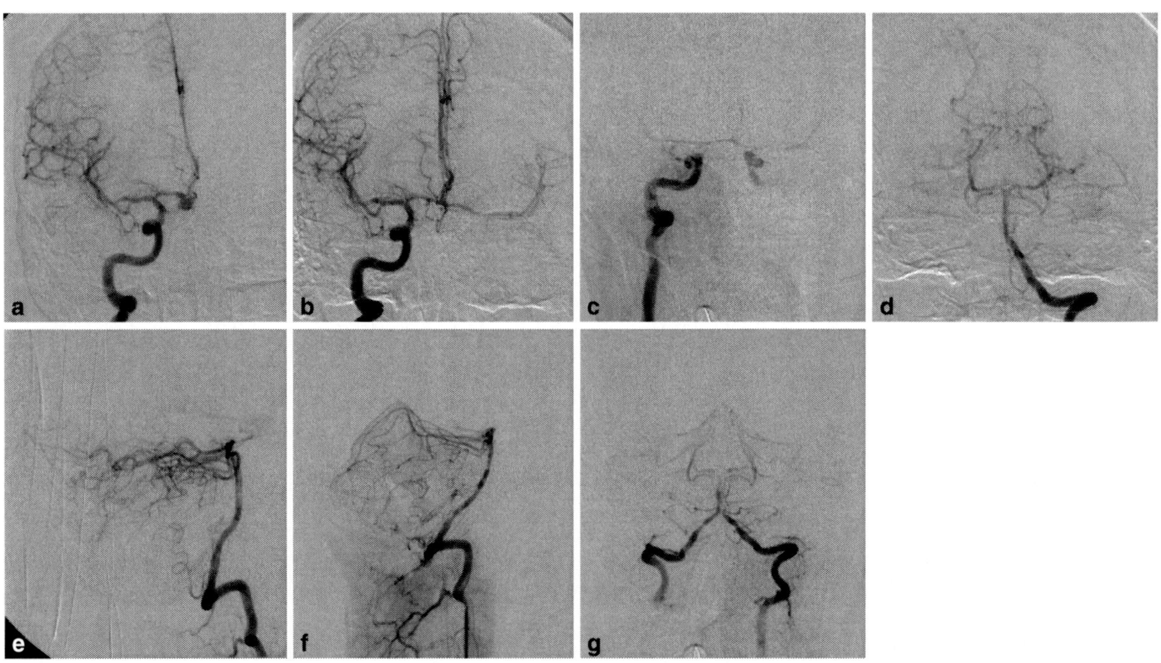

Fig. 6 (**a**) Second day after SAH in a 29-year-old man with an aneurysm of the right ACA/ACOM, WFNS I. (**b**) Reconstructive total occlusion of aneurysm, no vasospasm, ACOM functions. (**c**) Worsening on a background of triple-H therapy on the seventh day after SAH, carotid vessels no any vessels visualized because of the vasospasm increasing and brain swelling. (**d**, **e**) Angiography of the posterior circulation on the second day after SAH (normal blood flow). (**f**, **g**) Angiography of the posterior circulation on the seventh day after SAH (total vasospasm and arteries position changing through the brain swelling and dislocation), fatal outcome

Acknowledgments The authors acknowledge Maryna Maranova for her thorough and detailed assistance in collecting, reviewing, and analyzing the clinical data related to this manuscript.

Conflict of Interest Statement We declare that we have no conflict of interest.

References

1. Feigin V, Rinkel J, Lawes C, Algra A, Bennett D, Gijn J, Anderson C (2005) Risk factors for subarachnoid hemorrhage: an updated systematic review of epidemiological studies. Stroke 36:2773–2780
2. Keedy A (2006) An overview of intracranial aneurysms. Mcgill J Med 9:141–146
3. Paoletti C, Dematons C, Bellec C, Ragguenea J, PayendelaGaranderie D, Lo L, Lot G, George B, Cophignon J, Merland J (1999) Medical management of vasospasm and hemodynamic alterations in the neurosurgical ICU. In: Interverntioanal neuroradiology. WB Saunders, Philadelphia, pp 602–612
4. Kassell N, Helm G, Simmons N, Phillips C, Cail W (1992) Treatment of cerebral vasospasm with intra-arterial papaverine. J Neurosurg 77:848–852
5. Clouston J, Numaguchi Y, Zoarski G, Aldrich E, Simard J, Zitnay K (1995) Intraarterial papaverine infusion for cerebral vasospasm after subarachnoid hemorrhage. AJNR Am J Neuroradiol 16:27–36
6. Zubkov Y, Nikiforov B, Shustin V (1984) Balloon catheter technique for dilatation of constricted cerebral arteries after aneurysmal SAH. Acta Neurochir (Wien) 70:65–79
7. Higashida R, Halbach V, Cahan L, Brant-Zawadzki M, Barnwell S, Dowd C, Hieshima G (1989) Transluminal angioplasty for treatment of intracranial arterial vasospasm. J Neurosurg 71:648–653
8. Zakharov A, Krylov V (1992) The angiographic diagnosis of vascular vasospasm in ruptured cerebral aneurysms. Zh Vopr Neirokhir Im N N Burdenko 6:3–5
9. Fisher C, Kistler J, Davis J (1980) Relation of cerebral vasospasm to subarachnoid hemorrhage visualized by computerized tomographic scanning. Neurosurgery 6:1–9
10. Teasdale G, Drake C, Hunt W, Kassell N, Sano K, Pertuiset B, De Villiers J (1988) A universal subarachnoid hemorrhage scale; report of a committee of the World Federation of Neurosurgical Societies. J Neurol Neurosurg Psychiatry 5:1457
11. Bonita R, Beaglehole R (1988) Modification of the Rankin Scale: Recovery of motor function after stroke. Stroke 19:1497–1500
12. Rankin J (1957) Cerebral vascular accidents in patients over the age of 60. Scott Med J 2:200–215
13. Osborn A (1994) Diagnostic neuroradiology. CV Mosby, St Louis
14. Dandy W (1938) Intracranial aneurysm of the internal carotid artery: cured by operation. Ann Surg 107:654–659
15. Serbinenko F (1974) Balloon catheterization and occlusion of major cerebral vessels. J Neurosurg 41:125–145
16. Scheglov V (1995) Endosaccular detachable balloon catheter treatment of cerebral saccular aneurysms. In: Endovascular Interventional Neuroradiology, (Ed) Robert NN, Holtzman, Bennett, Stein, Meidi Winston. Springer Verlag, New York, Inc. pp 298–311
17. Hilal S (1988) Synthetic fiber coated platinum coils successfully used for the endovascular treatment of arteriovenous malformations, aneurysms, and direct arteriovenous fistulae of the central nervous system. AJNR Am J Neuroradiol 9:1030
18. Guglielmi G, Vinuela F, Dion J, Duckwiler G (1991) Electrothrombosis of saccular aneurysms via endovascular approach. Part 2: Preliminary clinical experience. J Neurosurg 75:8–14
19. Murayama Y, Nien Y, Duckwiler G, Gobin Y, Jahan R, Frazee J, Martin N, Vinuela F (2003) Guglielmi detachable coiled embolization of cerebral aneurysms: 11 years' experience. J Neurosurg 98:959–966

Prospective Factors of Temporary Arterial Occlusion During Anterior Communicating Artery Aneurysm Repair

Antônio Santos de Araújo Júnior, Paulo Henrique Pires de Aguiar, Mirella Martins Fazzito, Renata Simm, Marco Antonio Stefani, Carlos Alexandre Zicarelli, and Apio Claudio Antunes

Abstract *Introduction*: This study was undertaken to determine variables that could predict, in the perioperative period of anterior communicating artery (ACom) aneurysms surgeries, the likelihood of postoperative sequelae and complications, after temporary arterial occlusion (TAO).

Patients and Methods: In a universe of 32 patients submitted to ACom aneurysm repair in the last 7 years, 21 needed TAO intraoperatively, and had their data examined retrospectively.

Results: Aneurysms larger than 7 mm were more likely to be treated with longer TAO time than small aneurysms, ($p<0.0001$). There was no statistical correlation between time of occlusion and outcome. Age, Glasgow Coma Scale at initial evaluation, and Fisher scale at first CT scanning were independent factors of unfavorable outcome ($p<0.001$). Meanwhile gender, tobacco addiction, obesity, arterial hypertension, dyslipidemia, location of TAO (A1 or A2), intraoperative rupture (IR) and the aneurysm size were not identified as independent prognostic factors.

During follow-up period, two thirds of the patients had a favorable outcome, accomplishing normal daily life activities without major complications. Most patients developed clinical vasospasm (66.6 %), with 19 % of the patients harboring a severe disease. Delayed ischemic neurological deficit was observed in 28.5 %, without any statistical correlation to time of TAO or IR.

Conclusion: TAO during ACom aneurysm repair does not seem to add more morbidities to the procedure, and is not an independent prognostic factor.

Keywords Anterior communicating artery aneurysm • Brain aneurysm • Vascular neurosurgery

A.S. de Araújo Júnior, MD (✉)
Division of Post Graduation in Surgery, Federal University of Rio Grande do Sul, Porto Alegre, Brazil
e-mail: dr.antonioaraujojr@gmail.com

P.H.P. de Aguiar, MD, PhD
Division of Post Graduation in Surgery, Federal University of Rio Grande do Sul, Porto Alegre, Brazil

Intensive Care Unit, Santa Paula Hospital, São Paulo, Brazil

M.M. Fazzito, MD • R. Simm, MD • C.A. Zicarelli, MD
Intensive Care Unit, Santa Paula Hospital, São Paulo, Brazil

M.A. Stefani, MD, PhD • A.C. Antunes, MD, PhD
Division of Neurosurgery, Federal University of Rio Grande do Sul, Porto Alegre, Brazil

Introduction

Anterior communicating artery (AComm) aneurysms are the most common intracranial aneurysms, accounting for approximately 30–37 % of intracranial aneurysms [8, 17].

AComm aneurysms are also the most complex aneurysms of the anterior circulation due to the angioarchitecture and flow dynamics of the AComm region, frequent anatomical variations, deep interhemispheric location, and danger of severing the perforators with ensuing neurologic deficits [10].

AComm aneurysms are most commonly found at the A1-A2 junction on the dominant side [1]. The angle of the arteries at the bifurcation and the direction of blood flow are factors of hemodynamic stress in the apical region where these aneurysms often develop. They exist at the bifurcation of dominant A1, A2 and AComm and usually point in the direction away from the dominant A1 [1].

Worldwide the endovascular therapy is gaining an increasing role in the treatment of AComm aneurysms [9], but has not yet overwhelmed the microneurosurgical management, and seem to accomplish the same outcome in a long-term follow-up of ruptured cases [4, 15]. In everyday clinical practice and decision making, coiling and clipping are to be considered equivalent in the long term [4], but treatment options should be tailored case-to-case.

A variety of operative approaches to the anterior communicating complex for intracranial aneurysms have been

DOI 10.1007/978-3-319-04981-6_39, © Springer International Publishing Switzerland 2015

described [2, 17], but the most commonly used is the pterional approach best described by Yasargil and Fox [22].

The advantages of the pterional approach are as followed: neurosurgeons are familiar and comfortable with it; it provides a rapid access to the basal cisterns; it allows exposure to the proximal A1 segment to proximal control, and other common aneurysm locations when multiple ipsilateral aneurysms are present; it provides an anterolateral trajectory to the Acomm region that allows for easier visualization of perforating vessels supplying the septal region and chiasm [17].

However, the pterional approach may present some disadvantages. This is a unilateral approach to a midline structure. Sometimes retraction of the frontal lobe cannot be achieved adequately without widely opening the sylvian fissure, increasing the temporal lobe, insula, draining veins and middle cerebral artery dissection trauma [17]. Bone removal is required to minimize brain retraction and can be cosmetically disfiguring because temporalis muscle atrophy and risk of damage to the frontalis branch of the facial nerve [17].

To prevent some of these previous disadvantages, the anterior subfrontal [13, 17, 21] and the lateral supraorbital [10, 11] approaches for AComm aneurysm clipping were proposed. Up to now there is no optimal approach for AComm aneurysms clipping, and all seem to be feasible, being the choice of the approach an option of the surgeon. Despite its technical nuances the timing of treatment is still a controversial matter.

The ideal timing of clipping after aneurysmal subarachnoid hemorrhage (SAH) was unknown up to the International Subarachnoid Aneurysm Trial, which assessed differences in incidence of delayed cerebral ischemia and clinical outcome between different timings of treatment [7]. The risk for poor outcome was highest when treatment was performed after day 10; postponing treatment in patients who were eligible for treatment between days 5–10 after SAH was not recommended [7].

AComm aneurysms present frequently with SAH at small size [10]. Furthermore, unruptured AComm aneurysm may have increased risk of rupture regardless of size, also as an associated aneurysm, and require treatment. They demonstrate the highest incidence of post-operative morbidity among anterior circulation aneurysms [1].

The aim in microneurosurgical management of an AComm aneurysm is total occlusion of the aneurysm sac with preservation of flow in all branching and perforating arteries [10]. Precise dissection in the anatomy of the AComm complex and perforators requires not only experience and skill but patience to work the dome and base under repeated protection of temporary clips [10].

Elective use of temporary clips (ETC) prevents intraoperative anterior circulation aneurysmal rupture (IAR). Dhandapani et al. [6] have found a 4.5 % of IAR in patients who had ETC vs. 55.3 % of IAR without ETC ($p<0.001$). They have also demonstrated that IAR had significant association with unfavorable outcome (38 % vs. 24 %) ($p=0.02$) [6]. In addition, the use of ETC ($p=0.027$) and total temporary clipping less than 20 min ($p=0.049$) were noted to result in significantly better outcome, independent of other factors [6].

In Leipzig et al. [14] study, posteroinferior cerebellar artery and anterior and posterior communicating artery aneurysms were more liable to rupture intraoperatively. The IAR rate was greater in ruptured than unruptured aneurysms (10.7 versus 1.2 %, $p<0.0001$). There was a lower rate of IAR in operations using temporary arterial occlusion (3.1 versus 8.6 %, $p<0.0001$) [14].

According to Salary et al. outcome after aneurysmal SAH is related to the following triad of well-established clinical factors: Hunt and Hess grade, age, and clinical vasospasm [18].

Despite intraoperative aneurysmal rupture been recognized a factor of unfavorable outcome according to Dhandapani et al. [6], up to now there was no multivariate study to validate the use of temporary clipping or other epidemiological data as a independent factor of outcome.

Anesthetic Considerations

It is highly advisable the best anesthesiology practicing in neurosurgical treatment of intracranial aneurysms.

Standard American Society of Anesthesiologists monitoring and invasive arterial monitoring is necessary during surgery. Whether central venous pressure or pulmonary artery pressure should be monitored depends on several factors including patient medical history, size and location of the intracranial aneurysms, use of inotropic agents, and the anesthesiologist's discretion [3].

Induction of general anesthesia and intubation should be accomplished in a smooth and controlled manner. Small doses of anxiolytics like midazolam can help to decrease patient anxiety preoperatively, although one should be aware that this can change neurologic evaluation and create suspicion of deteriorating mental status postoperatively, especially in elderly patients [3].

Pinning the head in a Mayfield surgical frame is associated with a high sympathetic discharge, systemic hypertension, and potential aneurysm rupture. A bolus of opioids, such as sufentanil, or fentanyl, and scalp infiltration with a local anesthetic attenuates the hemodynamic changes during head pinning [3].

The surgical decision to use temporary clipping should prompt the anesthesia team to consider measures for brain protection, because temporary clipping can cause a period of reversible focal cerebral ischemia [3].

Communication between the surgeon and anesthesiologist about timing of application and release of the temporary clip is one of the most important factors in achieving optimal oxygenation and perfusion of the brain during this critical period [3].

If temporary clips are used before placement of the permanent aneurysm clip, the anesthesiologist can decrease the CMRO2 (cerebral metabolic rate for oxygen) by giving a bolus of IV anesthetic while blood pressure is maintained. A moderate decrease in blood pressure can help the surgeon manipulate the artery for placement of the temporary clip. After temporary clip placement, however, a higher blood pressure is needed to promote collateral perfusion to the ischemic area [3].

The Intraoperative Hypothermia For Aneurysm Surgery Trial showed that short-duration intraoperative hypothermia did not improve 3-month neurologic outcome after craniotomy for good-grade patients with aneurysmal subarachnoid hemorrhage [20]. Hypothermia is also associated with arrhythmias and cardiac ischemia, decreased platelet activity, prolonged coagulation, and increased infection rate [20].

Hyperglycemia also has a deleterious effect on recovery from ischemic brain injury [12, 16]. The prophylactic use of calcium antagonists like nimodipine in patients with SAH reduces the risk of brain damage [5]. The efficacy of magnesium in preventing delayed ischemic neurologic deficits in patients with SAH seems to be comparable with nimodipine [19].

Methods

In a universe of 92 patients submitted to AComm aneurysm clipping between 2000 and 2013 by the senior author, 32 were operated in the last 7 years. Among these patients, 21 needed temporary arterial occlusion during surgical aneurysm repair, and had their data examined retrospectively.

The admission characteristics of the patients are summarized in Table 1. All patients underwent diagnostic cerebral angiography, and had their data regarding the aneurysm morphology summarized in Table 2.

The surgical case characteristics and details regarding postoperative course were reviewed and are summarized in Table 3. The clinical outcome of the patients was assessed at 1-year follow-up by "Glasgow Outcome Scale – GOS", as defined: GOS 5 – good recovery (resumption of normal life despite deficits); GOS 4 – moderate disability (disabled but independent); GOS 3 – severe disability (conscious but disabled); GOS 2 – persistent vegetative state; and GOS 1 – death.

Results

Aneurysms larger than 7 mm were more likely to be treated with longer temporary clipping time than small aneurysms, <7 mm (11.3 ± 4.1 vs. 22 ± 5.7, *t*-Test, $p<0.0001$). There was no statistical correlation between time of occlusion and outcome ($r=0.92$, Pearson, $p>0.08$). There was also no statistical difference in outcome between patients submitted to intraoperative temporary clipping during more or less than 20 min.

Age, Glasgow Coma Scale (GCS) at initial evaluation, and Fisher scale at first CT scanning were independent factors of unfavorable outcome (Glasgow Outcome Scale ≤ 3) (cox-regression, $p<0.001$). Among variable factors, being older than 50 years, an initial GCS under 13, and a Fisher grade III or IV resulted in worse outcome.

Meanwhile gender, tobacco or alcohol addiction, obesity, arterial hypertension, dyslipidemia, location of temporary occlusion (A1 or A2), intraoperative rupture and the aneurysm size were not identified as independent prognostic factors.

During follow-up period, two thirds of the patients had a favorable outcome (GOS ≥ 4), accomplishing normal daily life activities without major complications. Among nine patients with unruptured aneurysms 100 % had a favorable outcome at 1-year follow-up (GOS ≥ 4), meanwhile, among 12 patients with ruptured aneurysms only 41.6 % had a favorable outcome.

Fifty-two percent of patients evolved with hydrocephalus, despite of routinely fenestration of the lamina terminalis, performed in 71.4 % of procedures. Most patients also developed clinical vasospasm (66.6 %), with 29 % of the patients harboring a severe disease. Delayed ischemic neurological deficit was observed in 28.5 %, secondary to severe vasospasm and without any statistical correlation to time of temporary occlusion or intraoperative aneurysm rupture.

Discussion

Despite Dhandapani et al. [6] findings, we were not able to demonstrate any statistical difference in outcome of patients submitted to ETC, even with time longer than 20 min, neither among whom IAR was observed. It may be explained because we had only four cases of ETC longer than 20 min, and just three cases of IAR.

Nevertheless we have taken statistically longer time of ETC in aneurysms greater than 7 mm, perhaps due some difficult to dissect the dome and base from larger aneurysms, and to locate all perforating branches before permanent closure of the aneurysm.

Table 1 Clinical characteristics of patients with AComm aneurysms

Characteristics*	
Total number of patients	21
Sex	
Male	6 (29)
Female	15 (71)
Male/female rate	0.4
Mean age (years)	52.8 ± 16.5
Range (years)	19–78
Presentation	
Unruptured	9 (43)
Ruptured	12 (57)
Fisher grade	
1	
2	6 (50)
3	5 (42)
4	1 (8)
Glasgow Coma Scale	
13–15	20 (95)
8–12	1 (5)
<8	0 (0)
Comorbidities	
Hypertension	16 (76)
Smoker	14 (66)
Alcohol	7 (33)
Obesity	8 (38)
Dyslipidemia	8 (38)

*Values represent number of patients, with percentages given in parentheses

Table 2 Summary of aneurysm morphological characteristics

Characteristics*	
Aneurysm size	
Small (<10 mm)	21 (100)
Large (10–25 mm)	0 (0)

*Values represent number of patients, with percentages given in parentheses

Our results are quite similar to those obtained by Salary et al. [18], which revealed unfavorable outcome following SAH related to age older than 50 years. Other independent factors of unfavorable outcome were Fisher grade III or IV and Glasgow Coma Scale under 13 at admission.

From all epidemiological comorbidities, such as tobacco or alcohol addiction, obesity, arterial hypertension or dyslipidemia, none has revealed as independent factor of unfavorable outcome.

Table 3 Summary of surgical case characteristics and post-operative course

Characteristics*	
Intraoperative aneurysm rupture	3 (14)
Temporary clipping performed	21 (100)
Average clip duration	13.8 ± 6.4
Lamina terminalis opening	15 (71)
Complications	
Vasospasm	14 (66)
Mild	10 (71)
Severe	4 (29)
Delayed ischemic deficit	6 (28)
Hydrocephalus	11 (52)
GOS 1-year follow-up	
GOS 5	8 (38)
GOS 4	6 (28)
GOS 3	2 (9)
GOS 2	3 (14)
GOS 1	2 (9)

*Values represent number of patients, with percentages given in parentheses

Despite the severity of the illness, two thirds of patients evolved with favorable outcome (GOS ≥4). However, in the group of ruptured cases, only 41.6 % patients evolved well.

Conclusion

Temporary clipping during ACom aneurysm repair does not seem to add more morbidities to the procedure, and is not an independent prognostic factor. However, age, initial GCS and Fisher grade are associated to unfavorable outcome.

Conflict of Interest Statement We declare that we have no conflict of interest.

References

1. Agrawal A, Kato Y, Chen L, Karagiozov K, Yoneda M, Imizu S, Sano H, Kanno T (2008) Anterior communicating artery aneurysms: an overview. Minim Invasive Neurosurg 51(3):131–135
2. Andaluz N, Zuccarello M (2008) Anterior communicating artery aneurysm surgery through the orbitopterional approach: long-term follow-up in a series of 75 consecutive patients. Skull Base 18(4):265–274
3. Avitsian R, Schubert A (2007) Anesthetic considerations for intraoperative management of cerebrovascular disease in neurovascular surgical procedures. Anesthesiol Clin 25(3):441–463

4. Bakker NA, Metzemaekers JD, Groen RJ, Mooij JJ, Van Dijk JM (2010) International subarachnoid aneurysm trial 2009: endovascular coiling of ruptured intracranial aneurysms has no significant advantage over neurosurgical clipping. Neurosurgery 66(5):961–962
5. Barker FG, Ogilvy CS (1996) Efficacy of prophylactic nimodipine for delayed ischemic deficit after subarachnoid hemorrhage: a metaanalysis. J Neurosurg 84:405–414
6. Dhandapani S, Pal SS, Gupta SK, Mohindra S, Chhabra R, Malhotra SK (2013) Does the impact of elective temporary clipping on intraoperative rupture really influence neurological outcome after surgery for ruptured anterior circulation aneurysms?-A prospective multivariate study. Acta Neurochir (Wien) 155(2):237–246
7. Dorhout Mees SM, Molyneux AJ, Kerr RS, Algra A, Rinkel GJ (2012) Timing of aneurysm treatment after subarachnoid hemorrhage: relationship with delayed cerebral ischemia and poor outcome. Stroke 43(8):2126–2129
8. El-Noamany H, Nakagawa F, Hongo K, Kakizawa Y, Kobayashi S (2001) Low anterior interhemispheric approach – a narrow corridor to aneurysms of the anterior communicating artery. Acta Neurochir (Wien) 143(9):885–891
9. Guglielmi G, Viñuela F, Duckwiler G, Jahan R, Cotroneo E, Gigli R (2009) Endovascular treatment of 306 anterior communicating artery aneurysms: overall, perioperative results. J Neurosurg 110(5):874–879
10. Hernesniemi J, Dashti R, Lehecka M, Niemelä M, Rinne J, Lehto H, Ronkainen A, Koivisto T, Jääskeläinen JE (2008) Microneurosurgical management of anterior communicating artery aneurysms. Surg Neurol 70(1):8–28
11. Hernesniemi J, Ishii K, Niemela M, Smrcka M, Kivipelto L, Fujiki M et al (2005) Lateral supraorbital approach as an alternative to the classical pterional approach. Acta Neurochir Suppl (Wien) 94:17–21
12. Kagansky N, Levy S, Knobler H (2001) The role of hyperglycemia in acute stroke. Arch Neurol 58:1209–1212
13. Kikuchi K, Watanabe K (1993) Modified bifrontal interhemispheric approach to aneurysms of the anterior communicating artery with the use of a trephine craniotomy. A review of personal experience with 25 cases. Acta Neurochir (Wien) 125:127–131
14. Leipzig TJ, Morgan J, Horner TG, Payner T, Redelman K, Johnson CS (2005) Analysis of intraoperative rupture in the surgical treatment of 1694 saccular aneurysms. Neurosurgery 56(3):455–468
15. Molyneux AJ, Kerr RS, Birks J, Ramzi N, Yarnold J, Sneade M, Rischmiller J, ISAT Collaborators (2009) Risk of recurrent subarachnoid haemorrhage, death, or dependence and standardised mortality ratios after clipping or coiling of an intracranial aneurysm in the International Subarachnoid Aneurysm Trial (ISAT): long-term follow-up. Lancet Neurol 8(5): 427–433
16. Pasternak JJ, McGregor DG, Schroeder DR, Lanier WL, Shi Q, Hindman BJ, Clarke WR, Torner JC, Weeks JB, Todd MM, IHAST Investigators (2008) Hyperglycemia in patients undergoing cerebral aneurysm surgery: its association with long-term gross neurologic and neuropsychological function. Mayo Clin Proc 83(4):406–417
17. Petraglia AL, Srinivasan V, Moravan MJ, Coriddi M, Jahromi BS, Vates GE et al (2011) Unilateral subfrontal approach to anterior communicating artery aneurysms: a review of 28 patients. Surg Neurol Int 2:124
18. Salary M, Quigley MR, Wilberger JE Jr (2007) Relation among aneurysm size, amount of subarachnoid blood, and clinical outcome. J Neurosurg 107(1):13–17
19. Schmid-Elsaesser R, Kunz M, Zausinger S et al (2006) Intravenous magnesium versus nimodipine in the treatment of patients with aneurysmal subarachnoid hemorrhage: a randomized study. Neurosurgery 58:1054–1065
20. Todd MM, Hindman BJ, Clarke WR et al (2005) Mild intraoperative hypothermia during surgery for intracranial aneurysm. N Engl J Med 352:135–145
21. Wakai S (1991) Subfrontal-basal interhemispheric approach for anterior communicating artery aneurysms. Technical note. Acta Neurochir (Wien) 108:78–80
22. Yasargil MG, Fox JL (1975) The microsurgical approach to intracranial aneurysms. Surg Neurol 3:7–14

Neurocritical Care

Critical Care of Aneurysmal Subarachnoid Hemorrhage: State of the Art

Alejandro A. Rabinstein

Abstract Subarachnoid hemorrhage (SAH) from a ruptured aneurysm is a very complex disease. The brain can be injured from the immediate effects of the acute bleeding, but can also be threatened by secondary insults hours and days later. Early and delayed systemic complications are common and can be very serious. This brief paper summarizes key practical concepts regarding the neurocritical care of patients with aneurysmal SAH (aSAH). It proposes as a framework the division of the time course of the disease into a first phase (from aneurysm rupture to aneurysm treatment) of resuscitation and stabilization and a second phase (from aneurysm treatment to the end of the acute hospitalization) of prevention and treatment of secondary insults. The main mechanisms of cerebral injury and the principal systemic complications are discussed and diagnostic and therapeutic advice is provided based on a combination of available evidence and clinical experience.

Keywords Aneurysmal subarachnoid hemorrhage • Vasospasm Ischemia • Hydrocephalus • Neurocritical care • Intensive care

Because of its neurological and systemic complexity, aneurysmal subarachnoid hemorrhage (aSAH) represents one of the paradigmatic challenges for a neurointensivist. Comprehensive reviews on the neurocritical care of aSAH have been published [1], and recent guidelines provide information on the management of the entire scope of the disease [2–4]. Instead, this brief paper will attempt to highlight key clinical points and convey some teaching messages I have learned over the years at the bedside.

The first of these points is that neurocritical care matters for patients with aSAH. Several studies have shown that when these patients are treated by a dedicated team with expertise in neurocritical care, their outcomes are better. They have shorter length of stay in the intensive care unit and in the hospital, they are more often discharged home or to rehabilitation facilities, and their functional outcomes are more favorable [5–7]. The improved outcomes observed in centers with higher case volumes of aSAH are further proof that expertise is crucial when treating this disease [8].

Time Course

The clinical course of aSAH can be basically divided into two main phases. The first phase is dominated by the impact of the primary injury (i.e., the aneurysm rupture) and encompasses the time from the bleeding to the treatment of the aneurysm. The goal of treatment during this phase is the acute neurological and systemic resuscitation and stabilization so that the procedure to secure the aneurysm can be safely performed. The second phase starts after the aneurysm is secured and generally spans 10–14 days from the aneurysm rupture. During this phase, the main objective of medical therapy is to prevent secondary brain injury and to treat it when present. Both phases can be punctuated by systemic complications, which vary depending on the time of the disease. Table 1 lists the most common neurological and systemic complication of both phases of SAH.

First Phase: Resuscitation and Stabilization

The characteristics of this period are markedly different depending on the clinical grade of the aSAH. Patients with aSAH of good clinical grade (World Federation of Neurosurgical Societies (WFNS) or Hunt and Hess I–III) present with adequate levels of alertness and often they have

A.A. Rabinstein, MD
Department of Neurology, Mayo Clinic,
200 First Street SW, Mayo W8B, Rochester, MN 55905, USA
e-mail: rabinstein.alejandro@mayo.edu

DOI 10.1007/978-3-319-04981-6_40,

Table 1 Main neurological and systemic complications in the early and delayed phases of aSAH

Neurological complications	Systemic complications
Early phase	
Aneurysm rebleeding	Stress-induced cardiomyopathy
Acute hydrocephalus	Pulmonary edema (neurogenic, cardiogenic)
Seizures	Cardiac arrhythmias
Global edema/intracranial hypertension	Acute hypertension
Delayed phase	
Vasospasm	Fever (central or infectious)
Seizures	Hyponatremia/hypernatremia
Delayed hydrocephalus	Anemia
Cortical spreading depolarizations	Infections (meningitis/ventriculitis, pulmonary, urinary)
Intracranial hypertension	Venous thromboembolism

no major early cardiopulmonary complications, with the exception of acute hypertension. However, these patients can deteriorate rapidly because of development of hydrocephalus, seizures, or the occurrence of rebleeding. Thus, they demand close neurological monitoring. Patients with poor clinical grade aSAH (WFNS or Hunt and Hess IV–V) present with stupor or coma and their prevalence of neurogenic cardiopulmonary injury is high. They generally require mechanical ventilation and may need acute treatment because of global brain edema with or without hydrocephalus.

The first step of management is to ensure that they have a secure airway, adequate ventilation and oxygenation, and an effective circulation. Isotonic fluids, analgesia, and antiemesis should be provided. Acute hypertension is very prevalent and it is recommended to reduce the systolic blood pressure below 160 mmHg based on observational data indicating that patients with higher systolic pressures have higher rates of rebleeding. However, blood pressure should be lowered gradually because sudden reduction can compromise the cerebral perfusion pressure, especially if the intracranial pressure is high.

Pulmonary edema is a common early complication and, consequently, patients with aSAH should have a chest X-ray and be monitored with pulse oximetry. When present, pulmonary edema may be neurogenic, cardiogenic, or share both mechanisms. Ventilation with positive end-expiratory pressure can lead to resolution of pure neurogenic pulmonary edema, but diuretics are necessary when a cardiogenic component is at play. Electrocardiographic changes (especially affecting repolarization, such as prolongation of the QTc interval or diffuse changes in the T waves) and small elevations in serum troponin concentrations are quite prevalent and often inconsequential. However, patients with poor-grade aSAH – particularly postmenopausal women – can develop stress-induced cardiomyopathy with depressed ventricular ejection function and manifestations of acute heart failure. Although the most common echocardiographic expression of stress-induced cardiomyopathy affects predominantly the apex and spares the base (thus known as apical ballooning syndrome or takotsubo cardiomyopathy), other forms of regional wall motion disturbances can occur. Coronary angiography is generally not necessary when the diagnosis of stress-induced cardiomyopathy is suspected in patients with severe aSAH and no antecedent coronary artery disease.

Hydrocephalus (communicating or obstructive) can be present upon presentation, but often develops during the first few hours. As it develops, the patient becomes less responsive, but the change is not sudden. Hypertension and bradycardia are common. Downward gaze can be seen as an expression of tectal compression from the dilated third ventricle. Although communicating hydrocephalus can be treated with lumbar drainage if preferred, obstructive cases demand ventriculostomy. Unlike the relatively silent and gradual manifestations of hydrocephalus, rebleeding presents much more dramatically. Posturing is common and often confused with seizures. Marked hypertension is associated first with tachycardia because of the massive sympathetic discharge, and then with bradycardia secondary to the intracranial hypertension.

True seizures can also occur in this acute phase, either upon aneurysm rupture or within the following hours. Estimates of seizure frequency vary across studies, but they are unquestionably much more common among patients with poor-grade aSAH. Prophylactic anticonvulsants are generally not recommended. If they are used, it is better to avoid phenytoin because of its association with poorer cognitive outcomes and its interaction with nimodipine.

Pharmacological treatment during this initial phase should include nimodipine for prevention of delayed ischemic damage [9]. Administration of an antifibrinolytic agent (tranexamic acid or aminocaproic acid) can reduce the risk of rebleeding if started promptly after aneurysm rupture and it is a safe therapy if only used for up to 72 h [10].

Second Phase: Prevention and Treatment of Secondary Insults

Following aneurysm treatment, patients often experience a short "honeymoon period" of relative stability after which secondary insults can occur. During this period, careful monitoring of neurological and hemodynamic functions is essential. Unfortunately, there are no ideal methods to achieve these goals.

Table 2 Multimodality monitoring: available bedside methods

Method	Physiological parameter	Spatial resolution
Ventriculostomy or intraparenchymal pressure probe[a]	Intracranial pressure	Global
Electroencephalography	Cortical electrical activity	Global
Depth electroencephalography[a]	Cortical electrical activity	Regional
Jugular bulb oximetry[a]	Hemispheric oxygenation	Global
Near-infrared spectroscopy	Cortical oxygenation	Regional
Brain tissue oxygen probe[a] (Licox®)	Interstitial brain oxygen	Regional
Transcranial Doppler	Cerebral blood flow velocities	Global
Xenon-133 flow measurement[b]	Hemispheric blood flow	Global
Laser Doppler flowmetry[a]	Cortical blood flow	Regional
Thermal diffusion flowmetry[a] (Hemedex®)	Cortical blood flow	Regional
Microdialysis	Cerebral metabolism	Regional

[a]Invasive
[b]Limited to investigational use because it requires injection of a radioactive tracer

We remain convinced that the neurological examination (when performed by an experience and attentive examiner) is the most reliable method to diagnose secondary brain insults in patients with aSAH. Consequently, we always try to maintain our ability to perform a complete neurological examination if at all feasible. That means we try to extubate patients early whenever the pulmonary condition allows weaning and we avoid sedation and minimize the use of opiates as much as possible. Multimodality monitoring is an appealing and pathophysiologically sound alternative in comatose patients. Multiple parameters can be monitored, as shown on Table 2. However, it is important to bear in mind that there is no evidence that treatment guided by the monitoring of any of these parameters (or any combination of them) improves outcomes in aSAH.

Although there is consensus that hemodynamic monitoring is important is aSAH with the goal of maintaining a normal intravascular volume, there is no optimal way of assessing the volume status of the intravascular compartment at the bedside. Fluid balance remains the most commonly followed parameter. Yet, it has been shown to be a poor indicator of the volemia [11]. Methods that use transpulmonary thermodilution (such as the PICCO system) are becoming increasingly popular, despite some limitations.

Table 3 Possible pathophysiological mechanisms of delayed cerebral damage in aSAH

Vasospasm (large and small vessels)
Intracranial hypertension
Disturbed autoregulation
Seizures (clinical and subclinical)
Cortical spreading depolarizations
Microthrombosis
Microembolism
Delayed axonal degeneration

Delayed cerebral ischemia has been traditionally attributed to vasospasm. However, recent research indicates that various other mechanisms apart from vasospasm may contribute to the development of delayed ischemia (Table 3). Also, treatments that reduce angiographic vasospasm (and should lessen vasospasm in small vessels), such as the endothelin antagonist clazosentan, have failed to improve clinical outcomes [12]. Whether this phenomenon can be explained by the impact of other mechanisms of delayed brain damage unaffected by the antispasm therapy or could be related to the negative side effects of the treatment remains to be elucidated [13].

That said, delayed vasospasm is a major cause of cerebral morbidity in aSAH. Monitoring with transcranial Doppler can be useful to detect it early, but the sensitivity and specificity of this method are suboptimal and highly variable across centers. We have found CT perfusion to be useful when we suspect early signs of vasospasm. Combined with CT angiography, its positive and negative predictive values are high when interpreted by trained specialists. However, the exposure to iodinated contrast and radiation limit the number of investigations that can be performed safely and the need to transport the patient out of the intensive care unit is also a drawback. Conventional angiography continues to be the most accurate method to evaluate the status of the intracranial circulation and offers the alternative of endovascular therapy, but the diagnostic information it provides is solely anatomic.

The medical treatment of vasospasm relies on hemodynamic augmentation. In practice, it consists of trying to ensure that the patient does not have intravascular volume contraction and, most importantly, raising the blood pressure with vasopressors. A fluid bolus may be useful to gain time until the vasopressor reaches full effect, but repeated boluses are ineffective and may cause volume-related complications (such as pulmonary edema). Inotropic support may be necessary in some instances. When medical treatment is insufficient to reverse the symptoms of cerebral ischemia, the patient should be promptly taken to the angiographic suite for endovascular therapy. Balloon angioplasty is preferable when the vasospasm affects the major intracranial branches. Selective intraarterial infusion of vasodilators (such as nicardipine or verapamil) has a shorter-lasting effect, but may still be helpful when the vasospasm is more distal.

It is true that hemodynamic augmentation has never been formally tested for the treatment of delayed symptomatic vasospasm in aSAH. However, experienced clinicians agree with our experience that frank clinical improvement usually follows the timely implementation of induced hypertension. Meanwhile, endovascular treatment options are not necessarily a better option. Their prophylactic use has been proven ineffective to improve outcomes and these invasive interventions can cause vessel damage and periprocedural strokes.

Various systemic complications can occur during this second phase of aSAH. Hyponatremia is very prevalent and most often caused by cerebral salt wasting syndrome, although inappropriate secretion of antidiuretic hormone can also occur. Avoidance of hypotonic solutions (including lactated Ringer's) and administration of fludrocortisone can reduce the risk of hyponatremia [14]. Hypertonic saline is necessary once hyponatremia is established. Hypernatremia is less common, but carries worse prognosis.

The incidence of fever is high in aSAH. Central fever is common in these patients, particularly in those with vasospasm [15]. However, it is always necessary to exclude infections. The cerebrospinal fluid must be examined in patients with ventriculostomy catheters or lumbar drains. Pulmonary and urinary tract infections are also relatively frequent. Because fever can worsen outcomes, it is advisable to try to maintain normothermia as long as this can be achieved without inducing excessive shivering. When the fever is refractory to the usual interventions, surface or intravascular cooling devices can be used.

Anemia is also common in aSAH and its presence has been shown to be associated with worse clinical outcomes in various studies [16]. However, transfusions have also been noticed to be associated with unfavorable outcomes [17]. At present, the optimal cut-off for transfusion in aSAH is not known.

Conflict of Interest Statement No pertinent conflicts of interest.

References

1. Rabinstein AA, Lanzino G, Wijdicks EF (2010) Multidisciplinary management and emerging therapeutic strategies in aneurysmal subarachnoid haemorrhage. Lancet Neurol 9:504–519
2. Diringer MN, Bleck TP, Claude Hemphill J III, Menon D, Shutter L, Vespa P, Bruder N, Connolly ES Jr, Citerio G, Gress D, Hänggi D, Hoh BL, Lanzino G, Le Roux P, Rabinstein AA, Schmutzhard E, Stocchetti N, Suarez JI, Treggiari M, Tseng MY, Vergouwen MD, Wolf S, Zipfel G, Neurocritical Care Society (2011) Critical care management of patients following aneurysmal subarachnoid hemorrhage: recommendations from the Neurocritical Care Society's Multidisciplinary Consensus Conference. Neurocrit Care 15:211–240
3. Connolly ES Jr, Rabinstein AA, Carhuapoma JR, Derdeyn CP, Dion J, Higashida RT, Hoh BL, Kirkness CJ, Naidech AM, Ogilvy CS, Patel AB, Thompson BG, Vespa P, American Heart Association Stroke Council; Council on Cardiovascular Radiology and Intervention; Council on Cardiovascular Nursing; Council on Cardiovascular Surgery and Anesthesia; Council on Clinical Cardiology (2012) Guidelines for the management of aneurysmal subarachnoid hemorrhage: a guideline for healthcare professionals from the American Heart Association/American Stroke Association. Stroke 43:1711–1737
4. Steiner T, Juvela S, Unterberg A, Jung C, Forsting M, Rinkel G (2013) European stroke organization guidelines for the management of intracranial aneurysms and subarachnoid haemorrhage. Cerebrovasc Dis 35:93–112
5. Suarez JI, Zaidat OO, Suri MF, Feen ES, Lynch G, Hickman J, Georgiadis A, Selman WR (2004) Length of stay and mortality in neurocritically ill patients: impact of a specialized neurocritical care team. Crit Care Med 32:2311–2317
6. Varelas PN, Schultz L, Conti M, Spanaki M, Genarrelli T, Hacein-Bey L (2008) The impact of a neuro-intensivist on patients with stroke admitted to a neurosciences intensive care unit. Neurocrit Care 9:293–299
7. Josephson SA, Douglas VC, Lawton MT, English JD, Smith WS, Ko NU (2010) Improvement in intensive care unit outcomes in patients with subarachnoid hemorrhage after initiation of neurointensivist co-management. J Neurosurg 112:626–630
8. McNeill L, English SW, Borg N, Matta BF, Menon DK (2013) Effects of institutional caseload of subarachnoid hemorrhage on mortality: a secondary analysis of administrative data. Stroke 44:647–652
9. Dorhout Mees SM, Rinkel GJ, Feigin VL, Algra A, van den Bergh WM, Vermeulen M, van Gijn J (2007) Calcium antagonists for aneurysmal subarachnoid haemorrhage. Cochrane Database Syst Rev (3):CD000277
10. Hillman J, Fridriksson S, Nilsson O, Yu Z, Saveland H, Jakobsson KE (2002) Immediate administration of tranexamic acid and reduced incidence of early rebleeding after aneurysmal subarachnoid hemorrhage: a prospective randomized study. J Neurosurg 97:771–778
11. Hoff R, Rinkel G, Verweij B, Algra A, Kalkman C (2009) Blood volume measurement to guide fluid therapy after aneurysmal subarachnoid hemorrhage: a prospective controlled study. Stroke 40:2575–2577
12. Macdonald RL, Higashida RT, Keller E, Mayer SA, Molyneux A, Raabe A, Vajkoczy P, Wanke I, Bach D, Frey A, Marr A, Roux S, Kassell N (2011) Clazosentan, an endothelin receptor antagonist, in patients with aneurysmal subarachnoid haemorrhage undergoing surgical clipping: a randomised, double-blind, placebo-controlled phase 3 trial (CONSCIOUS-2). Lancet Neurol 10:618–625
13. Rabinstein AA (2011) Secondary brain injury after aneurysmal subarachnoid haemorrhage: more than vasospasm. Lancet Neurol 10:593–595
14. Rabinstein AA, Bruder N (2011) Management of hyponatremia and volume contraction. Neurocrit Care 15:354–360
15. Rabinstein AA, Sandhu K (2007) Non-infectious fever in the neurological intensive care unit: incidence, causes and predictors. J Neurol Neurosurg Psychiatry 78:1278–1280
16. Rosenberg NF, Koht A, Naidech AM (2013) Anemia and transfusion after aneurysmal subarachnoid hemorrhage. J Neurosurg Anesthesiol 25:66–74
17. Festic E, Rabinstein AA, Freeman WD, Mauricio EA, Robinson MT, Mandrekar J, Zubair AC, Lee AS, Gajic O (2013) Blood transfusion is an important predictor of hospital mortality among patients with aneurysmal subarachnoid hemorrhage. Neurocrit Care 18:209–215

Detection of Delayed Cerebral Ischemia (DCI) in Subarachnoid Haemorrhage Applying Near-Infrared Spectroscopy: Elimination of the Extracerebral Signal by Transcutaneous and Intraparenchymatous Measurements in Parallel

Emanuela Keller, J. Froehlich, D. Baumann, C. Böcklin, C. Sikorski, M. Oberle, and M. Muser

Abstract *Background:* Detection of delayed cerebral ischemia (DCI) in high-grade subarachnoid haemorrhage (SAH) is an unsolved issue. Conventional near-infrared spectroscopy (NIRS) with optodes applied over the skin is controversial because the NIRS signal is contaminated by extracerebral tissue. The objective is to quantify and subtract the contribution from extracerebral tissue from the signal by using measurements in parallel with a NIRS brain tissue probe and conventional NIRS.

Methods: In a patient with high-grade SAH, two approaches for NIRS were applied. First, a conventional brain tissue probe for intracranial pressure (ICP) monitoring, supplied by optical fibres, was placed into the brain tissue 2 cm deep from the dura. Second, for conventional NIRS, a plaster-based patch carrying optodes (one emitter, two detectors) was attached to the skin. Central venous injections of 0.3 mg/kg body weight (bw) indocyanine green (ICG) were performed. ICG dye dilution curves obtained with the probe and patch were collected simultaneously and analysed for blood flow values.

Results: Twelve measurements in parallel with the probe and patch were performed. Mean cerebral blood flow (CBF) for the probe was higher (24.8 ± 9.1 ml/100 g/min) compared with the values obtained with the patch (for detector 1, extracerebral blood flow [ECBF] mean 5.1 ± 1.8 ml/100 g/min; $p = 0.002$; for detector 2, 6.6 ± 2.1 ml/100 g/min; $p = 0.002$). CBF values obtained with the probe correlated with blood flow values obtained with the patch (for CBF vs. ECBF detector 1, $r = 0.72$ [$p = 0.008$]; ECBF detector 2, $r = 0.79$ [$p = 0.002$]).

Conclusions: Blood flow values obtained with conventional NIRS correlated significantly with absolute CBF values obtained directly within the brain tissue. Simultaneous measurements with the NeMo Probe and NeMo Patch allow quantification and subtraction of the contribution from extracerebral tissues from the signal obtained with conventional NIRS.

Keywords Subarachnoid haemorrhage • Near-infrared spectroscopy • Cerebral blood flow • Neuromonitoring

Introduction

Detection of delayed cerebral ischemia (DCI), especially in unconscious patients with high-grade subarachnoid haemorrhage (SAH), remains an unsolved issue. New techniques combining near-infrared spectroscopy (NIRS) and indocyanine green (ICG) dye dilution to estimate cerebral blood flow (CBF) are available [2, 10, 12]. Transcutaneous NIRS with optodes applied over the skin, however, is controversial because the NIRS signal is contaminated by extracerebral tissues (skin, skull, cerebrospinal fluid layer) [5, 7, 8, 11, 15, 16]. To obtain measurement values directly from the brain tissue, a conventional probe for intracranial pressure (ICP) has recently been supplied with optical fibres for NIRS [9]. By measuring in parallel with the NIRS brain tissue probe and conventional NIRS through the skull, the objective is to develop algorithms to quantify and subtract the contribution from extracerebral tissues from the signal obtained by transcranial NIRS.

E. Keller, MD (✉) • C. Sikorski
Neurocritical Care Unit, Department of Neurosurgery, University Hospital Zurich, Frauenklinikstrasse 10, Zuerich CH-8091, Switzerland
e-mail: emanuela.keller@usz.ch

J. Froehlich • C. Böcklin
Laboratory for Electromagnetic Fields and Microwave Electronics, ETH, Zurich, Switzerland

D. Baumann
Laboratory for Electromagnetic Fields and Microwave Electronics, ETH, Zurich, Switzerland

NeMoDevices, Zurich, Switzerland

M. Oberle • M. Muser
NeMoDevices, Zurich, Switzerland

J. Fandino et al. (eds.), *Neurovascular Events After Subarachnoid Hemorrhage*, Acta Neurochirurgica Supplement, Vol. 120,
DOI 10.1007/978-3-319-04981-6_41,

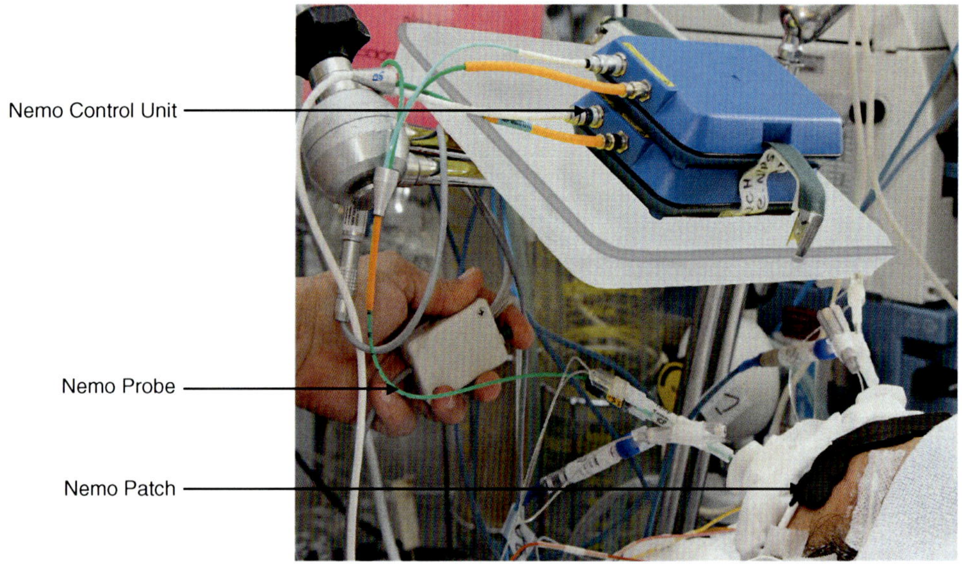

Fig. 1 Two NeMo control units (NIRS instruments) are connected to the sensors NeMo Patch (plaster-based patch, strictly noninvasive approach) and NeMo Probe (brain tissue probe, minimally invasive approach)

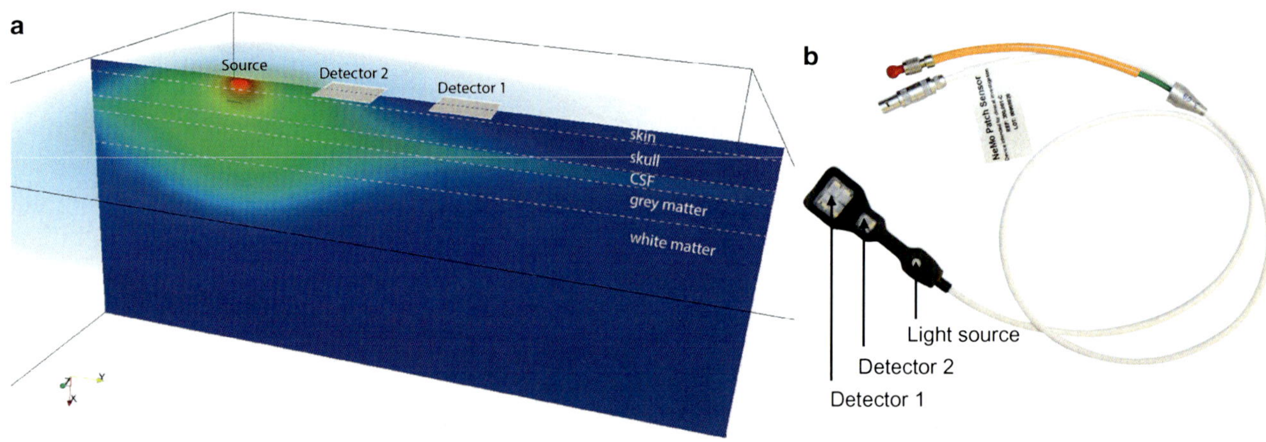

Fig. 2 Monte Carlo simulation of light propagation at 800 nm in a layered head model (**a**). The light intensity is shown in a logarithmic scale. Light guiding occurs in the cerebrospinal fluid layer, which has a slightly higher refractive index than the surrounding tissue. On a plaster-based patch, two detectors are placed at different distances from the laser source (detector 1, 4 cm; detector 2, 2 cm away from the light source) (**b**)

Methods

The study was approved by the Ethics Committee of the University of Zurich. Measurements were performed in a patient with severe SAH, Hunt and Hess grade 5, Fisher grade 4, with ruptured aneurysm of the anterior communicating artery. Because of occlusive hydrocephalus, a ventricular catheter (Bactiseal, Codman; Johnson & Johnson, USA) was inserted to drain cerebrospinal fluid. After coiling the ruptured aneurysm, the patient developed brain oedema, and ICP monitoring with an intraparenchymal probe was needed.

For NIRS two approaches were applied. (1) A conventional brain tissue probe for ICP monitoring, supplied with optical fibres (NeMo Probe, NeModevices AG, Switzerland) was inserted through a support bolt (Integra Life Sciences, Plainsboro, NJ) from a burr hole (Fig. 1). The probe was placed into the brain tissue 2 cm deep from the dura. Applying NIRS, in addition to the parameters of ICP and brain temperature, the concentration of oxygenated and deoxygenated haemoglobin (Hboxy and Hbdeoxy), as well as CBF and cerebral blood volume (CBV), were measured. (2) For conventional NIRS a plaster-based patch carrying optodes (one emitter, two detectors) was attached to the skin (NeMo Patch) (Fig. 2b). For spatially resolved spectroscopy (SRS) two detectors are placed at different distances from the laser source (distance from detector 1, 2 cm; from detector 2, 4 cm). Monte Carlo simulation of light propagation at 800 nm in a layered head model was performed with the same optode distances [1]. Two NIRS instruments, one connected to the probe, the other to the patch, specifically constructed for the measurement mode (NeMo Control Unit, NeMoDevices, Zurich, Switzerland) include the light

Table 1 Mean measurement values for the mean transit time of ICG (mtt_{ICG}), cerebral blood flow (CBF) and cerebral blood volume (CBV) obtained with the probe, as well as for the mean transit time of ICG ($Emtt_{ICG}$), blood flow (ECBF) and blood volume (ECBV) obtained with the patch including extracerebral tissue

		NeMo Patch (n=12)	
	NeMo Probe (n=12)	Detector 1	Detector 2
Mtt_{ICG} mean (s)	9.1±1.3		
$Emtt_{ICG}$ mean (s)		15.9±3.2	15.4±1.9
CBV mean (ml/100 g)	3.7±1.0		
ECBV mean (ml/100 g)		1.3±0.3	1.6±0.4
CBF mean (ml/100 g/min)	24.8±9.1		
ECBF mean (ml/100 g/min)		5.1±1.8	6.6±2.1

sources, the hardware for data collection and the software to analyse the NIRS data (Fig. 1).

Regular measurements were performed daily and repeated after 15 min under stable clinical conditions (unchanged ICP, mean arterial pressure and arterial partial pressure CO_2). Central venous injections of 0.3 mg/kg body weight (bw) ICG were performed into a tube leading into an antecubital vein, followed by 10 ml glucose 5 % flush. ICG dye dilution curves obtained with the probe and patch were collected simultaneously and analysed for blood flow values (NeMoSystem®, NeMoDevices, Zurich) based on published algorithms [10]. Measurement values are expressed in mean and standard deviation (SD). Measurement values are compared applying Wilcoxon matched pairs and calculating the correlation coefficient (Pearson; 2-tailed).

Results

In a first patient, 12 measurements in parallel with the probe and patch were performed. Mean measurement values for the mean transit time of ICG (mtt_{ICG}), cerebral blood flow (CBF) and cerebral blood volume (CBV) obtained with the probe, as well as for the mean transit time of ICG ($Emtt_{ICG}$), blood flow (ECBF) and blood volume (ECBV) obtained with the patch including signals from extracerebral tissue are given in Table 1. Mean values for the mtt_{ICG} obtained with the probe were significantly shorter compared with those obtained with the patch (for detector 1, $p=0.002$; for detector 2, $p=0.002$). Mean CBV obtained with the probe was significantly higher compared with the values obtained with the patch (for detector 1, $p=0.002$; detector 2, $p=0.002$). The corresponding values for CBF were higher for the probe compared with those obtained with the patch (for detector 1, $p=0.002$; for detector 2, $p=0.002$). There were no significant differences between $Emtt_{ICG}$ obtained with the patch detectors 1 and 2. However, ECBV and ECBF values obtained with detector 1 were slightly but significantly lower than those obtained with detector 2 (for ECBV, $p=0.003$; for ECBF, $p=0.004$).

The Monte Carlo simulations (Fig. 2a) show that, close to the source, light received by detector 2 is strongly reflected by the cerebrospinal fluid. At a larger distance from the source, most of the light that is received by detector 1 comes from the grey matter and a small portion from the white matter. CBF values obtained with the probe correlated significantly with blood flow values obtained with the patch (for CBF vs. ECBF detector 1, $r=0.72$ ($p=0.008$); ECBF detector 2, $r=0.79$ ($p=0.002$)).

Figure 3 shows dye dilution curves after ICG injection in optical density (OD) and in ICG concentration performed in parallel with the probe and patch. The maximum of the amplitude of the dye dilution curve measured with the probe occurs earlier and the amplitude is higher compared with NIRS measurements obtained with the patch through the scalp.

Discussion

Although NIRS seems to reflect significant changes in intracerebral vessels [11], it has not been demonstrated so far that these changes can be reliably distinguished from changes in extracerebral tissue [4, 15]. With the present study, for the first time, measurements in parallel with transcutaneous NIRS and a brain tissue probe with the tip in the white matter could be performed. The ECBF values obtained with conventional NIRS correlate significantly with CBF values obtained with the probe. The values for blood volume and flow from the NeMo Patch, however, were significantly lower compared with those from the NeMo Probe. ECBF values between 5.1 and 6.6 ml/100 g/min measured with the patch correspond with blood flow values measured in the extracerebral tissue with the intravenous ^{133}xenon dilution technique estimated to be 5–8 ml/100 g/min [3]. Monte Carlo simulations, furthermore, show that the cumulative NIRS signal obtained by optodes over the skin is strongly influenced by extracerebral tissue [1, 14].

For SRS it has been suggested that applying one light emitter and two detectors allows subtraction of the extracerebral contamination from the cumulative NIRS signal obtained by optodes applied over the skin [6, 13]. Our measurement values obtained from the two detectors, 1 and 2

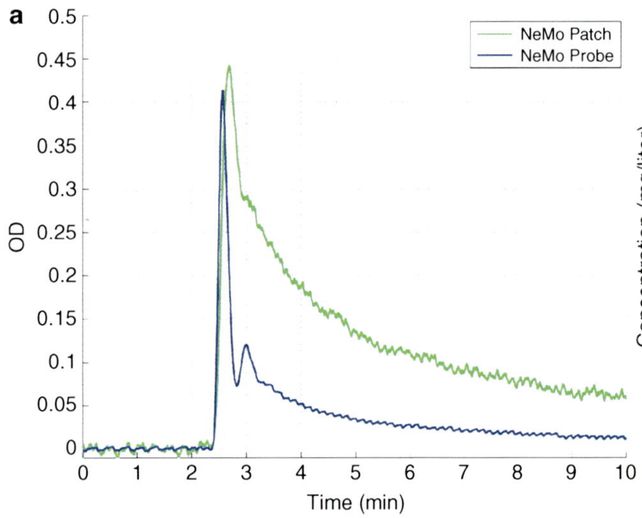

Fig. 3 Dye dilution curves after ICG injection in (**a**) optical density (OD) and (**b**) in ICG concentration in milligrams per litre (mg/l) performed in parallel with probe and patch

(4- and 2-cm apart from the light source) do not support this hypothesis. Inter-individual variability of anatomical structures (bone thickness, extracerebral vasculature, liquid space, etc.) may restrict the reliability of SRS. Furthermore, the composition of the extracerebral tissue in neurosurgical patients will change during the illness course, especially after craniotomy.

Dye dilution curves after ICG injection performed in parallel with the NeMo Probe and the NeMo Patch showed different specific characteristics for probe and patch measurements, reflecting lower blood flow within extracerebral tissue. The maximum of the amplitude of the dye dilution curve measured with the probe typically occurs earlier reflecting a faster transit time of the dye. The amplitude of the curve obtained with the probe compared with the patch is higher, corresponding to a higher concentration of ICG in the brain tissue than in extracerebral structures.

Conclusions

For the first time it was demonstrated that blood flow values obtained with conventional transcutaneous NIRS correlate significantly with absolute CBF values obtained directly within the brain tissue. With simultaneous measurements with the probe and patch, improved algorithms can be developed to quantify and subtract the contribution from extracerebral tissues from the signal obtained with conventional NIRS. This allows calculation of absolute values for CBF and oximetry data and definition of critical thresholds for ischemia not only for the NeMo Probe but also for the NeMo Patch.

Source of Funding This project was supported by the Swiss Innovation Promotion Agency (CTI) project no. 13553.1PFFLM-LS and the Eurostars project no. E!6526 OPTO-BRAIN, as well as by the Velux foundation. NeMoDevices provided technical equipment for this clinical trial.

Disclosures E. Keller, J. Froehlich, D. Baumann, M. Oberle and M. Muser have financial interests as founder, and staff members of NeMoDevices, AG.

References

1. Boecklin C, Baumann D, Keller E, Froehlich J (2012) Determining light distribution in human head using 3D Monte Carlo simulations. Optical interactions with tissue and cells XXIII. Proc SPIE 8221:17
2. Colacino JM, Grubb B, Jobsis FF (1981) Infra-red technique for cerebral blood flow: comparison with xenon 133 clearance. Neurol Res 3:17–31
3. Friberg L, Kastrup J, Hansen M, Bulow J (1986) Cerebral effects of scalp cooling and extracerebral contribution to calculated blood flow values using the intravenous 133Xe technique. Scand J Clin Lab Invest 46:375–379
4. Germon TJ, Evans PD, Barnett NJ, Wall P, Manara AR, Nelson RJ (1995) Optode separation determines sensitivity of near infrared spectroscopy to intra- and extracranial oxygenation changes. J Cereb Blood Flow Metab 15:S617
5. Germon TJ, Evans PD, Barnett NJ, Wall P, Manara AR, Nelson RJ (1999) Cerebral near infrared spectroscopy: emittor-detector separation must be increased. Br J Anaesth 82:831–837
6. Germon TJ, Evans PE, Barnett NJ, Lewis TT, Wall P, Nelson RJ (1997) Changes in tissue oxyhemoglobin concentration measured using multichannel near infrared spectroscopy during internal carotid angiography. J Neurol Neurosurg Psychiatry 63:660–664
7. Germon TJ, Kane NM, Manara AR, Nelson RJ (1994) Near-infrared spectroscopy in adults: effects of extracranial ischemia and intracranial hypoxia on estimation of cerebral oxygenation. Br J Anaesth 73:503–506

8. Hopton P, Walch TS, Lee A (1999) Measurement of cerebral blood volume using near-infrared spectroscopy and indocyanine green elimination. J Appl Physiol 87:1981–1987
9. Keller E, Froehlich J, Muroi C, Sikorski C, Muser M (2011) Neuromonitoring in intensive care: a new brain tissue probe for combined monitoring of intracranial pressure (ICP) cerebral blood flow (CBF) and oxygenation. Acta Neurochir Suppl 110:217–220
10. Keller E, Nadler A, Alkhadi H, Kollias S, Yonekawa Y, Niederer P (2003) Non invasive measurement of regional cerebral blood flow and regional cerebral blood volume by near infrared spectroscopy and indocyanine green dye dilution. Neuroimage 20:828–839
11. Kuebler WM, Sckell A, Habler O, Kleen M, Kuhnle GEH, Welte M, Messmer K, Goetz AE (1998) Noninvasive measurement of regional cerebral blood flow by near-infrared spectroscopy and indocyanine green. J Cereb Blood Flow Metab 18:445–456
12. McCormick PW, Stewart M, Goetting MG, Dujovny M (1991) Noninvasive cerebral optical spectroscopy for monitoring cerebral oxygen delivery and hemodynamics. Crit Care Med 19:89–97
13. Miwa M, Ueda Y, Chance B (1995) Development of time resolved spectroscopy system for quantitative non-invasive tissue measurement. Proc SPIE 2389:142–149
14. Mudra R, Nadler A, Niederer P, Keller E (2006) Analysis of near-infrared spectroscopy and indocyanine green dye dilution with Monte Carlo simulation of light propagation in the adult brain. J Biomed Opt 11:044009–044013
15. Owen-Reece H, Elwell CE, Wyatt JS, Delpy DT (1996) The effect of scalp ischemia on measurement of cerebral blood volume by near-infrared spectroscopy. Physiol Meas 17:279–286
16. Schwarz G, Litscher G, Kleinert R, Jobstmann R (1996) Cerebral oximetry in dead subjects. J Neurosurg Anesthesiol 8:189–193

Impaired Cerebrovascular Reactivity in the Early Phase of Subarachnoid Hemorrhage in Good Clinical Grade Patients Does Not Predict Vasospasm

Leodante da Costa, David Houlden, Gordon Rubenfeld, Michael Tymianski, Joseph Fisher, and Jorn Fierstra

Abstract *Objective:* Subarachnoid hemorrhage (SAH) alters cerebrovascular reactivity (CVR) to carbon dioxide (CO_2), which may be related to an increased risk of delayed ischemic neurological deficits (DINDs). We report the results of bedside CVR testing in the acute phase of SAH in good clinical grade patients without established vasospasm or signs of DIND.

Materials and Methods: Eighteen patients with SAH and 26 healthy subjects underwent CVR testing using transcranial Doppler with standardized changes in CO_2. None of the patients had clinical or radiological evidence of vasospasm or DIND at time of testing. A CVR index was calculated as the change in the middle cerebral artery blood flow velocity (MCAv) divided by the change in the end-tidal CO_2 partial pressure (PCO_2), Δ MCAv/Δ PCO_2, and values were compared with controls.

Results: SAH patients had lower CVR when compared with normal controls ($p=0.0001$ and $p=0.0094$, respectively). Impaired CVR was not correlated with future vasospasm ($p=0.2$).

Conclusions: Patients with SAH had significantly lower CVR indexes compared with healthy controls. Although impaired CVR was present in 50 % of the patients early after SAH, no correlation with later occurrence of DINDs was found.

Keywords Subarachnoid hemorrhage • CO_2 reactivity Delayed ischemic neurological deficit • Transcranial Doppler Vasospasm

L. da Costa, MD (✉)
Division of Neurosurgery, Department of Surgery,
Sunnybrook Health Sciences Centre, University of Toronto,
2075 Bayview Avenue, Room A1-37,
Toronto, ON M4N 3M5, Canada

Department of Medical Imaging, Sunnybrook Hospital,
University of Toronto, Toronto, ON, Canada
e-mail: leo.dacosta@sunnybrook.ca

D. Houlden, PhD
Department of Neuromonitoring, Medical Imaging,
The Ottawa Hospital, University of Ottawa, Toronto, ON, Canada

G. Rubenfeld, MD, MSc
Interdepartmental Division of Critical Care, Sunnybrook Hospital,
University of Toronto, Toronto, ON, Canada

M. Tymianski, MD, PhD
Division of Neurosurgery, Department of Surgery,
Toronto Western Hospital and University Health Network,
University of Toronto, Toronto, ON, Canada

J. Fisher, MD
Department of Anesthesia,
Toronto General Hospital and University Health Network,
University of Toronto,
Toronto, ON, Canada

J. Fierstra, MD, PhD
Department of Neurosurgery, University Hospital Zürich,
Zürich, Switzerland

Introduction

Vasospasm and delayed ischemic neurological deficits (DINDs) are serious consequences of subarachnoid hemorrhage (SAH). Vasospasm is demonstrated angiographically in approximately 70 % of patients, and approximately 35 % have DINDs [1]. Transcranial Doppler (TCD) was introduced by Aaslid et al. [2] for monitoring the development of vasospasm after SAH. It has become a routine bedside monitoring technique in the management of these patients, aiming at early detection of hemodynamic disturbances and timely institution of rescue measures, either medical or interventional. Despite the widespread use, sensitivity, and specificity of TCD for vasospasm, diagnoses are not robust [3]. CVR studies with patients in the acute and delayed phases after SAH showed conflicting results [4, 5], and, although

J. Fandino et al. (eds.), *Neurovascular Events After Subarachnoid Hemorrhage*, Acta Neurochirurgica Supplement, Vol. 120,
DOI 10.1007/978-3-319-04981-6_42, © Springer International Publishing Switzerland 2015

intuitively appealing, the test is not recommended as a monitoring modality for patients with SAH [6]. The aims of this study were to (a) evaluate the feasibility of using TCD to perform quantitative CVR measurements to CO_2 testing using a new standardized end-tidal CO_2 targeting system in the acute phase of SAH, (b) compare the CVR of patients to that in a healthy cohort, and (c) to evaluate whether impaired CVR in good clinical grade patients would be predictive of development of future vasospasm.

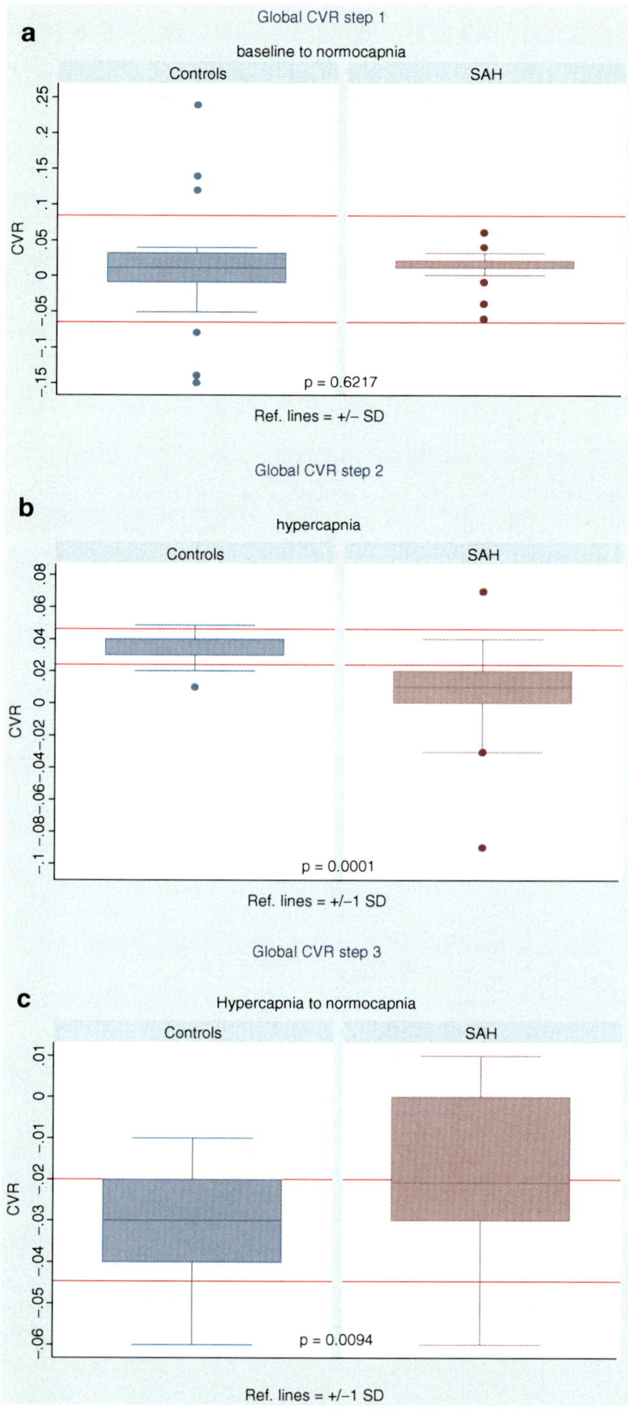

Fig. 1 Average global cerebrovascular reactivity index (*CVR*) in SAH patients and controls. (**a**) Step 1, normocapnia; (**b**) Step 2, hypercapnia; and (**c**) Step 3, return to normocapnia

Materials and Methods

Subjects

The study was approved by our institutional Research Ethics Board. Eighteen patients with documented SAH were prospectively recruited between November 2008 and December 2009. For this pilot clinical series, we included only good clinical grade patients (World Federation of Neurosurgical Societies (WFNS) score 1, 2, or 3), early in the course of their SAH (<7 days after initial bleed), who did not have clinical or radiological evidence of vasospasm or DIND at the time of the test. The control cohort consisted of 26 healthy volunteers who underwent the same study protocol.

Definition of Terms

For the purposes of this paper, vasospasm is the radiological demonstration of intracranial vessel narrowing of at least 50 % compared with previous imaging and/or increased middle cerebral artery blood flow velocity (MCAv) above 160 cm/s or a Lindegaard ratio ≥3, and DIND is the ischemic manifestation likely related to vasospasm after SAH. CO_2 manipulation is divided into four "phases" (2 min each, steady CO_2 levels) with three "steps" for the changes (Fig. 1).

Study Protocol

After the aneurysm was secured with the patient in stable clinical condition, continuous bilateral TCDs were performed using a PMD 100 Transcranial Doppler System and a 2-MHz transducer fixed in a standard head frame (Spencer Technologies, Seattle, USA). The middle cerebral artery (MCA) was insonated bilaterally through temporal bone windows. Tests were performed in a standard hospital bed with the head elevated at 30°. Once the temporal windows were located, the proper transducer position and angulation were noted and the bilateral probes were fixed on the head frame to prevent motion. The MCA was identified using established TCD criteria: depth from 30 to 60 mm, flow direction toward the transducer, flow velocities from 46 to 86 cm/s, and the anatomic relationship with the internal carotid artery (ICA) bifurcation.

End-tidal CO_2 ($PETCO_2$) values were precisely targeted for cerebrovascular reactivity (CVR) measurements using the method of prospective end-tidal targeting previously described by Slessarev et al. [7]. Blood pressure cuffs or arterial lines, when available, were used to record the blood pressure. After a short acclimatization period, subjects' $PETCO_2$ levels were set to 40 mmHg for 2 min (normocapnia; Step 1), 45 mmHg for 2 min (hypercapnia; Step 2), and then back to 40 mmHg (normocapnia; Step 3). The fraction of inspired oxygen (FIO_2) was kept at 100 %.

Data Analysis

MCAv was recorded bilaterally for each phase of the test. A global MCAv was generated averaging the means of both hemispheres. MCAv, pulsatility index (PI), end-tidal CO_2 and O_2 levels, heart rate (HR), blood pressure (BP), and intracranial pressure (ICP), when available, were recorded. The absolute change and percentage change for $P_{ET}CO_2$ and MCAv between each step in the protocol were calculated. The CVR index was calculated by dividing the percentage change in MCAv by the absolute change in $PETCO_2$ (CVR = % Δ MCAv/1 mmHg Δ CO_2). Separate calculations were made for the right and left side for each step of the test, and both sides were averaged to generate a global CVR (gCVR) index. The mean plus and minus one standard deviation of the control group data were used to define a "normal CVR," against which the SAH data was compared. The groups were also compared using the definition of "normal CVR" by Marshall et al. [8] as an increase in MCAv of at least 2 % per mmHg of CO_2 change. The Mann-Whitney test was used to analyze the differences between MCAv and CO_2 levels between the phases and the CVR index between the two groups. To test the association between mean MCAv and CO_2 level, a general linear mixed model (CO_2 group – SAH versus Control – and interaction between CO_2 group) was used. A random intercept model was used to account for variability between patients at baseline and a random slope to account for the variability between patients in the association between MCAv and $PETCO_2$.

Results

All CVR studies were performed within 7 days after the initial SAH (counted as day 1). Patient demographics and aneurysm location and treatment are shown in Table 1. Baseline $P_{ET}CO_2$ levels (mean ± SD), as measured before any gas manipulation, in the SAH group were 32.82 mmHg (±3.73) compared with 37.91 mmHg (±2.83) in the control group ($p=0.0001$). There were significant different changes in global blood flow velocity between the two groups during CO_2 manipulation, with a dampened response in flow velocity to hypercapnia in the SAH group (Table 2). Global CVR indexes during hypercapnia and back to normocapnia were significantly different between controls and SAH patients (Fig. 1). SAH patients showed impaired reactivity both with hypercapnia (SAH CVR = 0.076 ± 0.034; control CVR = 0.0353 ± 0.011; $p=0.0001$), and with the following decrease in CO_2 back to normocapnia (baseline CO_2 of 40 mmHg; SAH CVR = −0.02 ± 0.018; control CVR = −0.0323 ± 0.013; $p=<0.01$).

Vasospasm (for definition, see the Methods section) was present in nine patients (50 %) with SAH. Fifteen patients (83 %) had an impaired global CVR index with

Table 1 Patient demographics and aneurysm characteristics

		No. of patients
Mean age	52.7 years	
Women	7 (39 %)	
WFNS Grade		
I		8
II		4
III		4
IV		1[a]
V		1[a]
Aneurysm location		
Acom		5
ICA		3
MCA		2
Basilar		1
PICA		2
No aneurysm		5
Aneurysm treatment		
Clipped		5
Coiled		8

[a]Both subjects improved to WFNS 2 after external ventricular drain (EVD) placement

Acom anterior communicating artery, *ICA* internal carotid artery, *MCA* middle cerebral artery, *Basilar* basilar artery, *PICA* posterior inferior cerebellar artery

Table 2 Absolute MCA blood flow velocity change values at each step of the test for SAH and controls

	SAH	Controls	*p* value[a]
Step 1	6.87 cm/s	0.52 cm/s	0.02
Step 2	3.91 cm/s	12.47 cm/s	<0.01
Step 3	−8.97 cm/s	−12.93 cm/s	0.02

Step 1 baseline target at normocapnia = 40 mmHg, *Step 2* target hypercapnia = 45 mmHg, *Step 3* return to baseline normocapnia

[a]Mann-Whitney test

Table 3 CVR indexes in each step of the CO_2 challenge

Variable	Overall ($n=18$)	Vasospasm ($n=10$)	No vasospasm ($n=8$)	p value
CVR Step 1 (median, RR)	1.09 (0.64, 3.34)	1.06 (−0.81, 2.33)	2.5 (0.87, 4.55)	0.16
CVR Step 2 (median, RR)	0.86 (0, 2.83)	1.28 (0.05, 3.19)	0.015 (−0.73, 1.67)	0.20
CVR Step 3 (median, RR)	0.95 (0, 2.22)	0.57 (−0.11, 1.8)	1.16 (0.27, 2.52)	0.57

RR relative risk

hypercapnia, and seven (38 %) during the step back to baseline normocapnia (Step 3). No relationship between the presence of early impairment of CVR in any of the steps and the later development of vasospasm was found (Table 3). With only one event of DIND, no attempt was made to analyze the influence of impaired CVR on the occurrence of DINDs.

Discussion

Our study shows that impairment of the intracranial vascular response to CO_2 occurs early in SAH, and that good clinical grade does not exclude the possibility of impaired CVR. Despite very similar absolute MCAv values at baseline between the two groups, the introduction of CO_2 challenge shows significant hemodynamic changes (Table 2). MCAv in awake, good clinical grade patients early after SAH did not increase with increasing levels of CO_2.

The novelty of our method is that this is the first time that TCD has been coupled with a precise method to control CO_2 levels, increasing reliability and reproducibility of the test and allowing changes in MCAv to be detected using a small change in $P_{ET}CO_2$. This is important, especially if the aim is to develop a bedside test that can be repeated routinely in this critically ill population.

Whether impaired CVR can be used a marker for future development of radiological vasospasm and/or DIND remains to be determined. We could not find any relationship between the presence of early impairment of CVR to CO_2 and later development of radiographic vasospasm or DIND in this small patient population. Other groups, such as Frontera et al. [5] found that impaired reactivity to CO_2 was a good predictor of symptomatic vasospasm, preceding symptoms in 78 % of the patients, with a good sensitivity and negative predictive value, but a poor specificity and positive predictive value. Carrera et al. [9] reported a trend toward decreased CO_2 reactivity assessed with TCD after SAH in patients who later evolved with DIND, where normalization of CVR was correlated with less likelihood of developing DINDs. A possible explanation for the discrepancy between our results and previous series is the fact that our study used a single measurement of CVR while the patients had no radiological evidence of vasospasm, while Frontera et al. [5] and Carrera et al. [9] performed repeated measurements at different days during hospital stay. Up to 75 % of patients with aSAH will have angiographic vasospasm at some point in their hospital stay [10] and changes in CVR demonstrated during the period patients are at risk could be a reflection of progressive narrowing of the large vessels in the Circle of Willis, leading to distal vasodilation and consequent impaired CVR. Without radiological documentation of the absence of vasospasm, clinical grade only is not an indication that the actual vessel diameter remains constant.

Study Limitations

Studies showing impaired CVR to CO_2 after SAH have already been published, although using different techniques and populations (intraoperative measurements, late or during vasospasm assessment). We performed only one measurement for each patient, which can be a source of error or provide incomplete information regarding the overall picture, especially in a dynamic situation such as CBF changes and care after SAH. However, daily measures would require concomitant imaging to exclude vasospasm, and this is not practical in a clinical setting. Additionally, measurements during the vasospasm window would not answer our question regarding the ability of CVR to predict the future development of vasospasm. We think that if CVR is to be called "a good predictor" for DIND or vasospasm, it should be measured before any evidence of angiographic vessel narrowing is present.

Conclusions

In this small patient population, our findings demonstrate that impaired CVR in the early phase of SAH in good clinical grade patients does not predict vasospasm. We also demonstrated the feasibility of a new method of investigating changes in CVR to CO_2 after SAH with controllable and reproducible stimuli.

Conflict of Interest Statement Joseph Fisher is senior scientist and Director of Thornhill Research, company that invented and produces the Respiract™.

References

1. Charpentier C, Audibert G, Guillemin F, Civit T, Ducrocq X, Bracard S, Hepner H, Picard L, Laxenaire MC (1999) Multivariate analysis of predictors of cerebral vasospasm occurrence after aneurysmal subarachnoid hemorrhage. Stroke 30(7):1402–1408
2. Aaslid R, Huber P, Nornes H (1984) Evaluation of cerebrovascular spasm with transcranial Doppler ultrasound. J Neurosurg 60(1):37–41
3. Creissard P, Proust F, Langlois O (1995) Vasospasm diagnosis: theoretical and real transcranial Doppler sensitivity. Acta Neurochir (Wein) 136(3–4):181–185
4. Schmieder K, Jarus-Dziedzic K, Wronski J, Harders A (1997) CO_2 reactivity in patients after subarachnoid haemorrhage. Acta Neurochir (Wien) 139(11):1038–1041
5. Frontera JA, Rundek T, Schmidt JM, Claassen J, Parra A, Wartenberg KE, Temes RE, Mayes RA, Mohr JP, Marshall RS (2006) Cerebrovascular reactivity and vasospasm after subarachnoid hemorrhage: a pilot study. Neurology 66(5):727–729
6. Sloan MA, Alexandrov AV, Tegeler CH, Spencer MP, Caplan LR, Feldmann E, Wechsler LR, Newel DW, Gomez CR, Babikian VL, Lefkowitz D, Goldman RS, Armon C, Hsu CY, Goodin DS (2004) Assessment: transcranial Doppler ultrasonography: report of the Therapeutics and Technology Assessment Subcommittee of the American Academy of Neurology. Neurology 62(9): 1468–1481
7. Slessarev M, Han J, Mardimae A, Prisman E, Preiss D, Volgyesi G et al (2007) Prospective targeting and control of end-tidal CO_2 and O_2 concentrations. J Physiol 581(Pt 3):1207–1219
8. Marshall RS, Rundek T, Sproule DM, Fitzsimmons BF, Schwartz S, Lazar RM (2003) Monitoring of cerebral vasodilatory capacity with transcranial Doppler carbon dioxide inhalation in patients with severe carotid artery disease. Stroke 34(4):945–949
9. Carrera E, Kurtz P, Badjatia N, Fernandez L, Claassen J, Lee K, Schmidt JM, Connolly ES, Marshall RS, Mayer SA (2010) Cerebrovascular carbon dioxide reactivity and delayed cerebral ischemia after subarachnoid hemorrhage. Arch Neurol 67(4): 434–439
10. Fletcher TM, Taveras JM, Pool JL (1959) Cerebral vasospasm in angiography for intracranial aneurysms. Incidence and significance in one hundred consecutive angiograms. Arch Neurol 1: 38–47

Application of Lumbar Drainage in Vasospasm After Spontaneous Subarachnoid Hemorrhage and Prevention of Late Cerebral Infarction

Hasan Emre Aydin, Zühtü Özbek, Nevin Aydin, Özge Bolluk, Murat Vural, Ali Arslantas, and Metin Ant Atasoy

Abstract Cerebral vasospasm, especially delayed cerebral ischemia following subarachnoid hemorrhage (SAH) is the most important complication that effects mortality and morbidity of patients with intracranial aneurysms. The presence of cerebral vasospasm has been correlated with an increase in mortality in the first 2 weeks after SAH. Despite clinical studies and research, the etiopathogenesis of cerebral vasospasm is not understood exactly and there is not yet an effective therapy. The aim of our study was to investigate the effect of application of lumber drainage on vasospasm and delayed cerebral infarction following SAH and to examine the incidence of complications. Patient groups were determined by retrospective screening of 70 patients who underwent a surgical operation at the Osmangazi University Medical Faculty Department of Neurosurgery between 2009 and 2013 after a diagnosis of ruptured aneurysmal SAH. After the application of lumbar drainage, the complications and mortality after aneurysm surgery was significantly decreased and correlated with the amount of hemorrhagic cerebrospinal fluid drainage.

Keywords Aneurysm surgery • Lumbar drainage • Subarachnoid hemorrhage • Vasospasm

H.E. Aydin (✉) • Z. Özbek • M. Vural
A. Arslantas • M.A. Atasoy
Department of Neurosurgery, Osmangazi University, Medical Faculty, Eskisehir 26480, Turkey
e-mail: dremreaydin@gmail.com

N. Aydin
Department of Radiology, Osmangazi University, Medical Faculty, Eskisehir 26480, Turkey

Ö. Bolluk
Department of Biostatic, Osmangazi University, Medical Faculty, Eskisehir 26480, Turkey

Introduction

Subarachnoid hemorrhage (SAH) is associated with high mortality and morbidity. In the etiology of SAH, trauma and ruptured intracranial aneurysms are the most common causes. Although the incidence varies between countries, the estimated average SAH rate is 6–7 in a population of 100,000, and 10–15 % of these patients die before medical intervention [11–13, 20]. Aneurysmal SAH incidence increases depending on age [3, 18, 22]. The average peak age range for aneurysmal SAH is 55–60 years, and it is 1.6 times more common in women than men [3, 11, 14]. Despite effective surgical treatment, 7 % of these patients die because of vasospasm [4, 9, 12, 24]. Aneurysms are often the result of high blood pressure, hyperlipidemia, smoking, genetic factors, and weakness in the blood vessel walls as a result of biomechanical stress [3, 5, 14].

Patients are usually admitted to the hospital with sudden onset of severe headache and neck stiffness [20]. Cranial computed tomography (CT) scan and lumbar puncture (LP) are the diagnostic procedures of SAH. CT has to be performed first to exclude the existence of intracerebral hematoma to prevent the risk of herniation before LP. If the diagnosis of SAH in CT results is unclear, LP must be performed. Despite the sensitivity of CT approaches, more than 95 %, for a definitive diagnosis, digital subtraction angiography (DSA) must be performed in SAH patients [12].

Vasospasm following SAH is divided into two types, clinical and radiological vasospasm [8]. Clinically, vasospasm is the late period of focal ischemic neurological deficit after SAH. Severe headache, decrease in consciousness, low-grade fever, and focal neurological deficits are the clinical symptoms of vasospasm. Radiological vasospasm is arterial contraction, as shown in cerebral angiography. Contraction occurs secondary to structural spasm of smooth muscle [25].

J. Fandino et al. (eds.), *Neurovascular Events After Subarachnoid Hemorrhage*, Acta Neurochirurgica Supplement, Vol. 120,
DOI 10.1007/978-3-319-04981-6_43,

Material and Methods

Clinical Ethics Committee approval of Osmangazi University Medical Faculty for nonpharmacological trials was obtained for the study. Seventy patients who were treated with aneurysm clipping between 2009 and 2013 at the Osmangazi University Medical Faculty Department of Neurosurgery with the diagnosis of ruptured aneurysmal SAH were evaluated by retrospective screening.

The Sigmastat 3.5 and SPSS 13.0 package program was used for statistical analysis of the data. The chi-square test was used to compare discontinuous variables such as staging among the groups. $P<0.05$ was considered as statistically significant. CT images were taken through the PACS (Picture Archiving and Communicating System) to provide standardization, and 5-mm sections were obtained from the skull base up to the vertex. SAH volume was measured in the interhemispheric fissure, bilateral sylvian fissures, suprasellar cistern, bilateral basal sylvian cisterns, and interpedicular and ambient cisterns [16].

A lumbar drainage catheter was placed for all patients in the operation room before surgery. Aneurysm clipping was performed with Sugita clips. Routinely, CT scans of the patients were obtained at the time of admission and after the surgery. The Glasgow Coma Scale (GCS) was used for clinical follow-up after surgery. During daily follow-up, if cerebrospinal fluid (CSF) was clear, drainage was not performed, however, if it was hemorrhagic, approximately 200 cc/day of CSF was drained until the day that the fluid became completely clear. Lumbar drainage was terminated on the 7th day after surgery.

The patients were divided into three groups. In the first group of patients, vasospasm did not develop during their stay in hospital. In the second group, vasospasm developed and the patients showed clinical benefit after treatment. In the third group, vasospasm developed and the patients did not respond to treatment.

The aim of this study was to determine the effectiveness of CSF removal by lumbar drainage on the development and treatment of clinical vasospasm in aneurysmal SAH patients.

Results

Clinical outcomes of 70 patients who underwent aneurysm clipping with aneurysmal SAH are presented. We evaluated the relation between SAH volumes measured on the initial CT scan and development of postoperative vasospasm despite effective vasospasm treatment. The average age of the patients was 59 years. The male to female ratio was 2:3. When evaluated according to Fisher and Hunt Hess grade, in accordance with the literature, mortality was significantly higher in patients with a high grade at admission (Fig. 1).

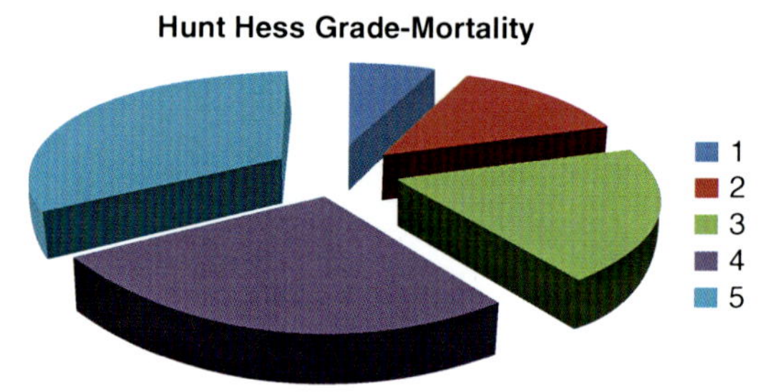

Fig. 1 Hunt and Hess grade at hospital admission and related mortality

The patients were divided into three groups. In the first group, vasospasm did not develop during the patient's stay in the hospital. In the second group, clinical vasospasm developed after surgery. In the early postoperative days, the CSF was hemorrhagic in these patients. After daily drainage (maximum 200 cc), the color of the CSF turned clear. The patients of the second group showed clinical benefits but there was no significant difference in mortality and morbidity when compared with the first group. The clinical improvement of the patients in group 2 may be interpreted as the effect of CSF drainage by removing the blood and blood products and cleaning the subarachnoid space. In the third group, clinical vasospasm developed after surgery and did not respond to medical and CSF drainage treatment. On daily drainage, CSF was permanently hemorrhagic and never became clear. In this group, patients developed permanent neurologic deficits. These poor neurologic consequences may be attributed to blood and blood products that cannot be removed from subarachnoid space by lumbar drainage. The mortality and the morbidity of the patients in group 3 were significantly higher when compared with group 1 (Table 1) (Fig. 2). Common complications such as hydrocephalus and increased intracranial pressure in patients with CSF drainage occurred less frequently in both groups when compared with literature values.

Discussion

There is currently an ongoing controversy regarding the diagnosis of vasospasm and SAH volume on initial CT scan. Although some studies show an increase in vasospasm based on initial CT scans because of SAH volume, others detect no significant difference [12, 16]. The amount of blood in the cisterns and fissures is known as an important risk factor in vasospasm [6, 9, 19, 23]. Although the Hunt and Hess classification and Glasgow Coma Scale are used for clinical staging, the Fisher Scale is used to determine the relationship between the amount of blood on CT scan and risk of vasospasm [10, 15]. The main determinant for the survey after SAH is the Fisher grade on the initial CT scan [13]. Severe neurologic status within the first 24 h after bleeding, old age, and the size of aneurysm are determining factors of mortality and morbidity after SAH. Early surgery is necessary to prevent rebleeding.

Table 1 CSF drainage and mortality

Lumbar drainage	Exitus, *n* (%)	Discharge, *n* (%)	Total (*n*)	Statistical count
Hemorrhagic	24 (80.0)	6 (20.0)	30	X^2: 28.82
Clear	3 (10.3)	26 (89.7)	29	*p*: 0.000

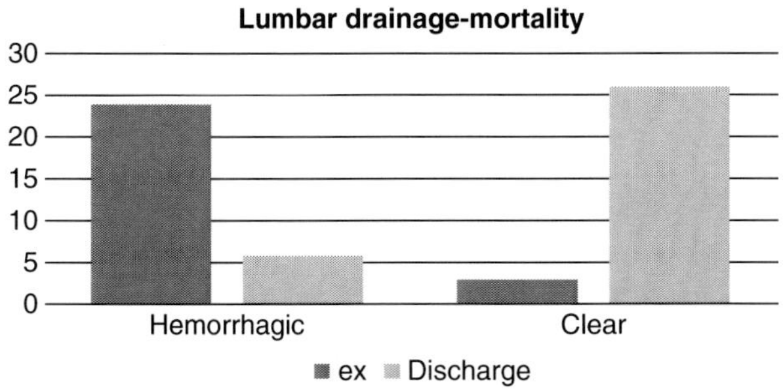

Fig. 2 Relationship between hemorrhagic cerebrospinal fluid and mortality

Vasospasm effects can be reduced by compensating for hypovolemia and severe anemia with hydration and blood transfusion in the postoperative period. Hypertensive therapy and calcium channel blockers may be particularly useful. Blood and blood products within the subarachnoid space play an important role in the development of cerebral vasospasm, which can be prevented by removing degrading products from the space via lumbar drainage [1, 6, 7, 9, 19]. Additionally, CSF drainage reduces the intracranial pressure and development of hydrocephalus, and a permanent shunt may be not necessary [21].

In the half of the cases, vasospasm appears as a delayed ischemic neurological deficit. These patients can be divided into two groups. In half, there is spontaneous resolution, and the remaining progress to cerebral infarction. In recent series, it has been reported that 15–20 % of these patients remain plegic or die despite all treatment options. Because symptomatic vasospasm causing delayed infarction may not present obvious symptoms in comatose patients, the smallest change in neurological examination should be approached with suspicion in this group of patients [11].

In a study of clinical and radiological vasospasm among a cohort of 921 patients, 17 % of patients had symptomatic vasospasm and 28 % had radiological vasospasm [8, 24]. Radiological vasospasm can be detected nearly 70 % of the SAH cases in DSA in the first week and only one-third of the cases were symptomatic that were proven in DSA [17].

Conclusion

In conclusion, 1-week follow-up with application of lumbar drainage and CSF drainage seems to reduce the risk for SAH complications such as vasospasm. This may reduce the morbidity and mortality of the disease.

Conflict of Interest Statement We declare that we have no conflict of interest

References

1. Al-Tamimi YZ, Bhargava D, Feltbower RG et al (2012) Lumbar drainage of cerebrospinal fluid after aneurysmal subarachnoid hemorrhage: a prospective, randomized controlled trial. Stroke 43(3):677–682
2. Barker FG, Ogilvy CS (1996) Efficacy of prophylactic nimodipine for delayed ischemic deficit after subarachnoid hemorrhage: a metaanalysis. J Neurosurg 84:405–414
3. Bınatlı OA, Ulug E, Ozhan I, Bardakcı S, Ozdamar N (2008) Spontaneous subarachnoid hemorrhage: a retrospective study of 273 cases. J Turk Cerebrovasc Dis 14(2):33–39
4. Cai J, Sun Y, Yuan F, Chen L, He C et al (2012) A novel intravital method to evaluate cerebral vasospasm in rat models of subarachnoid hemorrhage: a study with synchrotron radiation angiography. Plos One. doi:10.1371/journal.pone.0033366
5. Cebral JR, Rachi M (2013) Suggested connections between risk factors of intracranial aneurisms: a review. Ann Biomed Eng 41(7):1366–1383
6. Cook DA (1995) Mechanisms of cerebral vasospasm in subarachnoid hemorrhage. Pharmacol Ther 66:259–284
7. Ecker A, Riemenschenider PA (1951) Arteriographic demonstration of spasm of the intracranial arteries. J Neurosurg 8:660–667
8. Ellis JA, Goldstein H, Meyers PM et al (2013) Post subarachnoid hemorrhage vasospasm in patients with primary headache disorders. Neurocrit Care 18(3):362–367
9. Erdi FM, Guney O, Kiyici A, Esen H (2011) The effects of alpha lipoic acid on cerebral vasospasm following experimental subarachnoid hemorrhage in the rabbit. Turk Neurosurg 21(4):527–533
10. Fisher CM, Kistler JP, Davis JM (1980) Relation of cerebral vasospasm to subarachnoid hemorrhage visualized by computerized tomographic scanning. Neurosurgery 6(1):1–9
11. Gijn VJ, Rinkel GJE (2001) Subarachnoid hemorrhage: diagnosis, causes and management. Brain 124:249–278
12. Greenberg MS (2010) Handbook of neurosurgery. Thieme, New York
13. Guler MT, Kocaeli H, Korfalı E (2009) Subarachnoid hemorrhage: prevalence, risk factors and prognosis. Turk Sci J Neurosurg 2(2):9–14
14. Hidetoshi M, Uemura A, Fujii M et al (2013) Morphological and clinical risk factors for the rupture of anterior communicating artery aneurysms. J Neurosurg 118(5):978–983
15. Hunt WE, Hess RM (1968) Surgical risk as related to time of intervention in the repair of intracranial aneurysms. J Neurosurg 28:14–20
16. Jung SW, Lee CY, Man BY (2012) The relationship between subarachnoid hemorrhage volume and development of cerebral vasospasm. J Cerebrovasc Endovasc Neurosurg 14(3):186–191
17. Kassel NF, Sasaki T, Colohan ART (1985) Cerebral vasospasm following aneurysmal subarachnoid hemorrhage. Stroke 16: 562–572
18. Kaura V, Bonner S (2012) Subarachnoid hemorrhage: early clinical indicators and biomarkers. Trends Anaesth Crit Care 2:42–47
19. Khurana VG, Besser M (1997) Pathophysiological basis of cerebral vasospasm following aneurysmal subarachnoid hemorrhage. J Clin Neurosci 4(2):122–131

20. Korfali E, Zileli M (2010) Basic neurosurgery. Bulus, Ankara
21. Ormond DR, Dressler A, Kim S et al (2013) Lumbar drains may reduce the need for permanent CSF diversion in spontaneous subarachnoid haemorrhage. Br J Neurosurg 27(2):171–174
22. Ozdemir M, Bozkurt M, Kahilogulları G, Ugur HC, Egemen N (2011) Management of subarachnoid hemorrhage and complications: review. J Ankara Univ Med Faculty 64(1):52–55
23. Pluta MR, Jacob HS, Dreier J et al (2009) Cerebral vasospasm following subarachnoid hemorrhage: time for a new world of thought. Neurol Res 31(2):151–158
24. Siasios I, Kapsalaki EZ, Fountas KN (2013) Cerebral vasospasm pharmacological treatment: an update. Neurol Res Int. doi:10.1155/2013/571328
25. Wilkins RH (1988) Cerebral vasospasm. Contemp Neurosurg 10:18–21

Redefining Secondary Injury After Subarachnoid Hemorrhage in Light of Multimodal Advanced Neuroimaging, Intracranial and Transcranial Neuromonitoring: *Beyond Vasospasm*

Gregory Kapinos

Abstract The classic idea that arterial narrowing, called vasospasm (VSP), represents the hallmark of secondary injury after subarachnoid hemorrhage, has been challenged. The more complex and pleiotropic pathophysiological repercussions from the irruption of arterial blood into the subarachnoid layers go beyond the ascribed VSP. Putting adjectives in front of this term, such as "symptomatic," "microdialytic," or "angiographic" VSP, is misleading. Delayed cerebral ischemia (DCI) is a better term but remains restrictive to severe hypoperfusive injury and neglects oligemia, edema, and metabolic nonischemic injuries. In recognition of these issues, the international conference on VSP integrated "neurovascular events" into its name (www.vasospasm2013.com) and a multidisciplinary research group was formed in 2010 to study subgroups of DCI/VSP and their respective significance.

In three parts, this tiered article provides a broader definitional envelope for DCI and secondary neurovascular insults after SAH, with a rubric for each subtype of delayed neuronal dysfunction. First, it pinpoints the need for nosologic precision and covers current terminological inconsistency. Then, it highlights the input of neuroimaging and neuromonitoring in defining secondary injurious processes. Finally, a new categorization of deteriorating patients is proposed, going beyond a hierarchical or dichotomized definition of VSP/DCI, and common data elements are suggested for future trials.

Keywords Delayed cerebral ischemia • Blood-brain barrier permeability • Cerebral edema • Delayed ischemic neurologic deficit • Cerebral infarction • Perfusion • Vasoreactivity • Cerebral microdialysis • Cerebral oximetry • Electroencephalogram

G. Kapinos, MD, MS
Department of Neurosurgery, North Shore-LIJ Health System, 300 Community Drive, Tower, 9th floor, Manhasset, NY 11030, USA
e-mail: kapigreg@gmail.com

Preamble

In the world of aneurysmal subarachnoid hemorrhage (SAH),"looking beyond vasospasm" (VSP) [26] pertains not only to researchers on their secondary injury etiopathogenetic quest, but is also very relevant to clinicians because different definitions of VSP and delayed cerebral ischemia (DCI) are portentous of different prognostic significance [21, 71, 72] and carry different therapeutic implications [10]. A paradigm shift [9, 26, 46] surged from a clearer understanding of multiple pathophysiological processes occurring both in the acute and subacute phases that are responsible for both the initial and delayed multiform injuries onto the vessels and directly onto the cerebral parenchyma [59].

Part I: Common Data Elements are Needed for Nosologic Consistency with Each Subtype of Delayed Cerebral Ischemia and Vasospasm After Subarachnoid Hemorrhage

Introduction

The International Multidisciplinary Research Group aiming at defining DCI after SAH [71, 72] advocated for a separation of DCI from VSP after SAH [20, 72]. Nevertheless, recent randomized clinical trials (RCT) still mention VSP as the gold standard by catheter-guided digital subtraction angiography (DSA) or as a composite endpoint along with clinicoradiologic ischemic findings. They use different criteria to define deterioration; delayed ischemic neurologic deficit (DIND); permanent neurologic deficit (PND); symptomatic, sonographic, or angiographic VSP; and delayed infarcts.

DOI 10.1007/978-3-319-04981-6_44,

Methods

Similar to our prior efforts to highlight terminological variance in RCT [34, 35], we systematically reviewed the 38 RCT listed in the American Heart Association (AHA) guidelines for management of SAH [16] to extract the defining criteria and semantics used for endpoints corresponding to each subtype of ischemic or vasospastic events (IVE). IVE were again analyzed through our delineated 14 categories, focusing on the respective definitions in each RCT for clinical deterioration, method to ascribe the latter to an ischemic process or to an arterial narrowing, the persistence in time of the neurological deficit, its response to treatment, the definitions and imaging modality for detection of arterial narrowing (mainly computed tomographic angiography [CTA], transcranial doppler [TCD], or DSA) and of delayed infarctions (mainly CT and magnetic resonance imaging [MRI]), differential diagnoses for other injuries with etiological allocation, presence or absence of a method accounting for perfusion defects, and neurocognitive alterations.

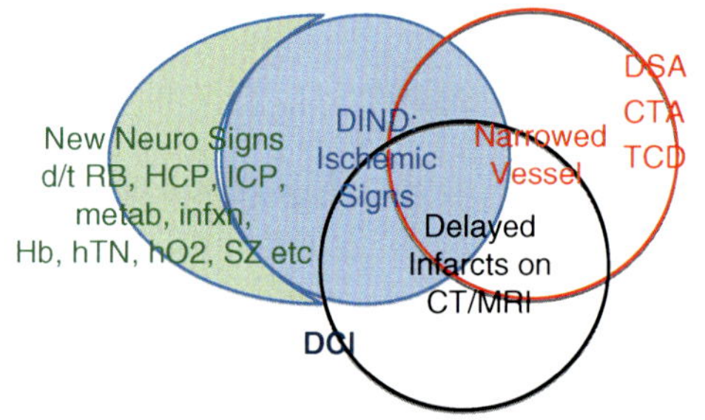

Fig. 1 Diagram depicting groups of SAH patients, with poor overlap of delayed ischemic neurologic deficits (*DIND*), vasospasm assessed by CTA, DSA, or TCD, and delayed cerebral ischemia (*DCI*) consisting of clinical ischemia (or DIND) and/or infarctions seen on CT or MRI scans. Classically, deteriorating patients may be considered ischemic if we exclude new neurological signs caused by rebleed (*RB*), hydrocephalus (*HCP*), intracranial pressure (*ICP*) crisis, metabolic or infectious causes, anemia (*Hb*), hypotension (*hTN*), hypoxemia (*hO2*), seizures (*SZ*), etc.

Results

Deterioration is defined in 16 RCT, 10 of which use a coma scale, whereas others prefer neurologic exams, either standardized (motor scores or National Institutes of Health Stroke Scale [NIHSS] in 4 RCT) or not, and some evoke clinical impression (classic deterioration between days 4 and 21 for 4 RCT or multidisciplinary adjudication upon discharge for 1 RCT).

DINDs (21 RCT) always imply neurologic clinical changes with the need to exclude causes other than delayed ischemia, but the list of excluding syndromes (at the least comprising rebleed and hydrocephalus and at the most also mentioning anemia, hypotension, seizures, and metabolic, respiratory, and infectious causes) differ significantly and concomitant processes may occur. Three RCT mention signs prompting hemodynamic optimization separate from DIND. Because DIND is difficult to appreciate in case of coma (one RCT) and the group of patients with DIND is known to poorly overlap with the vasospastic group (Fig. 1) [21, 71], even by the traditional gold standard of DSA, one can articulate that diffusion-weighted imaging (DWI) should be used to truly confirm ischemia [45], or that serial perfusion imaging [41, 76, 78, 81] would better detect clinical and subclinical hypoperfused patients (Fig. 2 and discussion below).

PND (four RCT) is neurologic deficit upon discharge, but "persistent neurologic deficit" (usually meaning DIND lasting >2 h, or, for some others, meaning persistent deficits after hemodynamic augmentation treatment) is not interchangeable for PND. Reversibility to hyperdynamic therapy versus angioplasty is also a relevant nuance (one RCT).

Symptomatic VSP (6 RCT) is misleadingly interchanged for "clinical VSP" (6 RCT). Thirteen RCT refer to actual DIND with (10 RCT) or without excluding other causes of neurologic decline, and 9 RCT mean DIND with or without concomitant evidence of narrowed vessel but ascribed to the latter, and only 3 RCT restrict this term to only DIND with objectivated narrowed vessel. Clinical impression (2 RCT) and hierarchical diagnosis (1 RCT) are oversimplifications of DCI/VSP with the sole goal of dichotomizing patients to measure potential prognostic significance [53], whereas the subgroups are fundamentally different because they depict completely different degrees of cerebral versus vascular injuries (see the discussion below regarding DCI).

Both *sonographic VSP* (13 RCT) and *angiographic VSP* (5 RCT) have poor concordance in thresholds and in severity stratification and are poorly sensitive and specific for DCI, infarcts, or DIND [20, 21, 72].

DCI is still often referred to as probable (clinical) or definite (clinicoradiologic), but this terminology lacks descriptiveness and again, the three subgroups of DCI (clinical, radiologic, or both) are fundamentally different because these different groups of patients are suffering or suffered completely different severities of cerebral and/or vascular injuries. Very misleadingly and varying between RCT, DCI is still sometimes used to refer to the ongoing injurious ischemic process (hypoperfusive injury captured by clinical exam or perfusion imaging) or to the outcome of a completed injury with irreversible lesion (seen on imaging). Capturing ischemia as an ongoing process with mild clinical reversible manifestation cannot mean the same as completed infarctions. Also to the contrary, some infarcts may be clinically silent in good clinical grade awake patients and not portentous

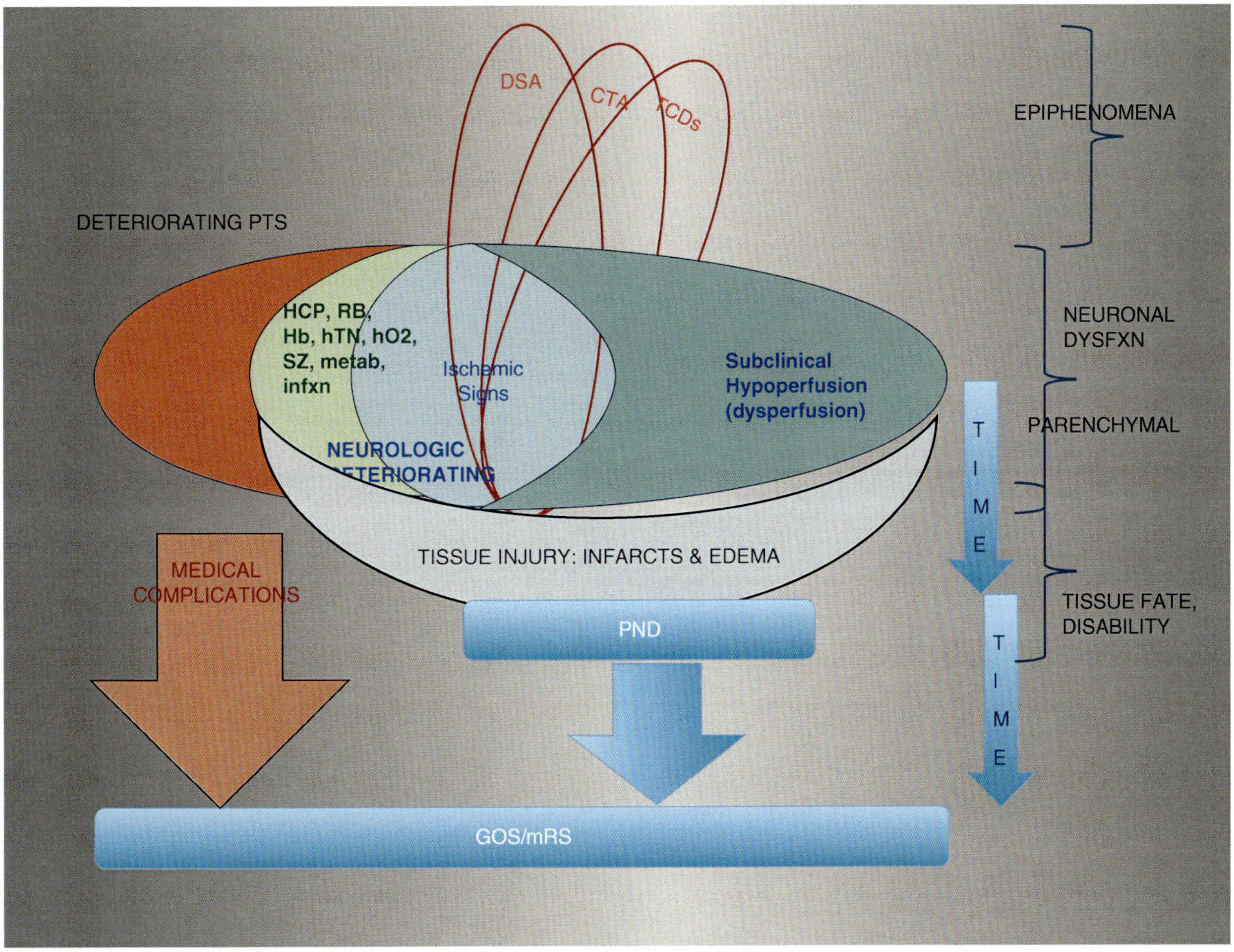

Fig. 2 Diagram depicting the pathophysiology in evolution for certain groups of worsening SAH patients. Some epiphenomena and causal processes can be detected with TCD, CTA, or DSA, or with assessment of autoregulation. However, neuronal dysfunction per se, caused by dysperfusion with ischemia or oligemia (or, on the other hand, with edema from blood-brain barrier opening) is to be measured at the *parenchymal* level while still *ongoing*, without permanent irreversible lesions. Finally, *time* and treatment interventions play a role. DCI, as defined recently (Frontera et al. and Vergouwen et al.) amalgamates ischemic signs on exam with permanent deficits and infarctions, whereas we prefer to keep ischemic and edematous *processes* at one level before the endpoint of *lesion* (tissue injury with completed infarctions or chronic edema). In our figure, we also point out that functional outcome (Glasgow Outcome Scale (*GOS*)) and disability (modified Rankin Scale (*mRS*)) endpoints are also greatly affected by nonpurely neurological processes such as medical complications [15]. Similar to other clinicians using DWI and CTP routinely during deterioration after SAH [10, 18, 45, 53, 70, 79, 81], we propose that perfusion imaging is the new gold standard for detection of delayed hypoperfusive injury/DCI, because subclinical hypoperfusion can be deleterious, and relying on completed infarctions to detect ischemia is dépassé. Using perfusion imaging or quantitative EEG, rather than excluding other causes of neurologic deterioration offers the advantage of eliminating the issue of concomitant processes and of silent deterioration in case of coma

of major disability, whereas small lesions difficult to discern on CT scans may be responsible for major clinical deficits and disability. The amalgamated entity of DCI seems not so judicious after all, even if it is a more relevant endpoint than VSP, with higher prognostic significance [20, 21, 71, 72].

Delayed lucencies have explicit etiologic process in only 7 of the 14 RCT listed in the guidelines. Causal allocation varies from simple adjudication into three groups, to multilevel diagnostic criteria accounting for timing, location, size, number, parent vessel, and timing of clinical correlate, creating 18 types. Ictal (or acute) infarcts [57] are accounted for in only four RCT. Perfusion deficits are analyzed in only four RCT. Only one RCT went beyond a classic neurologic exam at the bedside and measured neurocognitive sequelae.

Conclusion

There is inter-RCT inconsistency in the criteria used for each subgroup of DCI and for the disparate composite endpoint of DCI [35]. Frontera et al. highlighted the clinical relevance of each subtype of DCI/VSP, putting emphasis on clinical and radiological findings being more prognostically relevant than

TCD and DSA findings [21]. This was a major step forward and was embraced and verified by the community [19, 72]. However, we think that each subgroup of DCI (per Vergouwen's definition [72]) is still intrinsically different, mixing processes and outcomes. Furthermore, recent studies scrutinizing perfusion, permeability, and vasoreactivity, as well as electrographic, spectroscopic, and intracortical probing, push the envelope of DCI even further to better delineate each category of delayed neuronal dysfunction with metabolic disarray.

Part II: Avant Garde Neuroimaging and Neuromonitoring Revolutionize Prediction, Diagnosis, and Prognosis of Delayed Cerebral Ischemia After Subarachnoid Hemorrhage

Introduction

RCT use dissimilar criteria to define VSP and DCI after SAH [34].

Methods

We systematically reviewed the last 20 years of English medical literature for the input of multimodal neuroimaging in understanding VSP and DCI after SAH [29, 31]. We hereby did the same to add the input of intracranial and transcranial neuromonitoring, focusing on vasoreactivity, continuous quantitative electroencephalography (EEG), cerebral oximetry (PbtO2 by Licox) flowmetry (CBF probing by Hemedex), and microdialysis (CMD), as well as near-infrared spectroscopy (NIRS). We condensed the recent qualitative and quantitative data suggesting a role for structural, sonographic, angiographic, diffusive, perfusive, dispersive, permeabilitic, and metabolic neuroimaging as well as neuromonitoring in the prediction and detection of VSP and DCI. Compiled evidence is given in the form of questions and answers.

Results

What constitutes acute brain injuries (ABI)?

Noncontrast CT [12, 57], DSA [4, 6, 47], CT perfusion (CTP) [30, 41, 44, 50, 53, 58, 70], MR perfusion (MRP) [76], DWI [24, 27, 56, 61–65, 75, 77], T2 [37], permeability [3], metabolic and spectroscopic data [25, 52, 80] colocalizing with microdialytic data [54], all together suggest cerebral ischemia/oxidative distress caused by global severe hypoperfusion [58], especially in deep watershed territories [48, 76], pial microthrombotic events [43, 51], diffuse blood-brain barrier disruption [3, 69], early global vasogenic edema [2, 3], and, rarely, ultra-early vasospasm [4].

Can we quantify ABI and correlate their severity to neurological presentation and development of DCI and also predict outcome?

Acute noncontrast CT [12, 42, 48, 57], CTP [1, 17, 41, 44, 53, 58, 70, 78, 79], MRP [23, 76, 80], DWI [57, 75–77], and T2 [37] can quantify the injury, classify patterns of infarcts [42, 48] and edema [12], and correlate with survival rates. Two Japanese studies in poor clinical grade patients use DWI to refuse aneurysmal obliteration to severely infarcted elderly patients [61–64].

Can perfusion imaging in the acute and subacute phase detect VSP/DCI earlier than clinical exam and even predict DCI?

Delayed infarcts can be predicted by the following thresholds: mean transit time (MTT) >7 s or cerebral blood flow (CBF) <34 mL/100 g/min or cerebral blood volume (CBV)<3 mL/100 g [41] or time-to-peak (TTP) interhemispheric difference (IHD) >1.0 s [44]. Early acute perfusion imaging can predict DCI with the following thresholds: CBV <1.7 [53] or CBV interhemispheric ratio (IHR) <0.77 [70] or CBF <25 [53] or CBF IHR <0.72 [70] or MTT >5.5 s [53] or MTT IHD >0.87 s or TTP IHD >1.0 s [70].

Does the magnitude of perfusion defects correlate with the severity of angiographic VSP and impending infarction?

Perfusive defects substantiate ongoing ischemia as cause of deterioration with the following diagnostic thresholds: MTT>5.9 s [18, 19] or 6.4 s [78] or MTT IHD >1.1 s [18, 19]. Perfusive defects substantiate significant ischemia mandating resorting to endovascular treatment with the following thresholds: MTT >7.6 s or CBF<39. [79, 81]

What other advanced neuroimaging and neuromonitoring techniques are studied in DCI?

Diffusion [45, 76] and perfusion [7, 10, 39, 68], and also flow heterogeneity with relative dispersion [40] and bedside spectroscopy [60] all hold promise for prediction of neurologic worsening, refining categorization of DCI with therapeutic repercussions [5, 19, 28, 38].

Loss of cerebrovascular reactivity [8] can also be detected by TCD and seems to precede DIND [22, 36] and DCI [11]. As a correlate, relative dispersion can be measured and seems to portent poorer outcome [40]. Cerebroximetric probing measures brain parenchymal oxygen tension, with low values being associated with poorer outcomes [49]. Transcranially in the bitemporal regions,

NIRS can measure the cortical parenchymal amount of oxyhemoglobin, reflecting the adequacy of CBF variations. Declining values have been correlated with ischemic events and NIRS is used by some clinicians to detect DCI after SAH [8, 60].

CMD alerts clinicians to commencing metabolic distress [2], whether from ischemia, edema, or inflammation. Its sensitive detection of relative imbalance in energetic supply/demand/use has been shown to have diagnostic value during the acute and subacute phases after SAH [60, 66]. Patterns of ABI on CMD differ from those of DCI [54]. Microdialytic ischemic patterns have very good positive predictive values for both DIND and delayed infarctions [66]. Bridging CMD to clinical and neuroimaging correlates, colocalization has even been demonstrated between regions of interest with relative metabolic disarray on CMD (but without ischemia per CBF thresholds) and both relative hypoxia per positron imaging and clinical deficits in patients with DIND [55]. This corroborates earlier findings leading one to think that not all DIND patients suffer from ischemia per se; a few may experience some type of nonischemic metabolic distress, echoing the metabolic penumbra paradigm in TBI and ICH [73].

EEG: The gradual diminishment of regional cortical neuronal function (caused by ischemia, edema, inflammation, or oxidative disarray from any cause) can be detected by loss of fast frequencies and increases in slow frequencies by continuous EEG, even before visible clinical impairment. Scalp EEG seems to suffice to detect ischemic patterns with quantitative measurements such as the relative alpha variability (RAV) and alpha/delta ratio (ADR). Indeed, early detection of DCI can be performed by detecting a decrease in RAV [74] and, more recently, a drop in ADR was shown to precede DIND and infarcts after SAH by many hours [14]. Intracortical EEG, even with a single probe placed in a bundle with CMD and PbtO2, can also reveal any depreciation in neuronal function through an attenuation in electric regional power, with a significant drop in ADR a few days before documented vasospasm in ischemic SAH patients [67].

Finally, EEG is not only helpful in SAH for detecting seizures and early ischemic changes, but the presence of periodic epileptiform discharges and the absence of normal reactivity, variability, and sleep architecture are also dramatically correlated to a poorer outcome [13].

Conclusions

Robust neuroimaging data and preliminary but consistent, salient, and appealing electrographic and neuromonitoring data offer new support for diagnostic and prognostic refinements in SAH. Neurosurgeons and neurointensivists ought to become keen neurophysiologists acquainted with these new techniques and nuanced pathophysiological processes devastating their patients. Some of these modalities are already used by some groups to manage complex SAH patients [5, 8, 10, 11, 17, 28, 81]. Given the disconcerting negative results in many recent large RCT in SAH with traditional DCI/VSP definitions and endpoints, it is a necessity for our neurosurgical critical care community to devise surrogate endpoints for upcoming trials, integrating some advanced electrographic, neuroimaging, and transcranial and intracranial neuromonitoring parameters to finely depict the heterogeneity and complexity of all subgroups of deteriorating patients. Some of these parameters will surely be integrated in the common data elements efforts of the NIH and other consortiums (such as IMPACT) caring for all types of severe brain injuries [33].

Part III: Progressive Nosology for Delayed Neurovascular Insults After Aneurysmal Subarachnoid Hemorrhage

Objectives

We propose a novel classification of secondary injuries after aneurysmal SAH with better nosological terminology based on best descriptiveness of the objective clinical impairment, probed physiological disturbance, or imaged abnormality [32].

Background

We previously highlighted the terminological inconsistencies in the 38 RCT listed in the 2009 guidelines from the AHA for management of aSAH. There remains intra- and inter-RCT inconsistency in the terminology and specific criteria used for each category of DCI and VSP, even in the 2011 Neurocritical Care Society [71] and 2012 AHA guidelines [16].

Methods

Etymologic precision and rigorous adherence to purely objective description of the impairment on exam and/or abnormality documented by EEG, neuroimaging, or cerebral probing guided our new nomenclature, inspired from the RCT listed in the recent guidelines.

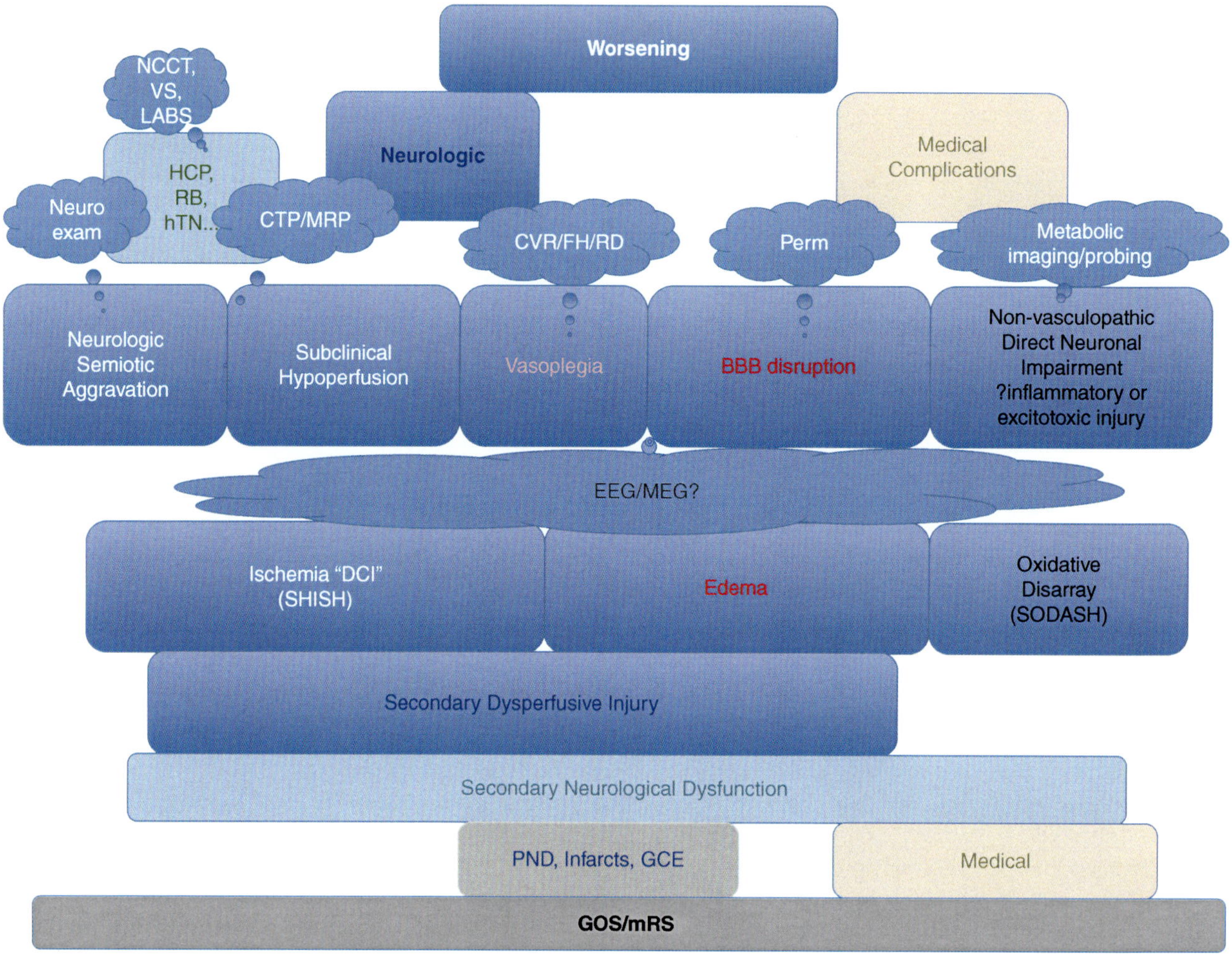

Fig. 3 Noncontrast CT (*NCCT*), vital signs (*VS*), and laboratory results allow clinicians to find obvious other causes for deterioration. Ischemic patients on clinical exam (semiotic neurological aggravation) can be aggregated with subclinical hypoperfused patients and captured all together by perfusion imaging. We suggest secondary hypoperfusive injury after SAH (*SHISH*) as a better term than *ischemia* because hypoperfusion may not always lead to overt infarction, even if sustained after SAH, as opposed to acute ischemic stroke models. Perfusion imaging also offers the possibility of measuring excessive perfusion and leakiness of the blood-brain barrier (*BBB*), because some patients suffer from global cerebral edema and can benefit from radically different treatment options than the classic first-line therapy consisting of hemodynamic augmentation. We also propose a distinct group for patients with metabolic derangement leading to neuronal dysfunction without any perfusive abnormality (secondary oxidative disarray after SAH (*SODASH*)). This group of nonvasculopathic patients may benefit the most from neuroprotective agents. Finally, cerebral infarctions and chronic edema are at a different level of endpoints. This *tissue* or *lesional* level integrates time and interventions, on the path down toward the ultimate functional endpoints, materialized into the GOS and mRS, which are affected also by medical factors

Results

Abandoned terms are Symptomatic VSP, Clinical VSP, DCI (probable and definite), TCD VSP, Microdialytic and EEG VSP, Ictal Infarctions, and Surgery-Related Infarctions. Remaining terms are Deterioration, DIND, Persistent Neurologic Deficit, PND, Rebleed, Hydrocephalus, Angiographic VSP, Ischemic Lesion, Perfusion Defects, Delayed Infarctions, and Retraction Injury. Proposed new terms are Semiotic as a nuance to Symptomatic, Aggravation as a nuance to Deterioration, Secondary replaces Delayed, Hypoperfusion and Relative Dispersion (RD) are nuances to Ischemia, Vasculopathy is a nuance to VSP, Hyperveloce State replaces Sonographic VSP, Loss of Flow Heterogeneity (FH) adds to Loss of Cerebral Autoregulation (or CVR), and Early Cerebral Infarctions replaces Ictal Infarcts. More importantly, hypoperfusion, edema, and oxidative disarray finally capture the entire spectrum of secondary neurologic dysfunction. Hypoperfusion and metabolic derangement now account for the ongoing injurious process, rather than relying on completed infarctions to detect ischemia [32]. Indeed, one should conceive of the evolution of post-SAH injurious processes leading to secondary injury and lesions on at least three levels (Fig. 2). Figure 3 summarizes the gross categories of patients with the specific modality to be used to detect the injurious process of each subgroup.

Conclusion

Finer clinical exam, TCD with pulsatility index and vasoreactivity, CMD, interstitial cerebroximetry (PbtO2) and interstitial flowmetry (CBF), NIRS, cortical and surface EEG, as well as multimodal imaging with diffusion, perfusion, relative dispersion, permeability, flow heterogeneity, positron emission, and spectroscopy shine some light onto injurious processes and hold promise for earlier detection of all types of secondary injury after SAH. Umbrella terms such as VSP and aggregated rubrics such as DCI ought to be abandoned, whereas precise terminology can describe the exact abnormality for each subtype of worsening patients. It is of utmost importance to recognize these subgroups, because of therapeutic implications. Focal versus global ischemia may not be addressed by the same therapeutic tools; edematous or intracranial hypertensive patients may not benefit from regular ischemia-targeting treatment options; loss of autoregulation and its localization might be a separate entity for a special armamentarium; and, finally, neuroprotective agents may be better suited as unique tools for the patients with no vascular impairment but with parenchymal metabolic derangement. Tailored individualized therapies may be guided by a more rigorous understanding of the specific injurious process by subgroup. A bigger impact from novel therapies may now be detectable if we use correct surrogate endpoints rather than applying global broad-spectrum multifaceted therapies and looking at an amalgamated composite endpoint of "DCI/VSP."

Conflict of Interest Statement Dr. Kapinos declares that he has no conflict of interest. The articulated interpretations in this article represent solely his personal views.

References

1. Aralasmak A, Akyuz M, Ozkaynak C, Sindel T, Tuncer R (2009) CT angiography and perfusion imaging in patients with subarachnoid hemorrhage: correlation of vasospasm to perfusion abnormality. Neuroradiology 51:85–93
2. Asgari S, Vespa P, Hu X (2013) Is there any association between cerebral vasoconstriction/vasodilatation and microdialysis lactate to pyruvate ratio increase? Neurocrit Care 19:56–64
3. Baik SK, Kim YS, Lee HJ, Park J, Kim GC (2008) Immediate CT findings following embolization of cerebral aneurysms: suggestion of blood-brain barrier or vascular permeability change. Neuroradiology 50:259–266
4. Baldwin ME, Macdonald RL, Huo D, Novakovic RL, Goldenberg FD, Frank JI, Rosengart AJ (2004) Early vasospasm on admission angiography in patients with aneurysmal subarachnoid hemorrhage is a predictor for in-hospital complications and poor outcome. Stroke 35:2506–2511
5. Beck J, Raabe A, Lanfermann H, Berkefeld J, De Rochemont RM, Zanella F, Seifert V, Weidauer S (2006) Effects of balloon angioplasty on perfusion- and diffusion- weighted magnetic resonance imaging results and outcome in patients with cerebral vasospasm. J Neurosurg 105:220–227
6. Bederson JB, Levy AL, Ding WH, Kahn R, DiPerna CA, Jenkins AL 3rd, Vallabhajosyula P (1998) Acute vasoconstriction after subarachnoid hemorrhage. Neurosurgery 42:352–360
7. Binaghi S, Colleoni ML, Maeder P, Uské A, Regli L, Dehdashti AR, Schnyder P, Meuli R (2007) CT angiography and perfusion CT in cerebral vasospasm after subarachnoid hemorrhage. Am J Neuroradiol 28:750–758
8. Budohoski KP, Czosnyka M, Kirkpatrick PJ, Smielewski P, Steiner LA, Pickard JD (2013) Clinical relevance of cerebral autoregulation following subarachnoid haemorrhage. Nat Rev Neurol 9:152–163
9. Cahill J, Zhang JH (2009) Subarachnoid hemorrhage: is it time for a new direction? Stroke 40:S86–S87
10. Carlson AP, Yonas H (2009) Radiographic assessment of vasospasm after aneurismal subarachnoid hemorrhage: the physiological perspective. Neurol Res 31:593–604
11. Carrera E, Kurtz P, Badjatia N, Fernandez L, Claassen J, Lee K, Schmidt JM, Connolly ES, Marshall RS, Mayer SA (2010) Cerebrovascular carbon dioxide reactivity and delayed cerebral ischemia after subarachnoid hemorrhage. Arch Neurol 67:434–439
12. Claassen J, Carhuapoma JR, Kreiter KT, Du EY, Connolly ES, Mayer SA (2002) Global cerebral edema after subarachnoid hemorrhage: frequency, predictors, and impact on outcome. Stroke 33:1225–1232
13. Claassen J, Hirsch LJ, Frontera JA, Fernandez A, Schmidt M, Kapinos G, Wittman J, Connolly ES, Emerson RG, Mayer SA (2006) Prognostic significance of continuous EEG monitoring in poor-grade subarachnoid hemorrhage patients. Neurocrit Care 4:103–112
14. Claassen J, Hirsch LJ, Kreiter KT, Du EY, Connolly ES, Emerson RG, Mayer SA (2004) Quantitative continuous EEG for detecting delayed cerebral ischemia in patients with poor-grade subarachnoid hemorrhage. Clin Neurophysiol 115:2699–2710
15. Claassen J, Vu A, Kreiter KT, Kowalski RG, Du EY, Ostapkovich N, Fitzsimmons BF, Connolly ES, Mayer SA (2004) Effect of acute physiologic derangements on outcome after subarachnoid hemorrhage. Crit Care Med 32:832–838
16. Connolly ES Jr, Rabinstein AA, Carhuapoma JR, Derdeyn CP, Dion J, Higashida RT, Hoh BL, Kirkness CJ, Naidech AM, Ogilvy CS, Patel AB, Thompson BG, Vespa P; American Heart Association Stroke Council; Council on Cardiovascular Radiology and Intervention; Council on Cardiovascular Nursing; Council on Cardiovascular Surgery and Anesthesia; Council on Clinical Cardiology (2012) Guidelines for the management of aneurysmal subarachnoid hemorrhage: a guideline for healthcare professionals from the American Heart Association/American Stroke Association. Stroke 43:1711–1737
17. Dankbaar JW, de Rooij NK, Rijsdijk M, Velthuis BK, Frijns CJ, Rinkel GJ, van der Schaaf IC (2010) Diagnostic threshold values of cerebral perfusion measured with computed tomography for delayed cerebral ischemia after aneurysmal subarachnoid hemorrhage. Stroke 41:1927–1932
18. Dankbaar JW, de Rooij NK, Velthuis BK, Frijns CJ, Rinkel GJ, van der Schaaf IC (2009) Diagnosing delayed cerebral ischemia with different CT modalities in patients with subarachnoid hemorrhage with clinical deterioration. Stroke 40:3493–3498
19. Dankbaar JW, Rijsdijk M, van der Schaaf IC, Velthuis BK, Wermer MJ, Rinkel GJ (2009) Relationship between vasospasm, cerebral perfusion, and delayed cerebral ischemia after aneurysmal subarachnoid hemorrhage. Neuroradiology 51:813–819

20. Etminan N, Vergouwen MD, Macdonald RL (2013) Angiographic vasospasm versus cerebral infarction as outcome measures after aneurysmal subarachnoid hemorrhage. Acta Neurochir Suppl 115:33–40
21. Frontera JA, Fernandez A, Schmidt JM, Claassen J, Wartenberg KE, Badjatia N, Connolly ES, Mayer SA (2009) Defining vasospasm after subarachnoid hemorrhage: what is the most clinically relevant definition? Stroke 40:1963–1968
22. Frontera JA, Rundek T, Schmidt JM, Claassen J, Parra A, Wartenberg KE, Temes RE, Mayer SA, Mohr JP, Marshall RS (2006) Cerebrovascular reactivity and vasospasm after subarachnoid hemorrhage: a pilot study. Neurology 66:727–729
23. Griffiths PD, Wilkinson ID, Mitchell P, Patel MC, Paley MN, Romanowski CA, Powell T, Hodgson TJ, Hoggard N, Jellinek D (2001) Multimodality MR imaging depiction of hemodynamic changes and cerebral ischemia in subarachnoid hemorrhage. Am J Neuroradiol 22:1690–1697
24. Hadeishi H, Suzuki A, Yasui N, Hatazawa J, Shimosegawa E (2002) Diffusion-weighted magnetic resonance imaging in patients with subarachnoid hemorrhage. Neurosurgery 50:741–748
25. Handa Y, Kimura H, Arishima H, Ishida M, Ishii H, Kubota T (2001) Changes in neuronal metabolites in brain following subarachnoid haemorrhage evaluated by proton MR spectroscopy. Acta Neurochir Suppl 77:135–138
26. Hansen-Schwartz J, Vajkoczy P, Macdonald RL, Pluta RM, Zhang JH (2007) Cerebral vasospasm: looking beyond vasoconstriction. Trends Pharmacol Sci 28:252–256
27. Hattingen E, Blasel S, Dettmann E, Vatter H, Pilatus U, Seifert V, Zanella FE, Weidauer S (2008) Perfusion-weighted MRI to evaluate cerebral autoregulation in aneurysmal subarachnoid haemorrhage. Neuroradiology 50:929–938
28. Hertel F, Walter C, Bettag M, Mörsdorf M (2005) Perfusion-weighted magnetic resonance imaging in patients with vasospasm: a useful new tool in the management of patients with subarachnoid hemorrhage. Neurosurgery 56:28–35
29. Hoang A, Kapinos G, Sanelli PC (2011) Multimodal Neuroimaging perusal refines diagnostic and prognostic accuracy for delayed cerebral ischemia after subarachnoid hemorrhage. Neurology 76(9)(S4):A315
30. Huang AP, Arora S, Wintermark M, Ko N, Tu YK, Lawton MT (2010) Perfusion computed tomographic imaging and surgical selection with patients after poor-grade aneurysmal subarachnoid hemorrhage. Neurosurgery 67:964–974
31. Kapinos G (2011) Advanced neuroimaging revolutionizes diagnosis and prognosis for delayed cerebral ischemia after subarachnoid hemorrhage. J Neuroimaging 21(1):97–98
32. Kapinos G, Hoang A, Sanelli PC (2011) Novel classification of secondary injuries after aneurysmal subarachnoid hemorrhage. Neurology 76(9)(S4):A148.
33. Kapinos G, Hemphill JC 3rd (2013) Clinicoradiologic acute monitoring after intracerebral hemorrhage: Toward standards? Neurology 81:1–2
34. Kapinos G, Hoang A, Sanelli PC (2011) Terminological variance for each subtype of delayed cerebral ischemia and vasospasm after aneurysmal subarachnoid hemorrhage. Neurosurg Focus 30(2):A25–26
35. Kapinos G, Sanelli PC, Hoang A, Segal AZ, Rosengart AJ, Fink ME (2010) Terminological variance for each subtype of delayed cerebral ischemia and vasospasm after aneurysmal subarachnoid hemorrhage. Crit Care Med 38(12):A322
36. Lam JM, Smielewski P, al-Rawi P, Griffiths P, Yu AL, Pickard JD, Kirkpatrick PJ (2000) Prediction of cerebral ischaemia during carotid endarterectomy with preoperative CO2-reactivity studies and angiography. Br J Neurosurg 14:441–448
37. Liu Y, Soppi V, Mustonen T, Könönen M, Koivisto T, Koskela A, Rinne J, Vanninen RL (2007) Subarachnoid hemorrhage in the subacute stage: elevated apparent diffusion coefficient in normal-appearing brain tissue after treatment. Radiology 242:518–525
38. Majoie CB, van Boven LJ, van de Beek D, Venema HW, van Rooij WJ (2007) Perfusion CT to evaluate the effect of transluminal angioplasty on cerebral perfusion in the treatment of vasospasm after subarachnoid hemorrhage. Neurocrit Care 6:40–44
39. Moftakhar R, Rowley HA, Turk A, Niemann DB, Kienitz BA, Van Gomple J, Başkaya MK (2006) Utility of computed tomography perfusion in detection of cerebral vasospasm in patients with subarachnoid hemorrhage. Neurosurg Focus 21:E6
40. Mustonen T, Koivisto T, Vanninen E, Vanninen R (2006) Kuikka JT (2006) Cerebral perfusion heterogeneity and complexity in patients with acute subarachnoid haemorrhage. Nucl Med Commun 27:157–164
41. Nabavi DG, LeBlanc LM, Baxter B, Lee DH, Fox AJ, Lownie SP, Ferguson GG, Craen RA, Gelb AW, Lee TY (2001) Monitoring cerebral perfusion after subarachnoid hemorrhage using CT. Neuroradiology 43:7–16
42. Naidech AM, Bendok BR, Bassin SL, Bernstein RA, Batjer HH, Bleck TP (2009) Classification of cerebral infarction after subarachnoid hemorrhage impacts outcome. Neurosurgery 64:1052–1057
43. Ohkuma H, Manabe H, Tanaka M, Suzuki S (2000) Impact of cerebral microcirculatory changes on cerebral blood flow during cerebral vasospasm after aneurysmal subarachnoid hemorrhage. Stroke 31:1621–1627
44. Pham M, Johnson A, Bartsch AJ, Lindner C, Müllges W, Roosen K, Solymosi L, Bendszus M (2007) CT perfusion predicts secondary cerebral infarction after aneurysmal subarachnoid hemorrhage. Neurology 69:762–765
45. Phan TG, Huston J 3rd, Campeau NG, Wijdicks EF, Atkinson JL, Fulgham JR (2003) Value of diffusion-weighted imaging in patients with a nonlocalizing examination and vasospasm from subarachnoid hemorrhage. Cerebrovasc Dis 15:177–181
46. Pluta RM, Hansen-Schwartz J, Dreier J, Vajkoczy P, Macdonald RL, Nishizawa S, Kasuya H, Wellman G, Keller E, Zauner A, Dorsch N, Clark J, Ono S, Kiris T, Leroux P, Zhang JH (2009) Cerebral vasospasm following subarachnoid hemorrhage: time for a new world of thought. Neurol Res 31:151–158
47. Qureshi AI, Sung GY, Suri MA, Straw RN, Guterman LR, Hopkins LN (1999) Prognostic value and determinants of ultraearly angiographic vasospasm after aneurysmal subarachnoid hemorrhage. Neurosurgery 44:967–973
48. Rabinstein AA, Weigand S, Atkinson JL, Wijdicks EF (2005) Patterns of cerebral infarction in aneurysmal subarachnoid hemorrhage. Stroke 36:992–997
49. Ramakrishna R, Stiefel M, Udoetuk J, Spiotta A, Levine JM, Kofke WA, Zager E, Yang W, Leroux P (2008) Brain oxygen tension and outcome in patients with aneurysmal subarachnoid hemorrhage. J Neurosurg 109:1075–1082
50. Rijsdijk M, van der Schaaf IC, Velthuis BK, Wermer MJ, Rinkel GJ (2008) Global and focal cerebral perfusion after aneurysmal subarachnoid hemorrhage in relation with delayed cerebral ischemia. Neuroradiology 50:813–820
51. Romano JG, Forteza AM, Concha M, Koch S, Heros RC, Morcos JJ, Babikian VL (2002) Detection of microemboli by transcranial doppler ultrasonography in aneurysmal subarachnoid hemorrhage. Neurosurgery 50:1026–1030
52. Rowe J, Blamire AM, Domingo Z, Moody V, Molyneux A, Byrne J, Cadoux-Hudson T, Radda G (1998) Discrepancies between cerebral perfusion and metabolism after subarachnoid haemorrhage: a magnetic resonance approach. J Neurol Neurosurg Psychiatry 64:98–103
53. Sanelli PC, Jou A, Gold R, Reichman M, Greenberg E, John M, Cayci Z, Ugorec I, Rosengart A (2011) Using CT perfusion during the early baseline period in aneurysmal subarachnoid hemor-

rhage to assess for development of vasospasm. Neuroradiology 53:425–434
54. Sarrafzadeh A, Haux D, Sakowitz O, Benndorf G, Herzog H, Kuechler I, Unterberg A (2003) Acute focal neurological deficits in aneurysmal subarachnoid hemorrhage: relation of clinical course, CT findings, and metabolite abnormalities monitored with bedside microdialysis. Stroke 34:1382–1388
55. Sarrafzadeh AS, Nagel A, Czabanka M, Denecke T, Vajkoczy P, Plotkin M (2010) Imaging of hypoxic-ischemic penumbra with (18)F-fluoromisonidazole PET/CT and measurement of related cerebral metabolism in aneurysmal subarachnoid hemorrhage. J Cereb Blood Flow Metab 30:36–45
56. Sato K, Shimizu H, Fujimura M, Inoue T, Matsumoto Y, Tominaga T (2010) Acute-stage diffusion-weighted magnetic resonance imaging for predicting outcome of poor-grade aneurysmal subarachnoid hemorrhage. Journal of Cerebral Blood Flow & Metabolism 30:1110–1120
57. Schmidt JM, Rincon F, Fernandez A, Resor C, Kowalski RG, Claassen J, Connolly ES, Fitzsimmons BF, Mayer SA (2007) Cerebral infarction associated with acute subarachnoid hemorrhage. Neurocrit Care 7:10–17
58. Schubert GA, Seiz M, Hegewald AA, Manville J, Thomé C (2009) Acute hypoperfusion immediately after subarachnoid hemorrhage: a xenon contrast-enhanced CT study. J Neurotrauma 26:2225–2231
59. Sehba FA, Bederson JB (2006) Mechanisms of acute brain injury after subarachnoid hemorrhage. Neurol Res 28:381–398
60. Seule M, Muroi C, Sikorski C, Keller E (2013) Monitoring of cerebral hemodynamics and oxygenation to detect delayed ischemic neurological deficit after aneurysmal subarachnoid hemorrhage. Acta Neurochir Suppl 115:57–61
61. Shamoto H et al (2007) Management of severe subarachnoid hemorrhage with diffusion-weighted imaging in acute stage. Surg Cereb Stroke (Jpn) 35:276–281
62. Shimizu H et al (2005) Diffusion-weighted imaging in patients with severe subarachnoid hemorrhage (SAH): Relationship with delayed spasm and clinical outcome. Surg Cereb Stroke (Jpn) 33:109–112
63. Shimoda M, Hoshikawa K, Shiramizu H, Oda S, Yoshiyama M, Matsumae M (2010) Clinical implication of subarachnoid clots detected by diffusion-weighted imaging in the acute stage of aneurysm rupture. Neurol Med Chir (Tokyo) 50:192–199
64. Shimoda M, Hoshikawa K, Shiramizu H, Oda S, Yoshiyama M, Osada T, Matsumae M (2010) Early infarction detected by diffusion-weighted imaging in patients with subarachnoid hemorrhage. Acta Neurochir (Wien) 152:1197–1205
65. Shimoda M, Takeuchi M, Tominaga J, Oda S, Kumasaka A, Tsugane R (2001) Asymptomatic versus symptomatic infarct from vasospasm in patients with subarachnoid hemorrhage: Serial magnetic resonance imaging. Neurosurgery 49:1341–1348
66. Skjøth-Rasmussen J, Schulz M, Kristensen SR, Bjerre P (2004) Delayed neurological deficits detected by an ischemic pattern in the extracellular cerebral metabolites in patients with aneurysmal subarachnoid hemorrhage. J Neurosurg 100:8–15
67. Stuart RM, Waziri A, Weintraub D, Schmidt MJ, Fernandez L, Helbok R, Kurtz P, Lee K, Badjatia N, Emerson R, Mayer SA, Connolly ES, Hirsch LJ, Claassen J (2010) Intracortical EEG for the detection of vasospasm in patients with poor-grade subarachnoid hemorrhage. Neurocrit Care 13:355–358
68. Sviri GE, Britz GW, Lewis DH, Newell DW, Zaaroor M, Cohen W (2006) Dynamic perfusion computed tomography in the diagnosis of cerebral vasospasm. Neurosurgery 59:319–325
69. Uchiyama Y, Abe T, Hirohata M, Tanaka N, Kojima K, Nishimura H, Norbash AM, Hayabuchi N (2004) Blood brain-barrier disruption of nonionic iodinated contrast medium following coil embolization of a ruptured intracerebral aneurysm. Am J Neuroradiol 25:1783–1786
70. van der Schaaf I, Wermer MJ, van der Graaf Y, Velthuis BK, van de Kraats CI, Rinkel GJ (2006) Prognostic value of cerebral perfusion-computed tomography in the acute stage after subarachnoid hemorrhage for the development of delayed cerebral ischemia. Stroke 37:409–413
71. Vergouwen MD; Participants in the International Multi-Disciplinary Consensus Conference on the Critical Care Management of Subarachnoid Hemorrhage (2011) Vasospasm versus delayed cerebral ischemia as an outcome event in clinical trials and observational studies. Neurocrit Care 15:308–311
72. Vergouwen MD, Vermeulen M, van Gijn J, Rinkel GJ, Wijdicks EF, Muizelaar JP, Mendelow AD, Juvela S, Yonas H, Terbrugge KG, Macdonald RL, Diringer MN, Broderick JP, Dreier JP, Roos YB (2010) Definition of delayed cerebral ischemia after aneurysmal subarachnoid hemorrhage as an outcome event in clinical trials and observational studies: proposal of a multidisciplinary research group. Stroke 41:2391–2395
73. Vespa PM (2009) Metabolic penumbra in intracerebral hemorrhage. Stroke 40:1547–1548
74. Vespa PM, Nuwer MR, Juhász C, Alexander M, Nenov V, Martin N, Becker DP (1997) Early detection of vasospasm after acute subarachnoid hemorrhage using continuous EEG ICU monitoring. Electroencephalogr Clin Neurophysiol 103:607–615
75. Wartenberg KE, Sheth SJ, Michael Schmidt J, Frontera JA, Rincon F, Ostapkovich N, Fernandez L, Badjatia N, Sander Connolly E, Khandji A, Mayer SA (2011) Acute Ischemic Injury on Diffusion-Weighted Magnetic Resonance Imaging after Poor Grade Subarachnoid Hemorrhage. Neurocrit Care 14:407–415
76. Weidauer S, Lanfermann H, Raabe A, Zanella F, Seifert V, Beck J (2007) Impairment of cerebral perfusion and infarct patterns attributable to vasospasm after aneurysmal subarachnoid hemorrhage: A prospective MRI and DSA study. Stroke 38:1831–1836
77. Weidauer S, Vatter H, Beck J, Raabe A, Lanfermann H, Seifert V, Zanella F (2008) Focal laminar cortical infarcts following aneurysmal subarachnoid haemorrhage. Neuroradiology 50:1–8
78. Wintermark M, Dillon WP, Smith WS, Lau BC, Chaudhary S, Liu S, Yu M, Fitch M, Chien JD, Higashida RT, Ko NU (2008) Visual grading system for vasospasm based on perfusion CT imaging: comparisons with conventional angiography and quantitative perfusion CT. Cerebrovasc Dis 26:163–170
79. Wintermark M, Ko NU, Smith WS, Liu S, Higashida RT, Dillon WP (2006) Vasospasm after subarachnoid hemorrhage: Utility of perfusion CT and CT angiography on diagnosis and management. Am J Neuroradiol 27:26–34
80. Wong GK, Yeung DK, Ahuja AT, King AD, Lam CW, Chan MT, Gin T, Poon WS (2010) Intracellular free magnesium of brain and cerebral phosphorus-containing metabolites after subarachnoid hemorrhage and hypermagnesemic treatment: a ^{31}P–magnetic resonance spectroscopy study. Clinical article. J Neurosurg 113:763–769
81. Yonas H, Sekhar L, Johnson DW, Gur D (1989) Determination of irreversible ischemia by xenon-enhanced computed tomographic monitoring of cerebral blood flow in patients with symptomatic vasospasm. Neurosurgery 24:368–372

Early Diagnosis of Cerebral Ischemia in Cerebral Vasospasm by Oxygen-Pulse Near-Infrared Optical Topography

Yuichi Tanaka, Akira Ebihara, Masashi Ikota, Tomotaka Yamaguro, Haruna Kamochi, Gen Kusaka, Mami Ishikawa, Takehiko Konno, Toshihiro Mashiko, and Eiju Watanabe

Abstract *Purpose*: Early diagnosis of vasospasm is a key factor in the choice of treatment after subarachnoid hemorrhage (SAH). However, a noninvasive method of diagnosing delayed ischemic neurological deficit (DIND) has not been established. We therefore propose a new method of diagnosing cerebral ischemia using near-infrared optical topography (OT) with oxygen inhalation.

Materials and Methods: We used a 44-channel OT system that covers the bilateral frontotemporoparietal areas to assess 29 patients who underwent surgery within 72 h of the onset of SAH. The patients inhaled room air followed by oxygen for 2 min, and then peripheral oxygen saturation (SpO_2) was continuously monitored at the index fingertip. The patients were assessed by *N*-isopropyl-p-[^{123}I]iodoamphetamine (IMP)-SPECT and OT on the same day. Ischemic findings were confirmed using principal component analysis with reference to the systemic SpO_2 value.

Results: Seven of 29 patients developed DIND. Evidence of ischemia was identified by OT in all seven of these patients before the onset of DIND. The OT and SPECT findings agreed in 27 (93 %) of the 29 patients.

Discussion and Conclusions: Our method might detect cerebral ischemia before the onset of DIND and thus be clinically useful for assessing cerebral ischemia with vasospasm.

Keywords Near-infrared optical topography • Cerebral ischemia • Cerebral vasospasm • Oxygen inhalation • SPECT

Y. Tanaka (✉) • A. Ebihara • M. Ikota • T. Yamaguro
H. Kamochi • G. Kusaka • M. Ishikawa
Department of Neurosurgery,
Jichi Medical University Saitama Medical Center,
Saitama-Ken, Japan
e-mail: chinu@jichi.ac.jp

T. Konno • T. Mashiko • E. Watanabe
Department of Neurosurgery, Jichi Medical University,
Saitama-Ken, Japan

Introduction

Few drugs are available that can specifically and effectively treat cerebral vasospasm, which is a serious complication that affects the prognosis of subarachnoid hemorrhage (SAH). On the other hand, asymptomatic cerebral ischemia arises before delayed ischemic neurological deficits (DIND) manifest [8]. Therefore, the early diagnosis of cerebral ischemia caused by cerebral vasospasm is a key factor in the choice of treatment for cerebral vasospasm after SAH. However, a totally noninvasive diagnostic procedure for diagnosing cerebral ischemia caused by cerebral vasospasm has not yet been established. Cerebral hemodynamics are conventionally assessed using cerebral angiography, perfusion computed tomography (CT), magnetic resonance imaging angiography (MRA), single-photon emission computed tomography (SPECT), and positron emission tomography (PET). Although these modalities can evaluate cerebral perfusion deficits, they have several disadvantages, because they expose patients to physical stress and considerable invasiveness, and because assessment takes time [7, 14]. A less invasive method is needed that can repeatedly measure changes in cerebral hemodynamics, preferably at the bedside in real time.

Near-infrared spectroscopy (NIRS) can measure changes in the concentrations of oxygenated (HbOxy), deoxygenated (HbR), and total (HbTotal) hemoglobin in cerebral tissues, as well as changes in cerebral blood volume (CBV) [3–6, 12, 13]. Total hemoglobin is defined as the sum of HbOxy and HbR. Optical topography (OT) is a NIRS technique that provides spatial maps of hemodynamics and changes in oxygenation in cerebral tissues [6, 12, 13] and it is suitable for repeatedly measuring changes in cerebral oxygenation at bedside. We developed a new noninvasive method of diagnosing chronic cerebral ischemia using near-infrared OT with oxygen inhalation [2].

J. Fandino et al. (eds.), *Neurovascular Events After Subarachnoid Hemorrhage*, Acta Neurochirurgica Supplement, Vol. 120,
DOI 10.1007/978-3-319-04981-6_45, © Springer International Publishing Switzerland 2015

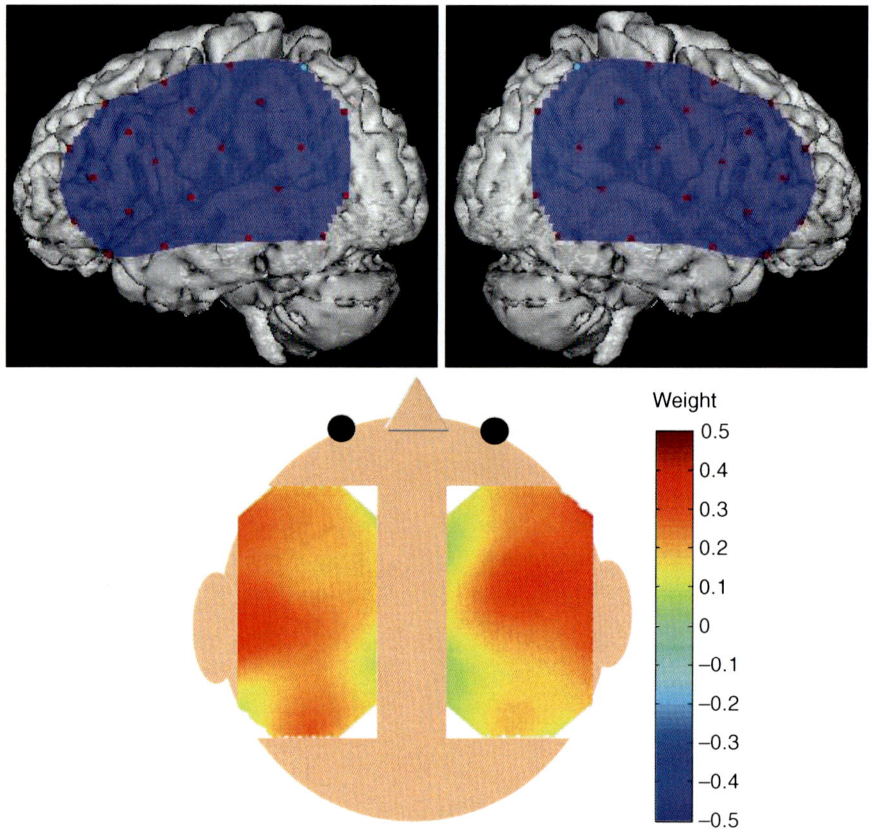

Fig. 1 Position of probes on brain surface and near infrared optical topogram of weight coefficients from a healthy volunteer

Materials and Methods

We assessed 29 patients with Hunt and Kosnik neurological grades 1–4 who were treated by surgical clipping or coiling at our hospital within 72 h of the onset of SAH between 2006 and 2010. Their average age was 53.9 years, and they had aneurysms located in the anterior cerebral (ACA; $n=17$), middle cerebral (MCA; $n=8$), internal carotid ($n=8$), and vertebral ($n=1$) arteries. Cerebral vasospasm in all patients was treated with fasudil and nitroglycerin for 14 days after clipping or coiling. Patients with acutely deteriorating DIND were assessed by cerebral angiography to determine whether an arterial infusion of fasudil would be beneficial. Cerebral ischemia caused by cerebral vasospasm was assessed in all patients using SPECT on days 6 or 8 and DIND was clinically diagnosed. Deterioration in consciousness level, the appearance of motor weakness, sensory deficits, or aphasia was defined as DIND if postoperative cerebral hematoma, hydrocephalus, recurrent SAH, and electrolyte disturbances were absent [9].

Measurement by OT and ^{123}I-IMP SPECT

The 29 patients were examined by OT on days 2, 4, 6, 8, 10, 12, and 14, and simultaneously by SPECT on days 6 or 8 on the same day as OT after the onset of SAH. The OT and *N*-isopropyl-p-[^{123}I]iodoamphetamine (^{123}I-IMP)-SPECT findings on either day 6 or day 8 were compared to assess whether cerebral ischemia was identified.

Evaluation of Optical Topography

The patients were assessed using an ETG4000 continuous-wave OT system (Hitachi Medical Corporation, Tokyo, Japan). Near-infrared light rays with wavelengths of 695 and 830 nm were guided by optical fiber bundles and transmitted into the cranium. Reflections of near-infrared rays were detected by receiver probes positioned on the scalp at 30 mm from transmitter probes. Both the scalp and cerebral hemodynamics influence OT signals because near-infrared light is absorbed by hemoglobin in the extracerebral and cerebral tissues. However, changes in cerebral hemodynamics and oxygenation caused by manipulating the type of inhaled gas can be detected using settings similar to those applied herein [3, 10].

Changes in hemoglobin concentrations in areas of the MCA were measured in supine patients by placing the probes on the scalp to cover the bilateral frontotemporoparietal area (Fig. 1). Measurements proceeded with a response rate of 10 Hz.

Patients breathed through an OX-135 oxygen face mask (Atom Medical Corporation, Tokyo, Japan) and peripheral oxygen saturation (SpO_2) was measured at the tip of the index finger using an OLV 3100 SpO_2 monitor (Nihon Koden Corporation, Tokyo, Japan). Air was delivered through the oxygen face mask at a flow rate of 8 L/min, and OT measurements were started.

After the OT values were stabilized, the patients inhaled air for 1 min, followed by oxygen at the same flow rate for 2 min, and then air once again at the same flow rate for 3 min. The SpO_2 changed in a trapezoidal manner under these conditions. Changes in HbOxy associated with oxygen inhalation in the cerebral tissues were measured using OT [1].

Analysis of OT Data

The time courses of HbOxy data were analyzed as follows. Data from OT were processed using MATLAB R14 (Math Works Inc., Natick, MA, USA) and principal component analysis (PCA) was applied to the data. Signal interference has been identified and removed from extracerebral tissues using this technique [11]. The weights are the coefficients of each channel for the synthesis of the principal component, and they reflect the degree to which the data in each channel contribute to the principal component data. Cross-correlations between each component and SpO_2 were calculated. The principal component with the highest correlation coefficient included changes in HbOxy associated with oxygen inhalation, and this was analyzed in detail. To evaluate the transmission of systemic SpO_2 changes to cerebral tissues, the weight coefficients of the principal components were calculated for each channel. Contour maps (topograms) were drawn using weight coefficients positioned at each measurement point (Fig. 1).

Evaluation of Cerebral Ischemia

The laterality of OT was determined by comparing the channel inspections in the symmetrical positions on the topogram. The side with a lower weight coefficient was defined as the ischemic side. Statistical significance was determined using the nonparametric Mann-Whitney *U* test. Differences with $P<0.05$ were considered significant. Two neurosurgeons and two radiologists determined the ischemic side on SPECT images. The ischemic sides in OT and SPECT were compared, and the possibility of identifying cerebral ischemia was investigated. The ischemic side of OT was compared with those of SPECT, and two neurosurgeons investigated the possibility of identifying ischemic findings and ischemic sides.

Results

Table 1 shows the results of the 29 patients who were assessed by OT and ^{123}I-IMP SPECT on the same day. DIND developed in 7 (24 %) of the patients who had concurrent ischemic findings on both images. However, ischemia was detected on OT before DIND. Early ischemic findings were not evident in OT images of 10 patients, and none of them developed DIND. In 22 patients who did not develop DIND, OT and ^{123}I-IMP SPECT image showed ischemic findings in 11 and 13 of them, respectively. Among the 13 patients with ischemic findings on ^{123}I-IMP SPECT images, 11(84.6 %) were concurrent with those of OT and all 9 patients without ischemic findings on ^{123}I-IMP SPECT images also had no ischemic findings on OT images. Among the 22 patients who did not develop DIND, the findings on OT and ^{123}I-IMP SPECT agreed in 20 (90.9 %) of them. Among all 29 patients, ^{123}I-IMP SPECT and OT images showed ischemic findings in 20 and 18 of them, respectively, and the findings were concurrent in 18 (90 %) of the 20 patients with such findings on ^{123}I-IMP SPECT images. Among all 29 patients, 9 patients had no ischemic findings on either ^{123}I-IMP SPECT or OT images. In total, the presence or absence of ischemia on OT and ^{123}I-IMP SPECT images concurred in 27 (93.1 %) of the 29 patients.

Seven of the 20 patients with evidence of ischemia on SPECT images developed DIND, whereas 9 without such evidence did not. On the other hand, DIND did not develop in 10 patients without evidence of early ischemia on OT. Among 19 patients with evidence of early ischemia on OT, 7 (36.8 %) developed DIND, whereas the ischemic findings on OT improved in the remaining 12 (63.2 %) patients and DIND did not arise.

Case Presentation

A 59-year-old woman was admitted to our hospital with sudden onset of severe headache and disturbed consciousness. Assessment by CT revealed moderate SAH and cerebral angiography revealed an anterior communicating artery aneurysm, which was surgically clipped on day 1. Ischemic findings or brain damage caused by the surgery were not evident on postoperative CT images and her level of consciousness improved. Laterality was essentially absent on OT images on day 2 (Fig. 2a), but evidence of ischemia appeared in the left sides of the topogram (Fig. 2b) and of the SPECT images on day 6 (Fig. 2b). However, DIND had not yet developed at this point. We determined that ischemia caused by vasospasm had started and we enhanced the systemic therapy for cerebral vasospasm. The topogram on day 11 indicated improved ischemia (Fig. 2c) and the absence of DIND.

Discussion

We developed a new method of diagnosing chronic cerebral ischemia using OT with oxygen inhalation [2]. This method can repeatedly evaluate cerebral oxygenation and detect cerebral ischemia at the bedside. The present study aimed to

Table 1 Patient characteristics

Case no.	Age	Sex	AN	Op	DIND	Ischemic side SPECT	Ischemic side OT	Early ischemia (OT)
1	35	M	Acom	Clip	–	N	N	–
2	62	F	MCA	Clip	–	R	R	+
3	63	F	Acom	Clip	+	L	L	+
4	40	M	MCA	Clip	–	R	N	+
5	52	F	ACA	Clip	–	L	L	+
6	24	M	ACA	Clip	–	N	N	–
7	63	F	ACA	Clip	–	N	N	–
8	51	F	MCA	Clip	+	R	R	+
9	55	F	MCA	Clip	–	R	R	+
10	65	F	ACA	Clip	+	L	L	+
11	51	F	MCA	Clip	–	N	N	–
12	60	F	ACA	Clip	–	L	L	–
13	57	F	MCA	Clip	–	N	N	–
14	45	M	ICA	Coil	–	N	N	–
15	47	F	ACA	Clip	–	R	R	+
16	70	F	ICA	Clip	–	L	L	+
17	57	M	ACA	Clip	–	N	N	+
18	54	M	ACA	Clip	–	N	N	–
19	66	F	VA	Clip	–	N	N	–
20	55	F	MCA	Clip	+	L	L	+
21	51	M	ACA	Clip	+	R	R	+
22	53	F	ACA	Clip	–	L	L	+
23	78	F	ICA	Coil	–	R	R	+
24	45	F	ACA	Clip	–	R	R	+
25	61	F	ACA	Clip	+	R	R	+
26	34	M	ACA	Clip	+	L	L	+
27	56	M	MCA	Clip	–	R	R	+
28	52	F	ACA	Clip	–	R	R	+
29	61	F	ACA	Clip	–	R	N	–

Columns labeled SPECT, OT, and Early ischemia (OT) indicate side with cerebral ischemia in each modality

ACA anterior cerebral artery, *Acom* anterior communicating artery, *AN* aneurysm, *Early ischemia (OT)* early ischemic finding on OT, *F* female, *ICA* internal carotid artery, *L* left, *M* male, *MCA* middle cerebral artery, *N* no laterality, *Op* operation, *OT* optical tomography, *R* right, *SPECT* single-photon emission computed tomography, *VA* vertebral artery

determine whether OT with oxygen inhalation can detect acute cerebral ischemia caused by cerebral vasospasm before the onset of DIND.

The concentration of HbOxy in cerebral tissue increases under oxygen inhalation and decreases under room air inhalation. However, concentrations of HbOxy induced by oxygen inhalation change less in ischemic than in normal regions [2]. We developed a new method of diagnosing chronic cerebral ischemia using OT with oxygen inhalation [2]. This method detects changes in the HbOxy concentration of brain tissue, and thus chronic cerebral ischemia in patients with conditions such as unilateral internal carotid artery occlusion [2].

Here, we investigated whether our method could detect acute ischemic states caused by cerebral vasospasm before the onset of DIND. We assessed 29 patients by OT and CT on either day 6 or day 8 after surgery within 72 h of the onset of SAH. We investigated the occurrence of DIND and the detection of early ischemia on OT images from all 29 patients. We found DIND in seven of them and the OT and SPECT findings of ischemia agreed in all of them. Early ischemic findings were detected by OT before DIND devel-

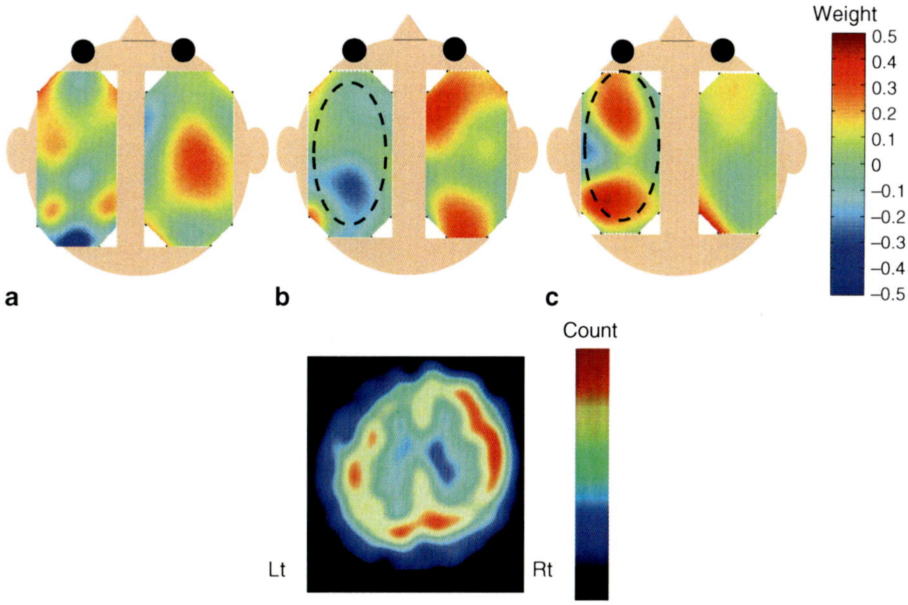

Fig. 2 Optical topograms of patient 1 on days 2, 6, and 10, and SPECT on day 6. Laterality of weight coefficients is essentially absent on day 2 (**a**). Ischemic findings are evident in the left frontal lobe on OT (*dotted circle*) and in SPECT (**b**). Ischemic findings on day 10 are improved by additional enhanced treatment for cerebral vasospasm (*dotted circle*) (**c**)

oped in these seven patients. Ten patients with no evidence of ischemia on OT images did not develop DIND. These results suggest that OT could detect cerebral ischemia before the onset of DIND and as well as SPECT after the onset of DIND. On the other hand, DIND did not occur in the other 22 patients. Among these 22 patients, ischemic findings were evident on ^{123}I-IMP SPECT images from 13 of them, 11 (84.6 %) concurred with those of OT. However, OT did not detect ischemic findings in two patients. These results suggest that the sensitivity of detecting cerebral ischemia is lower for OT than for SPECT [2]. Among the 22 patients who did not develop DIND, the findings on OT and ^{123}I-IMP SPECT concurred in 20 (90.9 %) of the cases. In total, the findings on OT and ^{123}I-IMP SPECT concurred in 27 (93.1 %) of the 29 patients. This 93.1 % rate of diagnostic agreement with SPECT suggests that our method could help to diagnose cerebral ischemia during the acute phase of SAH.

Optical topography uncovered evidence of ischemia in 19 patients, among whom 7 developed DIND. However, ischemic findings improved in 12 (63 %) of the 19 patients because of additional enhanced treatment, and none of them developed DIND. Thus, enhanced treatment for vasospasm improved ischemia in 63 % of patients in whom OT detected early ischemic findings and DIND consequently did not develop. These results suggest that the enhanced systemic treatment for vasospasm that started soon after OT prevented DIND. However, ischemic findings did not improve in the remaining seven (37 %) patients despite additional treatment and all of them developed DIND.

Our method could detect ischemia before DIND occurred and 63 % of patients in whom ischemia was detected by OT received enhanced treatment for vasospasm and did not develop DIND. These results suggest that our method could be applicable to the early diagnosis of cerebral ischemia caused by vasospasm.

Conclusion

We developed a practical method of detecting cerebral oxygenation that could detect cerebral ischemia and identify its location before DIND onset. Thus, the method might be clinically applicable as a real-time, noninvasive means of assessing cerebral ischemia with a view to treating cerebral vasospasm.

Conflict of Interest Statement We declare that we have no conflict of interest.

References

1. Cooper RJ et al (2012) The utility of near-infrared spectroscopy in the regression of low-frequency physiological noise from functional magnetic resonance imaging data. Neuroimage 59(4):3128–3138
2. Ebihara A, Tanaka Y, Konno T, Kawasaki S, Fujiwara M, Watanabe E (2012) Evaluation of cerebral ischemia using near-infrared spectroscopy with oxygen inhalation. J Biomed Opt 17(9):096002
3. Germon TJ et al (1998) Sensitivity of near infrared spectroscopy to cerebral and extra-cerebral oxygenation changes is determined by emitter-detector separation. J Clin Monit Comput 14:353–360
4. Hillman EM et al (2007) Optical brain imaging in vivo. Techniques and applications from animal to man. J Biomed Opt 12(5):051402
5. Kannan RP et al (2002) Non-invasive assessment of language lateralization by transcranial near-infrared optical topography and functional MRI. Hum Brain Mapp 16(3):183–189
6. Koh PH, Elwell CE, Delpy DT (2009) Development of a dynamic test phantom for optical topography. Adv Exp Med Biol 645:141–146
7. Komiyama M et al (1998) Prospective analysis of complications of catheter cerebral angiography in the digital subtraction angiography and magnetic resonance era. Neurol Med Chir 38(9):534–540
8. Ohkuma H, Suzuki A, Habler O et al (2003) Cortical blood flow during cerebral vasospasm after aneurysmal subarachnoid hemorrhage: three-dimensional N-isopropyl-[123]iodoamphetamine single photon emission CT findings. AJNR Am J Neuroradiol 24:444–450
9. Shibuya M et al (1992) Effect of AT 877 on cerebral vasospasm after aneurysmal subarachnoid hemorrhage. J Neurosurg 76(4):571–577

10. Terborg C et al (2003) Non invasive monitoring of cerebral oxygenation during vasomotor reactivity tests by a new near-infrared spectroscopy device. Cerebrovasc Dis 16(1):36–41
11. Virtanen J, Noponen T, Merilainen P (2009) Comparison of principal and independent component analysis in removing extracerebral interference from near-infrared spectroscopy signals. J Biomed Opt 14(5):054032
12. Watanabe E et al (1996) Non-invasive functional mapping with multi-channel near infra-red spectroscopic topography in humans. Neurosci Lett 205(1):41–44
13. Watanabe E et al (2000) Noninvasive cerebral blood volume measurement during seizures using multichannel near-infrared spectroscopic topography. J Biomed Opt 5(3):287–290
14. Wintermark M et al (2005) Accuracy of dynamic perfusion CT with deconvolution in detecting acute hemispheric stroke. AJNR Am J Neuroradiol 26(1):104–112

Clot-Clearance Rate in the Sylvian Cistern Is Associated with the Severity of Cerebral Vasospasm After Subarachnoid Hemorrhage

Tomikatsu Toyoda, Ichiro Yonekura, Akira Iijima, Munehisa Shinozaki, and Takeo Tanishima

Abstract Rapid clot removal and clearance has been proposed as an effective tool for preventing cerebral vasospasm after subarachnoid hemorrhage (SAH). We examined the relationship between clot-clearance rate and the severity of cerebral vasospasm in 110 consecutive patients with aneurysmal SAH. We measured clot-clearance rates per day in the basal and Sylvian cisterns, and evaluated the presence of symptomatic vasospasm based on changes in clinical symptoms and the appearance of a new low-density area on a computed tomography (CT) scan. The severity of symptomatic cerebral vasospasm was associated with age and the SAH grade on admission; however, we observed no significant difference between these variables in patients with urokinase irrigation or fasudil hydrochloride treatment. The mean clot-clearance rates per day for patients with asymptomatic and permanent delayed ischemic neurological deficit were 41.9 and 41.5 %, respectively, in the basal cistern ($P=0.7358$) and 37.7 and 23.9 %, respectively, in the Sylvian cistern ($P=0.0021$). The reduced clot-clearance rate in the Sylvian cistern increased the risk of vasospasm-related infarction ($P=0.0093$) and markedly reduced unfavorable outcomes ($P=0.0115$).

Keywords Subarachnoid hemorrhage • Cerebral vasospasm • Delayed ischemic neurological deficit • Clot-clearance rate

T. Toyoda, MD (✉) • I. Yonekura
M. Shinozaki • T. Tanishima
Department of Neurosurgery,
JCHO Tokyo Shinjuku Medical Center,
5-1 Tsukudocho Shinjuku, Tokyo, 162-8543, Japan
e-mail: ttoyoda-tky@umin.net

A. Iijima
Department of Neuroendovascular Treatment,
JCHO Tokyo Shinjuku Medical Center,
5-1 Tsukudocho Shinjuku, Tokyo, 162-8543, Japan

Introduction

Cerebral vasospasm after subarachnoid hemorrhage (SAH) is a major cause of morbidity and mortality. Although numerous reports describe the pathogenesis and mechanisms of vasospasm, these factors remain a matter of debate. Improved clinical management, such as triple-H (hypertension, hypervolemia, and hemodilution) therapy, endovascular techniques, and vasodilatory drug (e.g., nimodipine) administration has reduced the frequency of severe vasospasm. Nevertheless, these methods have not decreased the overall incidence of vasospasm [2]. Subarachnoid clot is an important contributing factor in the development of vasospasm, and rapid clot removal coupled with cisternal irrigation therapy and/or the "head-shaking" method reduces the incidence of cerebral vasospasm and improves the clinical outcome after aneurysmal SAH [3]. Furthermore, a quantitative analysis of clot clearance indicated that initial clot volume and clot-clearance rate are independent predictors of vasospasm [1, 4]. In the present study, we examined the clot-clearance rate per day in 110 patients after acute-stage surgery. We hypothesized that cisternal irrigation therapy would clear clots in the basal cistern but not the Sylvian cistern because of the placement of inflow and outflow catheters in the ventricle and basal cistern, respectively. We also evaluated the difference in the clot-clearance rates between the basal and Sylvian cisterns, and determined how these rates affect the degree of vasospasm, the incidence of vasospasm-related infarction, and the clinical outcome.

Materials and Methods

We performed a retrospective review of the medical records of consecutive patients with aneurysmal SAH admitted to Tokyo Koseinenkin Hospital between April 2005 and December 2012. The eligibility criterion for the study was an SAH treated surgically within 48 h of onset. A total of 110 consecutive

DOI 10.1007/978-3-319-04981-6_46,

patients were included in the study. Among these 110 patients, 91 had undergone cerebrospinal fluid (CSF) irrigation with urokinase after surgery, and 50 had received fasudil hydrochloride treatment. The mean age was 59.0 years (range, 33–79 years), and 64 patients were women. The assigned World Federation of Neurosurgical Societies (WFNS) grade was good (Grades 1–3) for 81 patients and poor (Grades 4–5) for 29 patients. We analyzed the CT scans using image analysis software, and calculated the initial clot volume and changes in the clot volume within the lesion (basal and Sylvian cisterns). The clot-clearance rate per day was calculated as a percentage ([lesion volume in postoperative CT lesion volume at admission/postoperative day] × 100). A diagnosis of symptomatic vasospasm was made on the basis of the criteria defined by Haley et al. [2]. The vasospasm was evaluated and classified according to severity using the following scale: asymptomatic (Grade 0), transient delayed ischemic neurological deficit (tDIND, Grade 1), and persistent delayed ischemic neurological deficit (pDIND, Grade 2). Angiographic vasospasm was assessed by angiogram (including magnetic resonance angiography (MRA)). The severity of angiographic vasospasm was considered to be absent or mild if a 0–33 % decrease in arterial diameter was observed on angiogram, moderate if there was a 34–66 % decrease, or severe if there was a decrease in arterial diameter >66 %. Cerebral infarction caused by vasospasm was diagnosed from imaging studies. Patient outcome was assessed at 3 months postoperatively using the modified Rankin Scale (mRS) and clinic records. Outcome was classified as favorable (mRS 0–2) or unfavorable (mRS 3–6) for the purpose of statistical analysis. Variables are presented as mean ± SD. Multiple regression analysis was used to assess the relationship between the severity of vasospasm and each factor; a probability value of 0.05 or less was considered significant.

Results

Symptomatic vasospasm developed in 63 of the 110 patients (57 %), including tDIND in 35 patients (32 %) and pDIND in 28 patients (25 %). No symptomatic vasospasm was observed in 47 patients (43 %). Angiographic vasospasm was classified as none/mild in 65 (59 %) of the patients, moderate in 12 (11 %), and severe in 33 (29 %). The severity of vasospasm correlated significantly with age ($P<0.05$) and poor WFNS SAH grade on admission ($P<0.01$). Treatment of the aneurysm and cisternal irrigation therapy with urokinase were not significant factors related to the severity of vasospasm. Fasudil hydrochloride treatment suppressed angiographic cerebral vasospasm ($P<0.01$), but this treatment was ineffective for symptomatic vasospasm or patient outcome. The mean initial clot volume was 9.0 ± 4.5 ml in asymptomatic patients, 8.8 ± 4.5 ml in tDIND patients, and 11.0 ± 5.8 ml in pDIND patients; there were no significant differences among these groups ($P=0.3795$). Respectively, the clot-clearance rates in the each group were 41.9 ± 20.7 %, 38.3 ± 17.7 %, and 43.1 ± 25.8 % in the basal cistern, and 37.7 ± 17.6 %, 29.6 ± 12.7 %, and 24.1 ± 18.2 % in the Sylvian cistern. The clot-clearance rate in the Sylvian cistern was significantly associated with the severity of symptomatic vasospasm ($P=0.0027$) and angiographic vasospasm ($P=0.0001$). The results of the univariate analyses for symptomatic vasospasm are shown in Table 1. Vasospasm-related infarction was seen in 34 patients (29 %), and 30 (88 %) of these infarcts occurred in patients with severe vasospasm. Significant differences were observed for age ($P<0.01$), poor WFNS grade ($P<0.05$), initial clot volume ($P<0.05$), and clot-clearance rate per day in the Sylvian cistern ($P<0.05$). Regarding clinical outcome, 74 of the 110 patients had reached an independent status (mRS 0–2, 67 %), whereas 36 patients showed an unfavorable status (mRS 3–6, 33 %) by the 3-month follow-up examination. Variables that independently predicted poor outcome were an older age ($P<0.01$), poor WFNS grade ($P=0.0001$), initial SAH clot volume ($P=0.0001$), and clot-clearance rate per day in the Sylvian cistern ($P<0.05$; Table 2). We observed that symptomatic vasospasm ($P=0.0024$) and vasospasm-related infarction ($P=0.0001$) were independent factors leading to an unfavorable outcome.

Discussion

Few studies have quantified subarachnoid clot volume using image analysis [1, 4]. Reilly et al. reported a method for quantitatively analyzing subarachnoid clots and noted that clot volume and clearance rate were significant predictors of vasospasm [4]. Here, we demonstrate an association between the severity of symptomatic vasospasm and clot clearance in the basal and Sylvian cisterns in 110 patients with aneurysmal SAH. We observed increased risks for severe vasospasm and vasospasm-related infarction among patients with insufficient clot washout in the Sylvian cistern. In contrast, the clot-clearance rate in the basal cistern did not affect the severity of vasospasm or the incidence of vasospasm-related infarction. Therefore, our data suggest that the clot-clearance rate in the Sylvian cistern, but not that in the basal cistern, is a significant factor in increasing the risk of severe vasospasm and vasospasm-related infarction.

Conclusion

This study demonstrates that clot-clearance rate in the Sylvian cistern is strongly associated with the degree of vasospasm, vasospasm-related infarction, and clinical outcomes.

Conflict of Interest Statement We declare that we have no conflict of interest.

Table 1 Factors related to severity of symptomatic vasospasm

Symptomatic vasospasm	No vasospasm (Grade 0)	Transient DIND (Grade 1)	Persistent DIND (Grade 2)	*P*
Mean age	50.2 years	58.9 years	64.8 years	*0.0101*
SAH grade (WFNS)				
1–3	40 patients	26 patients	15 patients	
4–5	7 patients	9 patients	13 patients	*0.0017**
Aneurysmal treatment				
Clipped	45 patients	33 patients	23 patients	0.0936
Coiled	2 patients	2 patients	5 patients	
Urokinase irrigation therapy	41 patients	30 patients	20 patients	0.2091
Fasudil hydrochloride treatment	14 patients	16 patients	10 patients	0.2796
Initial clot volume	8.2 ± 3.7 ml	8.4 ± 4.3 ml	9.5 ± 4.7 ml	0.3795
Clot clearance ratio/day in the basal cistern	41.9 ± 20.7 %	38.3 ± 17.7 %	41.5 ± 26.5 %	0.7358
Clot clearance ratio/day in the Sylvian cistern	37.7 ± 17.6 %	29.6 ± 12.7 %	23.9 ± 17.9 %	**0.0021***

DIND delayed ischemic neurological deficit, *SAH* subarachnoid hemorrhage, *WFNS* World Federation of Neurosurgical Societies
Data are presented as means ± standard deviations where appropriate
*$P<0.05$

Table 2 Factors associated with increased risk of unfavorable outcome in 110 patients with aneurysmal subarachnoid hemorrhage

Outcomes	Favorable ($n=74$)	Unfavorable ($n=36$)	*P*
Mean age	54.7 years	64.6 years	*0.0003**
Gender	32 men/42 women	14 men/22 women	0.6634
SAH grade (WFNS)			
1–3	63 patients	18 patients	
4–5	11 patients	18 patients	*0.0001**
Aneurysm treatment			
Clipped	70 patients	31 patients	
Coiled	4 patients	5 patients	0.1277
Urokinase irrigation	63 patients	28 patients	0.3458
Fasudil hydrochloride treatment	27 patients	13 patients	0.9289
Initial clot volume	8.2 ± 3.9 ml	11.9 ± 5.7 ml	*0.0001**
Clot clearance ratio/day in the basal cistern	41.5 ± 21.2 %	38.7 ± 21.6 %	0.5249
Clot clearance ratio/day in the Sylvian cistern	34.5 ± 16.5 %	25.7 ± 17.0 %	*0.0115**
Vasospasm-related infarction	8 patients	26 patients	*0.0001**

SAH subarachnoid hemorrhage, *DIND* delayed ischemic neurological deficit, *WFNS* World Federation of Neurosurgical Societies
Data are presented as means ± standard deviations where appropriate
*$P<0.05$

References

1. Friedman JA, Goersss SJ, Meyer FB (2002) Volumetric quantification of Fisher Grade 3 aneurysmal subarachnoid hemorrhage: a novel method to predict symptomatic vasospasm on admission computerized tomography scans. J Neurosurg 97:401–407
2. Haley EC Jr, Kassell NF, Tornoer JC (1993) A randomized trial of nicardipine in subarachnoid hemorrhage: angiographic and transcranial Doppler ultrasound results. A report of the Cooperative Aneurysm Study. J Neurosurg 78:537–546
3. Kodama N, Sasaki T, Kawakami M, Sato M, Asari J (2000) Cisternal irrigation therapy with urokinase and ascorbic acid for prevention of vasospasm after aneurysmal subarachnoid hemorrhage. Outcome in 217 patients. Surg Neurol 53:110–118
4. Reilly C, Amidei C, Tolentino J, Jahromi BS, Macdonald RL (2004) Clot volume and clearance rate as independent predictors of vasospasm after aneurysmal subarachnoid hemorrhage. J Neurosurg 101:255–261

Clinical Trials

Intrathecal Application of the Nimodipine Slow-Release Microparticle System EG-1962 for Prevention of Delayed Cerebral Ischemia and Improvement of Outcome After Aneurysmal Subarachnoid Hemorrhage

Nima Etminan, R. Loch Macdonald, Cara Davis, Kevin Burton, Hans-Jakob Steiger, and Daniel Hänggi

Abstract The effective reduction of delayed cerebral ischemia (DCI), a main contributor for poor outcome following aneurysmal subarachnoid hemorrhage (SAH), remains challenging. Previous clinical trials on systemic pharmaceutical treatment of SAH mostly failed to improve outcome, probably because of insensitive pharmaceutical targets and outcome measures, small sample size, insufficient subarachnoid drug concentrations and also detrimental, systemic effects of the experimental treatment per se. Interestingly, in studies that are more recent, intrathecal administration of nicardipine pellets following surgical aneurysm repair was suggested to have a beneficial effect on DCI and neurological outcome. However, this positive effect remained restricted to patients who were treated surgically for a ruptured aneurysm. Because of the favorable results of the preclinical data on DCI and neurological outcome in the absence of neurotoxicity or systemic side effects, we are initiating clinical trials. The PROMISE (Prolonged Release nimOdipine MIcro particles after Subarachnoid hemorrhage) trial is designed as an unblinded, nonrandomized, single-center, single-dose, dose-escalation safety and tolerability phase 1 study in patients surgically treated for aSAH and will investigate the effect of intracisternal EG-1962 administration. The NEWTON (Nimodipine microparticles to Enhance recovery While reducing TOxicity after subarachNoid hemorrhage) trial is a phase 1/2a multicenter, controlled, randomized, open-label, dose-escalation, safety, tolerability, and pharmacokinetic study comparing EG-1962 and nimodipine in patients with aneurysmal SAH.

Keywords Subarachnoid hemorrhage • Intrathecal application • EG-1962 microparticle system • Delayed cerebral ischemia

Introduction

The case fatality rate during the course of aneurysmal subarachnoid hemorrhage (SAH) is 35 % [1]. The main reasons for the poor prognosis after SAH can be roughly separated into pathomechanisms related to primary or early brain injury caused by the initial rupture of the aneurysm and various pathomechanisms contributing to delayed cerebral ischemia (DCI). The latter is a multifactorial phenomenon, with macrovascular spasm (formerly angiographic vasospasm (VSP)), microvascular spasm, microthromboembolism, and cortical spreading depolarization/ischemia as the main proischemic pathomechanisms [2–6]. Although therapeutic targets to limit the extent of early brain injury are fairly limited, previous clinical trials were mainly designed to pharmaceutically target macrovascular spasm or inflammation, most of which failed to improve neurological outcome [7, 8]. Interestingly, to date, nimodipine remains the only drug proven to reduce the incidence of poor outcome, regardless of macrovascular spasm [9]. There are several reasons why many drugs have not seemed to improve outcome in previous trials or have had minimal benefits, but one hypothesis is that the drugs had detrimental systemic side effects, such as arterial hypotension (e.g., for nicardipine or nimodipine) or pulmonary edema (e.g., for clazosentan), that counteracted the beneficial

N. Etminan, MD (✉) • H.-J. Steiger, MD • D. Hänggi, MD
Department of Neurosurgery, Medical Faculty, Heinrich-Heine-University, Moorenstr.5, 40225 Düsseldorf, Germany
e-mail: etminan@uni-duesseldorf.de

R.L. Macdonald, MD, PhD
Division of Neurosurgery, St. Michael's Hospital, 30 Bond St., Toronto, ON M5B 1W8, Canada

Department of Surgery, Institute of Medical Science, University of Toronto, Toronto, ON Canada

Labatt Family Centre of Excellence in Brain Injury and Trauma Research, Keenan Research Centre of the Li Ka Shing Knowledge Institute of St. Michael's Hospital, Toronto, ON Canada

C. Davis, MS • K. Burton, PhD
Evonik Industries, Birmingham, AL, USA

J. Fandino et al. (eds.), *Neurovascular Events After Subarachnoid Hemorrhage*, Acta Neurochirurgica Supplement, Vol. 120,
DOI 10.1007/978-3-319-04981-6_47, © Springer International Publishing Switzerland 2015

effects of the drug [8, 10–12]. Therefore, some studies aim to design drugs for intrathecal application to reduce the incidence of systemic side and DCI and to ultimately improve outcome after SAH. Here, we review data of the intrathecal application of a nimodipine slow-release microparticle system EG-1962 for improvement of outcome and prevention of DCI after SAH.

Dihydropyridines for SAH

Two main dihydropyridines are used in patients with SAH, nimodipine and nicardipine. In Europe and in North America, patients with aSAH are typically treated with the oral (USA, Canada, and Europe) and/or intravenous (Europe) 1,4-dihydropyridine-derivative calcium channel blocker, nimodipine. Nimodipine is a highly lipophilic drug that binds to the α_1 subunit of L-type calcium channel, inhibits calcium influx through this channel, and, therefore, inhibits vasoconstriction and increases cerebral blood flow [13]. Nimodipine was primarily designed to reduce VSP but, in previous clinical trials, nimodipine was not shown to have a meaningful effect on VSP. However, regardless of the lack of reduction of VSP, nimodipine was proven to significantly reduce the incidence of poor outcome [9]. More recently, it became clear that DCI is a multifactorial phenomenon and that, even though 70 % of patients develop VSP, only 30 % of these patients develop clinical features of DCI [7]. This suggests that even though VSP is certainly associated with DCI, it may not be the best surrogate for the effectiveness of a pharmaceutical therapy against DCI. Thus, the beneficial effect of nimodipine may be related to the reduction of microvascular spasm, and inhibition of cortical spreading ischemia and microthromboemboli [6, 14]. This is supported by data on the fibrinolytic activity of nimodipine [14]. Additionally, nimodipine is suspected to exert neuroprotective effects through reduced neuronal injury by inhibition of neuronal Ca^{2+} influx. Nevertheless, in therapeutic doses, orally or intravenously administered nimodipine is associated with arterial hypotension in up to 50 % of patients [15, 16].

The use of nicardipine for SAH patients is more established in Asia, especially in Japan, where nimodipine is not commercially available. Similar to nimodipine, nicardipine is also a dihydropyridine L-type calcium channel inhibitor that is less lipid soluble than nimodipine, is a cerebral vasodilator and has been studied in different trials upon systemic (intravenous), intraarterial, and intrathecal application [17–23]. Briefly, the systemic administration of nicardipine was not shown to reduce the incidence of poor outcome (death or dependence) in the majority of randomized trials but was shown to have some beneficial effect on the incidence of secondary ischemia (clinical and radiological features of DCI). Whether the lack of evidence of an overall beneficial effect of systemic nicardipine application truly originated in the pharmacological characteristics, as opposed to the trial design and sample size in previous trials, remains unclear.

Intrathecal Application of Dihydropyridines

The main motivations for the intrathecal administration of dihydropyridines are primarily (a) increased CSF concentrations of these drugs, with (b) lower systemic concentrations and (c) lower systemic side effects, primarily hypotension. Here, some studies administered liquid intrathecal dihydropyridine solutions either via ventricular or cisternal drains or via lumbar catheters [21, 22, 24–26]. In summary, the results of these studies illustrated some beneficial effects but were also limited by the practicability of the administration method (continuous intrathecal irrigations via external ventricular drains (EVDs)) and study designs (lack of placebo-controlled or randomized study designs) [26]. Data more recently obtained on the local delivery of sustained-release formulations of dihydropyridines, such as nicardipine, into the subarachnoid space onto cerebral arteries provide evidence that the incidence of DCI is markedly reduced and neurological outcome improved [17, 19, 20]. A prospective, clinical trial randomized 32 patients with aSAH to undergo aneurysm clipping with ($n = 16$) or without ($n = 16$) intracisternal administration of up to 40 mg nicardipine in poly(D,L-LACTIDE-CO-glycolide) (PLGA) pellets [17]. Here, angiographic VSP was significantly reduced in patients treated with pellets (73 % control versus 7 % with pellets). Patients treated with pellets also had a lower incidence of delayed ischemic lesions (47 % control versus 14 % with pellets), better outcome on the modified Rankin scale (mRS) and National Institutes of Health stroke scale (NIHSS), and significantly lower mortality (38 % control versus 6 % with pellets). A limitation of the pellets is that an increasing proportion of patients are undergoing endovascular repair of ruptured aneurysms, nicardipine pellets cannot easily be put in the basal cisterns in these patients. Another study investigated the feasibility and efficacy of intraventricular application of nicardipine pellets via EVDs in patients undergoing surgical or endosvascular repair of ruptured aneurysms [27]. Here, the efficacy of nicardipine pellets did not differ compared with control, because intraventricular

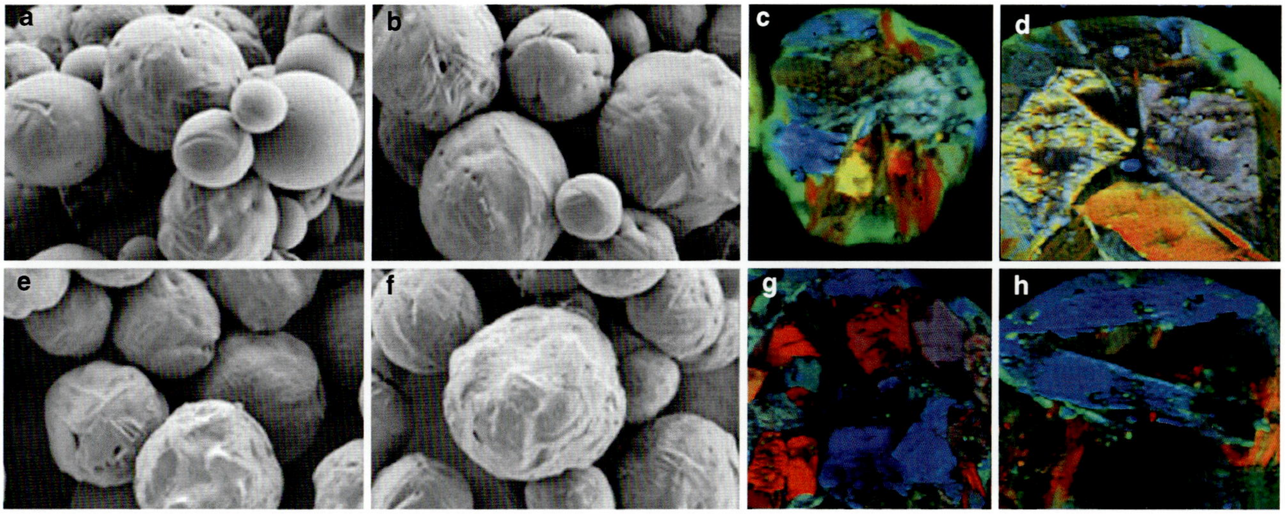

Fig. 1 Scanning electron microscopy and Raman spectroscopy of an example of one formulation of nimodipine microparticles. Scanning electron microscopy (**a**, **b**) and Raman spectroscopy (**c**, **d**, *red* is form 1 of nimodipine, *green* is amorphous nimodipine, and *blue* is form 2 of nimodipine) at baseline. After attempted forced degradation at 30–35 °C for 30 days, the microparticles showed very slight polymer melt (scanning electron microscopy (**e**, **f**), and Raman spectroscopy (**g**, **h**), where *red* is form 1 of nimodipine, *green* is amorphous nimodipine, and *blue* is form 2 of nimodipine), which was avoided after optimization of the formulation

application of the pellets did not improve functional outcome in patients undergoing endovascular coiling, as compared with patients receiving intraventricular pellets and undergoing surgical aneurysm repair. It was concluded that one of the possible explanations for the limited efficacy of intraventricular pellet application in the endovascular group is that the lamina terminalis is not opened in these patients, which may inhibit the distribution of nicardipine in the subarachnoid space.

Rationale for Development of Nimodipine Microparticles

As aforementioned, one of the strongest arguments to develop a potent method to deliver a dihydropyridine intrathecally is to achieve a high CSF concentration in the absence of systemic side effects, and preferably applicable for both treatment modalities to repair ruptured aneurysms. Nimodipine was selected because it is more lipophilic than nicardipine and thus may permeate subarachnoid clots more effectively. At present, nicardipine pellets have not been prepared according to good manufacturing practices and they also are prepared with the neurotoxin dichloromethane [28]. Because of the aforementioned beneficial effects of nimodipine on neurological outcome and probably different pathomechanisms contributing to DCI and the limitations of the pellets per se, the ideal drug vehicle would then be a more lipid-soluble formulation of the dihydropyridine nimodipine embedded in PLGA (Evonik Corporation and Edge Therapeutics, Inc.®) with hyaluronic acid as a diluent.

Formulation of EG-1962

The microparticles were designed as 70 μm in diameter (range 20–125 μm), because very small microparticles would be removed more rapidly by macrophages, whereas larger microparticles are not practical for minimally invasive injection (Fig. 1) [17, 19, 29, 30]. Additionally, the drug loading was maximized (to 65 wt. %) to reduce the injection volume and account for the projected dose requirements for intraventricular injection. Also, assuming that the highest potential dose in patients would be 400 mg, the initial burst of drug release within the first 24 h was chosen to be less than 25 %, equaling 100 mg nimodipine potentially released into the systemic circulation, which would be expected to produce plasma concentrations that would remain below those that can cause hypotension. Finally, the formulation characteristics were designed to release nimodipine over 21 days to equal the duration of oral nimodipine treatment. This pharmacokinetic design would then ensure sufficient nimodipine doses, because it extends to beyond the time when DCI develops [31]. For perioperative application, we tested stability following gamma irradiation and found that there were no changes in drug content, main peak purity, and mean particle size after sterilization with 27 kGy radiation (Fig. 2).

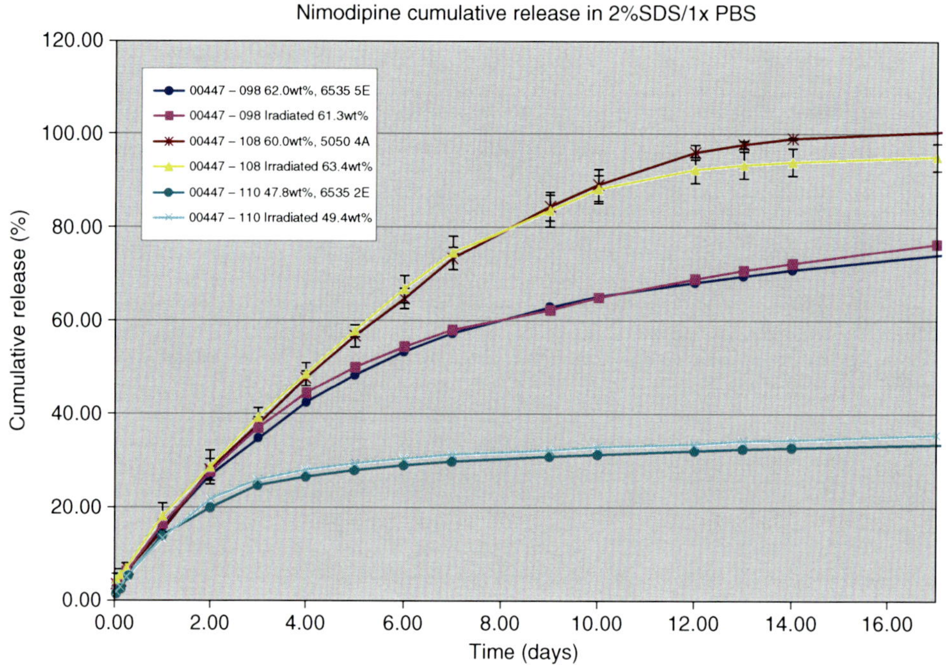

Fig. 2 Nimodipine cumulative release in vitro from several different formulations of microparticles showing the ability to synthesize formulations with different release characteristics and that there is no change in the release characteristics after gamma irradiation with 27 kilogray radiation

Preclinical Studies on Release Characteristics and Toxicity

Release characteristics of different formulations or neat nimodipine were tested different in vitro and in different models [32–34]. More recently, we tested this in Wistar rats at subcutaneous doses of 20 or 200 mg/kg and buffer or plasma nimodipine concentrations, which were measured daily. We found sustained nimodipine release for all doses and formulations, including the neat nimodipine, which was likely because of its high lipid solubility within subcutaneous fat (Fig. 3).

Because nimodipine microparticles in hyaluronic acid have never been injected into the subarachnoid or intraventricular CSF, potential toxicity was investigated in rats and beagles in escalating doses up to threefold times the estimated human dosage (1,200 mg). All animals survived until their sacrifice and there were no EG-1962-related toxicity findings in clinical observations, neurobehavioral evaluations, body weight, food consumption, ophthalmoscopy, hematology, coagulation, clinical chemistry, urinalysis, organ weight, or macroscopic pathology.

Future Perspective

We are initiating two clinical trials. The PROMISE (Prolonged Release nimOdipine MIcro particles after Subarachnoid hemorrhage) trial will be designed as an unblinded, non-randomized, single-center, single-dose, dose-escalation safety and tolerability phase 1 study in patients neurosurgically treated for aSAH at the Department of Neurosurgery, Medical Faculty of the Heinrich-Heine University, Düsseldorf, Germany, and will solely investigate the effect of intracisternal EG-1962 administration. The NEWTON (Nimodipine microparticles to Enhance recovery While reducing TOxicity after subarachNoid hemorrhage) trial will be a phase 1/2a multicenter, controlled, randomized, open-label, dose escalation, safety, tolerability, and pharmacokinetic study comparing EG-1962 and nimodipine in patients with aneurysmal SAH treated by neurosurgical clipping or endovascular coiling. In this study, EG-1962 will be administered by intraventricular catheter that would be in place as part of standard of care in eligible patients.

Conclusion

Due to the promising preclinical data, there is a strong rationale to investigate the effects of EG-1962 in patients suffering from high-grade SAH. Therefore, we are initiated two clinical trials on intracisternal and intraventricular EG-1962 application.

Conflict of Interest Statement N. Etminan and D. Hänggi are scientific advisors for Edge Therapeutics, Inc. R.L. Macdonald is chief scientific officer of Edge Therapeutics, Inc. Cara Davis and Kevin Burton are employess of Evonik.

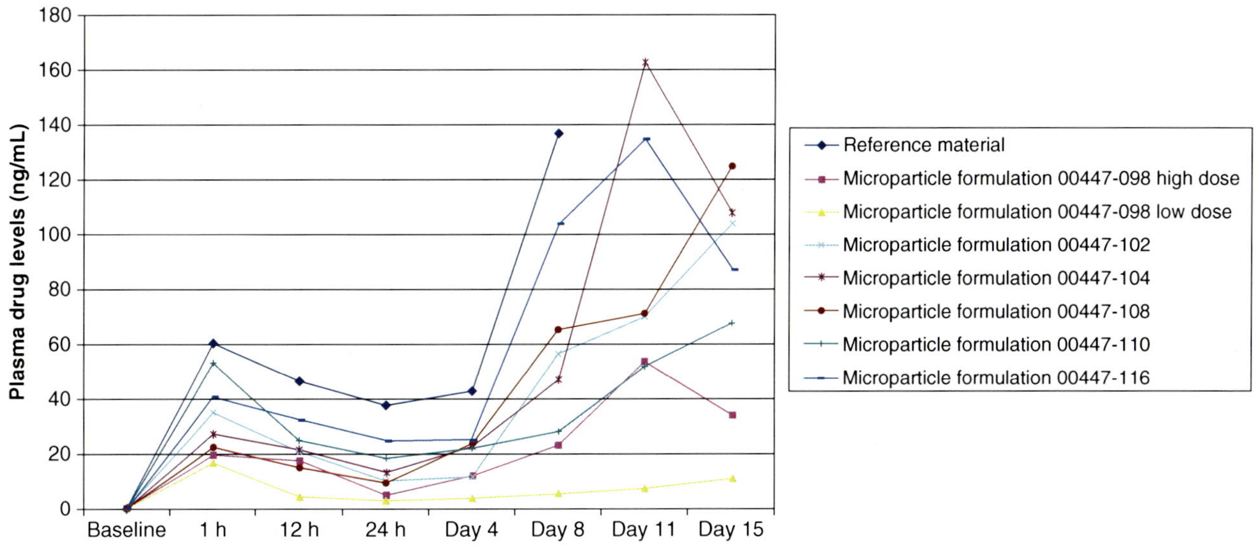

Fig. 3 Release characteristics in vivo in the subcutaneous space of rats of neat nimodipine (reference material) or six different formulations of microparticles containing nimodipine. The release characteristics can be varied to alter the initial burst release at 1 h as well as the time course of release over 15 days

References

1. Lovelock CE, Rinkel GJ, Rothwell PM (2010) Time trends in outcome of subarachnoid hemorrhage: population-based study and systematic review. Neurology 74:1494–1501
2. Dreier JP, Major S, Manning A, Woitzik J, Drenckhahn C, Steinbrink J et al (2009) Cortical spreading ischaemia is a novel process involved in ischaemic damage in patients with aneurysmal subarachnoid haemorrhage. Brain 132:1866–1881
3. Ohkuma H, Manabe H, Tanaka M, Suzuki S (2000) Impact of cerebral microcirculatory changes on cerebral blood flow during cerebral vasospasm after aneurysmal subarachnoid hemorrhage. Stroke 31:1621–1627
4. Park KW, Metais C, Dai HB, Comunale ME, Sellke FW (2001) Microvascular endothelial dysfunction and its mechanism in a rat model of subarachnoid hemorrhage. Anesth Analg 92:990–996
5. Vergouwen MD, Ilodigwe D, Macdonald RL (2011) Cerebral infarction after subarachnoid hemorrhage contributes to poor outcome by vasospasm-dependent and -independent effects. Stroke 42:924–929
6. Vergouwen MD, Vermeulen M, Coert BA, Stroes ES, Roos YB (2008) Microthrombosis after aneurysmal subarachnoid hemorrhage: an additional explanation for delayed cerebral ischemia. J Cereb Blood Flow Metab 28:1761–1770
7. Etminan N, Vergouwen MD, Ilodigwe D, Macdonald RL (2011) Effect of pharmaceutical treatment on vasospasm, delayed cerebral ischemia, and clinical outcome in patients with aneurysmal subarachnoid hemorrhage: a systematic review and meta-analysis. J Cereb Blood Flow Metab 31:1443–1451
8. Etminan N, Vergouwen MDI, Macdonald RL (2013) Angiographic vasospasm versus cerebral infarction as outcome measures after subarachnoid hemorrhage. Acta Neurochir Suppl 115:33–40
9. Dorhout Mees SM, Rinkel GJ, Feigin VL, Algra A, van den Bergh WM, Vermeulen M, et al (2007)) Calcium antagonists for aneurysmal subarachnoid haemorrhage. Cochrane Database Syst Rev (3):CD000277
10. Feigin VL, Rinkel GJ, Algra A, Vermeulen M, van Gijn J (1998) Calcium antagonists in patients with aneurysmal subarachnoid hemorrhage: a systematic review. Neurology 50:876–883
11. Macdonald RL, Kassell NF, Mayer S, Ruefenacht D, Schmiedek P, Weidauer S et al (2008) Clazosentan to overcome neurological ischemia and infarction occurring after subarachnoid hemorrhage (conscious-1): randomized, double-blind, placebo-controlled phase 2 dose-finding trial. Stroke 39:3015–3021
12. Vergouwen MD, Etminan N, Ilodigwe D, Macdonald RL (2011) Lower incidence of cerebral infarction correlates with improved functional outcome after aneurysmal subarachnoid hemorrhage. J Cereb Blood Flow Metab 31:1545–1553
13. Tomassoni D, Lanari A, Silvestrelli G, Traini E, Amenta F (2008) Nimodipine and its use in cerebrovascular disease: evidence from recent preclinical and controlled clinical studies. Clin Exp Hypertens 30:744–766
14. Vergouwen MD, Vermeulen M, de Haan RJ, Levi M, Roos YB (2007) Dihydropyridine calcium antagonists increase fibrinolytic activity: a systematic review. J Cereb Blood Flow Metab 27:1293–1308
15. Radhakrishnan D, Menon DK (1997) Haemodynamic effects of intravenous nimodipine following aneurysmal subarachnoid haemorrhage: implications for monitoring. Anaesthesia 52:489–491
16. Dankbaar JW, Slooter AJ, Rinkel GJ, Schaaf IC (2010) Effect of different components of triple-h therapy on cerebral perfusion in patients with aneurysmal subarachnoid haemorrhage: a systematic review. Crit Care 14:R23
17. Barth M, Capelle HH, Weidauer S, Weiss C, Munch E, Thome C et al (2007) Effect of nicardipine prolonged-release implants on cerebral vasospasm and clinical outcome after severe aneurysmal subarachnoid hemorrhage: a prospective, randomized, double-blind phase IIa study. Stroke 38:330–336
18. Haley EC Jr, Kassell NF, Torner JC, Truskowski LL, Germanson TP (1994) A randomized trial of two doses of nicardipine in aneurysmal subarachnoid hemorrhage. A report of the cooperative aneurysm study. J Neurosurg 80:788–796
19. Kasuya H, Onda H, Sasahara A, Takeshita M, Hori T (2005) Application of nicardipine prolonged-release implants: analysis of 97 consecutive patients with acute subarachnoid hemorrhage. Neurosurgery 56:895–902, discussion 895–902
20. Kasuya H, Onda H, Takeshita M, Okada Y, Hori T (2002) Efficacy and safety of nicardipine prolonged-release implants for preventing vasospasm in humans. Stroke 33:1011–1015

21. Rosenberg N, Lazzaro MA, Lopes DK, Prabhakaran S (2011) High-dose intra-arterial nicardipine results in hypotension following vasospasm treatment in subarachnoid hemorrhage. Neurocrit Care 15:400–404
22. Shibuya M, Suzuki Y, Enomoto H, Okada T, Ogura K, Sugita K (1994) Effects of prophylactic intrathecal administrations of nicardipine on vasospasm in patients with severe aneurysmal subarachnoid haemorrhage. Acta Neurochir (Wien) 131:19–25
23. Webb A, Kolenda J, Martin K, Wright W, Samuels O (2010) The effect of intraventricular administration of nicardipine on mean cerebral blood flow velocity measured by transcranial doppler in the treatment of vasospasm following aneurysmal subarachnoid hemorrhage. Neurocrit Care 12:159–164
24. Hanggi D, Beseoglu K, Turowski B, Steiger HJ (2008) Feasibility and safety of intrathecal nimodipine on posthaemorrhagic cerebral vasospasm refractory to medical and endovascular therapy. Clin Neurol Neurosurg 110:784–790
25. Hanggi D, Eicker S, Beseoglu K, Behr J, Turowski B, Steiger HJ (2009) A multimodal concept in patients after severe aneurysmal subarachnoid hemorrhage: results of a controlled single centre prospective randomized multimodal phase I/II trial on cerebral vasospasm. Cen Eur Neurosurg 70:61–67
26. Zhang YP, Shields LB, Yao TL, Dashti SR, Shields CB (2013) Intrathecal treatment of cerebral vasospasm (2012). J Stroke Cerebrovasc Dis 22(8):1201–1211
27. Barth M, Pena P, Seiz M, Thome C, Muench E, Weidauer S et al (2011) Feasibility of intraventricular nicardipine prolonged release implants in patients following aneurysmal subarachnoid haemorrhage. Br J Neurosurg 25:677–683
28. Kasuya H (2011) Clinical trial of nicardipine prolonged-release implants for preventing cerebral vasospasm: multicenter cooperative study in Tokyo. Acta Neurochir Suppl 110:165–167
29. Lemperle G, Morhenn VB, Pestonjamasp V, Gallo RL (2004) Migration studies and histology of injectable microspheres of different sizes in mice. Plast Reconstr Surg 113:1380–1390
30. Nicholas AP, McInnis C, Gupta KB, Snow WW, Love DF, Mason DW et al (2002) The fate of biodegradable microspheres injected into rat brain. Neurosci Lett 323:85–88
31. Toyota BD (1999) The efficacy of an abbreviated course of nimodipine in patients with good-grade aneurysmal subarachnoid hemorrhage. J Neurosurg 90:203–206
32. Bege N, Renette T, Endres T, Beck-Broichsitter M, Hanggi D, Kissel T (2013) In situ forming nimodipine depot system based on microparticles for the treatment of posthemorrhagic cerebral vasospasm. Eur J Pharm Biopharm 84:99–105
33. Cook DJ, Kan S, Ai J, Kasuya H, Macdonald RL (2012) Cisternal sustained release dihydropyridines for subarachnoid hemorrhage. Curr Neurovasc Res 9:139–148
34. Hanggi D, Perrin J, Eicker S, Beseoglu K, Etminan N, Kamp MA et al (2012) Local delivery of nimodipine by prolonged-release microparticles-feasibility, effectiveness and dose-finding in experimental subarachnoid hemorrhage. PLoS One 7:e42597

Effect of Human Albumin on TCD Vasospasm, DCI, and Cerebral Infarction in Subarachnoid Hemorrhage: The ALISAH Study

Jose I. Suarez, R.H. Martin, E. Calvillo, E.M. Bershad, and C.P. Venkatasubba Rao

Abstract *Background and Purpose*: The neuroprotective effects of human albumin have been studied in animal models of stroke and in humans with various intracranial disorders. We investigated the effect of 25 % human albumin (ALB) on mean cerebral blood flow velocities (MCBFV), delayed cerebral ischemia (DCI), and cerebral infarction.

Methods: We studied patients from the Albumin in Subarachnoid Hemorrhage (ALISAH) pilot clinical trial. We collected data on MCBFV as measured by transcranial Doppler ultrasound (TCD), incidence of DCI, and cerebral infarctions on head computed tomography (CT) scan at 90 days.

Results: TCD showed vasospasm in 75 % ($n=15$), 55 % ($n=11$), and 29 % ($n=2$) of subjects in dosage tiers 1, 2, and 3, respectively. DCI was present in 20 % ($n=4$), 15 % ($n=3$), and 14 % ($n=1$) of subjects in dosage tiers 1, 2, and 3, respectively. Cerebral infarctions were seen in 45 % (5 of 9), 27 % (3 of 18), and 25 % (1 of 4) of subjects who had follow-up head CT scans in dosage tiers 1, 2, and 3, respectively.

Conclusions: Higher dosages of ALB were associated with a lower incidence of TCD vasospasm, DCI, and cerebral infarction at 90 days in a dose-dependent manner.

Keywords Subarachnoid hemorrhage • Human albumin • Clinical trials • Delayed cerebral ischemia • Transcranial Doppler ultrasound

The ALISAH Investigators

J.I. Suarez, MD(✉) • E. Calvillo, RN • E.M. Bershad, MD
C.P. Venkatasubba Rao, MD
Division of Vascular Neurology and Neurocritical Care,
Baylor College of Medicine, Baylor St Luke's Medical Center,
6501 Fannin ST, NB:302, Houston, TX 77030, USA
e-mail: jisuarez@bcm.edu

R.H. Martin, PhD
Division of Biostatistics and Epidemiology, Medical University of South Carolina, Charleston, SC, USA

Introduction

Subarachnoid hemorrhage (SAH) is a devastating disease and neurological emergency that represents about 5 % of all strokes. However, SAH accounts for 27 % of all stroke-related years of potential life lost before the age of 65 years [10]. In addition, many survivors report impaired mood or cognitive function. These statistics underlie the importance of finding newer therapeutic approaches to improve outcome of SAH patients. The only medication that has shown modest efficacy in SAH is nimodipine [3]. Recent clinical trials have failed to demonstrate any benefit of compounds targeting various cellular pathways [4, 6]. We have completed the Albumin In Subarachnoid Hemorrhage (ALISAH) pilot clinical trial [7, 8]. The objective of the present analysis was to determine the effect of 25 % human albumin (ALB) on mean cerebral blood flow velocities (MCBFV) as determined by transcranial Doppler ultrasound (TCD), delayed cerebral ischemia (DCI), and cerebral infarctions in patients enrolled in the ALISAH study.

Materials and Methods

Study Design

The detailed design of the ALISAH Pilot Clinical Trial was described elsewhere [8]. Briefly, ALISAH was designed to investigate the safety and treatment effect of four different dosages of ALB of increasing magnitude (0.625, 1.25, 1.875, and 2.5 g/kg; tiers 1, 2, 3, and 4, respectively). Each dosage was to be administered to 20 adult subjects daily for 7 days. We found that ALB up to 1.25 g/kg/day × 7 days was tolerated by SAH patients with improved outcomes. The study was stopped after 47 subjects were enrolled (20 in tier 1, 20 in tier 2, and 7 in tier 3) [7] because of severe cardiovascular side effects in dosage tier 3. Subjects were

J. Fandino et al. (eds.), *Neurovascular Events After Subarachnoid Hemorrhage:* Acta Neurochirurgica Supplement, Vol. 120,
DOI 10.1007/978-3-319-04981-6_48, © Springer International Publishing Switzerland 2015

monitored in the ICU during the acute phase (study days 1–7) with daily TCD.

ALISAH was approved by the Institutional Review/Ethics Committee of each participating institution, all participants provided written, informed consent, and procedures and treatments followed were in accordance with study protocol and institutional guidelines.

Outcomes

The outcomes for the current analysis included TCD vasospasm, DCI, and cerebral infarctions on head CT scans at 90 days [8]. TCD vasospasm was defined as MCBFV > 120 cm/s, and Lindegaard ratio > 3 in either middle cerebral artery (MCA) [9]. DCI was defined as any neurological deterioration (e.g., hemiparesis, aphasia, altered consciousness) presumed related to ischemia that persisted for more than an hour and could not be explained by other diagnoses on imaging studies, electrophysiological, or laboratory findings, and that occurred within 4–14 days after SAH [3, 8]. Cerebral infarctions were classified as new or old, compared with postaneurysm treatment on head CT, and the territory of infarction was determined. All head CT scans were interpreted by a central board-certified neuroradiologist blinded to the treatment tier.

Statistical Analysis

The statistical analysis for the data presented is primarily descriptive. Subject assignment to each treatment tier was not randomized, but done sequentially by dose-escalation following clearance by the Data and Safety Monitoring Board (DSMB). Data are presented as means ± standard deviation, median and range, or numbers and proportion as appropriate.

Results

Of the 47 subjects enrolled in the ALISAH study, 2 (1 in tier 1 and 1 in tier 3) died and 2 (1 in tier 1 and 1 in tier 2) withdrew consent. However, these events occurred after study day 7, which allowed the collection of TCD data during the treatment phase for all subjects. We also have complete data collection for DCI events. Head CT scan at 90 days was voluntary and available for 33 patients; 11 for tier 1, 18 for tier 2, and 4 for tier 3.

As previously reported, most subjects were women (72 %), white (87 %), and the median age was 51 years [7]. Most subjects (62 %) were current smokers and all were independent before SAH. There were more current smokers in tier 1 (75 %), compared with tiers 2 (55 %) and 3 (43 %). Ruptured aneurysms were mostly located in the anterior circulation, and located more on the right side (22/47) compared with the left side (12/47), both sides (5/47), and midline (8/47). Aneurysms were treated within 24 h of symptom onset, mostly with coiling (72 %).

In Table 1, we present the outcomes investigated for this report. We found that subjects in higher ALB dosage tiers experienced less TCD vasospasm, DCI, and cerebral infarctions. We also present the MCBFV trends during the treatment period in Fig. 1. MCBFVs for subjects in tier 2 were lower overall, particularly in the left MCA compared with tiers 1 and 3. MCBFV for dosage tier 3 was higher at baseline and remained higher, mostly because of 1 subject who experienced severe elevation (>200 cm/s) in both MCAs.

Discussion

ALB has been shown to be neuroprotective in animal models of cerebral ischemia [1, 2]. In addition, there is some preliminary data indicating improved clinical outcome in patients with ischemic stroke [5]. We have shown that ALB dosages up to 1.25 g/kg/day × 7 days are well tolerated and may improve outcome in SAH patients [7]. This finding extends the applicability of ALB to clinical entities other than ischemic stroke.

The mechanisms by which ALB accomplish its salutatory effects on the brain are still under investigation but may include several actions [5, 7]. ALB administration can produce an increase in the serum oncotic pressure, which draws interstitial fluid and ameliorates organ perfusion. Moreover, ALB has significant antioxidant properties and can improve microcirculatory blood flow while decreasing leukocyte adherence with resultant anti-inflammatory effects.

Conclusion

Although exploratory in nature, increasing doses of ALB may be associated with lower rates of TCD vasospasm, DCI, and cerebral infarctions. The current report suggests that one possible mechanism for the improved outcome seen in SAH subjects may be related to improved cerebral blood flow with resultant decreased events of DCI and cerebral infarctions. Further investigation of this finding is needed.

Table 1 Outcomes according to treatment tier

Outcome	Tier 1 (0.625 g/kg)	Tier 2 (1.25 g/kg)	Tier 3 (1.875 g/kg)	All groups
TCD vasospasm	15/20 (75 %)	11/20 (55 %)	2/7 (28.6 %)	28/47 (59.6 %)
DCI	4/20 (20 %)	3/20 (15 %)	1/7 (14.3 %)	8/47 (17 %)
Cerebral infarction	5/11 (45 %)	3/18 (16 %)	1/4 (25 %)	9/33 (27 %)
New	3/11 (27 %)	3/18 (16 %)	0	6/33 (18 %)
Old	2/11 (18 %)	0	1/4 (25 %)	3/33 (9 %)
Vascular territory	All MCA	1 MCA, 2 ACA	MCA	7 MCA, 2 ACA

TCD transcranial Doppler ultrasound, *DCI* delayed cerebral infarction, *MCA* middle cerebral artery, *ACA* anterior cerebral

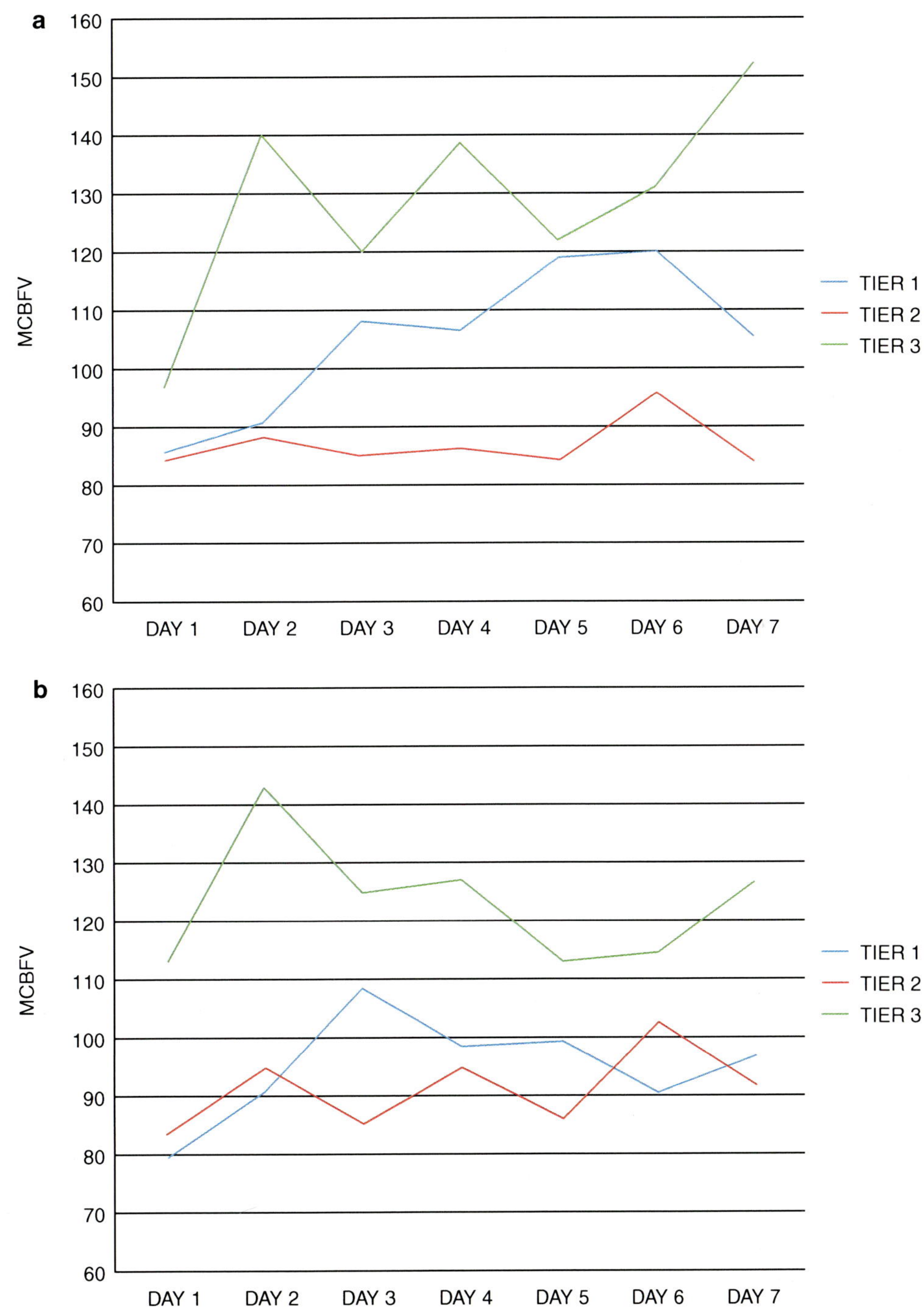

Fig. 1 Distribution of MCBFV by treatment tier. (**a**) Left MCA. (**b**) Right MCA. *MCA* middle cerebral artery, *MCBFV* mean cerebral blood flow velocity

Acknowledgments and Sources of Funding ALISAH was funded by the NIH/NINDS (R01NS049135; PI: Suarez JI).

ALB was provided by GRIFOLS International (Barcelona, Spain) at no cost to the study.

Clinical Trial Registration – URL: http://www.clinicaltrials.gov. Unique identifier: NCT00283400.

Disclosures None.

Conflict of Interest Statement We declare that we have no conflict of interest.

References

1. Belayev L, Liu Y, Zhao W, Busto R, Ginsberg MD (2001) Human albumin therapy of acute ischemic stroke: marked neuroprotective efficacy at moderate doses and with a broad therapeutic window. Stroke 32:553–560
2. Belayev L, Zhao W, Pattany PM, Weaver RG, Huh PW, Lin B (1998) Diffusion-weighted magnetic resonance imaging confirms marked neuroprotection efficacy of albumin therapy in focal cerebral ischemia. Stroke 29:2587–2599
3. Diringer MN, Bleck TP, Claude Hemphill J 3rd, Menon D, Shutter L, Vespa P et al (2011) Critical Care Management of patients following aneurysmal subarachnoid hemorrhage: recommendations from the Neurocritical Care Society's Multidisciplinary Consensus Conference. Neurocrit Care 15:211–240
4. Dorhout Mees SM, Algra A, Vandertop WP, van Kooten F, Kuijsten HA, Boiten J et al (2012) Magnesium for aneurysmal subarachnoid hemorrhage (MASH-2): a randomized placebo-controlled trial. Lancet 380:44–49
5. Hill MD, Martin RH, Palesch YY, Tamariz D, Waldman BD, Ryckborst KJ et al (2011) The Albumin in Acute Stroke Part 1 trial: an exploratory efficacy analysis. Stroke 42:1621–1625
6. Macdonald RL, Higashida RT, Keller E, Mayer SA, Molyneux A, Raabe A et al (2012) Randomized trials of clazosentan in patients with aneurysmal subarachnoid hemorrhage undergoing endovascular coiling. Stroke 43:1463–1469
7. Suarez JI, Martin RH, Calvillo E, Dillon C, Bershad EM, Macdonald RL et al (2012) The Albumin In Subarachnoid Hemorrhage (ALISAH) multicenter pilot clinical trial: safety and neurologic outcomes. Stroke 43:683–690
8. Suarez JI, Martin RH (2010) Treatment of subarachnoid hemorrhage with human albumin: ALISAH study. Rationale and design. Neurocrit Care 13:262–277
9. Suarez JI, Qureshi AI, Yahia AB, Parekh PD, Tamargo RJ, Williams MA et al (2002) Symptomatic vasospasm diagnosis after subarachnoid hemorrhage: evaluation of transcranial Doppler ultrasound and cerebral angiography as related to compromised vascular distribution. Crit Care Med 30:1348–1355
10. Suarez JI, Tarr RW, Selman WR (2006) Aneurysmal subarachnoid hemorrhage. N Engl J Med 354:387–396

Risk Factors for Vasospasm-Induced Cerebral Infarct When Both Clipping and Coiling Are Equally Available

Kenji Kanamaru, Hidenori Suzuki, and Waro Taki

Abstract *Introduction*: Vasospasm-induced cerebral infarct is still a significant cause of poor outcome after aneurysmal subarachnoid hemorrhage (SAH).

Materials and Methods: In 537 patients of the Prospective Registry of Subarachnoid Aneurysms Treatment cohort, ruptured aneurysms were treated either microsurgically or endovascularly judged by the attending neurosurgeon to be appropriate for the individual patient within 3 days of onset. Factors for vasospasm-induced cerebral infarct were examined.

Results: Clipping (273 patients) was preferably performed for middle cerebral artery aneurysms, while coiling (264 patients) was preferred for larger, internal carotid artery and posterior circulation aneurysms. After aneurysmal obliteration, cerebrospinal fluid drainage was performed more in clipped patients, and antithrombotic treatment was performed more in coiled patients. Vasospasm-induced cerebral infarct occurred in 17.7 %, and multivariable logistic regression showed that vasospasm-induced cerebral infarct increased the odds of poor outcome by a factor of 5.2 (adjusted odds ratio, 5.2; 95 % confidence interval, 2.8–9.8; $P<0.001$). Multivariate analyses showed that vasospasm-induced cerebral infarct was significantly associated with admission World Federation of Neurosurgical Societies grade IV–V, Fisher computed tomography (CT) group 3–4, and ruptured middle cerebral artery aneurysms.

Conclusions: New treatment strategies for vasospasm-induced cerebral infarct are needed, especially for ruptured middle cerebral artery aneurysm cases associated with massive SAH.

Keywords Cerebral aneurysm • Cerebral vasospasm • Cerebral infarct • Endovascular treatment • Microsurgery • Subarachnoid hemorrhage

Introduction

Aneurysmal subarachnoid hemorrhage (SAH) remains a devastating neurological disorder [11]. Recent studies provided evidence that cerebral infarction had the strongest association with poor outcomes, and therefore multidisciplinary research groups recommended that SAH clinical trials should only use cerebral infarction and functional outcome as the primary outcome measures [1, 16]. Clinical deterioration caused by delayed cerebral ischemia and angiographic vasospasm should only be secondary outcome measures [16]. However, few studies have investigated predictors for severe vasospasm or vasospasm-induced cerebral infarct, although many predictors have been reported for the incidence of cerebral vasospasm [3, 6]. Thus, the aim of this study was to examine predictors for vasospasm-induced cerebral infarct and its impact on outcomes after SAH at the period when both clipping and coiling are equally available.

K. Kanamaru, MD, PhD
Department of Neurosurgery, Suzuka Kaisei Hospital, Suzuka, Japan

H. Suzuki, MD, PhD (✉)
Department of Neurosurgery, Mie University Graduate School of Medicine, 2-174 Edobashi, Tsu, Mie 514-8507, Japan

Research Center for Matrix Biology, Mie University Graduate School of Medicine, 2-174 Edobashi, Tsu, Mie 514-8507, Japan
e-mail: suzuki02@clin.medic.mie-u.ac.jp

W. Taki, MD, PhD
Department of Neurosurgery, Mie University Graduate School of Medicine, 2-174 Edobashi, Tsu, Mie 514-8507, Japan

J. Fandino et al. (eds.), *Neurovascular Events After Subarachnoid Hemorrhage*, Acta Neurochirurgica Supplement, Vol. 120,
DOI 10.1007/978-3-319-04981-6_49, © Springer International Publishing Switzerland 2015

Materials and Methods

Patient and Clinical Variables

This study used data from a prospective cohort study (Prospective Registry of Subarachnoid Aneurysms Treatment) performed at 29 tertiary referral centers in Japan that provide both microsurgical clipping and endovascular coiling, depending on the characteristics of each case, between March 2006 and February 2007 [12–15]. The Institutional Ethics Committee approved the study. Of 760 SAH patients who reached the centers, 614 patients met the following inclusion criteria: ≥20 years of age at onset, SAH on computed tomography (CT) scans or lumbar puncture, saccular aneurysm as the cause of SAH confirmed on three-dimensional CT angiography (3D-CTA) or digital subtraction angiography (DSA), and aneurysmal obliteration by clipping or coiling within 14 days of onset. Excluded from the study were patients with ruptured fusiform, dissecting, traumatic, mycotic, and arteriovenous malformation-related aneurysms or SAH of unknown etiology, and patients who were treated using medical instruments or drugs that were not approved by the Japanese Ministry of Health, Labor and Welfare; thus, none of the patients in this series were treated with nimodipine, surface-modified or bioactive coils, or intracranial stents. Because 26 patients did not give written informed consent, the remaining 588 patients were registered to the data center within 2 days of the initial treatment. For the purpose of this study, nine cases of missing data of vasospasm and 42 cases of no aneurysmal obliteration within 3 days of onset were excluded. Thus, 537 cases were eligible for this study. Timing of aneurysmal obliteration, selection of clipping or coiling, and other medical management or treatment were decided by site investigators and not limited.

Baseline demographic and clinical data included age, gender, World Federation of Neurosurgical Societies (WFNS) grade on admission [2], Fisher CT group on admission [4], interval from ictus to aneurysmal obliteration, modality used for aneurysmal obliteration, and location and size of the ruptured aneurysm. The aneurysms were classified into four groups: small size/small neck, small size/wide neck, large, and giant. Small size/small neck aneurysms were defined as aneurysms having a maximum aneurysmal diameter (A) <10 mm, neck size (N) <4 mm and $A/N \geq 1.5$; small size/wide neck as $A < 10$ mm, $N \geq 4$ mm and $A/N < 1.5$; large as $A \geq 10$ mm but <25 mm; and giant as $A \geq 25$ mm.

Data on other treatments and complications included cerebrospinal fluid (CSF) drainage, antiplatelet administration, endovascular therapy for vasospasm, symptomatic vasospasm, and vasospasm-induced cerebral infarction. Ventricular, cisternal, or spinal CSF drainage was established to control acute hydrocephalus or to promote subarachnoid blood clearance. Antiplatelets were administered to prevent overthrombosis after coiling or to prevent symptomatic vasospasm. Symptomatic vasospasm was defined as otherwise unexplained clinical deterioration (i.e., a new focal deficit, decrease in the level of consciousness, or both) or a new infarct on CT that was not visible on admission or immediate postoperative scan (vasospasm-induced cerebral infarction), or both. Other potential causes of clinical deterioration, such as hydrocephalus, rebleeding, or seizures, were rigorously excluded. Determination of these complications was made at each center, and the organizing and protocol committee qualified them [13]. Outcome was blindly assessed using the modified Rankin Scale (mRS) [7] at 3 and 12 months after SAH.

Statistics

Categorical variables were reported as a proportion and percentile and were analyzed using the chi-square or Fisher's exact test, as appropriate. Continuous variables were reported as a mean ± standard deviation and compared using the unpaired t test. The impact of each variable on vasospasm-induced cerebral infarction or poor outcome was determined by multivariate unconditional logistic regression analyses using the dichotomous status (presence or absence) as the dependent variable. All variables were considered independent variables regardless of the significance on univariate analysis, although only the variable with the smallest probability value was used as a candidate variable among similar clinical variables that were intercorrelated. Adjusted odds ratios (ORs) with 95 % confidence intervals (CIs) were calculated and independence of variables was tested using the likelihood ratio test on reduced models. Two-tailed probability values <0.05 were considered significant.

Results

Characteristics of Patients and Aneurysms Treated with Clipping or Coiling

Clipping ($n = 273$) was preferably performed for middle cerebral artery (MCA) aneurysms (clip vs. coil = 106 cases [38.8 %] vs. 16 [6.1], $P < 0.001$), while coiling ($n = 264$) was preferred for larger dome-sized (6.1 ± 3.2 mm vs. 6.9 ± 3.9, $P < 0.025$), internal carotid artery (69 cases [25.3 %] vs. 92 [34.8], $P < 0.025$) and posterior circulation (11 cases [4.0 %] vs. 58 [22.0], $P < 0.001$) aneurysms. Patient age, gender, WFNS grade and Fisher CT group on admission, aneurysm neck size, and classification were not

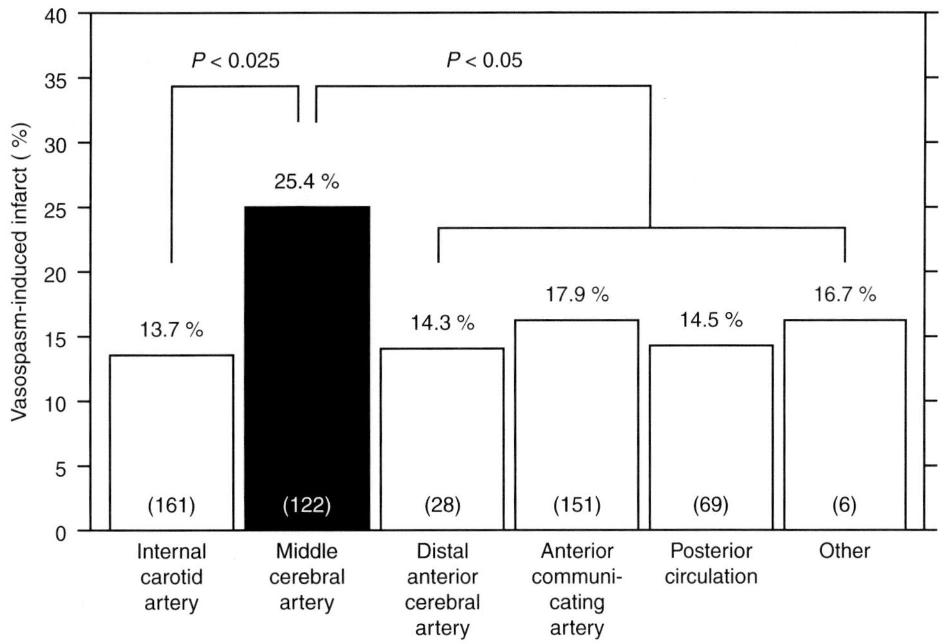

Fig. 1 Incidence of vasospasm-induced cerebral infarct stratified by aneurysm location. *()* number of cases, *P* value chi-square test

significantly different between the treatment modalities. After aneurysmal obliteration, CSF drainage was performed more in clipped patients (207 cases [75.8 %] vs. 158 [59.8], $P<0.001$), and antithrombotic treatment was performed more in coiled patients (22 cases [8.1 %] vs. 107 [40.5], $P<0.001$).

Vasospasm and Outcome

The incidence of symptomatic vasospasm (66 cases [24.2 %] vs. 50 [18.9]) and endovascular therapy for vasospasm (33 cases [12.1 %] vs. 24 [9.1]) was not significantly different between clipping and coiling. Vasospasm-induced cerebral infarct occurred more frequently after clipping than coiling (57 cases [20.9 %] vs. 38 [14.4], $P<0.05$). Multivariate analyses showed that Fisher CT group 3–4 (OR, 3.663; 95 % CI, 1.502–8.935; $P=0.004$), admission WFNS grade IV–V (1.958; 1.201–3.193; $P=0.007$), and MCA aneurysm (1.786; 1.013–3.151; $P=0.045$) were significant factors for vasospasm-induced cerebral infarction, when patient age, gender, admission WFNS grade (I–III or IV–V), Fisher CT group (1–2 or 3–4), aneurysm location (MCA or non-MCA), dome size, neck size, treatment modality (clipping or coiling), antiplatelet therapy, and CSF drainage (with/without irrigation) were used in the analyses. The difference in the incidence of vasospasm-induced cerebral infarct between clipping and coiling was explained by the fact that the majority of MCA aneurysms were treated by clipping (Fig. 1).

With regard to outcomes (Table 1), the incidence of independent survival (mRS 0–2) was similar between clipping and coiling at both 3 (62.6 vs. 67.3 %) and 12 (67.3 vs. 71.4 %) months after SAH. Multivariate logistic regression with poor outcome (1-year mRS 3–6) as a binary outcome demonstrated vasospasm-induced cerebral infarct to be a significant prognostic factor when patient age, gender, admission WFNS grade, Fisher CT group, aneurysm location, dome size, neck size, pretreatment aneurysm rerupture (in hospital, $n=41$, 7.6 %), treatment modality, antiplatelet therapy ($n=129$, 24.0 %), CSF drainage (with/without irrigation, $n=365$, 68.0 %), vasospasm-induced cerebral infarct ($n=95$, 17.7 %), shunt-dependent hydrocephalus ($n=101$, 18.8 %), epilepsy ($n=26$, 4.8 %), infection (sepsis, pneumonia, etc.; $n=48$, 8.9 %), noninfectious cardiopulmonary complications ($n=35$, 6.5 %), clipping-related complications ($n=84$, 15.6 %), and coiling-related complications ($n=52$, 9.7 %) were used in the analyses (Table 2).

Discussion

This prospective registry study showed that vasospasm-induced cerebral infarct remains a significant causative factor for poor outcome after SAH when ruptured aneurysms were treated either microsurgically or endovascularly based on the judgment of the attending neurosurgeon to be appropriate for the individual patient within 3 days of onset. Multivariate analyses showed that admission WFNS grade

IV–V, Fisher CT group 3–4, and ruptured MCA aneurysms were independent factors for the development of vasospasm-induced cerebral infarct. Treatment modalities did not significantly affect the incidence of vasospasm-induced cerebral infarct, although this was not a randomized study and the characteristics of patients and postprocedural management were different between clipping and coiling.

Table 1 Modified Rankin Scale (mRS) at 3 and 12 months after subarachnoid hemorrhage

Variable	Clip (*n*=273)	Coil (*n*=264)	*P* value[a]
mRS at 3 months	*n*=270	*n*=263	
0	86 (31.9)	131 (49.8)	<0.001
1	39 (14.4)	24 (9.1)	ns
2	44 (16.3)	22 (8.4)	<0.01
3	19 (7.0)	11 (4.2)	ns
4	37 (13.7)	28 (10.6)	ns
5	22 (8.1)	21 (8.0)	ns
6	23 (8.5)	26 (9.9)	ns
0–1	125 (46.3)	155 (58.9)	<0.005
0–2	169 (62.6)	177 (67.3)	ns
mRS at 12 months	*n*=263	*n*=255	
0	105 (39.9)	145 (56.9)	<0.001
1	36 (13.7)	25 (9.8)	ns
2	36 (13.7)	12 (4.7)	<0.001
3	21 (8.0)	13 (5.1)	ns
4	25 (9.5)	17 (6.7)	ns
5	14 (5.3)	14 (5.5)	ns
6	26 (9.9)	29 (11.4)	ns
0–1	141 (53.6)	170 (66.7)	<0.005
0–2	177 (67.3)	182 (71.4)	ns

Number of cases (%)
ns not significant
[a]Chi-square test

Younger age, worse clinical grade on admission, more blood volume on the initial CT scan, acute hydrocephalus, transcranial Doppler (TCD) ultrasound values, and the modality of aneurysm treatment have been suggested as predictors for the incidence of cerebral vasospasm [6]. However, it remains unclear whether vasospasm severity can be predicted. Jabbarli et al. [6] reported that significant predictors for severe vasospasm were younger age (<51 years of age) and early onset of mean flow velocities >160 cm/s on TCD ultrasound in a retrospective study including 70 consecutive patients with aneurysmal SAH, most of which were treated endovascularly. Fergusen et al. [3] reported that predictors associated with cerebral infarction in the tirilazad data set, in which all ruptured aneurysms were treated by clipping, were increasing age, history of hypertension or diabetes mellitus, worse WFNS grade, larger aneurysm size, symptomatic vasospasm, temperature higher than 38 °C at 8 days after SAH, and use of prophylactically or therapeutically induced hypertension. Cerebral infarction was strongly associated with poor outcome after aneurysmal SAH, and the most important potentially treatable factor associated with infarction was symptomatic vasospasm [3]. Regarding aneurysm location, the effects of poor outcome are obscure and variable depending on studies. Ruptured MCA aneurysms associated with massive Sylvian hematoma cause acute cerebral swelling, which may aggravate vasospasm and the resultant cerebral infarct, leading to poor outcome [9, 10].

Recently, early brain injury has attracted considerable attention as a cause of delayed brain injury after SAH other than vasospasm [5]. Naidech et al. [8] reported that some cerebral infarctions occurred by day 2 or associated with no angiographic vasospasm. In a multivariate analysis, cerebral infarction was significantly related to worse WFNS grade and SAH–Physiologic Derangement Score >2 on admission. Global cerebral edema was also predictive of cerebral infarction [8]. These findings suggest that physiological derangement and cerebral edema may be clinical indicators of early brain injury and be worthwhile targets for intervention to

Table 2 Significant variables in multivariate logistic regression with poor outcome (1-year modified Rankin Scale 3–6) as a binary outcome

Variables	Odds ratio	95 % confidence interval	*P* value
Age	1.081	1.055–1.107	<0.001
WFNS grade IV	3.628	1.730–7.607	0.001
WFNS grade V	13.105	5.218–32.911	<0.001
Coiling-related complications	2.562	1.026–6.398	0.044
Vasospasm-induced cerebral infarct	5.190	2.751–9.792	<0.001
Shunt-dependent hydrocephalus	2.201	1.194–4.057	0.011

Age, sex, World Federation of Neurosurgical Societies (WFNS) grade on admission, Fisher computed tomography (CT) group, aneurysm location, dome size, neck size, pretreatment aneurysm rerupture (in hospital), treatment modality, antiplatelet therapy, cerebrospinal fluid drainage (with/without irrigation), vasospasm-induced cerebral infarct, shunt-dependent hydrocephalus, epilepsy, infection, cardiopulmonary complications, clipping-related complications, and coiling-related complications were used in multivariate logistic regression. Age and size were used as continuous variables decrease the occurrence and clinical impact of cerebral infarction after SAH, although this study did not address those issues.

Conclusion

In summary, this study showed that vasospasm-induced cerebral infarct still has a significant impact on poor outcome, and that new treatment strategies for vasospasm-induced cerebral infarct are needed, especially for ruptured MCA aneurysm cases associated with massive SAH. The next study should also clinically study impacts of early brain injury on delayed cerebral injury, cerebral infarct development, and poor outcome after SAH.

Conflict of Interest Statement We declare that we have no conflict of interest.

References

1. Diringer MN, Bleck TP, Hemphill JC III, Menon D, Shutter L, Vespa P, Bruder N, Connolly ES Jr, Citerio G, Gress D, Hanggi D, Hoh BL, Lanzino G, Roux PL, Rabinstein A, Schmutzhard E, Stocchetti N, Suarez JI, Treggiari M, Tseng M-Y, Vergouwen MDI, Wolf S, Zipfel G (2011) Critical care management of patients following aneurysmal subarachnoid hemorrhage: recommendations from the Neurocritical Care Society's Multidisciplinary Consensus Conference. Neurocrit Care 15:211–240
2. Drake CG (1988) Report of World Federation of Neurological Surgeons Committee on a universal subarachnoid hemorrhage grading scale. J Neurosurg 68:985–986
3. Fergusen S, Macdonald RL (2007) Predictors of cerebral infarction in patients with aneurysmal subarachnoid hemorrhage. Neurosurgery 60:658–667
4. Fisher CM, Kistler JP, Davis JM (1980) Relation of cerebral vasospasm to subarachnoid hemorrhage visualized by computerized tomographic scanning. Neurosurgery 6:1–9
5. Hou J, Zhang JH (2013) Does prevention of vasospasm in subarachnoid hemorrhage improve clinical outcome? No. Stroke 44(Suppl 1):S34–S36
6. Jabbarli R, Gläsker S, Weber J, Taschner C, Olschewski M, Van Velthoven V (2013) Predictors of severity of cerebral vasospasm caused by aneurysmal subarachnoid hemorrhage. J Stroke Cerebrovasc Dis 22:1332–1339
7. Lyden PD, Lau GT (1991) A critical appraisal of stroke evaluation and rating scales. Stroke 22:1345–1352
8. Naidech AM, Drescher J, Tamul P, Shaibani A, Batjer HH, Alberts MJ (2006) Acute physiological derangement is associated with early radiographic cerebral infarction after subarachnoid haemorrhage. J Neurol Neurosurg Psychiatry 77:1340–1344
9. Niikawa S, Kitajima H, Ohe N, Miwa Y, Ohkuma A (1998) Significance of acute cerebral swelling in patients with Sylvian hematoma due to ruptured middle cerebral artery aneurysm, and its management. Neurol Med Chir (Tokyo) 38:844–850
10. Smith ER, Carter BS, Ogilvy CS (2002) Proposed use of prophylactic decompressive craniectomy in poor-grade aneurysmal subarachnoid hemorrhage patients presenting with associated large Sylvian hematomas. Neurosurgery 51:117–124
11. Suarez JI, Tarr RW, Selman WR (2006) Aneurysmal subarachnoid hemorrhage. N Engl J Med 354:387–396
12. Suzuki H, Taki W, Prospective Registry of Subarachnoid Aneurysms Treatment (PRESAT) group (2013) Effect of aneurysm treatment modalities on cerebral vasospasm after aneurysmal subarachnoid hemorrhage. Acta Neurochir Suppl 115: 99–105
13. Taki W, Sakai N, Suzuki H, Prospective Registry of Subarachnoid Aneurysms Treatment (PRESAT) group (2011) Determinants of poor outcome following aneurysmal subarachnoid hemorrhage when both clipping and coiling are available: PRESAT in Japan. World Neurosurg 76:437–445
14. Taki W, Sakai N, Suzuki H, Prospective Registry of Subarachnoid Aneurysms Treatment (PRESAT) group (2012) Factors predicting retreatment and residual aneurysms at 1 year after endovascular coiling for ruptured cerebral aneurysms: PRESAT in Japan. Neuroradiology 54:597–606
15. Taki W, Sakai N, Suzuki H, Prospective Registry of Subarachnoid Aneurysms Treatment (PRESAT) group (2013) Importance of independently evaluated initial anatomic result after endovascular coiling for ruptured cerebral aneurysms. J Clin Neurosci 20: 527–531
16. Vergouwen MDI, Vermeulen M, van Gijn J, Rinkel GJE, Wijdicks EF, Muizelaar JP, Mendelow AD, Juvela S, Yonas H, Terbrugge KG, Macdonald RL, Diringer MN, Broderick JP, Dreier JP, Roos YBWEM (2010) Definition of delayed cerebral ischemia after aneurysmal subarachnoid hemorrhage as an outcome event in clinical trials and observational studies. Proposal of a Multidisciplinary Research Group. Stroke 41:2391–2395

Effectiveness of Intraarterial Administration of Fasudil Hydrochloride for Preventing Symptomatic Vasospasm After Subarachnoid Hemorrhage

Atsushi Saito, Mizuho Inoue, Hiroyuki Kon, Shunji Imaruoka, Kiyoshi Basaki, Hiroshi Midorikawa, Tatsuya Sasaki, and Michiharu Nishijima

Abstract *Objective*: We examined the effect of intraarterial administration of fasudil hydrochloride (IAFC), a Rho kinase inhibitor, for the prevention of symptomatic vasospasm after SAH by evaluating cerebral circulation.

Methods: We evaluated IAFC cases of 57 sides of 38 patients (12 men and 26 women, average age 60.2 years old) diagnosed with aneurysmal subarachnoid hemorrhage (SAH) from February 2012 to November 2012. All cases were treated by clipping or coil embolization within 48 h after onset. Indication for IAFC was the existence of a spastic change on follow-up digital subtraction angiography (DSA) compared with that of onset.

Results: Clipping was performed in 30 cases and coil embolization in 8 cases. IAFC was performed an average of 6.6 days after onset. Color gradient mapping demonstrated reduction of the circulation time after IAFC compared with before IAFC on 39 sides, no change on 15 sides, and extension on 3 sides. Average arterial circulation time before IAFC was 2.25 ± 0.57 s and after IAFC was 1.95 ± 0.55 s. IAFC significantly shortened average arterial circulation ($P = 0.005$). No case developed symptomatic vasospasm after IAFC.

Conclusion: IAFC significantly reduced the cerebral circulation time after aneurysmal SAH and might be effective for the prevention of symptomatic vasospasm.

Keywords Subarachnoid hemorrhage • Vasospasm • Fasudil hydrochloride • Circulation time

A. Saito, MD, PhD (✉) • M. Inoue • H. Kon • S. Imaruoka
K. Basaki • H. Midorikawa • T. Sasaki • M. Nishijima
Departments of Neurosurgery and Radiology,
Aomori Prefectural Central Hospital,
2-1-1 Higashitsukurimichi, Aomori 0308553, Japan
e-mail: satsushi2002@yahoo.co.jp

Introduction

Aneurysmal subarachnoid hemorrhage (SAH) is a major cause of stroke; approximately 3–15 % of all stroke cases are attributed to ruptured intracranial aneurysms [1, 15]. Outcome of treatment after SAH depends on several factors, including the severity of the initial event, peri-ictal medical management, various surgical variables, and incidence of SAH-related complications. Cerebral vasospasm is the most frequent and troublesome complication of SAH [15].

Various protein kinases, such as myosin light chain kinase, protein kinase C, and Rho kinase, have been reported to play a critical role in the signal transduction pathway underlying the development of cerebral vasospasm [4, 5, 10]. Therapy with fasudil, a Rho-kinase inhibitor (RKI), is effective for preventing cerebral vasospasm and subsequent ischemic injury after surgery for aneurysmal SAH [13]. Fasudil has been widely used in Japan for this indication since 1995 [16, 17]. Hydroxyfasudil, an active metabolite of fasudil, also inhibits Rho-kinase [14], and has a pharmacological profile similar to that of fasudil. Hydroxyfasudil improves hemodynamic function by increasing regional cerebral blood flow and by ameliorating endothelial damage/dysfunction; moreover, it prevents inflammatory responses by inhibiting neutrophil and monocyte infiltration [11, 12]. The area under the plasma concentration–time curve for hydroxyfasudil was estimated to be approximately 4.5 times more than that for fasudil in patients who had SAH and were receiving 30 mg of fasudil [17]. However, the precise mechanism of vasospasm development after SAH remains unclear and a definitive prevention therapy has not been established yet.

There are a number of methods for assessing the features of vasospasm and for predicting its occurrence. Measuring the cerebral circulation time (CCT), which is the transit time

DOI 10.1007/978-3-319-04981-6_50,

of a contrast dye from the arterial to the venous phase, is one of the methods to evaluate hemodynamic changes caused by vasospasm. Several studies have suggested that the CCT can be used to estimate the cerebral blood flow or cerebrovascular reserve, mean transit time, and oxygen ejection fraction on a positron emission tomographic scan [4, 19]. Further, some investigators have observed that CCT can be prolonged during vasospasm and improves after vasospasm treatment with papaverine and/or angioplasty [3, 6]. Udoetuk et al. focused on angiographic circulation time and reported that prolonged CCT, which suggests increased small vessel resistance, can be detected within 24 h after SAH and is associated with subsequent angiographic vasospasm [18].

In this study, we determined the effectiveness of intraarterial administration of fasudil hydrochloride (IAFC) for preventing symptomatic vasospasm after SAH by evaluating cerebral arterial circulation using digital subtraction angiography (DSA).

Methods

Patient population

From January 2008 to January 2013, 237 cases of aneurysmal SAH were treated in our institute. We focused on recent cases that received IAFC and the effect of IAFC was evaluated by cerebral circulation. Between February 2012 and November 2012, IAFC was performed on 57 sides of 38 patients (12 men and 26 women; average age, 60.2 years) who were diagnosed with aneurysmal SAH. All cases were treated by clipping or coil embolization within 48 h after onset. Location of the aneurysm was determined at onset and vasospasm was diagnosed 5–7 days after onset, both were determined using DSA. We performed multidisciplinary treatments for preventing vasospasm development after SAH, such as intraoperative irrigation with saline containing urokinase during the surgical maneuver, intrathecal administration of urokinase for remnant clots after obliteration of the aneurysm, intravenous administration of fasudil hydrochloride, and IAFC [2, 9]. IAFC was indicated by the existence of a spastic change on follow-up DSA compared with that at onset. An endovascular technique and 30 mg of fasudil hydrochloride were used for IAFC, which was performed from the ICA, the main trunks of the middle cerebral artery (MCA), or the anterior cerebral artery (ACA).

Evaluation of cerebral circulation

Arterial circulation time was determined by calculating the time from the appearance of the contrast medium in the terminal portion of the ICA to its appearance in the capillary phase and was analyzed quantitatively. This evaluation was performed by modifying the method previously reported in Udoetuk et al. [18].

Color gradient-mapping images showing cerebral arterial blood flow were visualized using AngioViz (GE Healthcare, France). AngioViz produces color-coded parametric images representing time to peak and maximum pixel opacification. The AngioViz imaging software (Innova3131IQ, GE Healthcare, France) can be used for DSA images of any region in the body and produces color-coded parametric images representing time to peak, maximum pixel opacification, and combinations of these parameters to assist in the visualization of vascular flow.

Results

Clipping was performed in 30 patients and coil embolization was performed in 8 patients. The Hunt and Kosnik grade was 2 for 27 patients, 3 for 8 patients, and 4 for 3 patients. The ruptured aneurysm was located in the ACA in 1 patient, the anterior communicating artery in 13 patients, the MCA in 11 patients, the ICA in 8 patients, and the posterior circulation in 4 patients. Angiographic vasospasm was found to occur 16 times in the A1 to A2 portion of the ACA, 13 times in the M1 to M2 portion of the MCA, and 3 times in the ICA (to ICA terminal portion). Peripheral dominant angiographic vasospasm, in which spastic findings were located distal to the A2 portion of the ACA or the M2 portion of the MCA, was observed 25 times.

Cerebral arterial circulation before and after IAFC

No significant difference was observed in the systolic blood pressure, diastolic blood pressure, and heart rate before and after IAFC. The average cerebral arterial circulation time was 2.25 ± 0.57 s and 1.95 ± 0.55 s before and after IAFC, respectively, as measured using DSA. Cerebral arterial circulation time from the appearance of the contrast at the ICA terminal to its appearance in the capillary phase was signifi-

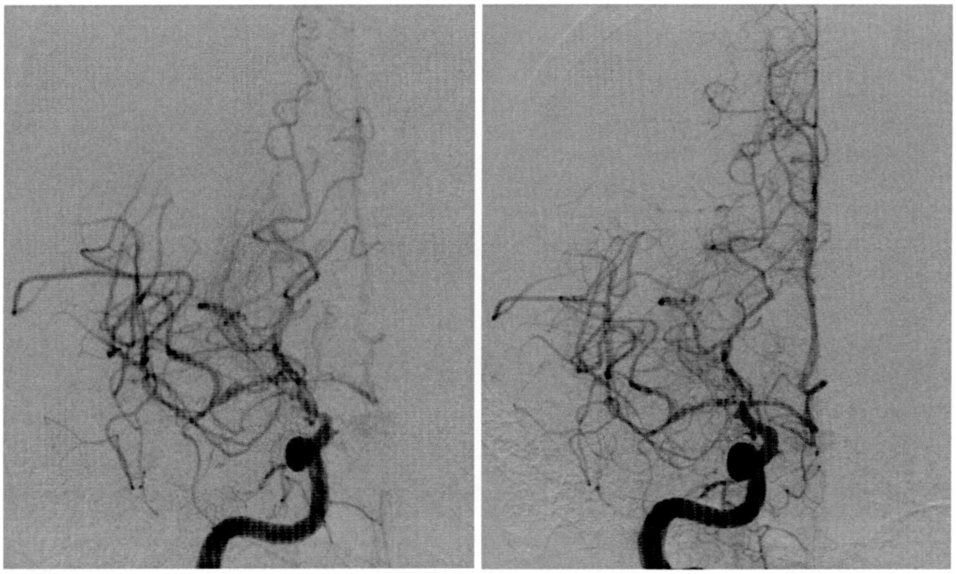

Fig. 1 A representative case of vasospastic improvement after intraarterial administration of fasudil hydrochloride (*IAFC*). Right internal carotid angiography showed severe vasospasm in the internal carotid artery (*ICA*) and the anterior cerebral artery (*ACA*) and moderate vasospasm in the middle cerebral artery before IAFC (*pre-IAFC*). Angiographic vasospasm in the ICA and ACA markedly dilated in response to IAFC, and phase of the peripheral vessels distal to ACA appeared earlier after IAFC (*Post-IAFC*) compared with (*post-IAFC*)

cantly shortened after IAFC ($P=0.005$); the difference between pre- and post-IAFC values was 0.30 ± 0.30 s.

Color gradient mapping showed remarkable improvement in cerebral arterial blood circulation after IAFC in most cases. After IAFC, the time to peak of contrast medium opacification in the main trunks of the ACA, the MCA, and the ICA changed faster in 39 sides, slower in 3 sides, and at the same speed in 15 sides. No symptomatic vasospasm was observed after IAFC and no complication occurred during the endovascular treatment (Figs. 1 and 2, Table 1).

Discussion

We analyzed the arterial circulation time on DSA performed 5–7 days after the onset of SAH in 38 patients. Patients who had factors that could skew the CCT, such as elevated intracranial pressure, mean arterial pressure, abnormal CO_2, or evidence of atherosclerotic stenosis or intracranial lesions, were excluded from our analysis. Our results demonstrate that arterial circulation time significantly shortened after IAFC and, in most cases, the time to peak of contrast medium reduced after IAFC. No patient developed symptomatic vasospasm after IAFC.

This single-center, retrospective study has several potential limitations. First, the number of patients was small, which means that these results should be considered to be preliminary. Second, the calculated arterial circulation time can be considered as an estimate, at best, because of the large time-frame intervals of the DSA equipment at our institution (images were acquired at 3.75 frames/s), although this method has been used and modified in previous studies on CCT [18].

The significance of arterial circulation time and the time to peak of contrast medium visualized on color gradient images has been reported previously. Prolonged circulation time is considered a measure of increased microcirculation resistance [6]. In part, this is based on the assumption that the time required by a contrast agent to pass from the cerebral arteries to the veins should be prolonged in patients with disorders of small vessels [8]. Arterial circulation time is shown to be prolonged in cases with vasospasm, poor clinical grade, or poor outcome [7, 18]. For example, similar to our observations, the findings of Ohkuma et al. indicated an inverse relationship between cerebral blood flow and arterial circulation time during vasospasm at 5–7 days after SAH and correlation between the severity of vasospasm and the arterial circulation time [6]. Our results might reflect the disturbed microcirculation caused by vasospasm and the recovery caused by reduction of microvascular resistance after IAFC.

Conclusion

IAFC significantly reduced the cerebral circulation time after aneurysmal SAH and might be effective for preventing symptomatic vasospasm after SAH.

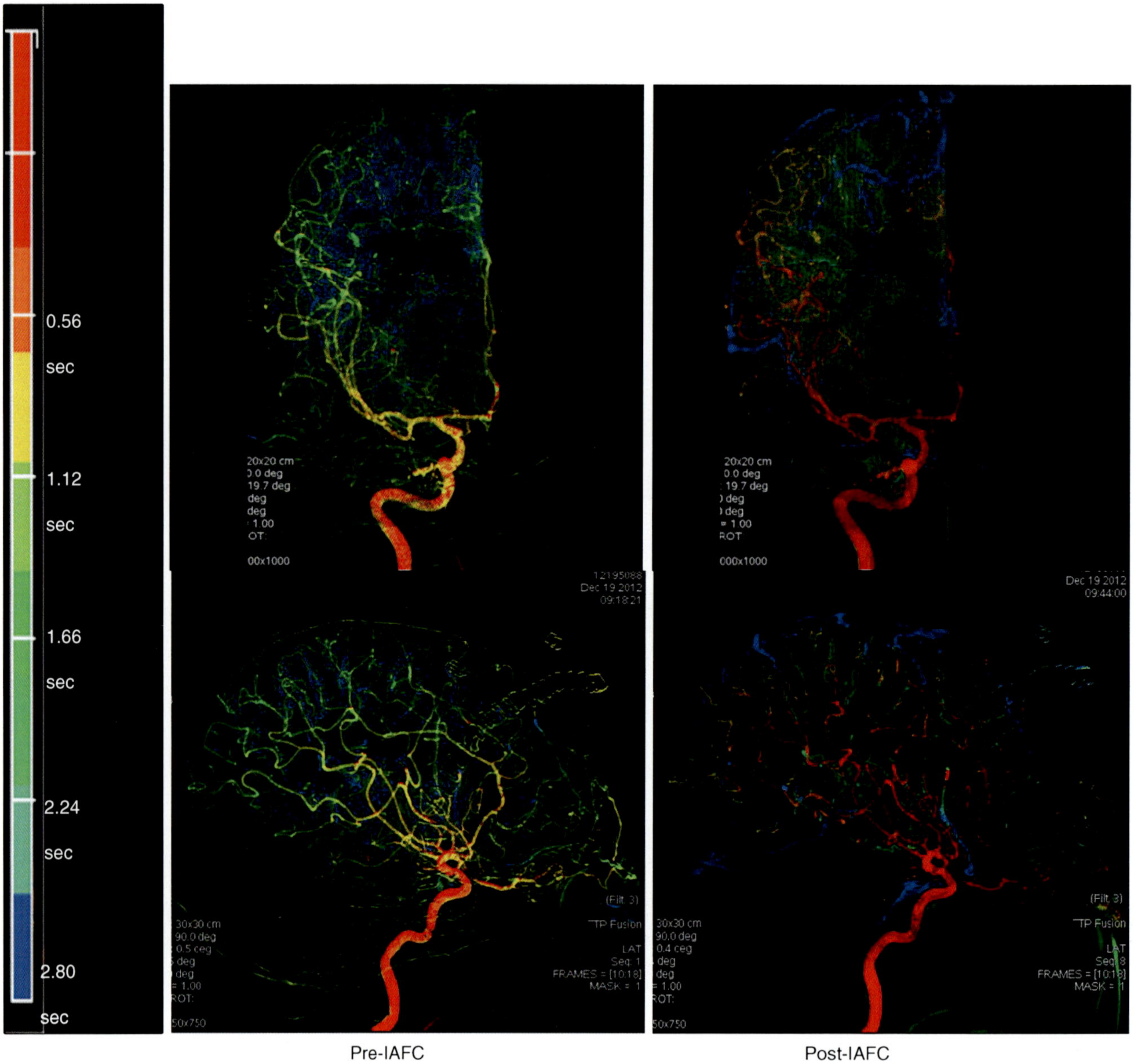

Fig. 2 A representative image of color gradient mappings of time to peak of the contrast medium. Color gradient images reconstituted from angiography of the right ICA showed that time to peak of circulating contrast medium reduced after IAFC (*post-IAFC*) compared with that before IAFC (*pre-IAFC*). The *color bar* shows the time scale

Table 1 Comparison of arterial circulation time with pre- and post-IAFC

	Average (s)	*P* value
Pre-IAFC	2.25 ± 0.57	
Post-IAFC	1.95 ± 0.55	0.005
Difference	0.30 ± 0.30	

Conflict of Interest Statement We declare that we have no conflict of interest.

References

1. Ingall T, Asplund K, Mahonen M, Bonita R (2000) A multinational comparison of subarachnoid hemorrhage epidemiology in the WHO MONICA stroke study. Stroke 31:1054–1061
2. Inoue M, Sasaki T, Takazawa H, Morita T, Narisawa A, Saito A, Midorikawa H, Nishijima M (2013) Symptomatic vasospasm in elderly patients with aneurysmal subarachnoid hemorrhage: comparison with nonelderly patients. Acta Neurochir Suppl 115:281–284
3. Iseda T, Nakano S, Yoneyama T, Ikeda T, Moriyama T, Sameshima T, Goya T, Wakisaka S (2000) Angiographic cerebral circulation time

before and after endovascular therapy for symptomatic vasospasm. Clin Radiol 55:679–683
4. Ito H, Inugami A, Shishido F, Okudera T, Ogawa T, Hatazawa J, Fujita H, Shimosegawa E, Kanno I, Fukuda H (1994) Circulation time determined by carotid angiography in patients with chronic internal carotid artery occlusion: Comparison with cerebral blood flow and oxygen metabolism measured by PET [in Japanese]. Kaku Igaku 31:1193–1199
5. Kim I, Leinweber BD, Morgalla M, Butler WE, Seto M, Sasaki Y, Peterson JW, Morgan KG (2000) Thin and thick filament regulation of contractility in experimental cerebral vasospasm. Neurosurgery 46:440–446
6. Ohkuma H, Manabe H, Tanaka M, Suzuki S (2000) Impact of cerebral microcirculatory changes on cerebral blood flow during cerebral vasospasm after aneurysmal subarachnoid hemorrhage. Stroke 31:1621–1627
7. Okawara SH, Kimura J, Hahn JY (1974) Cerebral circulation time with ruptured intracranial aneurysms. J Neurosurg 41:415–420
8. Pradilla G, Thai QA, Legnani FG, Hsu W, Kretzer RM, Wang PP, Tamargo RJ (2004) Delayed intracranial delivery of a nitric oxide donor from a controlled-release polymer prevents experimental cerebral vasospasm in rabbits. Neurosurgery 55:1393–1400
9. Sasaki T, Kodama N, Kawakami M, Sato M, Asari J, Sakurai Y, Watanabe K, Onuma T, Matsuda T (2000) Urokinase cisternal irrigation therapy for prevention of symptomatic vasospasm after aneurysmal subarachnoid hemorrhage: a study of urokinase concentration and the fibrinolytic system. Stroke 31: 1256–1262
10. Sato M, Tani E, Fujikawa H, Kaibuchi K (2000) Involvement of Rhokinase-mediated phosphorylation of myosin light chain in enhancement of cerebral vasospasm. Circ Res 87:195–200
11. Satoh S, Yamaguchi T, Hitomi A, Sato N, Shiraiwa K, Ikegaki I, Asano T, Shimokawa H (2002) Fasudil attenuates interstitial fibrosis in rat kidneys with unilateral ureteral obstruction. Eur J Pharmacol 455:169–174
12. Satoh S, Hitomi A, Ikegaki I, Kawasaki K, Nakazono O, Iwasaki M, Mohri M, Asano T (2010) Amelioration of endothelial damage/dysfunction is a possible mechanism for the neuroprotective effects of Rho-kinase inhibitors against ischemic brain damage. Brain Res Bull 81:191–195
13. Shibuya M, Suzuki Y, Sugita K, Saito I, Sasaki T, Takakura K, Nagata I, Kikuchi H, Takemae T, Hidaka H (1992) Effect of AT877 on cerebral vasospasm after aneurismal subarachnoid hemorrhage. J Neurosurg 76:571–577
14. Shibuya M, Hirai S, Seto M, Satoh S, Ohtomo E (2005) Effects of fasudil in acute ischemic stroke: results of a prospective placebo-controlled double-blind trial. J Neurol Sci 238:31–39
15. Siasios I, Kapsalaki EZ, Fountas KN (2013) Cerebral vasospasm pharmacological treatment: an update. Neurol Res Int. doi:10.1155/2013/571328
16. Suzuki Y, Shibuya M, Satoh S, Sugimoto Y, Takakura K (2007) A postmarketing surveillance study of fasudil treatment after aneurismal subarachnoid hemorrhage. Surg Neurol 68:126–132
17. Suzuki Y, Shibuya M, Satoh S, Sugiyama H, Seto M, Takakura K (2008) Safety and efficacy of fasudil monotherapy and fasudil-ozagrel combination therapy in patients with subarachnoid hemorrhage: sub-analysis of the post-marketing surveillance study. Neurol Med Chir 48:241–248
18. Udoetuk JD, Stiefel MF, Hurst RW, Weigele JB, LeRoux P (2007) Admission angiographic cerebral circulation time may predict subsequent angiographic vasospasm after aneurismal subarachnoid hemorrhage. Neurosurgery 61:1152–1161
19. Yamamoto S, Watanabe M, Uematsu T, Takasawa K, Nukata M, Kinoshita N (2004) Correlation of angiographic circulation time and cerebrovascular reserve by acetazolamide-challenged single photon emission CT. AJNR Am J Neuroradiol 25:242–247

Cognitive Impairment in Aneurysmal Subarachnoid Hemorrhage Patients with Delayed Cerebral Infarction: Prevalence and Pattern

Alberto Chi Ho Chu, George Kwok Chu Wong, Sandy Wai Lam, Adrian Wong, Karine Ngai, Wai Sang Poon, and Vincent Mok

Abstract *Background*: Cognitive deficits commonly occur after aneurysmal subarachnoid hemorrhage (aSAH) and clinical understanding is important for treatment and rehabilitation. Delayed cerebral infarction was shown to be related to poor outcome. Data on delayed cerebral infarction-related cognitive impairment were lacking.

Objective: We investigated the prevalence and pattern of delayed cerebral infarction-associated cognitive impairment.

Methods: We carried out a prospective observational and diagnostic accuracy study in Hong Kong in patients aged 21–75 years with aSAH who had been admitted within 96 h of ictus. The domain-specific neuropsychological assessment battery at 1 year after ictus was used for cognitive assessments. A cognitive domain deficit was defined as a cognitive domain z score less than −1.65 (below the fifth percentile). Cognitive impairment was defined by two or more cognitive domain deficits. The current study is registered at ClinicalTrials.gov of the U.S. National Institutes of Health (NCT01038193).

Results: One hundred and twenty aSAH patients were recruited. Patients with delayed cerebral infarction (DCI) have cognitive impairment more frequently (22 % vs 11 %; odds ratio: 2.2, 0.6 to 7.8, $p=0.192$). Cognitive domain deficits commonly affected in aSAH patients with delayed cerebral infarction were verbal memory, language, and visuospatial memory and skill domains, and were relatively uncommon in aSAH patients without delayed cerebral infarction.

Conclusion: In patients with aSAH, delayed cerebral infarction was associated with a specific pattern of cognitive domain deficits. The pathophysiology should be further investigated.

Keywords Aneurysm • Cognitive impairment • Stroke Subarachnoid hemorrhage

Introduction

Aneurysmal subarachnoid hemorrhage (aSAH) accounts for 3 % of strokes. Estimated independence after aSAH varied between 36 and 60 % only [1, 10]. Global and focal neurological deficit in aSAH survivors has been well documented. Recent studies showed that cognitive impairment in aSAH patients might affect their functional outcomes and 27–44 % of patients who returned to the community exhibited cognitive dysfunction [11, 14, 15]. Thus, it is clinically important to better understand the pattern of cognitive dysfunction after aSAH.

The exact cause of cognitive impairment after SAH is not clear. It is postulated that the primary and secondary brain injury, such as delayed cerebral infarction, may contribute to the functional deficit of the patients. Reports in the literature have confirmed that delayed cerebral infarction is related to poor outcome [16, 17, 20]. However, data on the prevalence or pattern of delayed cerebral infarction-related cognitive impairment are lacking. With this in mind, we designed the current study.

A.C.H. Chu, MRCS • G.K.C. Wong, MD (✉) • S.W. Lam, BSocSc
K. Ngai, BSocSc • W.S. Poon, FRCS
Division of Neurosurgery, Department of Surgery,
Prince of Wales Hospital, The Chinese University of Hong Kong,
4/F Clinical Science Building, 30-32 Ngan Shing Street,
Shatin, NT, Hong Kong SAR, China
e-mail: georgewong@surgery.cuhk.edu.hk

A. Wong, PhD
Department of Psychological Studies,
The Hong Kong Institute of Education, 10 Lo Ping Road,
Tai Po, NT, Hong Kong

V. Mok, MD
Division of Neurology, Department of Medicine and Therapeutics,
Prince of Wales Hospital, The Chinese University of Hong Kong,
4/F Clinical Science Building, 30-32 Ngan Shing Street,
Shatin, NT, Hong Kong SAR, China

J. Fandino et al. (eds.), *Neurovascular Events After Subarachnoid Hemorrhage*, Acta Neurochirurgica Supplement, Vol. 120,
DOI 10.1007/978-3-319-04981-6_51,

Methods

This prospective observational study was performed in four neurosurgical centers in Hong Kong [16–18]. It is registered at ClinicalTrials.gov of the US National Institutes of Health (NCT01038193) and was approved by hospital ethics committees. This study conforms to the Declaration of Helsinki, and written informed consent was obtained from all of the participants or their next of kin.

The patient inclusion criteria were: (1) spontaneous SAH with angiography-confirmed etiology of intracranial aneurysm; (2) hospital admission within 96 h after ictus; (3) age between 21 and 75 years of age; (4) a speaker of Chinese (Cantonese); and (5) informed consent from the patients or their next of kin. The patient exclusion criteria were: (a) a history of previous cerebrovascular or neurological disease other than unruptured intracranial aneurysm or (b) a history of neurosurgical operation before ictus.

Assessments [17, 18]

Assessments were conducted 3 years after ictus by one of the two research assistants (psychology graduates) trained and supervised by a postdoctoral research psychologist. The battery of cognitive assessments had previously been reported in our local Chinese population [17–19]. The choice of the battery of cognitive assessments was based on: (a) previous cognitive studies in local Chinese patients and standard cognitive tests validated in the Cantonese-speaking population; and (b) a balanced battery covering verbal and visuospatial memory, attention and working memory, executive functions, psychomotor speed, and language.

A. Verbal memory domain
   1. Hong Kong List Learning Test (HKLLT) [3]. The HKLLT was developed based on the California Verbal Learning Test, which has been used in vascular cognitive impairment studies. It is a verbal learning and memory test that consists of two 16-word lists with three learning trials with immediate recall, 10-min delayed recall, and 30-min delayed recall and recognition for each list. The HKLLT has been validated in both healthy and pathological local populations.

B. Visuospatial skill and memory domain
   1. The Rey Osterrieth Complex Figure is a commonly used test for assessing visuospatial construction skills and visuospatial memory [5, 9].

C. Attention and working memory domain
   1. Verbal and visual digit span forward and backward from the Chinese Wechsler Memory Scale Third Edition for the examination of simple attention and working memory [6, 13]. Verbal and visual spans have been used as donor scales for composite psychometric measures.

D. Executive function and psychomotor speed domain
   1. Symbol–Digit Modalities Test. This brief, easy-to-administer, timed coding test is a variant of the Digit–Symbol Coding Task in the Wechsler Adult Intelligence Scale—Third edition. Timed coding tasks have been used in studies that involve subjects with suspected vascular cognitive impairment.
   2. Color Trails Test (CTT). This test originated from the Trail Making Test (TMT), which is used for the timed assessment of psychomotor speed and executive functions. Using colored numbers instead of the English alphabet, the CTT is considered to be an acceptable cultural substitute for the original TMT with similar psychometric properties [7].
   3. Animal Fluency. This test requires subjects to generate as many animal names as possible in 1 min. It is a simple timed test that sensitively measures speed and activation, as well as such executive processes as clustering, set shifting, and retrieval [4, 8].

E. Language domain
   1. Modified Boston Naming Test (mBNT). The Boston Naming Test is the most frequently used confrontation naming test for assessing language. Here, we have used a validated modified version that contains 15 stimuli appropriate for use in Chinese cultures.

Cognitive domain scores were computed by averaging the z scores of the respective test measures derived from the established age-matched and education-matched norms. A cognitive domain deficit was defined through a cognitive domain z score less than −1.65 (below the fifth percentile). We used the presence of two or more cognitive domain deficits rather than any cognitive domain deficits as the definition of cognitive impairment as in neuropsychological outcome study of the International Subarachnoid Aneurysm Trial (ISAT) [12].

Statistical Analysis

The statistical analyses were generated using IBM SPSS Statistics for Windows 21 (SPSS, Chicago, Illinois, USA). Categorical data are presented as number (percentages) and numerical data are presented as means ± standard deviations (SD), unless otherwise stated. Categorical data were analyzed using the chi-square test or Fisher's exact test, and continuous data were analyzed using the unpaired Student's t-test or Mann–Whitney U-test, as appropriate. Statistical significance was indicated by a two-tailed probability value of less than 0.05

Results

One hundred and twenty patients completed the neurocognitive assessment at 1 year. The patient cohort was previously reported [17]. In brief, the patient characteristics are shown in Table 1. One hundred and five (88 %) patients had favorable outcome as defined by the modified Rankin Scale (mRS) 0–2.

One or more cognitive domain deficits were found in 6 (32 %) patients with delayed cerebral infarction and 23 (23 %) patients without delayed cerebral infarction (odds ratio: 1.57, 0.54–4.58, $p=0.290$). Cognitive impairment (two or more domain deficits) was found in 4(21 %) patients with delayed cerebral infarction and 11(11 %) patients without delayed cerebral infarction (odds ratio: 2.18, 0.61–7.76, $p=0.192$).

Table 1 Patient profiles

	Patients assessed
	($n=120$)
Age, median (IQR)	51 years (46–61 years)
Women	82 patients (68 %)
Hypertension	41 patients (34 %)
Smoker	31 patients (26 %)
WFNS grade	
I	73 patients (61 %)
II	29 patients (24 %)
III	3 patients (2 %)
IV	11 patients (9 %)
V	4 patients (3 %)
Location of aneurysm	
Anterior cerebral artery	31 patients (26 %)
PComA	18 patients (15 %)
ICA other than PComA	23 patients (26 %)
Middle cerebral artery	31 patients (26 %)
Posterior circulation	16 patients (13 %)
Aneurysm treatment	
Coiling	59 patients (49 %)
Clipping	56 patients (47 %)
Delayed cerebral infarction	19 patients (16 %)
mRS	
0	36 patients (30 %)
1	21 patients (18 %)
2	48 patients (40 %)
3	13 patients (11 %)
4	1 patients (1 %)
5	1 patients (1 %)

IQR interquartile ranges, *PComA* posterior communicating artery, *ICA* internal carotid artery, *WFNS* World Federation of Neurosurgical Societies, *mRS* modified Rankin Scale

Cognitive domain deficits commonly affected in aSAH patients with delayed cerebral infarction were verbal memory (21 % vs 4 %; odds ratio: 6.47, 1.45–28.66, $p=0.021$), language (16 % vs 6 %; odds ratio: 2.97, 0.67–13.09, $p=0.152$), and visuospatial memory and skill (13 % vs 5 %; odds ratio: 2.42, 0.75–7.83, $p=0.126$) domains (Table 2).

Discussion

Functional outcome of patients with aSAH is usually assessed by mRS. Cognitive domain function can interact with the patient's physical ability in determining his or her real functional independence. This interaction also affects the potential and capability of patients in returning to their usual work and usual quality of life.

We showed that DCI worsened cognitive domain functions in aSAH patients and that verbal memory domain deficit was significantly associated with DCI. Verbal memory is predominantly mediated by the medial temporal lobes, including the hippocampus and parahippocampus network. A previous study showed significant reduction in bilateral hippocampal volumes among patients with aSAH [2]. A similar finding was observed in visuospatial memory and function domain and language domain.

The proportions of patients with executive and psychomotor speed domain deficit are similar in those with and without DCI. The executive function is predominantly mediated by the frontal lobes and it encompasses higher cortical function such as planning, inhibition, problem solving, attention, and decision making [1]. One possibility that two groups of patients have a similar prevalence of executive function domain deficit is that the executive and psychomotor speed domain function may be mainly affected by the primary hemorrhage.

There were limitations in the current study. First, although the domain-based neuropsychological battery we used has been validated in a Chinese population with established norm, it is possible that it was not sensitive enough to measure subtle cognitive changes. Second, the cognitive domain outcomes are dichotomized for analyses and the patient number did not allow matched analyses. Finally, fatigue can adversely affected performance because the battery of cognitive assessments is tiring.

Conclusion

In conclusion, our study showed a distinct pattern of cognitive domain deficits in a prospective observational SAH cohort. These findings should be further investigated in future multicenter prospective studies.

Table 2 Cognitive domain deficit in patients with and without delayed cerebral infarction (DCI)

	Patients with DCI (%) ($n=19$)	Patients with no DCI (%) ($n=101$)	Odds ratio (95 % CI)	p-value
Verbal memory domain deficit	4 (21)	4 (4)	6.47 (1.45–28.66)	0.021*
Visuospatial skill and memory domain deficit	5 (26)	13 (13)	2.42 (0.75–7.83)	0.126
Attention and working memory domain deficit	2 (10)	6 (6)	1.86 (0.35–10.01)	0.371
Language domain deficit	3 (16)	6 (6)	2.97 (0.67–13.09)	0.152
Executive function and psychomotor speed domain deficit	2 (11)	10 (10)	1.07 (0.22–5.32)	0.600
Cognitive impairment	4 (21)	11 (11)	2.18 (0.61–7.76)	0.192

DCI delayed cerebral infarction
*$p<0.05$

Conflict of Interest Statement/Financial Disclosure We declare that we have no conflict of interest.

References

1. Al-Khindi T, Macdonald RL, Schweizer TA (2010) Cognitive and functional outcome after aneurysmal subarachnoid hemorrhage. Stroke 41:e519–e536
2. Bendel P, Koivisto T, Hänninen T, Kolehmainen BM, Könönen M, Hurskainen H, Pennanen C, Vanninen R (2006) Subarachnoid hemorrhage is followed by temporomesial volume loss. Neurology 67:575–582
3. Chan AS, Kwok I (1999) Hong Kong list learning test: manual and preliminary norm. Department of Psychological and Clinical Psychology Center, Hong Kong
4. Dikmen S, Corrigan JD, Levin HS, Machamer J, Stiers W, Weisskopf MG (2009) Cognitive outcome following traumatic brain injury. J Head Trauma Rehabil 24:430–438
5. Lam CL, Gandek B, Ren XS, Chan MS (1998) Tests of scaling assumptions and construct validity of the Chinese (HK) version of the SF-36 health survey. J Clin Epidemiol 51:1139–1147
6. Lam CL, Lauder IJ, Lam TP, Gandek B (1999) Population based norming of the Chinese (HK) version of the SF-36 health survey. H K Pract 21:460–470
7. Lee TM, Chan CC (2000) Are trail making and color trails tests of equivalent constructs? J Clin Exp Neuropsychol 22:529–534
8. Lim PP, Ng LL, Chiam PC, Ong PS, Ngui FT, Sahadevan S (2000) Validation and comparison of three brief depression scales in an elderly Chinese population. Int J Geriat Psychiatry 15:824–830
9. Rey A (1941) L'examen psychologique dans les cas d'encephalopathie traumatique. Arch de Psychologie 28:296–302
10. Rinkel GJ, Algra A (2011) Long-term outcomes of patients with aneurysmal subarachnoid haemorrhage. Lancet Neurol 10:349–356
11. Schweizer TA, Al-Khindi T, Macdonald RL (2012) Mini-mental state examination versus Montreal cognitive assessment: rapid assessment tools for cognitive and functional outcome after aneurysmal subarachnoid hemorrhage. J Neurol Sci 316:137–140
12. Scott RB, Eccles F, Molyneux AJ, Kerr RS, Rothwell PM, Carpenter K (2010) Improved cognitive outcomes with endovascular coiling of ruptured intracranial aneurysms: neuropsychological outcomes from the International Subarachnoid Aneurysm Trial. Stroke 41:1743–1747
13. Wechsler D (2005) Wechsler Memory Scale III (Chinese): manual. Psychological Corporation, Taiwan
14. Wong GK, Wong R, Mok VC, Fan DS, Leung G, Wong A, Chan AS, Zhu CX, Poon WS (2009) Clinical study on cognitive dysfunction after spontaneous subarachnoid haemorrhage: patient profiles and relationship to cholinergic dysfunction. Acta Neurochir 151:1601–1607
15. Wong GK, Wong R, Mok VC, Wong A, Poon WS (2010) Natural history and medical treatment of cognitive dysfunction after spontaneous subarachnoid haemorrhage: review of current literature with respect to aneurysm treatment. J Neurol Sci 299:5–8
16. Wong GK, Lam SW, Ngai K, Wong A, Mok V, Poon WS, Cognitive Dysfunction after Aneurysmal Subarachnoid Haemorrhage Investigators (2012) Evaluation of cognitive impairment by the Montreal cognitive assessment in patients with aneurysmal subarachnoid haemorrhage: prevalence, risk factors and correlations with 3 month outcomes. J Neurol Neurosurg Psychiatry 83:1112–1117
17. Wong GK, Lam SW, Ngai K, Wong A, Poon WS, Mok V, Cognitive Dysfunction after Aneurysmal Subarachnoid Haemorrhage Investigators (2013) Cognitive domain deficits in patients with aneurysmal subarachnoid haemorrhage at 1 year. J Neurol Neurosurg Psychiatry 84:1054–1058
18. Wong GK, Lam SW, Wong A, Ngai K, Poon WS, Mok V (2013) Comparisons of Montreal Cognitive Assessment and Mini-Mental State Examination in evaluating cognitive domain deficit following aneurysmal subarachnoid haemorrhage. PLoS One 8(4):e59946
19. Wong GK, Ngai K, Wong A, Lam SW, Mok VC, Yeung J, Rainer T, Wong R, Poon WS (2011) Long-term cognitive dysfunction in patients with traumatic subarachnoid hemorrhage: prevalence and risk factors. Acta Neurochir 154:105–111
20. Wong GK, Poon WS (2013) Clinical, transcranial Doppler ultrasound, radiological features and prognostic significance. Acta Neurochir Suppl 113:9–11

Animal Models

Foreword Chapter Animal Models of SAH

Serge Marbacher

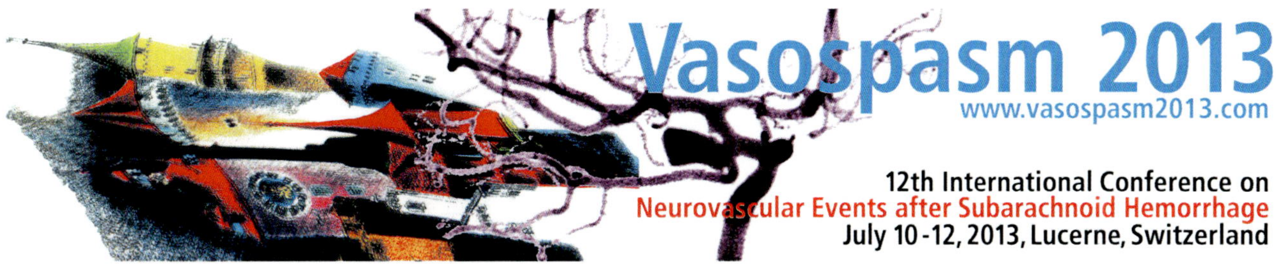

Dear Colleagues,

The workshop session "Animal Models for the Study of Delayed Cerebral Vasospasm and Early Brain Injury after Subarachnoid Hemorrhage" held during Vasospasm 2013 in Lucerne was a great success. The workshop offered the unique opportunity to share experiences and discuss current practices and future prospects of animal models in the field of subarachnoid hemorrhage (SAH) research.

Animal models provide a basis for clarifying the complex pathogenesis after SAH and for the evaluation of potential therapeutic strategies. Despite decades of effort, the translation of basic research into clinically effective treatment has remained poor. Lack of adequate and standardized SAH animal models is one reason for the lack of success.

The following chapter provides a review of technical details of established and novel SAH models in mice, rats, rabbits, dogs, and nonhuman primates. Discussion of parameters used, advantages and limitations, outcome measures, and applicability for the study of early brain injury and delayed cerebral vasospasm provide guidance for conducting experiments in the future.

The workshop aimed to serve as a starting point for discussions on more standardized performance of experimental SAH animal models. The ultimate goal would be to seek consensus on standards that would allow multicenter collaborative studies and comparison of data between different laboratories, optimizing both animal welfare and scientific validity.

In this spirit, we thank the cochairs, lecturers, and especially the participants for making this first workshop a resounding success, and we look forward to a collegial and cooperative continuation of the initiated discussions.

Serge Marbacher, MD

S. Marbacher, MD, MSc
Department of Neurosurgery, Kantonsspital Aarau, Aarau, Switzerland
e-mail: serge.marbacher@ksa.ch

J. Fandino et al. (eds.), *Neurovascular Events After Subarachnoid Hemorrhage*, Acta Neurochirurgica Supplement, Vol. 120,
DOI 10.1007/978-3-319-04981-6_52, © Springer International Publishing Switzerland 2015

Anterior Circulation Model of Subarachnoid Hemorrhage in Mice

Mohammed Sabri Attia and R. Loch Macdonald

Abstract Subarachnoid hemorrhage (SAH) remains one of the most morbid subtypes of stroke around the world and has been the focus of hemorrhagic stroke research for longer than five decades. Animal models have been instrumental in shaping the progress and advancement of SAH research, particularly models that allow for transgenic manipulation. The anterior circulation mouse model provides the research community with a rodent model that depicts very similar clinical findings of SAH; from the location of the hemorrhages to the secondary complications that arise after the hemorrhagic insult. The model allows for the recreation of clinically relevant findings such as large vessel vasospasm, oxidative stress, microcirculatory spasm and microthrombosis, and delayed neuronal injury – all of which appear in human cases of SAH. The model is also not technically demanding, is highly reproducible, and allows for an array of transgenic manipulation, which is essential for mechanistic investigations of the pathogenesis of SAH. The anterior circulation mouse model of SAH is one of a few models that are currently used in mice, and provides the research community with a relatively easy, reliable, and clinically relevant model of SAH – one that could be effectively be used to test for early brain injury (EBI) and delayed neurological injury after SAH.

Keywords Anterior circulation • Subarachnoid hemorrhage • Vasospasm • Mouse • Perichiasmatic • Early brain injury • Delayed brain injury • Animal models • SAH

Introduction of Model

The prechiasmatic animal model was first introduced by the group of Prunell et al. in 2002 when it was first constructed and used on rats for the induction of experimental subarachnoid hemorrhage (SAH) [2]. The prechiasmatic model focuses on using the anterior circulation and allows for the injection of autologous or nonautologous blood into the prechiasmatic cistern using an anterior approach. The model was first constructed as an experimental SAH model to approximate the clinical picture of SAH. Clinically speaking, approximately 80 % of aneurysms found in aSAH patients were often located in the anterior circulation and anterior fossa [1]. As a result, constructing a model with an anterior distribution of hemorrhage was thought to be beneficial and more translatable to the clinical picture. The model was then adapted to be used in mice, and some technical modifications were made to maximize the proximity of

M.S. Attia, MSc
Division of Neurosurgery, St. Michael's Hospital,
30 Bond Street, Toronto, ON M5B 1W8, Canada

Labatt Family Centre of Excellence in Brain Injury
and Trauma Research, Keenan Research Centre,
Li Ka Shing Knowledge Institute of St. Michael's Hospital,
Toronto, ON Canada

R.L. Macdonald, MD, PhD (✉)
Division of Neurosurgery, St. Michael's Hospital,
30 Bond Street, Toronto, ON M5B 1W8, Canada

Labatt Family Centre of Excellence in Brain Injury
and Trauma Research, Keenan Research Centre,
Li Ka Shing Knowledge Institute of St. Michael's Hospital,
Toronto, ON Canada

Department of Surgery, Institute of Medical Science,
University of Toronto, Toronto, ON Canada
e-mail: macdonaldlo@smh.ca

Disclosures
M. Sabri has no disclosures. R. L. Macdonald receives grant support from the Physicians Services Incorporated Foundation, Brain Aneurysm Foundation, Canadian Stroke Network and the Heart and Stroke Foundation of Ontario. R.L. Macdonald is a consultant for Actelion Pharmaceuticals and Chief Scientific Officer of Edge Therapeutics, Inc.

J. Fandino et al. (eds.), *Neurovascular Events After Subarachnoid Hemorrhage*, Acta Neurochirurgica Supplement, Vol. 120,
DOI 10.1007/978-3-319-04981-6_53, © Springer International Publishing Switzerland 2015

recreating a hemorrhagic event in mice [3]. Adapting the anterior model in mice was a big objective because it allows for the use of transgenic technology to further dissect the pathogenesis of SAH.

Model Techniques and Methodology

For our model and our studies, all experiments and protocols are approved by the Animal Care Committee associated with our hospital base and comply with all regulations of the Canadian council of animal care. Mice used in our experiments are randomized by gender and weigh between 17 and 25 g. Experimental model characteristics have been published by our laboratory in great detail [3]. In brief, animals can be anesthetized with either injectable anesthetics (ketamine 120 mg/kg and xylazine 30 mg/kg) or spontaneous inhalation of isofluorane. Body temperature is maintained at 37.0 ± 0.5 °C with a homeothermic heating pad and rectal temperature probe (Harvard apparatus, Holliston, MA, USA). The head is fixed in a stereotactic frame equipped with a mouse adaptor (Harvard apparatus) and stereotactic manipulators to hold the laser Doppler flow probe (BLT21, Transonics Systems, New York, NY, USA) and a spinal 27-gauge needle (BD Biosciences, San Jose, CA, USA). A simple incision is made midline of the anterior scalp to expose the skull and to visualize the sagittal sinus. A burr hole is drilled 4.5 mm anterior to the bregma and slightly lateral to the midline using a 0.9 mm STARRET drill (TRANSCAT, New York, NY, USA). The needle is angled ventrally at 35–40° (depending on the breed of mice), which allows the needle to advance between both hemispheres without penetrating any parenchyma or causing any brain damage (Fig. 1). Cerebral blood flow (CBF) is monitored on the contralateral aspect of the skull to monitor changes; recording times vary depending on experimental purposes. Once a stable recording is established, nonautologous blood from a donor animal or autologous blood is extracted from the mouse's tail artery and injected through the spinal needle. The spinal needle is advanced to the base of the skull until a fine resistance is detected; the needle is then pulled back (0.4–0.5 mm) to position the needle in the subarachnoid space in the prechiasmatic cistern. Either blood (experimental) or normal sterile saline (control) is injected at a steady speed, ranging from 5 to 15 s (depending on the model severity desired). The volume injected also depends on model severity desired and mouse breed, and usually varies from 50 to 100 μl. The needle is kept in this position for ~ 2 min to prevent backflow or CSF leakage.

Advantages and Disadvantages

Constructing the perfect model of any pathology requires a number of essential criteria to be considered efficient and useful. Schwartz et al. suggested a few criteria that may assist in the creation of an ideal model of SAH [4]. The model should be reproducible with very little variation, inexpensive, produce a documented and controlled volume of hemorrhage in the correct location, and reproduce the clinical complications and secondary sequelae of SAH. The anterior approach model of SAH was constructed and adapted in mice keeping all of these criteria in mind. The model provides the research community with a number of advantages and with ease of reproducibility, some of which are listed in Table 1.

The prechiasmatic anterior model has demonstrated to be reproducible, reliable, and have very little intergroup variability. This model would be classed under injectable SAH models, and it allows for controlling the volume and source of blood injected – allowing the severity of the hemorrhage to be controlled and the use of either autologous or nonautologous blood (donor animals of the same genetic background). The model also reliably recreates the Cushings reflex, with an increased intracranial pressure (ICP) and reduced CBF with the induction of SAH. The model has been used in our laboratory extensively, and reliably reproduced a number of essential secondary complications such as microthrombosis, microcirculatory spasm, neuronal degeneration and apoptosis, and large vessel vasospasm. This makes the anterior model one of the most flexible and reliable models available to the SAH community, and certainly one that could be used for research involving early brain injury (EBI) after SAH. Other models that exist in mice provide a number of advantages and disadvantages that are listed in Table 2.

Conclusions and Future Directions

The prechiasmatic anterior model adapted in mice provides the SAH community with a flexible model that is technically not challenging and that has been demonstrated to be increasingly reliable. Despite extensive research in our laboratory with this model, it is still in its early stages and requires further research and time-series analysis to truly understand whether this model is best used for EBI research, delayed-type complications research, or can effectively model both modalities of pathogenesis. Additionally, further work and research is needed to construct a model that truly encapsulates the pathogenesis of SAH and one that could take into account the multifactorial nature of this pathology.

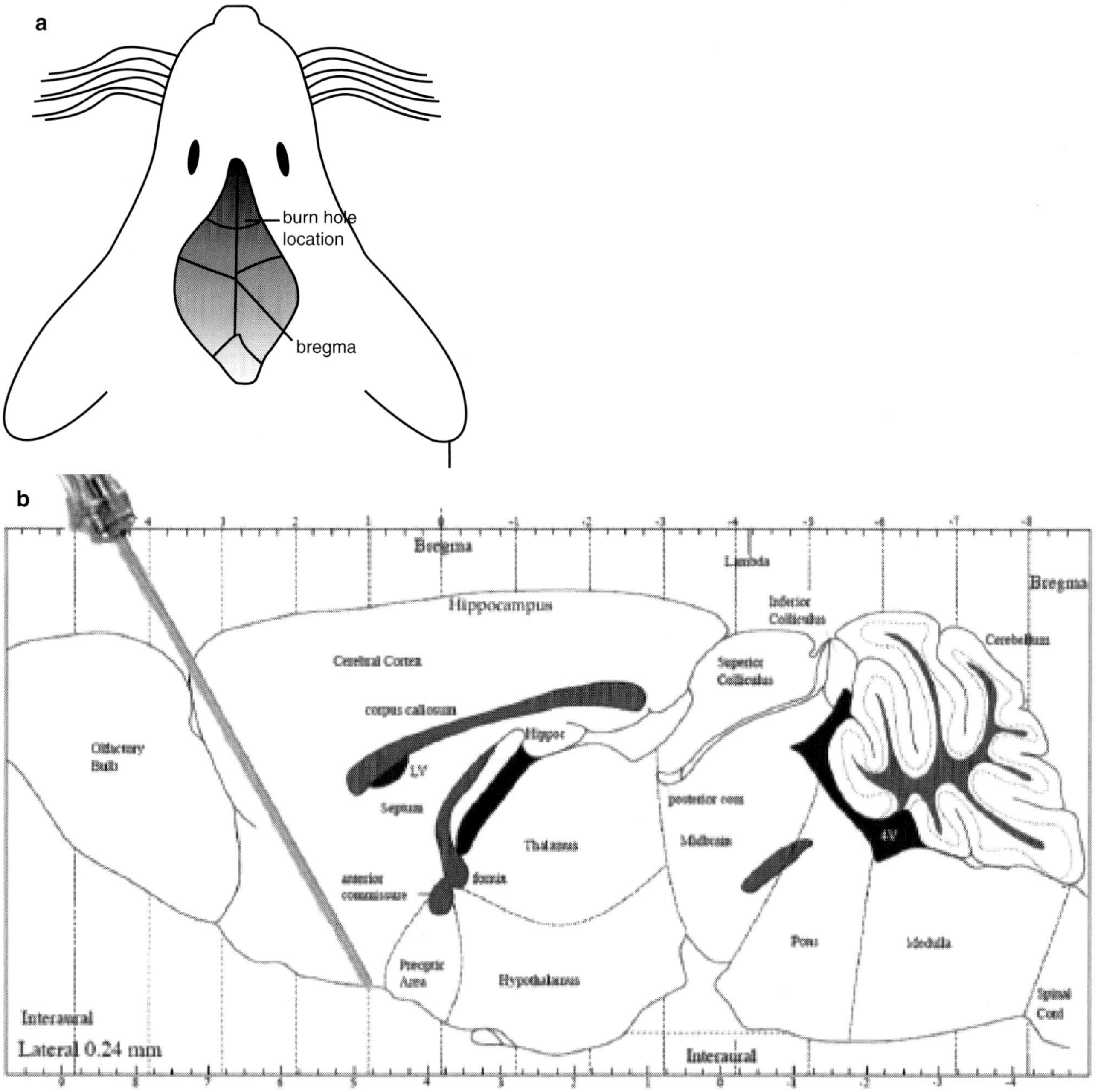

Fig. 1 (**a**) Location of the burr hole, at 4.5 mm from the bregma, slightly off midline. (**b**) Spinal needle is advanced at 40° to the base of the brain into the prechiasmatic cistern

Table 1 Summary of the advantages and disadvantages of the anterior circulation SAH model

Advantages	Disadvantages
Controlled volume of injected blood and reproducible	Does not recreate the natural aneurysmal rupture
Not challenging technically, with a low mortality	Difficult to monitor blood pressure (mouse tail cannulation)
Nonautologous or autologous sources of blood can be used	
Recreates an ICP spike	
Recreates primary complications of SAH	
Recreates secondary complications of SAH	

Table 2 Summary table of experimental SAH models and the advantages and disadvantages associated with each

Model	Advantages	Disadvantages
Endovascular perforation		Uncontrolled blood volume
		Variable severity
		High mortality/ morbidity
	Mimics spontaneous rupture of aneurysm	No experimental control
Blood injection models (basal cistern injection)	Severity controlled, volume of blood controlled	Location and distribution of blood not clinically similar
	Experimental controls exist	Does not mimic spontaneous rupture
Vein puncture	Mimics spontaneous rupture of aneurysm	Uncontrolled blood volume
		Variable severity
		Venous blood
		No experimental control
Hypertension and vascular fragility model	Mimics spontaneous rupture of aneurysm	SAH data does not exist yet
		Variable blood volume and severity
		No proper experimental control

Conflict of Interest Statement We declare that we have no conflict of interest.

References

1. Kassell NF, Torner JC, Haley EC Jr, Jane JA, Adams HP, Kongable GL (1990) The International Cooperative Study on the Timing of Aneurysm Surgery. Part 1: Overall management results. J Neurosurg 73:18–36
2. Prunell GF, Mathiesen T, Svendgaard NA (2002) A new experimental model in rats for study of the pathophysiology of subarachnoid hemorrhage. Neuroreport 13:2553–2556
3. Sabri M, Jeon H, Ai J, Tariq A, Shang X, Chen G, Macdonald RL (2009) Anterior circulation mouse model of subarachnoid hemorrhage. Brain Res 1295:179–185
4. Schwartz AY, Masago A, Sehba FA, Bederson JB (2000) Experimental models of subarachnoid hemorrhage in the rat: a refinement of the endovascular filament model. J Neurosci Methods 96:161–167

Mouse Model of Subarachnoid Hemorrhage: Technical Note on the Filament Perforation Model

Carl Muroi, Masayuki Fujioka, Serge Marbacher, Javier Fandino, Emanuela Keller, Katsunori Iwasaki, and Kenichi Mishima

Abstract Experiments using genetically engineered mice are regarded as indispensable to gaining a better understanding of the molecular pathophysiology in neuronal injury after subarachnoid hemorrhage (SAH). Therefore, mouse SAH models are becoming increasingly important. The circle of Willis perforation (cWp) model is the most frequently used mouse SAH model. We report and discuss the technical surgical approach, results, and difficulties associated with the cWp model, with reference to the existing literature. Our results largely confirmed previously published results. This model may be the first choice at present, because important pathologies can be reproduced in this model and most findings in the literature are based on it.

C. Muroi, MD (✉)
Department of Neuropharmacology, Faculty of Pharmaceutical Sciences, Fukuoka University, Fukuoka, Japan

Department of Neurosurgery, Kantonsspital Aarau, Tellstrasse, CH-5001, Aarau, Switzerland

Neurocritical Care Unit, Department of Neurosurgery, University Hospital Zurich, Zurich, Switzerland

Department of Intensive Care Medicine, University and University Hospital Bern, Bern, Switzerland
e-mail: carl.muroi@ksa.ch

M. Fujioka • K. Iwasaki • K. Mishima
Department of Neuropharmacology, Faculty of Pharmaceutical Sciences, Fukuoka University, Fukuoka, Japan

J. Fandino, MD • S. Marbacher, MD, MSc
Department of Neurosurgery, Kantonsspital Aarau, Aarau, Switzerland

E. Keller, MD
Neurocritical Care Unit, Department of Neurosurgery, University Hospital Zurich, Zurich, Switzerland
e-mail: emanuela.keller@usz.ch

Keywords Subarachnoid hemorrhage • Mouse • Mouse model • Vasospasm • Early brain injury

Introduction

Neuronal injury remains a challenging issue and is associated with a poor outcome after aneurysmal subarachnoid hemorrhage (SAH). Neuronal injury might be cerebral vasospasm (CVS) dependent or independent [16]. A variety of factors at the molecular level have been implicated in the pathogenesis of neuronal injury and/or CVS. These include cytokines and chemokines, leukocyte and platelet adhesion molecules, transcription factors, and upregulated receptors [3, 15, 16]. In this context, experiments using genetically engineered animals might be regarded as indispensable to obtain a better understanding of the molecular pathophysiology. The number of publications using mouse SAH models has been rapidly increasing during the past few years (Fig. 1a). Reviewing the literature up to 2012, the circle of Willis perforation (cWp) model is the most frequently used model (Fig. 1b). However, reports providing a detailed step-by-step surgical guide for the cWp model were not found. In this brief anecdotal report, we describe the detailed technical surgical approach and summarize our experience and observations.

Material and Methods

Animals

Experiences and observations presented are based on experiments performed using ddY (10–12 weeks, 21–26 g, Kyudo Co Ltd., Japan) as well as C57BL/6N (10–12 weeks, 21–26 g, Kyudo Co Ltd., Japan) mice.

J. Fandino et al. (eds.), *Neurovascular Events After Subarachnoid Hemorrhage*, Acta Neurochirurgica Supplement, Vol. 120, DOI 10.1007/978-3-319-04981-6_54, © Springer International Publishing Switzerland 2015

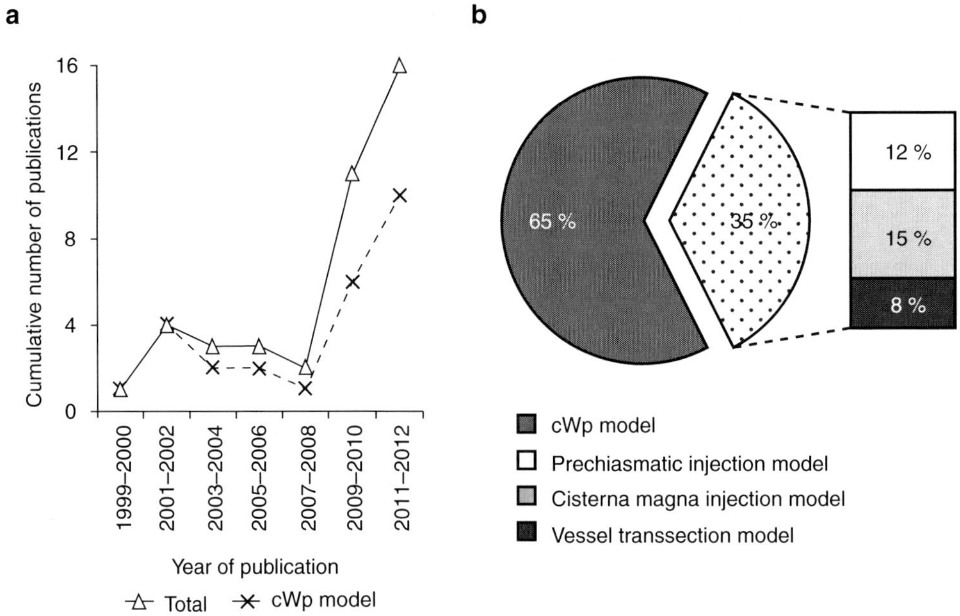

Fig. 1 (**a**) Cumulative number of publications with mouse SAH models, listed by year of publication. (**b**) Diagram showing the shares of the models in %

Perioperative Management

Standard microsurgical instruments including a bipolar forceps were used. The operating microscope had a 7- to 45-fold magnification (Arms Systems Co. Ltd., Japan). Mice were anesthetized with isoflurane (Escain, Mylan Co. Ltd., Japan): 5 % induction, 1.5 % maintenance, using a facemask. A thermostatically regulated, feedback-controlled heating pad (NS-TC10, Neuroscience Inc., Japan) was used to maintain body temperature at 37.5 °C. Intracranial pressure was measured using a fiber-optic micro pressure transducer (Samba Sensors AB, Goteborg, Sweden). In prone position, the tip of the sensor was placed on the left scull base.

Surgical Procedure

The mice were placed in a supine position. A midline incision was made in the neck. The underlying subcutaneous tissue was separated in a blunt fashion and the submaxillary glands were gently pushed aside. A triangle formed by the sternohyoid/omohyoid, sternocleidomastoid, and posterior belly of the digastric muscle was visualized (Fig. 2a). By dissecting the triangle, the neurovascular bundle consisting of the common carotid artery (CCA), vagal nerve, and internal jugular vein was visualized in the depth (Fig. 2b). The CCA was isolated, marked, and gently lifted with a holding thread. The CCA was traced cranially until the bifurcation. At the bifurcation, the occipital artery (OA)—the first branch of the external carotid artery (ECA)—could be seen beside the internal carotid artery (ICA). The ECA was traced in a cranial direction after the digastric muscle was pushed laterally (Fig. 2b). The ECA was traced until its further branching, preserving the ECA segment as long as possible. After a ligation, the ECA was coagulated and cut. Then, the OA was sacrificed. Afterwards, the ICA, which runs in an inferior-medial direction (point of view), was traced. The removal of the carotid body might be necessary because it might hamper the view. Next, the pterygopalatine artery (PPA) arising from the extracranial section of the ICA was identified (Fig. 2b). The tiny branches from the glossopharyngeal nerve lying on the ICA/PPA bifurcation were gently pushed cranially to gain an adequate view. Once the paths of the ICA and PPA were visible, the PPA was sacrificed (Fig. 2c). If the PPA was not sacrificed, the filament tended to take a *via falsa* toward the PPA instead of the ICA. A ligation was prepared on the most proximal part of the ECA stump. Mini clips (Roboz Surgical Instrument Co., Inc., USA) were placed at the ICA and CCA. An arteriotomy was performed on the distal part of the ECA stump (Fig. 2c). A 5-0 nylon filament (0.1-mm diameter, Ethilon, Ethicon Inc., USA) was pushed through the arteriotomy toward the ICA (Fig. 2d) until the tip reached the occluded part by the distal clip. One might consider rotating the ECA stump in the inferior direction before inserting the filament, so that the path for the filament would be straight. However, the tip of the filament can get stuck at the bifurcation while it is being advanced. Therefore, we inserted the filament at a more "physiological" angle ≤90° (Fig. 2d). Once the tip overcame the bifurcation, the stump with the filament was rotated inferiorly (Fig. 2e). The clips were removed and the filament was pushed further cranially. After removal of the clips, retrograde bleeding might occur. Gentle tightening of the prepared ligation avoids this. This inconvenience might be further avoided if the proximal clip was left

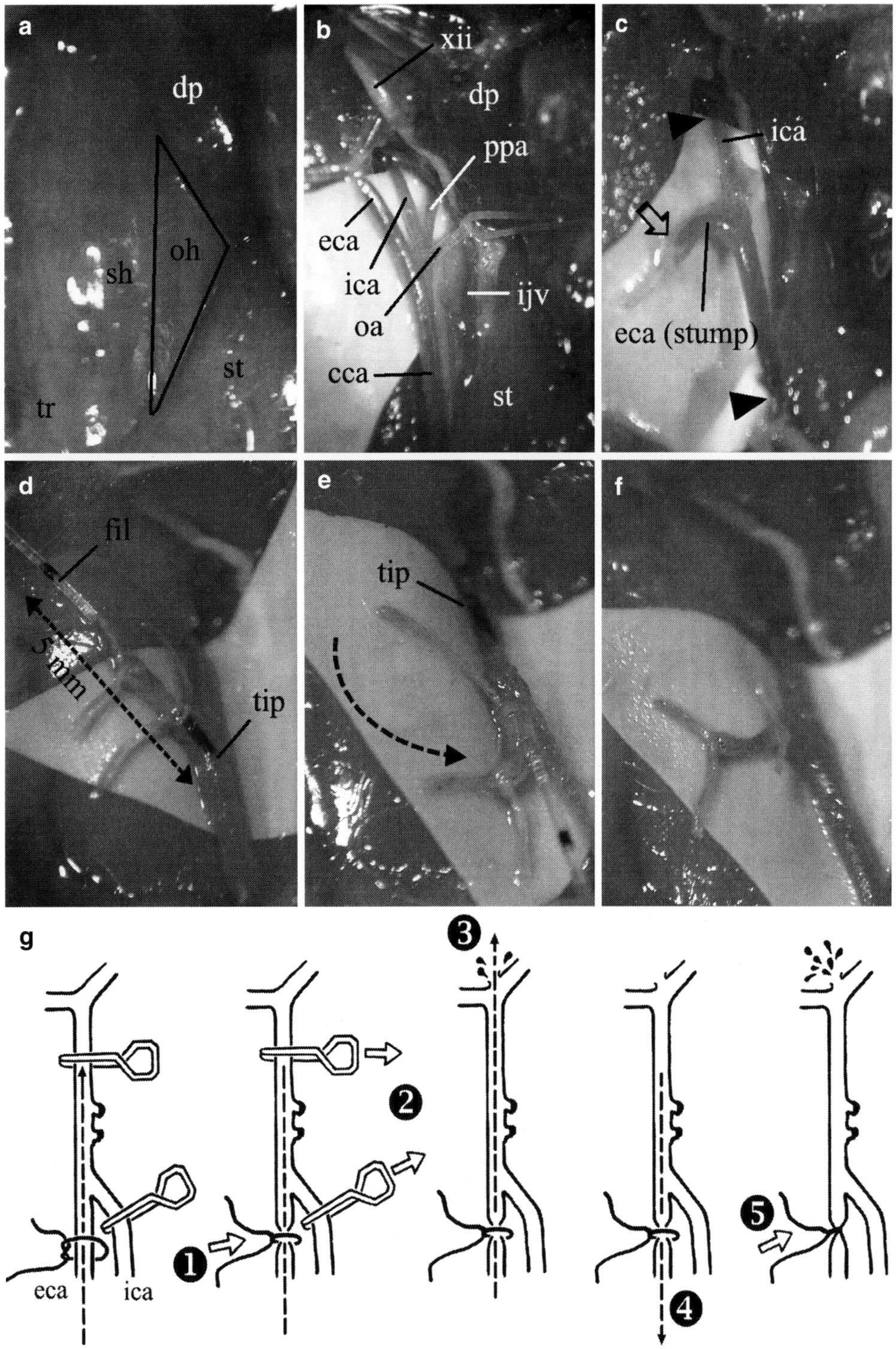

Fig. 2 Step-by-step illustration of the cWp model. (**a**) The triangle formed by the sternohyoid (*sh*)/omohyoid (*oh*), sternocleidomastoid (*st*), and posterior belly of the digastric muscle (*dp*) is shown. tr trachea. (**b**) the neurovascular bundle including the common carotid artery (*cca*) and internal jugular vein (*ijv*) is visualized. *eca* external carotid artery, *ica* internal carotid artery, *oa* occipital artery, *ppa* pterygopalatine artery, *xii* hypoglossal nerve. (**c**) A stump of the *eca* is created. The *oa* and *ppa* are sacrificed. The *Arrowheads* indicate the point where the clips are placed. The *arrow* indicateds the location of the arteriotomy. (**d**) The filament (*fil*) is pushed through the arteriotomy toward the *ica*. Note the phsiological angle between *eca* and *ica*/*cca*. *tip* tip of the filament. (**e**) The stump with the filament is rotated inferiorly once the tip overcome the bifurcation. (**f**) After perforation, the filament is withdrawn quickly and the prepared ligature tightened

in place and removed at the end of the procedure, i.e., after the perforation and complete withdrawal of the filament and ligation. However, accumulated experience revealed that the latter maneuver decreases the degree of success and volume of SAH, possibly because of rapid activation of the coagulation cascade. Therefore, we recommend the procedure as shown in Fig. 2g. The filament was gently pushed forward (~5 mm) until some resistance was felt. The filament was pushed an additional ~1 mm further to perforate the vessel. The filament was withdrawn quickly and the prepared ligature tightened (Fig. 2f). After ensuring hemostasis, the wound was adapted and sutured.

Evaluation of SAH and Histological Examinations

To evaluate the degree of hemorrhage, animals were killed at day 0, 1, and 2 after SAH. The brains were quickly removed and photographed under the operating microscope. For histological examination, euthanasia was performed by transcardial perfusion–fixation at day 2 after SAH. The brains were removed, postfixed and paraffin embedded. The blocks were sliced into 7-µm sections using a microtome (Leitz 1512 Microtome, Wetzlar Germany). Hematoxylin and eosin (HE) staining was performed for overview and CVS identification. For the assessment of neuronal injury, Fluoro-Jade C (FJC) staining (Merck Millipore, USA) was performed as previously described [21]. To evaluate the occurrence of apoptotic neurons, terminal deoxynucleotidyl transferase dUTP nick labeling (TUNEL) staining was performed (Roche Diagnostics, Germany). The numbers of FJC- and TUNEL-positive cells were determined in randomly selected regions of interest in the hippocampal region and cerebral cortex. Because microthrombosis has been discussed more recently as an additional explanation for neuronal injury after SAH, we investigated the occurrence of microthrombosis by immunohistochemistry (sheep anti-fibrinogen antibody; LifeSpan, BioSciences, USA).

Results

General Observations

The perforation caused a sharp increase in ICP. After withdrawal of the filament, the full reperfusion through the ICA caused a further increase in ICP, reflecting a full-scale SAH. We could clearly observe brief decreases in the respiration and pulse frequency in this phase, presumably reflecting a Cushing reflex, as in previous reports [4, 8]. The distance until vessel perforation was achieved varied by 1–3 mm among the cases. In our experience, this distance cannot be standardized by any means. The distance might vary 1~2 mm depending on the site of the arteriotomy, or on several other factors, such as the positioning of the animal's head. Therefore, ICP monitoring is probably the method of choice to confirm a successful induction of SAH [4]. However, with accumulating experience, one might successfully perform it without the need for monitoring, because animals clearly showed a Cushing reflex.

The presence of subarachnoid blood could be verified at all examined time points. The volume of subarachnoid blood varied among the cases. The amount of blood decreased gradually over time (Fig. 3a). Closer inspection of the ventral surface of the brains revealed that the filament perforated the circle of Willis in the vicinity of the ICA/posterior communicating artery (PcomA) bifurcation. In the literature, the majority of reports claimed to have caused a perforation in the vicinity of the anterior cerebral artery (ACA) [2, 5, 6, 8, 10–14, 17, 20, 22–24]. Taking the anatomical considerations and the stiffness of the filament into account, the ability to achieve a perforation at the ACA might be considered somewhat doubtful. However, because successful SAH could be induced, the exact location of the perforation might be irrelevant.

The surgical procedure is technically challenging because it requires a meticulous microvascular technique. At the outset, our success rate was approximately 50 %, with a high intraoperative morality (surgery-related death before SAH induction) of 25 %. After accumulating experience (20~30 cases), the success rate increased to >90 % and intraoperative mortality decreased to <5 %. Overall SAH-related mortality was 22 % in our series. In the literature, a mortality rate of 10 to ~30 % within the first 3 days seems to be a reliable figure for the cWp model [2, 5, 6, 8, 10–14, 17, 20, 22–24].

Histological Examinations

Presence of blood could be histologically verified (Fig. 3b). Morphological signs of CVS could be clearly seen in animals subjected to SAH (Fig. 3b). Degenerative neurons were visible in the ipsilateral cortex (parietal and temporal) and hippocampus. Apoptotic cells, which appeared to be neurons, were found in the ipsilateral cortex on day 2 and 3 after SAH (Fig. 3c). Presence of microthrombi could be observed in animals subjected to SAH (Fig. 3c).

Discussion

We successfully reconstructed and established the cWp SAH model, showing important pathologies such as vessel rupture, ICP increase, Cushing reflex, microthrombosis, CVS and neuronal injury, hence confirming previous studies. This mouse model was derived from the rat filament perforation model and was reported for the first time by Kamii et al. in 1999 [8]. The first paper dedicated to the model itself was published by Parra et al. in 2002 [17]. Another paper dedicated to the model itself followed in 2010 [4]. In the latter, suitable intraoperative parameters for the controlled and standardized induction of SAH were described.

It is common sense to consider that the initial amount of hemorrhage influences the degree of brain injury. Further, the time period during which erythrocytes break down and blood disappears from the CSF compartment closely mirrors the onset and resolution of CVS. The compartmental inflammatory response, which might contribute to CVS-dependent or -independent neuronal injury, is triggered by erythrocyte breakdown and also by hemoglobin release [15]. Therefore, the size of the hematoma and the kinetics of its resorption are

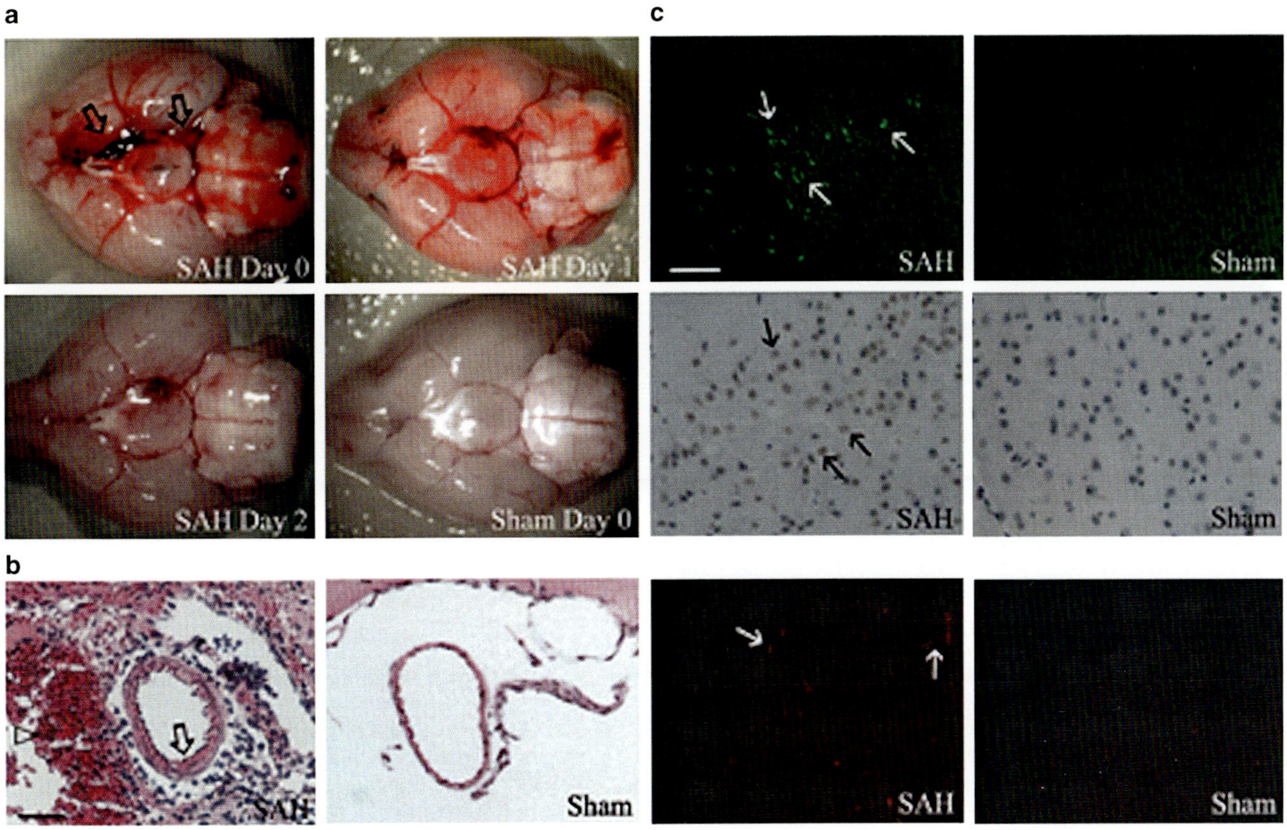

Fig. 3 (**a**) Representative brain specimens. Subarachnoid blood in the basal cisterns is clearly visible at day 0 (*arrows*). The amount of blood decreased with time. No SAH was seen in sham animals. (**b**) Representative image sections of the distal ICA showing morphological signs of CVS with thickened vessel wall in SAH (*arrow*). Note the subarachnoid blood (*arrowhead*). Bar: 50 μm. (**c**) *Upper row*: FJC-positive neurons after SAH (*arrows*). *Middle row*: TUNEL-positive cells after SAH (*arrows*). *Bottom row*: Fibrinogen-positive microthrombi after SAH (*arrows*). Bar: 100 μm

of interest. It is well accepted that in smaller animals (e.g., lissencephalic rodents), the clearance of the clot is more rapid than in larger animals (e.g., gyrenecephalic primates) [9]. However, detailed information about the rate of clot clearance in mouse SAH is rare in the literature. A detailed description is available for the cisterna magna injection model. One hour after SAH, a large diffuse blood clot was described in the subarachnoid space; on day 1, the clot was thinner, but still clearly visible around the major cerebral arteries; on day 3 or 4, the cisternal blood clot was essentially absent [9]. Our observations indicated a similar kinetic in hematoma resorption. The latter might explain the early onset of CVS in the mouse SAH model, which, in turn, might compromise the discrimination between the effects of early brain injury and CVS.

At this point, the impossibility of controlling the degree of SAH has to be mentioned again as the most crucial disadvantage of the cWp model, as already discussed in the literature [4, 9]. Advantages and disadvantages of the cWp model compared with other models have been discussed in detail elsewhere [1, 4, 10, 19]. In brief, the cWp model is technically (surgically) the most challenging model. Further, differentiation between the effects of SAH per se and effects of intracranial hypertension is not possible [18]. However, the model replicates the human pathophysiology satisfactorily, including vessel rupture and endothelial damage, which might be important features. No model other than the cWp model reflects the latter aspect. Furthermore, the superiority of the cWp model to reproduce early platelet–leukocyte–endothelial cell interactions after SAH has been described more recently [7].

Conclusions

Mice models are becoming increasingly popular, as better understanding of SAH-induced brain injury at the molecular level, using genetically engineered animals, is needed. The cWp model is the most frequently used SAH model in mice. The model replicates the important pathophysiology satisfactorily.

Acknowledgments CM has been supported by a personal research grant from the Swiss Foundation for Grants in Biology and Medicine and F. Hoffmann-La Roche Ltd., Basel, Switzerland.

Conflict of Interest Statement We declare that we have no conflict of interest.

References

1. Altay T, Smithason S, Volokh N, Rasmussen PA, Ransohoff RM, Provencio JJ (2009) A novel method for subarachnoid hemorrhage to induce vasospasm in mice. J Neurosci Methods 183:136–140
2. Borel CO, McKee A, Parra A, Haglund MM, Solan A, Prabhakar V, Sheng H, Warner DS, Niklason L (2003) Possible role for vascular cell proliferation in cerebral vasospasm after subarachnoid hemorrhage. Stroke 34:427–433
3. Chaichana KL, Pradilla G, Huang J, Tamargo RJ (2010) Role of inflammation (leukocyte-endothelial cell interactions) in vasospasm after subarachnoid hemorrhage. World Neurosurg 73:22–41
4. Feiler S, Friedrich B, Scholler K, Thal SC, Plesnila N (2010) Standardized induction of subarachnoid hemorrhage in mice by intracranial pressure monitoring. J Neurosci Methods 190:164–170
5. Gao J, Wang H, Sheng H, Lynch JR, Warner DS, Durham L, Vitek MP, Laskowitz DT (2006) A novel apoE-derived therapeutic reduces vasospasm and improves outcome in a murine model of subarachnoid hemorrhage. Neurocrit Care 4:25–31
6. Han BH, Vellimana AK, Zhou ML, Milner E, Zipfel GJ (2012) Phosphodiesterase 5 inhibition attenuates cerebral vasospasm and improves functional recovery after experimental subarachnoid hemorrhage. Neurosurgery 70:178–186
7. Ishikawa M, Kusaka G, Yamaguchi N, Sekizuka E, Nakadate H, Minamitani H, Shinoda S, Watanabe E (2009) Platelet and leukocyte adhesion in the microvasculature at the cerebral surface immediately after subarachnoid hemorrhage. Neurosurgery 64:546–553, discussion 553–544
8. Kamii H, Kato I, Kinouchi H, Chan PH, Epstein CJ, Akabane A, Okamoto H, Yoshimoto T (1999) Amelioration of vasospasm after subarachnoid hemorrhage in transgenic mice overexpressing CuZn-superoxide dismutase. Stroke 30:867–871, discussion 872
9. Lin CL, Calisaneller T, Ukita N, Dumont AS, Kassell NF, Lee KS (2003) A murine model of subarachnoid hemorrhage-induced cerebral vasospasm. J Neurosci Methods 123:89–97
10. Liu S, Tang J, Ostrowski RP, Titova E, Monroe C, Chen W, Lo W, Martin R, Zhang JH (2007) Oxidative stress after subarachnoid hemorrhage in gp91phox knockout mice. Can J Neurol Sci 34:356–361
11. McGirt MJ, Lynch JR, Parra A, Sheng H, Pearlstein RD, Laskowitz DT, Pelligrino DA, Warner DS (2002) Simvastatin increases endothelial nitric oxide synthase and ameliorates cerebral vasospasm resulting from subarachnoid hemorrhage. Stroke 33:2950–2956
12. McGirt MJ, Parra A, Sheng H, Higuchi Y, Oury TD, Laskowitz DT, Pearlstein RD, Warner DS (2002) Attenuation of cerebral vasospasm after subarachnoid hemorrhage in mice overexpressing extracellular superoxide dismutase. Stroke 33:2317–2323
13. Mesis RG, Wang H, Lombard FW, Yates R, Vitek MP, Borel CO, Warner DS, Laskowitz DT (2006) Dissociation between vasospasm and functional improvement in a murine model of subarachnoid hemorrhage. Neurosurg Focus 21:E4
14. Mino M, Kamii H, Fujimura M, Kondo T, Takasawa S, Okamoto H, Yoshimoto T (2003) Temporal changes of neurogenesis in the mouse hippocampus after experimental subarachnoid hemorrhage. Neurol Res 25:839–845
15. Muroi C, Mink S, Seule M, Bellut D, Fandino J, Keller E (2011) Monitoring of the inflammatory response after aneurysmal subarachnoid haemorrhage in the clinical setting: review of literature and report of preliminary clinical experience. Acta Neurochir Suppl 110:191–196
16. Muroi C, Seule M, Mishima K, Keller E (2012) Novel treatments for vasospasm after subarachnoid hemorrhage. Curr Opin Crit Care 18:119–126
17. Parra A, McGirt MJ, Sheng H, Laskowitz DT, Pearlstein RD, Warner DS (2002) Mouse model of subarachnoid hemorrhage associated cerebral vasospasm: methodological analysis. Neurol Res 24:510–516
18. Sabri M, Ai J, Lakovic K, D'Abbondanza J, Ilodigwe D, Macdonald RL (2012) Mechanisms of microthrombi formation after experimental subarachnoid hemorrhage. Neuroscience 224:26–37
19. Sabri M, Jeon H, Ai J, Tariq A, Shang X, Chen G, Macdonald RL (2009) Anterior circulation mouse model of subarachnoid hemorrhage. Brain Res 1295:179–185
20. Saito A, Kamii H, Kato I, Takasawa S, Kondo T, Chan PH, Okamoto H, Yoshimoto T (2001) Transgenic CuZn-superoxide dismutase inhibits NO synthase induction in experimental subarachnoid hemorrhage. Stroke 32:1652–1657
21. Schmued LC, Stowers CC, Scallet AC, Xu L (2005) Fluoro-Jade C results in ultra high resolution and contrast labeling of degenerating neurons. Brain Res 1035:24–31
22. Sozen T, Tsuchiyama R, Hasegawa Y, Suzuki H, Jadhav V, Nishizawa S, Zhang JH (2009) Role of interleukin-1beta in early brain injury after subarachnoid hemorrhage in mice. Stroke 40:2519–2525
23. Suzuki H, Sozen T, Hasegawa Y, Chen W, Zhang JH (2009) Caspase-1 inhibitor prevents neurogenic pulmonary edema after subarachnoid hemorrhage in mice. Stroke 40:3872–3875
24. Wakade C, King MD, Laird MD, Alleyne CH Jr, Dhandapani KM (2009) Curcumin attenuates vascular inflammation and cerebral vasospasm after subarachnoid hemorrhage in mice. Antioxid Redox Signal 11:35–45

The Rat Endovascular Perforation Model of Subarachnoid Hemorrhage

Fatima A. Sehba

Abstract The rat endovascular perforation model is considered the closest replica of human condition. Since its development, this model has been extensively used to study early brain injury after subarachnoid hemorrhage (SAH). However, like any other animal model, it has advantages and limitations. The following is a brief review of the rat endovascular perforation SAH model. One section is dedicated to technical considerations that can be used to overcome the model limitations.

Keywords Animal model • Subarachnoid hemorrhage • Rat Endovascular perforation model

Background

The rat endovascular perforation model of SAH was introduced in 1995 by Bederson and colleagues [1]. It is a noncraniotomy model in which SAH is created by perforating the intracranial bifurcation of the internal carotid artery (ICA). This model closely replicates the events that occur at and soon after SAH [6, 13, 14]. For this reason, the rat endovascular perforation model is particularly suited to study early brain injury after SAH.

Technique

Rats are anesthetized, such as with ketamine and xylazine (50 mg/kg + 5 mg/kg administered intraperitoneally), and placed on a homeothermic blanket (Harvard Apparatus) linked to a rectal temperature probe set to maintain body temperature at 37 °C. Rats are further transorally intubated, ventilated, and maintained on inspired isoflurane (1–2 % in 21 % oxygen-supplemented room air). The right femoral artery is cannulated for blood gas and mean arterial blood pressure (MABP) monitoring. A PE-50 catheter (Intermedics Inc.) is inserted into the cisterna magna for continuous intracranial pressure (ICP) measurement (Fig. 1b). A laser Doppler flowmetry (LDF) probe (0.8-mm diameter, model P-433; Vasamedics Inc.) is placed at a location immediately adjacent to the coronal suture and 5-mm lateral to the right of midline, over the territory of the middle cerebral artery and away from large meningeal vessels, for cerebral blood flow (CBF) measurement. For SAH induction, the right external carotid artery (ECA) is identified and exposed to its origin at the common carotid artery bifurcation. After distal ligation of the ECA, a temporary aneurysm clip is placed at the origin of the ECA while ensuring the patency of the ICA. A 3'0 prolene suture is advanced retrogradely through the ligated right ECA, and distally through the ICA until the suture perforates the intracranial bifurcation of the ICA. SAH is confirmed by a rapid rise in ICP and fall in CBF. The filament is then withdrawn into the ECA, reperfusing the ICA [1].

F.A. Sehba, PhD
Departments of Neurosurgery and Neurosciences,
Mount Sinai School of Medicine,
1 Gustave L. Levy Place, New York, NY 10029, USA
e-mail: fatima.sehba@mssm.edu

Advantages/Limitations

Advantages

A number of advantages have made the endovascular perforation model a favorite for studying early injury after SAH, such as:

Replicates early hallmark events of SAH: Accumulation of blood in the subarachnoid space, rapid rise in ICP, fall in CBF, a transient increase in MABP (Cushing response), and

J. Fandino et al. (eds.), *Neurovascular Events After Subarachnoid Hemorrhage*, Acta Neurochirurgica Supplement, Vol. 120,
DOI 10.1007/978-3-319-04981-6_55, © Springer International Publishing Switzerland 2015

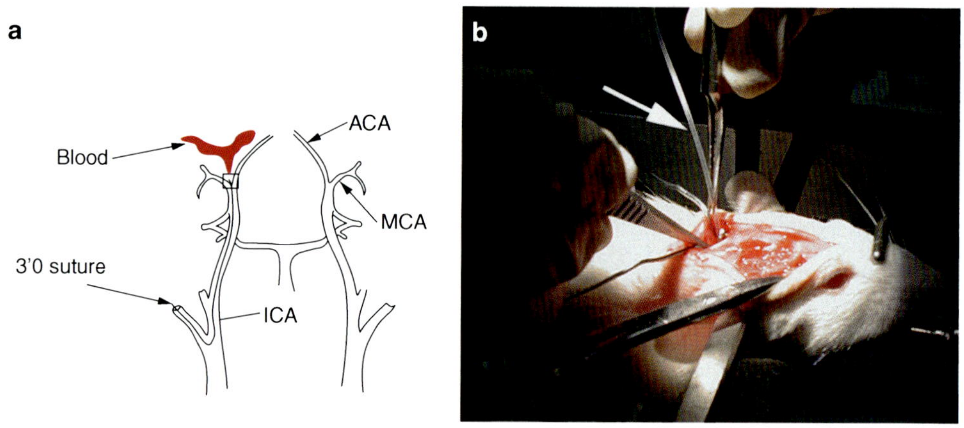

Fig. 1 Rat endovascular perforation model of SAH. (**a**) The technique used for SAH induction (Adapted from Bederson et al. [1]); (**b**) SAH surgery; *arrow* cannula placed in the cisterna magna for ICP recording

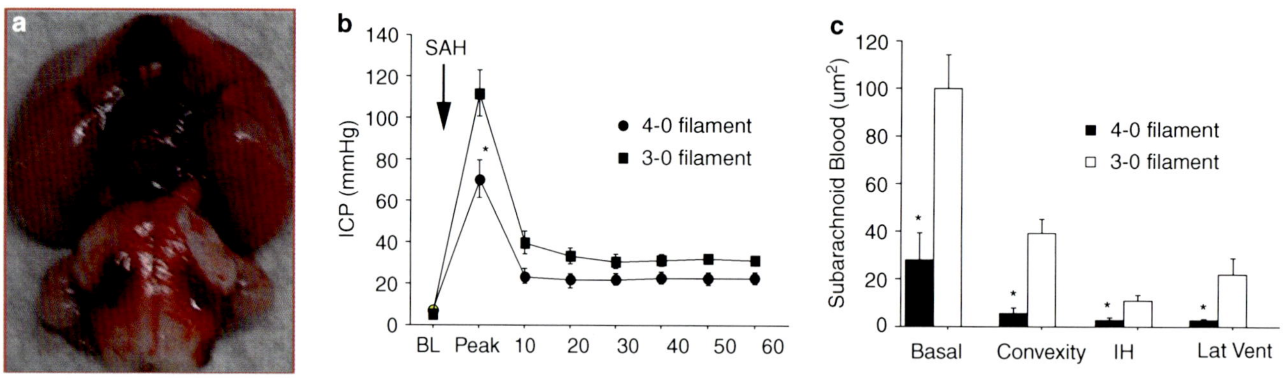

Fig. 2 Controlling and establishing severity of SAH. (**a**) Representative image showing blood accumulation in brain after SAH. In (**b**) and (**c**), note that filament size can be manipulated to create SAH of different severities; ICP rise and blood accumulation are greater when the ICA is perforated by 3'0 as compared with 4'0 suture. Data is from five animals per filament group. * Significantly different at $P < 0.05$

fall in cerebral perfusion pressure (CPP) are acute hallmark events of SAH. Because of the sudden nature of the injury, in patients, these hallmark events are mostly observed during rebleed. A major advantage of the endovascular perforation model is that it replicates all acute hallmark events of SAH.

Allows real-time recording of early physiological changes after SAH: This helps determine the intensity of hemorrhage and prevents pooling data from animals with different SAH intensity, which might lead to large standard deviations, making results difficult to accurately analyze. As described above, in the endovascular perforation model, catheters placed in the cisterna magna measure ICP (Figs. 1b and 2a); laser Doppler flowmeters placed on the temporal side of the skull, away from the large vessels, measure changes in CBF; and catheters placed in the femoral artery measure changes in MABP (for review see [1, 8]) after SAH.

Replicates mechanical trauma: Flooding of subarachnoid space with blood after aneurysm rupture exposes the brain and cerebral vasculature to mechanical trauma. Blood compresses adjacent cerebral arteries, stretches subarachnoid space, and obstructs the passage of CSF. Because SAH in the endovascular perforation model is induced by rupturing/perforating an intracranial artery (see above), it replicates the mechanical trauma experienced by the brain tissue and cerebral vasculature during SAH because blood is released under pressure and pools in basal cisterns [10].

Limitations

SAH surgery: A major limitation of the endovascular perforation model is that it requires complicated and extensive surgery. Hence, extensive hands-on training is required to master the procedure. Animal mortality in this model is as high as in SAH patients (45 % within the first 48 h).

Hemorrhage severity: Another major limitation is the inability to control the amount of bleeding and hemorrhagic severity, which, as explained above, can lead to wide standard deviations, making it difficult to draw firm conclusions when evaluating the effects of therapeutic agents [7, 8]. One reason underlying this limitation is that the severity of the bleed depends on the speed and force used to perforate the artery, which can vary from surgery to surgery and from surgeon to surgeon. However, with training, a surgeon's hand gets settled and he/she can begin to produce SAHs that have ICP rises of similar intensity.

Lack of proper sham control: The sham control in the endovascular perforation model is an animal that undergoes all the procedures that are performed in a SAH animal, including introducing a monofilament into the ICA, except for the perforation [8]. What makes this sham a poor control is that, unlike the sham control in an injection model, the sham control in this case does not experience any change in physiology.

Technical considerations

A number of considerations can help a surgeon master the endovascular perforation SAH model and reduce acute deaths. Some are as follows:

Acute death: The rapid rise in ICP at the time of SAH can increase the pressure at the respiratory centers to the point that the animal may stop breathing spontaneously. Use of a respiratory support, such as intubation or placement of a nose cone, ensures that the animal continues to breathe and does not die as SAH is induced [9].

Injury to brain tissue: Brain injury may occur because of the stabbing of the brain tissue by the filament used to perforate the artery. This injury occurs if the surgeon continues to advance the filament after the artery is perforated and can be avoided if a conscious attempt is made to retract the endovascular filament as soon as the artery is perforated. The event of perforation is felt by the surgeon and is confirmed by the rise in ICP; hence a quick look at the real-time ICP recording will confirm that artery is perforated and that the endovascular filament needs be retracted.

Controlling severity of SAH: Several methods to control the severity of SAH have been attempted. Veelken et al. [15] tried occluding the ipsilateral common carotid artery or left the endovascular filament in place to control SAH severity [15]. This mechanism however, hinders normal perfusion through the ipsilateral ICA, and creates a superimposed regional ischemia. Schwartz et al. manipulated the size of the monofilament to control the size of the bleed and the SAH severity [7]. They succeeded in creating smaller bleeds and smaller ICP rises (a low-intensity SAH) with 4'0 instead of 3'0 suture (Fig. 2). We frequently use an unsharpened, blunt 3'0 suture to create a low-intensity (≤40 mmHg) and a sharpened 3'0 suture to create a high-intensity SAH (≥40 mmHg) in rats.

Establishing severity of SAH: Measurements frequently used to establish SAH severity include the degree of ICP rise, CBF recovery at 60 min, and the volume of blood around the circle of Willis [8]. Schwartz et al. demonstrated that ICP and subarachnoid blood volume are directly associated with SAH severity; the greater the ICP rise and volume of subarachnoid blood, the greater the SAH intensity [7]. In addition, Bederson and colleagues found that CBF recovery at 60 min after SAH is inversely associated with SAH severity; SAH is lethal when CBF is reduced to less than 40 % of baseline for 60 min after SAH [2]. The volume of blood around the circle of Willis has also been used to reflect the hemorrhage severity. A number of different methods are used for subarachnoid blood measurement. Schwartz et al. traced the blood in the basal subarachnoid space, cortical convexities, and interhemispheric fissure on images of whole coronal sections to establish the hemorrhage severity [7]. They demonstrated that blood distribution after SAH is greatest in basal cortex and that blood volume is directly proportional to the ICP rise at SAH (Fig. 2c). Sugawara et al. measured blood in the basal cistern to establish SAH severity [12]. They divided the basal cistern into six segments and allotted a grade from 0 to 3 to each segment, depending on the amount of subarachnoid blood clot, and summed all scores to yield a total score. A score of 0–7 represented mild, 8–12 represented moderate, and 13–18 represented severe SAH.

Applicability for the study of EBI and delayed CVS: The endovascular perforation model is mostly used to study acute or early brain injury after SAH. However, it has also been used for studying delayed vasospasm and injury. Gules and colleagues compared arterial constriction (basilar artery and posterior communicating artery) by the endovascular morel with that produce by single- and double-injection models and found it to be comparable with the former but not the latter [5]. The time course of major cerebral artery vasospasm in the endovascular model is also studied and it appears that severe vasospasm is present at 24-h and persists for 72 h after SAH [3]. Consequently, arterial constriction at 24 h in the endovascular model has been used to study delayed vasospasm, delayed complications, and their resolution [4, 11, 16].

Conclusion

The endovascular perforation model is considered the closest replica of human SAH. The surgery required to induce SAH through this model is complicated and challenging but can be mastered with training. This model is better suited and extensively used to study early brain injury after SAH.

Conflict of Interest Statement We declare that we have no conflict of interest.

References

1. Bederson JB, Germano IM, Guarino L (1995) Cortical blood flow and cerebral perfusion pressure in a new noncraniotomy model of subarachnoid hemorrhage in the rat. Stroke 26:1086–1091

2. Bederson JB, Levy AL, Ding WH, Kahn R, DiPerna CA, Jenkins AL, Vallabhajosyula P (1998) Acute vasoconstriction after subarachnoid hemorrhage. Neurosurgery 42:352–360
3. Cahill J, Calvert JW, Solaroglu I, Zhang JH (2006) Vasospasm and p53-induced apoptosis in an experimental model of subarachnoid hemorrhage. Stroke 37:1868–1874
4. Furnish EJ, Brophy CM, Harris VA, Macomson S, Winger J, Head GA, Shaver EG (2010) Treatment with transducible phosphopeptide analogues of the small heat shock-related protein, HSP20, after experimental subarachnoid hemorrhage: prevention and reversal of delayed decreases in cerebral perfusion. J Neurosurg 112:631–639
5. Gules I, Satoh M, Clower BR, Nanda A, Zhang JH (2002) Comparison of three rat models of cerebral vasospasm. Am J Physiol Heart Circ Physiol 283:H2551–H2559
6. Nornes H (1978) Cerebral arterial flow dynamics during aneurysm haemorrhage. Acta Neurochir 41:39–48
7. Schwartz AY, Masago A, Sehba FA, Bederson JB (2000) Experimental models of subarachnoid hemorrhage in the rat: a refinement of the endovascular filament model. J Neurosci Methods 96:161–167
8. Sehba F, Bederson JB (2006) Rodent models of hemorrhagic stroke. In: Tatlisumak T, Fisher MJ (eds) Handbook of experimental neurology: methods and techniques in animal research. Cambridge University Press, Cambridge, pp 345–365
9. Sehba FA, Pluta RM (2013) Aneurysmal subarachnoid hemorrhage models: do they need a fix? Stroke Res Treat 2013:615154
10. Sehba FA, Pluta RM, Zhang JH (2011) Metamorphosis of subarachnoid hemorrhage research: from delayed vasospasm to early brain injury. Mol Neurobiol 43:27–40
11. Shiba M, Suzuki H, Fujimoto M, Shimojo N, Imanaka-Yoshida K, Yoshida T, Kanamaru K, Matsushima S, Taki W (2012) Imatinib mesylate prevents cerebral vasospasm after subarachnoid hemorrhage via inhibiting tenascin-C expression in rats. Neurobiol Dis 46:172–179
12. Sugawara T, Ayer R, Jadhav V, Zhang JH (2008) A new grading system evaluating bleeding scale in filament perforation subarachnoid hemorrhage rat model. J Neurosci Methods 167:327–334
13. Trojanowski T (1984) Early effects of experimental arterial subarachnoid haemorrhage on the cerebral circulation. Part I: Experimental subarachnoid haemorrhage in cat and its pathophysiological effects. Methods of regional cerebral blood flow measurement and evaluation of microcirculation. Acta Neurochir 72:79–94
14. Trojanowski T (1984) Early effects of experimental arterial subarachnoid haemorrhage on the cerebral circulation. Part II: Regional cerebral blood flow and cerebral microcirculation after experimental subarachnoid haemorrhage. Acta Neurochir 72:241–255
15. Veelken JA, Laing RJ, Jakubowski J (1995) The Sheffield model of subarachnoid hemorrhage in rats. Stroke 26:1279–1283, discussion 1284
16. Zheng JS, Zhan RY, Zheng SS, Zhou YQ, Tong Y, Wan S (2005) Inhibition of NADPH oxidase attenuates vasospasm after experimental subarachnoid hemorrhage in rats. Stroke 36:1059–1064

Rat Cisterna Magna Double-Injection Model of Subarachnoid Hemorrhage – Background, Advantages/Limitations, Technical Considerations, Modifications, and Outcome Measures

Erdem Güresir, Patrick Schuss, Valeri Borger, and Hartmut Vatter

Abstract The pathophysiological changes following aneurysmal subarachnoid hemorrhage (SAH) are commonly divided into early consequences (developing shortly after the bleeding) and delayed consequences of the bleeding. The development of delayed injury mechanisms, e.g., reduced cerebral blood flow (CBF) caused by cerebral vasospasm (CVS) or development of delayed ischemic neurological deficits (DIND), seem mainly to depend on the amount and duration of the subarachnoid blood clot. CVS may progress to cerebral ischemia and infarction, and therefore lead to delayed neurological deterioration. The rat double-hemorrhage model reproduces the time course of the delayed pathophysiological consequences of CVS, which imitates the clinical setting more precisely than other rodent models. Furthermore, this model is adjustable via various technical considerations or modifications. Therefore, the double-hemorrhage model is predisposed to be used to mimic the delayed effects of SAH and to investigate the use of drugs on morphological ischemic, functional, and vasospastic effects.

Keywords Double hemorrhage • Rat • Experimental model • Subarachnoid hemorrhage

Introduction

Aneurysmal subarachnoid hemorrhage (SAH) compromises an initial acute phase after the bleeding and a phase of delayed consequences of the subarachnoid blood clot. Mechanisms of early brain injury (EBI) include elevated intracranial pressure (ICP), reduced cerebral perfusion, and cerebral blood flow (CBF); these are deemed responsible for poor outcome. These conditions may lead to subsequent cerebral ischemia resulting in EBI in the early phase after aneurysm rupture [1]. Additionally, up to 66 % of patients suffering from SAH develop cerebral vasospasm (CVS), which may progress to cerebral ischemia and infarction [2]. Therefore, delayed ischemic neurological deficits (DIND) may be, at least in part, the result of delayed CVS. However, recent investigations demonstrated prevention of angiographic CVS by an endothelin receptor antagonist without improved neurological outcome [3]. This signifies that the causes of delayed neurological deterioration continues to be poorly understood and supports the need for further experimental investigations for better understanding of histopathological, vascular, and molecular consequences underlying SAH. Therefore, there is a necessity to further investigate early and delayed changes after SAH, e.g., by the induction of experimental SAH in rodents. For this purpose, animal models of experimental SAH were developed and carried out using vessel perforation and blood injection models [4, 5]. For focusing on delayed pathophysiological effects of SAH, single- and double-blood injection models have been reported to better reflect the clinical situation in humans suffering from SAH [4, 6].

Concerning delayed consequences of SAH, the time course of delayed deficits (e.g., DIND) that, at least in part, are caused by CVS, is increased in double-hemorrhage models when compared with single-hemorrhage models [4]. In double-hemorrhage models, the maximum angiographic vasospasm of cerebral arteries occurs between day 3 and 5 after the initial bleeding. In addition to the clinical and angiographic time course of CVS, CBF decreased significantly on day 5 [7]. Accordingly, the rat double-hemorrhage model, which is described in the following, seems to be a suitable and assessable rodent model for investigations on the delayed pathological effects of SAH.

E. Güresir, MD, PhD (✉) • P. Schuss, MD • V. Borger, MD
H. Vatter, MD, PhD
Department of Neurosurgery, University-Hospital Bonn, Sigmund-Freud-Strasse, 53127 Bonn, Germany
e-mail: erdem.gueresir@ukb.uni-bonn.de

J. Fandino et al. (eds.), *Neurovascular Events After Subarachnoid Hemorrhage*, Acta Neurochirurgica Supplement, Vol. 120, DOI 10.1007/978-3-319-04981-6_56, © Springer International Publishing Switzerland 2015

Materials and Methods

Adult male Sprague–Dawley or Wistar rats, weighing 250–500 g, are commonly used for the double-hemorrhage model [7–9]. Rats are anesthetized using intraperitoneal application of midazolam (1 mg/kg body weight) and ketamine (100 mg/kg body weight) [7, 8, 10, 11] and are allowed to breathe spontaneously. Circulation parameters and CBF are stable using this medication [12, 13]. Alternatively, isoflurane [14], with or without additional chloral hydrate [4, 15], is used. The body temperature of the animals should be maintained at approximately 37 °C by a heating pad.

A tube (Portex® polythene tube; luminal diameter, 0.96 mm) is inserted into the left femoral artery for measurement of blood gas values, control of the circulation, and as the source of the later-injected autologous blood. Another tube is inserted into the left femoral vein for additional medication or infusions (crystalloids or hydroxyethyl–starch) to maintain a stable circulation during the procedure, and for the application of contrast agents for conventional angiography or perfusion-weighted magnetic resonance imaging. Both tubes are plugged after irrigation with saline infusion, stored under the skin, and left inside the vessels until the animals are killed.

After both vessels are cannulated and circulatory conditions are stable, animals are positioned in a stereotactic frame. After positioning of the rat, the skin and the muscles are infiltrated with local anesthetics (e.g., mepivacaine 1 %). The skin incision covers the suboccipital region and the arch of C1 (Fig. 1). The acromiotrapezius muscle is cut strictly in the midline to avoid bleeding. The splenius and rhomboid muscles can be displaced laterally using a dissector and held with a retractor. Next, the suboccipital region, the atlanto-occipital membrane, and the C1 arch are exposed. After a small incision of the atlanto-occipital membrane, a tube (Portex® polythene tube; luminal diameter, 0.28 mm) is inserted in the cisterna magna. First, 0.1 ml cerebrospinal fluid is withdrawn using a syringe. Thereafter, 0.2 ml autologous arterial blood from the femoral artery approach is injected into the cisterna magna through the suboccipital tube to induce the SAH (Fig. 2). Animals are moved into a head-down position immediately after the injection and kept in this position for approximately 15 min to ensure an optimal subarachnoid distribution of the autologous blood. After surgical closure of the wounds, 5 ml crystalloid solution and 0.0125 mg fentanyl is administered subcutaneously. The femoral tubes are plugged after irrigation with saline infusion and stored under the skin.

An identical surgical procedure is repeated 24 h after the initial SAH for induction of the second SAH. During the subsequent observation or treatment course, animals receive 5 ml crystalloid solution and 0.0125 mg fentanyl subcutaneously twice a day.

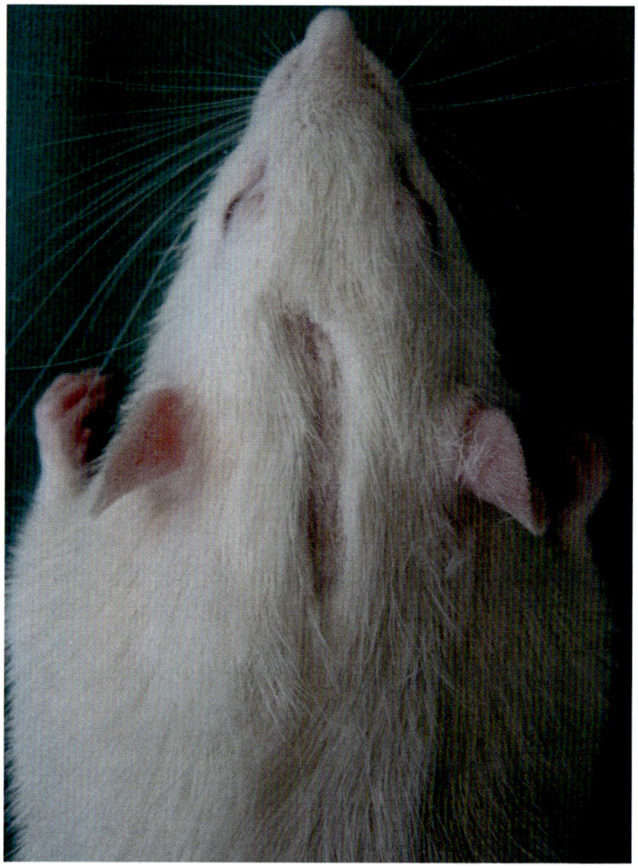

Fig. 1 The skin incision covers the suboccipital region and the arch of C1

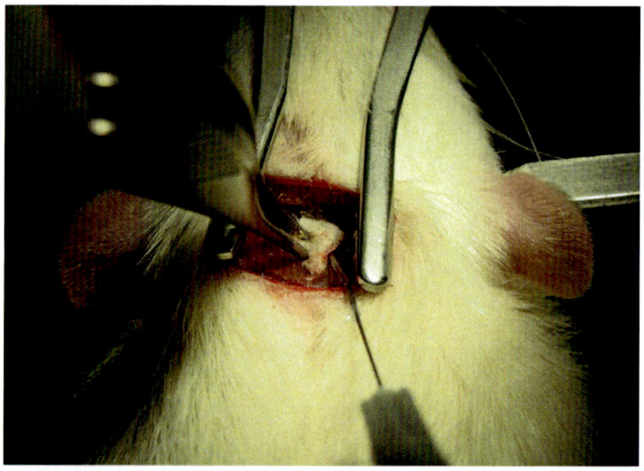

Fig. 2 Induction of subarachnoid hemorrhage by the injection of autologous arterial blood into the cisterna magna

Technical Considerations

An initial small skin incision ensures less surgical trauma and, therefore, a reduction of stress to the animals. The use of a flexible polythene tube for injection of autologous blood into the cisterna magna might minimize the risk of brainstem injuries. The leakage of injected arterial blood can be avoided by adding fibrillar haemostypticum patches (Tabotamp®) and cotton. The injected blood volume should not exceed 0.25 ml to avoid collateral damage.

Technical Modifications

Several technical modifications have been reported for the rat double-hemorrhage model. For instance, unilateral common carotid artery occlusion (CCAO) is known to cause moderate reduction of CBF in both cerebral hemispheres without asymmetrical perfusion [16]. A recent study demonstrated that CCAO deteriorates the effects of CVS in the rat double-hemorrhage model and therefore leads to an aggravation of CVS-related delayed brain tissue damage [17].

A modified rat double-hemorrhage model using a catheter-based blood injection into the cisterna magna through a parieto-occipital burr hole was suggested recently. This modification showed presumably lower mortality rate despite technical difficulties with the positioning of the catheter [18]. To reduce the confounding effects of surgical procedures, a modification using minimally invasive blood injection by a percutaneous, stereotactic injection technique has been reported [19].

Outcome Measures

Neurological Assessment

Delayed consequences of SAH are clinically diagnosed by the so-called delayed ischemic neurological deficit (DIND). Outcome measures include neurological scores, usually investigating motor deficits. For the rat double-hemorrhage model, scales by Ryba and Bederson were described and regularly used [20, 21]. Additionally, the rotating pole test allows prediction of functional motor deficits [22, 23]. Furthermore, Garcia reported a more detailed score for assessment of neurological deterioration in rats with middle cerebral artery occlusion [24]. Thereby, rats were scored from 0 to 3 in six neurobehavioral tests investigating spontaneous activity, symmetry in the movement of all four limbs, forepaw outstretching, climbing, body proprioception, and response to vibrissae touch.

Radiological Investigations

The gold standard in radiological investigations to detect CVS is digital subtraction angiography (DSA). The challenge in angiographic investigations of rat cerebral arteries because of the small vessel diameter has been discussed previously and several techniques have been investigated [15, 25, 26]. Selective catheterization of the vertebral artery (VA) shows the highest resolution in imaging the basilar artery (BA). However, multiple angiographic investigations contain a higher risk of cardiac abnormalities caused by the contrast medium. Therefore, the use of one selective DSA at the end of the experiment seems to represent a practical reference parameter for the quantitative determination of delayed CVS in the rat. The time course of the development of angiographic CVS in this model has already been characterized, and the maximum CVS was found to occur on day 5, in agreement with morphological investigations using immunohistochemistry [7, 8].

However, cerebral perfusion measurement by computed tomography (CT) or magnetic resonance (MR) imaging are becoming more important for diagnosis and monitoring of impaired CBF after SAH during the course of clinical treatment of patients with SAH. Accordingly, these tools have also been applied in the animal model [7, 27, 28].

Furthermore, determination of CBF and/or cerebral blood volume (CBV) is germane to detect delayed pathophysiological effects of CVS. The application of a noninvasive MR perfusion-weighted imaging (PWI) method was the first to characterize the decrease in CBF and CBV in the rat double-hemorrhage model in a semiquantitative fashion. Both CBV and CBF are reduced to approximately one-third of the control value on day 5 after the initial bleeding [7].

Histological Investigations

Histopathological investigations are used to investigate the morphological changes after SAH. Because of their known sensitivity to cerebral ischemia, vital neurons were counted in the hippocampus and adjoining cortex regions for the assessment of CVS-related cerebral ischemia [29–31]. Neurons were usually classified as nonvital or necrotic in the presence of pyknosis, karyorrhexis, karyolysis, cytoplasmic eosinophilia, or loss of affinity for hematoxylin [32]. In the rat double-hemorrhage model, a significantly decreased neuronal cell count was observed in the hippocampal regions and inner cortex layers as result of delayed cerebral damage caused by CVS on day 5 but not on day 3 [8].

Apoptosis as a result of delayed brain injury caused by CVS was detectable using the TUNEL-staining method in a histopathological investigation approximately 7 days after SAH [33]. Furthermore, the inner vessel diameter and wall thickness of the BA are commonly used as histological parameters to indicate CVS. Consistent with angiographic results, the reduction of the arterial diameter in histological investigations is approximately 50 % [7, 8, 34].

Functional Investigations

Functional investigations of the rat BA are performed to analyze cerebrovascular contractility or relaxation as well as drug effects. However, several investigations successfully provided functional data based on the rat double-hemorrhage model [11, 34–36].

Advantages and Limitations

This rat double-hemorrhage model has several limitations that have previously been discussed [14].

First, double-injection models seem less suitable to investigate the acute stage of SAH, including EBI [14]. However, Prunell et al. demonstrated a great variation in the amount of subarachnoid blood in the different injection and perforation models and a faster restoration of CBF after SAH induction in the injection models compared with the perforation models [37]. Although reflecting the clinical setting, great variation of subarachnoid blood volume might lead to the need for larger groups. The mortality rate in this rat double-hemorrhage model has been described to be up to 50 % in previous studies [7, 8, 11]. This mortality rate is even increased by the use of invasive procedures, such as DSA. The high mortality rate might have been criticized, but it also indicates the implementation of severe experimental SAH and is comparable to the outcome in humans.

Because of the known pronounced cortical collateralization in the rat, ischemic territorial infarctions do not occur [20]. Nevertheless, because of several advantages, the rat double-hemorrhage model is a feasible, effective, and customizable rodent model for experimental SAH. First, the experimental setting is cost effective, manageable, and can be established in most centers. Furthermore, this model provides a good imitation of the clinical setting and time course of delayed effects of CVS. Eventually, the degree of severity and characteristics of CVS as well as the reduction of CBF are more pronounced in the rat double-hemorrhage model when compared with single-injection models [5].

Conclusion

The aim of rat subarachnoid blood injection models is mainly to imitate CVS or delayed cerebral perfusion deficits after SAH. The rat double-hemorrhage model elongates the time course of the pathophysiological consequences of CVS, which imitates the clinical setting more precisely than single-hemorrhage models. The possibilities of extended investigations in this model, e.g., by in vivo evaluations such as MRI or DSA, considerably increases the complexity of the model but imitates the clinical course in humans more closely than other established rodent models. Therefore, the double-hemorrhage model is used to mimic the delayed effects of SAH and to investigate the use of drugs on morphological ischemic, functional, and vasospastic effects.

Conflict of Interest Statement We declare that we have no conflict of interest.

References

1. Sehba FA, Bederson JB (2006) Mechanisms of acute brain injury after subarachnoid hemorrhage. Neurol Res 28(4):381–398
2. Macdonald RL, Kassell NF, Mayer S, Ruefenacht D, Schmiedek P, Weidauer S, Frey A, Roux S, Pasqualin A, Investigators C– (2008) Clazosentan to overcome neurological ischemia and infarction occurring after subarachnoid hemorrhage (CONSCIOUS-1): randomized, double-blind, placebo-controlled phase 2 dose-finding trial. Stroke 39(11):3015–3021
3. Macdonald RL, Higashida RT, Keller E, Mayer SA, Molyneux A, Raabe A, Vajkoczy P, Wanke I, Bach D, Frey A, Marr A, Roux S, Kassell N (2011) Clazosentan, an endothelin receptor antagonist, in patients with aneurysmal subarachnoid haemorrhage undergoing surgical clipping: a randomised, double-blind, placebo-controlled phase 3 trial (CONSCIOUS-2). Lancet Neurol 10(7):618–625
4. Solomon RA, Antunes JL, Chen RY, Bland L, Chien S (1985) Decrease in cerebral blood flow in rats after experimental subarachnoid hemorrhage: a new animal model. Stroke 16(1):58–64
5. Gules I, Satoh M, Clower BR, Nanda A, Zhang JH (2002) Comparison of three rat models of cerebral vasospasm. Am J Physiol Heart Circ Physiol 283(6):H2551–H2559
6. Megyesi JF, Vollrath B, Cook DA, Findlay JM (2000) In vivo animal models of cerebral vasospasm: a review. Neurosurgery 46(2):448–460, discussion 460–441
7. Vatter H, Weidauer S, Konczalla J, Dettmann E, Zimmermann M, Raabe A, Preibisch C, Zanella FE, Seifert V (2006) Time course in the development of cerebral vasospasm after experimental subarachnoid hemorrhage: clinical and neuroradiological assessment of the rat double hemorrhage model. Neurosurgery 58(6):1190–1197, discussion 1190–1197
8. Güresir E, Raabe A, Jaiimsin A, Dias S, Raab P, Seifert V, Vatter H (2010) Histological evidence of delayed ischemic brain tissue damage in the rat double-hemorrhage model. J Neurol Sci 293(1–2): 18–22
9. Meguro T, Clower BR, Carpenter R, Parent AD, Zhang JH (2001) Improved rat model for cerebral vasospasm studies. Neurol Res 23(7):761–766
10. Dittmar MS, Fehm NP, Vatankhah B, Horn M (2004) Ketamine/xylazine anesthesia for radiologic imaging of neurologically impaired rats: dose response, respiratory depression, and management of complications. Comp Med 54(6):652–655
11. Güresir E, Vasiliadis N, Konczalla J, Raab P, Hattingen E, Seifert V, Vatter H (2013) Erythropoietin prevents delayed hemodynamic dysfunction after subarachnoid hemorrhage in a randomized controlled experimental setting. J Neurol Sci 332:128–135
12. Rousselle CH, Lefauconnier JM, Allen DD (1998) Evaluation of anesthetic effects on parameters for the in situ rat brain perfusion technique. Neurosci Lett 257(3):139–142

13. Lei H, Grinberg O, Nwaigwe CI, Hou HG, Williams H, Swartz HM, Dunn JF (2001) The effects of ketamine-xylazine anesthesia on cerebral blood flow and oxygenation observed using nuclear magnetic resonance perfusion imaging and electron paramagnetic resonance oximetry. Brain Res 913(2):174–179
14. Lee JY, Sagher O, Keep R, Hua Y, Xi G (2009) Comparison of experimental rat models of early brain injury after subarachnoid hemorrhage. Neurosurgery 65(2):331–343, discussion 343
15. Delgado TJ, Brismar J, Svendgaard NA (1985) Subarachnoid haemorrhage in the rat: angiography and fluorescence microscopy of the major cerebral arteries. Stroke 16(4):595–602
16. De Ley G, Nshimyumuremyi JB, Leusen I (1985) Hemispheric blood flow in the rat after unilateral common carotid occlusion: evolution with time. Stroke 16(1):69–73
17. Güresir E, Vasiliadis N, Dias S, Raab P, Seifert V, Vatter H (2012) The effect of common carotid artery occlusion on delayed brain tissue damage in the rat double subarachnoid hemorrhage model. Acta Neurochir (Wien) 154(1):11–19
18. Raslan F, Albert-Weissenberger C, Westermaier T, Saker S, Kleinschnitz C, Lee JY (2012) A modified double injection model of cisterna magna for the study of delayed cerebral vasospasm following subarachnoid hemorrhage in rats. Exp Transl Stroke Med 4(1):23
19. Dusick JR, Evans BC, Laiwalla A, Krahl S, Gonzalez NR (2011) A minimally-invasive rat model of subarachnoid hemorrhage and delayed ischemic injury. Surg Neurol Int 2:99
20. Bederson JB, Pitts LH, Tsuji M, Nishimura MC, Davis RL, Bartkowski H (1986) Rat middle cerebral artery occlusion: evaluation of the model and development of a neurologic examination. Stroke 17(3):472–476
21. Ryba MS, Gordon-Krajcer W, Walski M, Chalimoniuk M, Chrapusta SJ (1999) Hydroxylamine attenuates the effects of simulated subarachnoid hemorrhage in the rat brain and improves neurological outcome. Brain Res 850(1–2):225–233
22. Larsen CC, Povlsen GK, Rasmussen MN, Edvinsson L (2011) Improvement in neurological outcome and abolition of cerebrovascular endothelin B and 5-hydroxytryptamine 1B receptor upregulation through mitogen-activated protein kinase kinase 1/2 inhibition after subarachnoid hemorrhage in rats. J Neurosurg 114(4):1143–1153
23. Mattiasson GJ, Philips MF, Tomasevic G, Johansson BB, Wieloch T, McIntosh TK (2000) The rotating pole test: evaluation of its effectiveness in assessing functional motor deficits following experimental head injury in the rat. J Neurosci Methods 95(1):75–82
24. Garcia JH, Wagner S, Liu KF, Hu XJ (1995) Neurological deficit and extent of neuronal necrosis attributable to middle cerebral artery occlusion in rats. Statistical validation. Stroke 26(4):627–634, discussion 635
25. Longo M, Blandino A, Ascenti G, Ricciardi GK, Granata F, Vinci S (2002) Cerebral angiography in the rat with mammographic equipment: a simple, cost-effective method for assessing vasospasm in experimental subarachnoid haemorrhage. Neuroradiology 44(8):689–694
26. Weidauer S, Vatter H, Dettmann E, Seifert V, Zanella FE (2006) Assessment of vasospasm in experimental subarachnoid hemorrhage in rats by selective biplane digital subtraction angiography. Neuroradiology 48(3):176–181
27. Schambach SJ, Bag S, Groden C, Schilling L, Brockmann MA (2010) Vascular imaging in small rodents using micro-CT. Methods 50(1):26–35
28. Schambach SJ, Bag S, Schilling L, Groden C, Brockmann MA (2010) Application of micro-CT in small animal imaging. Methods 50(1):2–13
29. Soehle M, Heimann A, Kempski O (1998) Postischemic application of lipid peroxidation inhibitor U-101033E reduces neuronal damage after global cerebral ischemia in rats. Stroke 29(6):1240–1246, discussion 1246–1247
30. Hossmann KA (1998) Experimental models for the investigation of brain ischemia. Cardiovasc Res 39(1):106–120
31. Sugawara T, Lewen A, Noshita N, Gasche Y, Chan PH (2002) Effects of global ischemia duration on neuronal, astroglial, oligodendroglial, and microglial reactions in the vulnerable hippocampal CA1 subregion in rats. J Neurotrauma 19(1):85–98
32. Li F, Liu KF, Silva MD, Omae T, Sotak CH, Fenstermacher JD, Fisher M, Hsu CY, Lin W (2000) Transient and permanent resolution of ischemic lesions on diffusion-weighted imaging after brief periods of focal ischemia in rats: correlation with histopathology. Stroke 31(4):946–954
33. Lin CL, Dumont AS, Su YF, Dai ZK, Cheng JT, Tsai YJ, Huang JH, Chang KP, Hwang SL (2009) Attenuation of subarachnoid hemorrhage-induced apoptotic cell death with 17 beta-estradiol. Laboratory investigation. J Neurosurg 111(5):1014–1022
34. Vatter H, Konczalla J, Weidauer S, Preibisch C, Zimmermann M, Raabe A, Seifert V (2007) Effect of delayed cerebral vasospasm on cerebrovascular endothelin A receptor expression and function. J Neurosurg 107(1):121–127
35. Konczalla J, Mrosek J, Wanderer S, Schuss P, Güresir E, Seifert V, Vatter H, Platz J (2013) Functional effects of levosimendan in rat basilar arteries in vitro. Curr Neurovasc Res 10(2): 126–133
36. Schilling L, Vatter H, Mursch K, Ehrenreich H, Schmiedek P (2000) Characterization of the contractile and relaxant action of the endothelin-1 precursor, big endothelin-1, in the isolated rat basilar artery. Peptides 21(1):91–99
37. Prunell GF, Mathiesen T, Svendgaard NA (2004) Experimental subarachnoid hemorrhage: cerebral blood flow and brain metabolism during the acute phase in three different models in the rat. Neurosurgery 54(2):426–436, discussion 436–427

A Rabbit Cisterna Magna Double-Injection Subarachnoid Hemorrhage Model

Yuichiro Kikkawa

Abstract In recent years, the shift of research interest in the pathological condition after subarachnoid hemorrhage (SAH) from delayed cerebral vasospasm to early brain injury and the development of molecular genetic approaches in animal experiments has resulted in a diversification of animal SAH models. The properties of each animal SAH model thus need to be validated and the purpose of using each animal model should be clarified. This study presents the settings and technical procedures for a rabbit cisterna magna double-injection SAH model and discusses the advantages and limitations of using this model.

Keywords Rabbit • Subarachnoid hemorrhage • Cerebral vasospasm • Animal model

Introduction

In 1969, Offerhaus and van Gool reported the first rabbit model of subarachnoid hemorrhage (SAH) to investigate cardiac dysfunction after SAH [12]. In 1977, Svendgaard et al. reported increased reactivity of the isolated basilar artery after SAH using a rabbit SAH model [14]. In 1982, Edvinsson et al. first reported rabbit cerebral vasospasm (CVS) using a single-injection model [2]. Since the 1980s, rabbit SAH models have mainly been used for investigating CVS [10]. Volume-controlled blood injection via the cisterna magna is the most popular method of inducing SAH in the rabbit. On the other hand, Offerhaus and van Gool [12] and Marbacher et al. [9] reported blood pressure-controlled cisterna magna blood injection methods. The most common procedure for volume-controlled blood injection methods is to use 3 or 1 ml/kg of autologous blood injected into the cisterna magna per injection [10]. The frequency of blood injection ranges from one to three times, although the most commonly used method is one injection [10]. The double-injection method induces vasospasm that is more severe and prolonged than the single-injection method and is well established in dog models [15], and recently in a rat model [4]. In rabbits, the double-injection method reportedly produces vasospasm that is more severe and persistent [1, 16]. However, the double-injection method is not popular in rabbit models. One possible reason is because Spallone et al. reported the ineffectiveness of enhancement of CVS and a high mortality rate with the double-injection method [10, 13]. In the rabbit double-injection model, vasospasm peaks approximately 5 days after the first injection and persists for up to the next 2 days.

Rabbit Double-Injection SAH Model Procedure

Six-month-old male Japanese white rabbits (body weight, 2.5–3.0 kg) are anesthetized with an intramuscular injection of ketamine (40 mg/kg body weight) and placed into a restraining cage. Sodium pentobarbital (20 mg/kg body weight) is then injected into the marginal auricular vein as intravenous anesthesia. On day 0, 0.5–1.0 ml of cerebrospinal fluid (CSF) is aspirated percutaneously from the cisterna magna using a 23-gauge butterfly needle, and 2.5 ml of autologous arterial blood obtained from the central auricular artery is injected into the cistern magna over 1 min. The animal is then kept in a prone position with the head tilted down at 30° for 30 min. On day 2, a second injection of autologous

Y. Kikkawa, MD, PhD
Department of Neurosurgery, Graduate School of Medical Sciences, Kyushu University,
3-1-1 Maidashi, Higashi-ku, Fukuoka 812-8582, Japan
e-mail: ykikkawa@ns.med.kyushu-u.ac.jp

blood is similarly performed. CSF samples can be obtained just before injection of blood on days 0 and 2 and on the day of killing. On day 2, the CSF findings can confirm whether the first-injected blood has been properly injected into the cisterna magna.

Advantages and Limitations of Using the Rabbit Model

The rabbit model offers two main advantages. First, the size of the basilar artery in rabbits makes this vessel easy to handle. The basilar artery is easily hung on a wire for tension measurements and the thickness of the arterial wall is suitable for loading fluorescent dyes for calcium measurements. Second, a sufficient amount of basilar artery tissue for polymerase chain reaction (PCR) or immunoblot analysis can be obtained from a single animal. In our preparation, the wet weight of the entire length of the basilar artery is 8.6 mg on average. Approximately 70 mg of protein can be extracted from the basilar artery of one rabbit using a freezing/thawing method. For total RNA extraction, approximately 2.5 mg of RNA can be extracted from the basilar artery of one rabbit. This is equivalent to 80 PCRs, assuming that a total of 30 ng of RNA (in triplicate) is required for one reverse-transcription PCR (RT-PCR) assay. These two advantages are applicable to any large-animal model, such as dog, monkey, or pig. However, those animals are too large to handle as easily as rabbits and are much more expensive than rabbits. Rabbits are relatively inexpensive. Other benefits are that the central auricular artery and marginal auricular vein are safe, quick, minimally invasive, and offer highly reliable vascular access. Rabbits are relatively easy to restrain when using an appropriate restraining device, given their relatively docile nature. Intubation and respiratory support are not required in anesthesia.

There are two important limitations when using rabbits. First, useful antibodies for rabbit tissue are far less available than for tissues from other species. Many antibodies are not recommended for immunoreaction of rabbit tissue, because the rabbit is one of the most commonly used host species for raising antibodies. The second problem is the limited availability of genetically modified rabbits. Genetically modified rabbits, such as transgenic, knockout, conditional knockout, knock-in, and knockdown rabbits, are hard to obtain compared with mice, because of the difficulty in applying genetic modification techniques to rabbits. These may represent major problems for molecular biological approaches using rabbits.

Technical Considerations in Making the Double-Injection Rabbit SAH Model

Position, Head Fixation, and Puncture of the Cisterna Magna

The neck should be bent forward as much as possible to maximize the space between the foramen magnum and C1. We use perforated cardboard for head fixation while maintaining the bent-neck forward position (Fig. 1a). For accurate puncture, touching the inion and spinous process of C2 is important (Fig. 1b). For improved visualization, the posterior neck of the rabbit should be sprayed with alcohol or the hair of the posterior neck should be shaved. After injection of blood, rabbits are positioned by tilting them head-down by 30° for 30 min using an adjustable bed (Fig. 1c). Downward tilt is important to spread the blood cranially.

Causes of Death in the Procedure

Deaths occurring during the procedure are mainly caused by a failure of puncture and rapid elevation of intracranial pressure (ICP). Failure to achieve accurate puncture, such as brainstem needling or intraparenchymal blood injection, often leads to the death of the animal. To avoid puncture failure, the following factors may be important: having an appropriate posture, not evacuating too much CSF, and directing the needle slightly rostrally and puncturing as the tip of the needle runs through under the foramen magnum. A rapid increase in ICP causes respiratory arrest or cardiac arrest during the procedure. These problems tend to occur with the second injection. Pain stimulation or thoracic compression often restores respiration and cardiac rhythm. A slow injection is the most important factor to consider. We usually perform the injection over the course of 1 min. However, we sometimes take a much longer time for the injection, depending on the respiratory condition during the injection. We often encounter twitching of the roots of the ear when the injected blood reaches approximately 2.5–3.0 ml. This response may be caused by compression or stretching of the facial nerve by the injected blood. We consider this as a warning sign of reaching the maximum amount of blood able to be injected. A 2.5-ml syringe is appropriate for injection, because we can feel the resistance of the ICP through the syringe. After the injection of blood, observation of the respiratory condition for 10 min is important, because respiratory arrest mostly occurs in the first few minutes after injection.

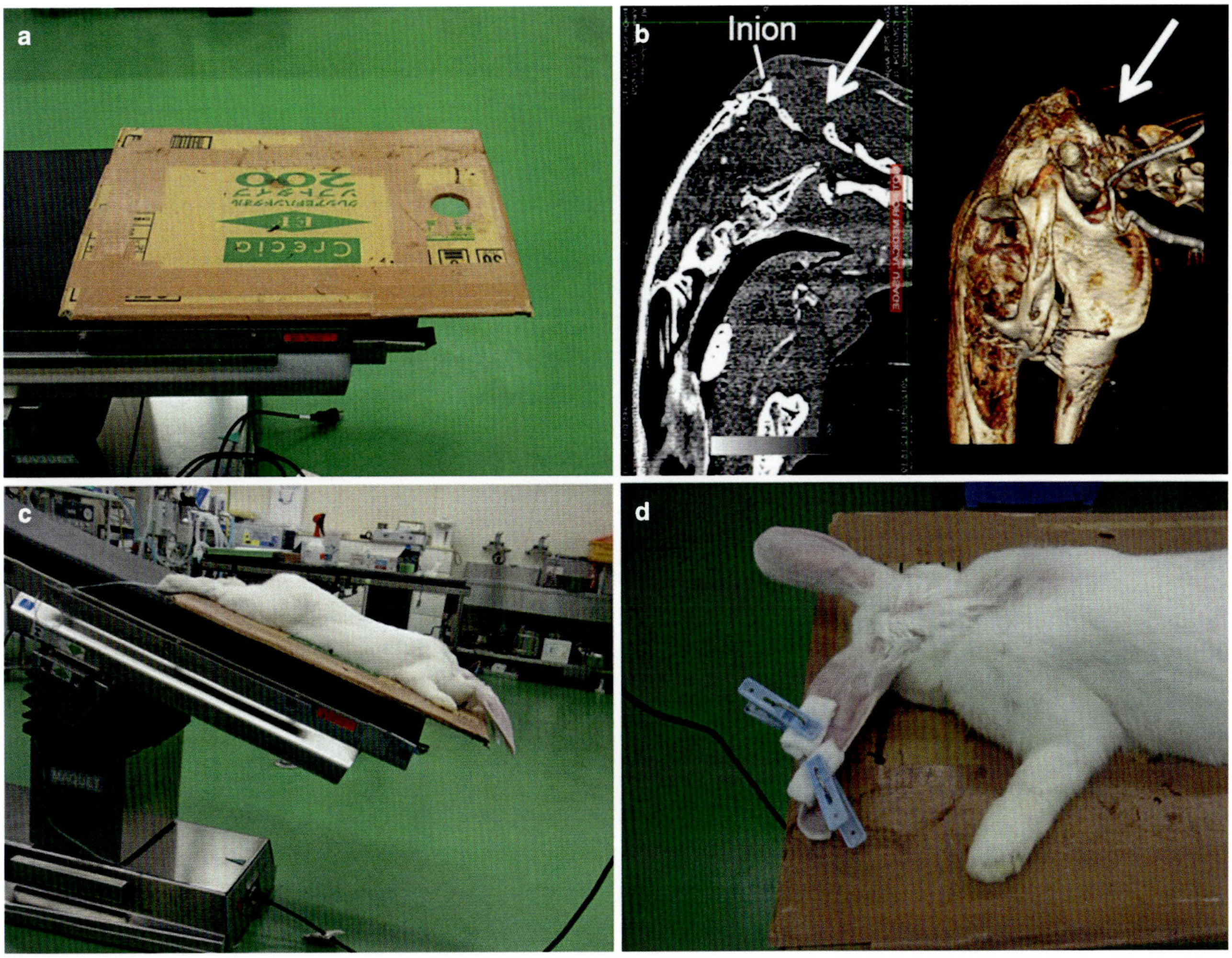

Fig. 1 Preparation of the rabbit subarachnoid hemorrhage model. (**a**) Cardboard with a hole for head fixation to keep a bent-neck forward position. (**b**) Sagittal section image and three-dimensional volume-rendering image of the rabbit head from computed tomography scan, showing the puncture point and direction of the needle (*white arrows*) for puncture of the cisterna magna. (**c**) Tilting the head 30° down on an adjustable bed with the feet of the rabbit strapped to the bed frame using silicone tubes. (**d**) Clothespin to stem bleeding from the central auricular artery and marginal auricular vein

Epidural, Subdural, and Intraparenchymal Hematomas

On rare occasions, blood is injected into spaces other than the subarachnoid space because of accidental movement of the needle chip induced by body movement, loss of traction of the subarachnoid membrane induced by excessive evacuation of CSF, or intense negative pressure during CSF evacuation. To avoid body movement, appropriate control of the depth of anesthesia is important, especially in our procedure, which does not require strict head fixation using instruments. Sodium pentobarbital regulates the depth of anesthesia. We confirm the depth of anesthesia by providing painful stimulation just before puncture. If the anesthesia is weak, finger pressure on the skin around the puncture point easily induces body movement. Deep anesthesia easily induces respiratory arrest following injection of blood.

After Blood Injection

Immediate withdrawal of the puncture needle causes leakage of injected blood with CSF from a pinhole in the dura mater. An indwelling venous catheter should also be maintained during the entire process in case additional anesthesia is required. It is therefore important to not withdraw all of the needles during the entire process. Preservation of the artery and vein in the ear is important, especially in the double-injection method, because we often use the same vessel repeatedly. After withdrawal of the needle, firm pressure

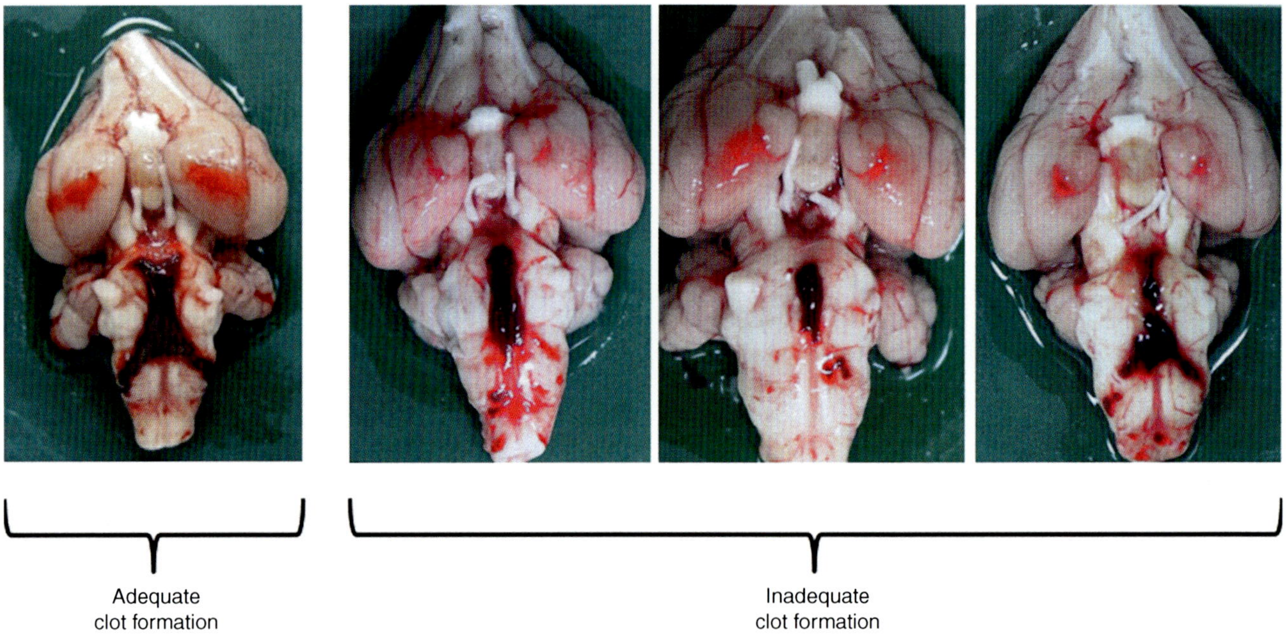

Fig. 2 Residual clots over the surface of the pons just after excising the whole brain. Onsite determination of the propriety of the subarachnoid hemorrhage model is based on residual clot formation just after sacrifice

should be applied on the pinhole to stem bleeding, so as to not damage the ear vessels by hematoma formation. We use clothespins to completely stem bleeding (Fig. 1d).

Outcome Measures

Blood clot formation, degree of vasospasm, cerebral perfusion, neurological and behavioral deficit, and appetite loss have been evaluated as outcome measures of the rabbit SAH model. Brief assessment of clot formation is important for onsite determination of the propriety of the SAH model just after sacrifice. A single report by Zhou et al. [16] described a scoring method of residual clots along the basilar artery of the rabbit SAH model. In our laboratory, when clots do not form sufficiently (Fig. 2), those models are excluded from the following experiments using the basilar artery. Expansion of clot formation can be evaluated quantitatively using imaging software [5]. For the evaluation of arterial narrowing, digital subtraction angiography (DSA), measurement of crosssectional area using a perfusion fixation sample, direct observation, and computed tomography (CT) angiography are available in rabbits. DSA and crosssectional area measurement are the most popular in rabbits [10]. Evaluation of the external diameter of the basilar artery through direct observation is readily applied on sacrifice day [6, 7]. A potential disadvantage of this method is underestimating arterial narrowing because the thickness of the arterial wall is included in the value. In our model, vasospasm occurs on day 3 after the first injection of blood and peaks on day 5 (data not shown). Recently, the usefulness of CT evaluation of vessel diameter and cerebral perfusion in rabbits has been reported [8, 11]. Few reports have described neurobehavioral scoring of the rabbit SAH model. The grading systems by Endo et al. [3] and Zhou et al. [16] are well known [3, 16]. Our rabbits show some slight loss of appetite on days 3 and 5, but rarely show neurological deterioration (data not shown), suggesting that the rabbit double-injection model does not tend to be symptomatic.

Applicability of the Rabbit Double-Injection Model for the Study of Early Brain Injury (EBI) and Delayed CVS (DCVS)

The rabbit double-injection method does not seem to be appropriate for the study of EBI for the following reasons. First, in the double-injection method, a second injection of blood may affect or mask early changes caused by the first injection. Second, ICP elevation is not sufficient in the volume-controlled blood injection method. Because elevated ICP is an important factor in EBI, pressure-controlled blood injection methods, such as endovascular perforation or extracranial–intracranial blood shunting, appear more appropriate than volume-controlled blood injection methods. For the study of DCVS, the double-injection method seems appropriate for the following reasons. First, the double-injection method in the rabbit SAH model causes delayed and prolonged vasospasm, such as that seen in SAH patients. Second, a wide body of research knowledge regarding CVS has been accumulated using rabbit basilar artery from previous studies. Third, evaluating narrowing of the cerebral artery is relatively easy in rabbits.

Conclusion

A rabbit double-injection SAH model seems more appropriate for the study of DCVS than for the study of EBI. Research using rabbits appears to encounter difficulties in molecular biological approaches because of the limited availability of suitable antibodies and the inapplicability of genetic modification techniques to rabbits.

Acknowledgment This research was supported by JSPS KAKENHI (Grant Numbers 24791510, 25670624 and 26462164).

Conflict of Interest Statement We declare that we have no conflict of interest.

References

1. Baker KF, Zervas NT, Pile-Spellman J, Vacanti FX, Miller D (1987) Angiographic evidence of basilar artery constriction in the rabbit: a new model of vasospasm. Surg Neurol 27:107–112
2. Edvinsson L, Egund N, Owman C, Sahlin C, Svendgaard NA (1982) Reduced noradrenaline uptake and retention in cerebrovascular nerves associated with angiographically visible vasoconstriction following experimental subarachnoid hemorrhage in rabbits. Brain Res Bull 9:799–805
3. Endo S, Branson PJ, Alksne JF (1988) Experimental model of symptomatic vasospasm in rabbits. Stroke 19:1420–1425
4. Gules I, Satoh M, Clower BR, Nanda A, Zhang JH (2002) Comparison of three rat models of cerebral vasospasm. Am J Physiol Heart Circ Physiol 283:H2551–H2559
5. Kameda K, Kikkawa Y, Hirano M, Matsuo S, Sasaki T, Hirano K (2012) Combined argatroban and anti-oxidative agents prevents increased vascular contractility to thrombin and other ligands after subarachnoid haemorrhage. Br J Pharmacol 165:106–119
6. Kikkawa Y, Kameda K, Hirano M, Sasaki T, Hirano K (2010) Impaired feedback regulation of the receptor activity and the myofilament Ca^{2+} sensitivity contributes to increased vascular reactiveness after subarachnoid hemorrhage. J Cereb Blood Flow Metab 30:1637–1650
7. Kikkawa Y, Matsuo S, Kameda K, Hirano M, Nakamizo A, Sasaki T, Hirano K (2012) Mechanisms underlying potentiation of endothelin-1-induced myofilament Ca^{2+} sensitization after subarachnoid hemorrhage. J Cereb Blood Flow Metab 32:341–352
8. Laslo AM, Eastwood JD, Pakkiri P, Chen F, Lee TY (2008) CT perfusion-derived mean transit time predicts early mortality and delayed vasospasm after experimental subarachnoid hemorrhage. AJNR Am J Neuroradiol 29:79–85
9. Marbacher S, Andereggen L, Neuschmelting V, Widmer HR, von Gunten M, Takala J, Jakob SM, Fandino J (2012) A new rabbit model for the study of early brain injury after subarachnoid hemorrhage. J Neurosci Methods 208:138–145
10. Marbacher S, Fandino J, Kitchen ND (2010) Standard intracranial in vivo animal models of delayed cerebral vasospasm. Br J Neurosurg 24:415–434
11. Murphy AM, Xenocostas A, Pakkiri P, Lee TY (2008) Hemodynamic effects of recombinant human erythropoietin on the central nervous system after subarachnoid hemorrhage: reduction of microcirculatory impairment and functional deficits in a rabbit model. J Neurosurg 109:1155–1164
12. Offerhaus L, van Gool J (1969) Electrocardiographic changes and tissue catecholamines in experimental subarachnoid haemorrhage. Cardiovasc Res 3:433–440
13. Spallone A, Pastore FS (1989) Cerebral vasospasm in a double-injection model in rabbit. Surg Neurol 32:408–417
14. Svendgaard NA, Edvinsson L, Owman C, Sahlin C (1977) Increased sensitivity of the basilar artery to norepinephrine and 5-hydroxytryptamine following experimental subarachnoid hemorrhage. Surg Neurol 8:191–195
15. Varsos VG, Liszczak TM, Han DH, Kistler JP, Vielma J, Black PM, Heros RC, Zervas NT (1983) Delayed cerebral vasospasm is not reversible by aminophylline, nifedipine, or papaverine in a "two-hemorrhage" canine model. J Neurosurg 58:11–17
16. Zhou ML, Shi JX, Zhu JQ, Hang CH, Mao L, Chen KF, Yin HX (2007) Comparison between one- and two-hemorrhage models of cerebral vasospasm in rabbits. J Neurosci Methods 159:318–324

The Rabbit Blood Shunt Subarachnoid Haemorrhage Model

Serge Marbacher, Ali Reza Fathi, Carl Muroi, Daniel Coluccia, Lukas Andereggen, Volker Neuschmelting, Hans Rudolf Widmer, Stephan M. Jakob, and Javier Fandino

Abstract The recently introduced rabbit blood shunt subarachnoid haemorrhage model is based on the two standard procedures of subclavian artery cannulation and transcutaneous cisterna magna puncture. An extracorporeal shunt placed in between the arterial system and the subarachnoid space allows examiner-independent SAH in a closed cranium. Despite its straightforwardness, it is worth examining some specific features and characteristics of the model. We outline technical considerations to successfully perform the model with minimal mortality and morbidity. In addition, we discuss outcome measures, advantages and limitations, and the applicability of the model for the study of early brain injury and delayed cerebral vasospasm after SAH.

Keywords Rabbit • Model • Subarachnoid haemorrhage Early brain injury • Delayed cerebral vasospasm

S. Marbacher, MD, MSc (✉) • A.R. Fathi, MD • J. Fandino, MD
Department of Neurosurgery, Kantonsspital Aarau,
Aarau, Switzerland
e-mail: serge.marbacher@ksa.ch; ali-reza.fathi@ksa.ch;
javier.fandino@ksa.ch

D. Coluccia
Department of Neurosurgery, Kantonsspital Aarau,
Aarau, Switzerland

Department of Intensive Care Medicine,
University and University Hospital Bern, Bern, Switzerland

C. Muroi, MD
Department of Neurosurgery, Kantonsspital Aarau,
Aarau, Switzerland

Department of Intensive Care Medicine,
University and University Hospital Bern, Bern, Switzerland

Department of Neuropharmacology,
Faculty of Pharmaceutical Sciences, Fukuoka University,
Fukuoka, Japan

Neurocritical Care Unit, Department of Neurosurgery,
University Hospital Zurich, Zurich, Switzerland
e-mail: carl.muroi@ksa.ch

L. Andereggen • H.R. Widmer
Department of Neurosurgery,
Bern University Hospital and University of Bern,
Bern, Switzerland
e-mail: lukas.andereggen@insel.ch; hansrudolf.widmer@insel.ch

V. Neuschmelting
Department of Neurosurgery, University Hospital Cologne,
Cologne, Germany
e-mail: volker.neuschmelting@uk-koeln.de

S.M. Jakob
Department of Intensive Care Medicine,
University and University Hospital Bern, Bern, Switzerland
e-mail: stephan.jakob@insel.ch

Background

The rabbit was introduced for the study of delayed cerebral vasospasm (DCVS) after subarachnoid haemorrhage (SAH) in the 1980s and has become one of the most widely used species in this field of research [12]. More than a dozen different rabbit SAH models have been described so far and almost all techniques are based on blood injections with a large range of associated parameters (delivery route, blood volumes, and injection time, speed, and pressure). Two SAH techniques that were more technically demanding, vessel puncture via left parasagittal [9] and transclival craniotomy [2], were proposed but did not become widespread. Nowadays, the standard for SAH induction is the single (and the increasingly used double) autologous blood injection into the cisterna magna [6, 12, 14, 20]. This technique has proved to induce consistent and reliable DCVS, although its suitability for the study of acute events after SAH remains a matter of debate.

We recently proposed a novel technique that aims to mimic the acute pathophysiology of SAH more closely. In this technique, the cisterna magna model has been adapted by connecting the arterial system (subclavian artery) and the cisterna magna via extracorporeal shunt. Blood flows under arterial pressure into the subarachnoid space in a closed cranium. The

J. Fandino et al. (eds.), *Neurovascular Events After Subarachnoid Hemorrhage*, Acta Neurochirurgica Supplement, Vol. 120,
DOI 10.1007/978-3-319-04981-6_58, © Springer International Publishing Switzerland 2015

blood flow is linked to the rabbit's physiology and driven by the pressure gradient between the arterial blood pressure and intracranial pressure (ICP). Although the blood shunt technique used for SAH induction is based on the standard procedures of subclavian artery cannulation and transcutaneous cisterna magna puncture, there are some specific features and characteristics important enough to be discussed in greater detail.

Materials and Methods

Anaesthesia, Perioperative Care, and Monitoring

General anaesthesia is induced in 3- to 4-month-old New Zealand White rabbits by subcutaneous administration of ketamine and xylazine and continued intravenously using the lateral ear vein. Lack of a toe-pinch reflex confirms that the rabbit is fully anaesthetised. The pectoral muscle is infiltrated with a local anaesthetic before dissection. The depth of anaesthesia is controlled every 20 min during surgery by monitoring respiratory rate, heart rate, and reaction to noxious stimulation (toe-pinch test). Postoperative pain relief is managed by subcutaneous administration of buprenorphine and transdermal fentanyl patches. Arterial blood gas status ($PaCO_2$, PaO_2) is analysed before angiography. Standard cardiovascular monitoring (invasive arterial blood pressure measurement, three-channel ECG) is performed throughout the experiment.

Angiography

Baseline digital subtraction angiography (DSA) is performed on day 0 before SAH and on day 3 after SAH. The rabbits are placed in a supine position. The surgical site is clipped, the skin cleaned with a suitable disinfectant, and the rabbit covered with sterile sheets. The rabbit's left or right subclavian artery is microsurgically exposed and cannulated using a 5.5-french pediatric three-lumen central venous catheter. DSA is performed by retrograde intra-arterial bolus injection of non-ionic Iopamidol. Images of the vertebrobasilar system are obtained using a rapid sequential angiographic technique.

SAH Induction

Following baseline DSA, the rabbit is repositioned from supine to prone with the head fixed in a head holder. The surgical site is clipped, the skin cleaned with a suitable disinfectant, and the rabbit covered with sterile sheets. Three burr holes are drilled in the frontal region of the skull according to outer skull landmarks [13]. The neuromonitoring equipment, including an intraparenchymal ICP tip and two intraparenchymal laser-Doppler flowmetry fine needle probes, is positioned and the burr holes are sealed with a thick plug of bone wax.

A 22G, 40-mm spinal access needle is inserted transcutaneously into the cisterna magna as described below. Correct positioning of the needle is confirmed by spontaneous dripping of cerebrospinal fluid with the head tilted down at 20° for a few minutes. The needle in the cisterna magna is then connected via a pressure tube (including an interposed ultrasound flow probe) to the previously catheterised subclavian artery used for DSA. "Spontaneous SAH" is performed by opening the connection between the subclavian artery and the cistern magna. ICP increases and reaches a plateau at diastolic blood pressure values. "Controlled SAH" can be performed by closing the shunt at any time point (e.g., at the desired level of ICP).

Technical Considerations

Age of the Rabbits

It has been shown that a single blood injection in older rabbits (20–40 months) results in a high mortality rate of 40 %, whereas mortality in younger (2–3 months) and adult (6–9 months) rabbits was 0 % [16]. Additionally, the time course and degree of vasospasm varies depending on the age of the rabbits examined. In young rabbits (2–3 months), arterial calibre has been shown to return almost to baseline values on day 7, whereas older rabbits (20–40 months) showed augmented continuous vasospasm with nearly maximal constriction even on day 7 after SAH [16]. In consideration of this data, we performed our experiments on 3- to 4-month-old animals.

Secure Ligatures of the Subclavian Artery

The subclavian artery is dissected and two ligatures are placed at the proximal and distal end of the exposed artery. After arteriotomy, retrograde cannulation, and catheter fixation, the distal ligature is also placed around the catheter, tied, and secured with a double knot (Fig. 1). This simple manoeuvre is of utmost importance first to prevent twisting or bending of the subclavian artery during repositioning from supine to prone position, and second, to prevent the artery from slipping and causing massive bleeding.

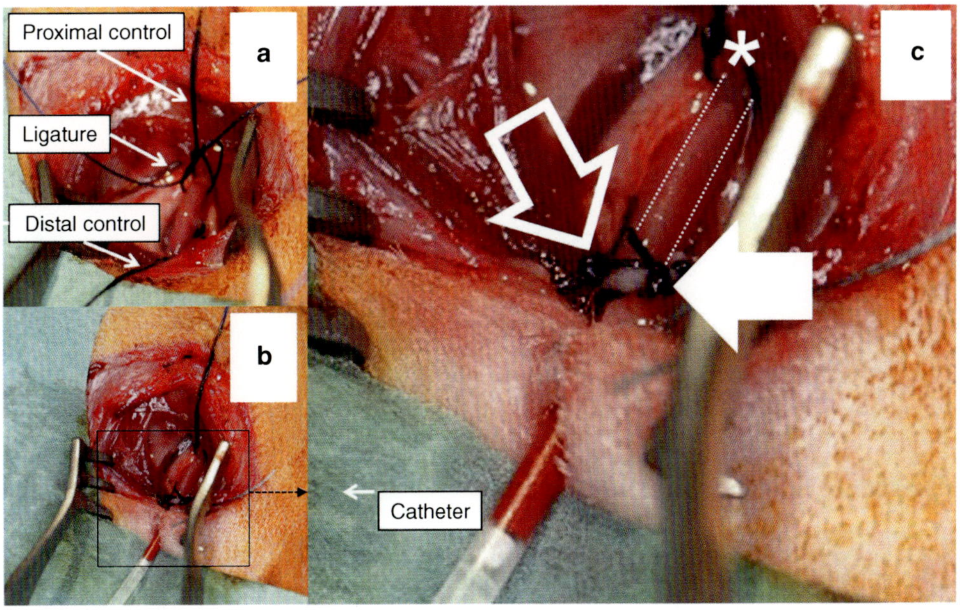

Fig. 1 Secure ligatures of the subclavian artery catheter. (**a**) The subclavian artery is dissected and secured with a proximal and distal ligature. One ligature is kept in place to secure the catheter. (**b**) After arteriotomy and retrograde cannulation, the catheter is fixed. (**c**) The catheter is fixed with one ligature (*hollow arrow*) and additionally secured and kept in placed by fixation to the distal ligature (*solid arrow*). The proximal ligature (*asterix*) is kept in place in case of slippage of the catheter during repositioning

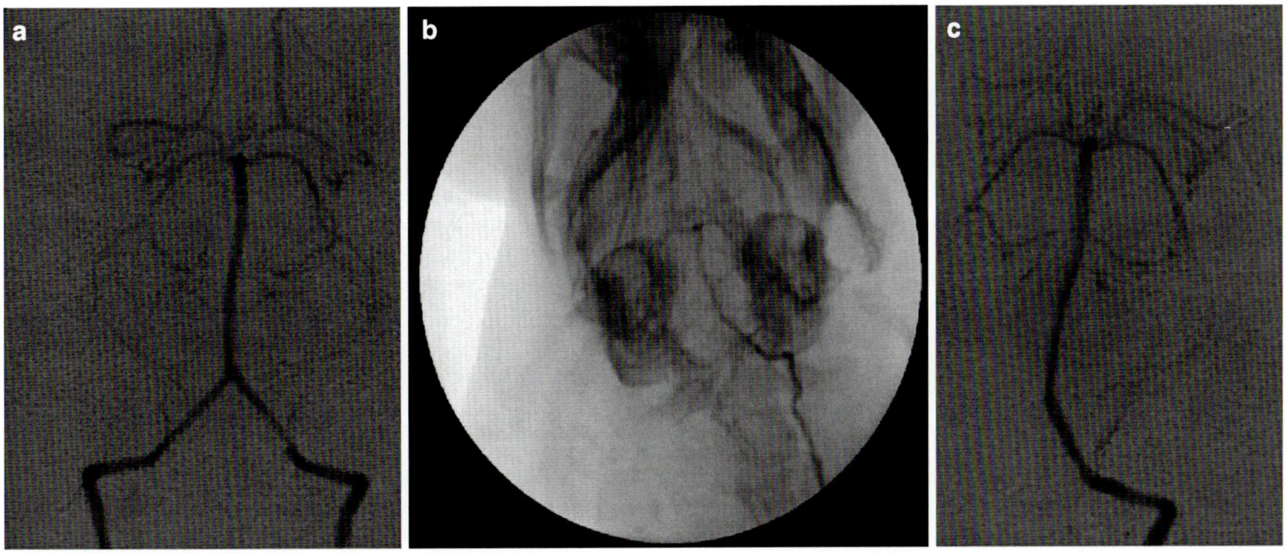

Fig. 2 Non-selective and selective angiography. (**a**) Non-selective angiography through retrograde intra-arterial bolus injection via subclavian artery. (**b**, **c**) Selective angiography through an angiographic catheter inserted into the rabbit's left vertebral artery

Angiography

Angiography can be either performed non-selectively through retrograde intra-arterial bolus injection of non-ionic Iopamidol, or selectively through an angiographic catheter inserted into the rabbit's left vertebral artery (Fig. 2). Each angiogram is calibrated according to an external sizing device (stainless steel skin stapler) placed over both mandible angles at the time of baseline DSA. Measurement of the vessel is performed three times (along a predefined length from the tip of the basilar artery) in a blinded fashion using automatic measurement analysis software, and mean values are determined (Fig. 3). Owing to these measures, we were able to keep intra- and inter-observer variability low.

Thirteen studies addressed the delayed occurrence of vasoconstriction after a single blood injection into the cisterna magna and showed maximal narrowing on day 2–4 [12]. In accordance with this body of literature, we performed follow-up angiography on day 3 after blood shunt-induced SAH on day 0. However, the exact time course using this novel approach remains to be determined by a study of serial DSA.

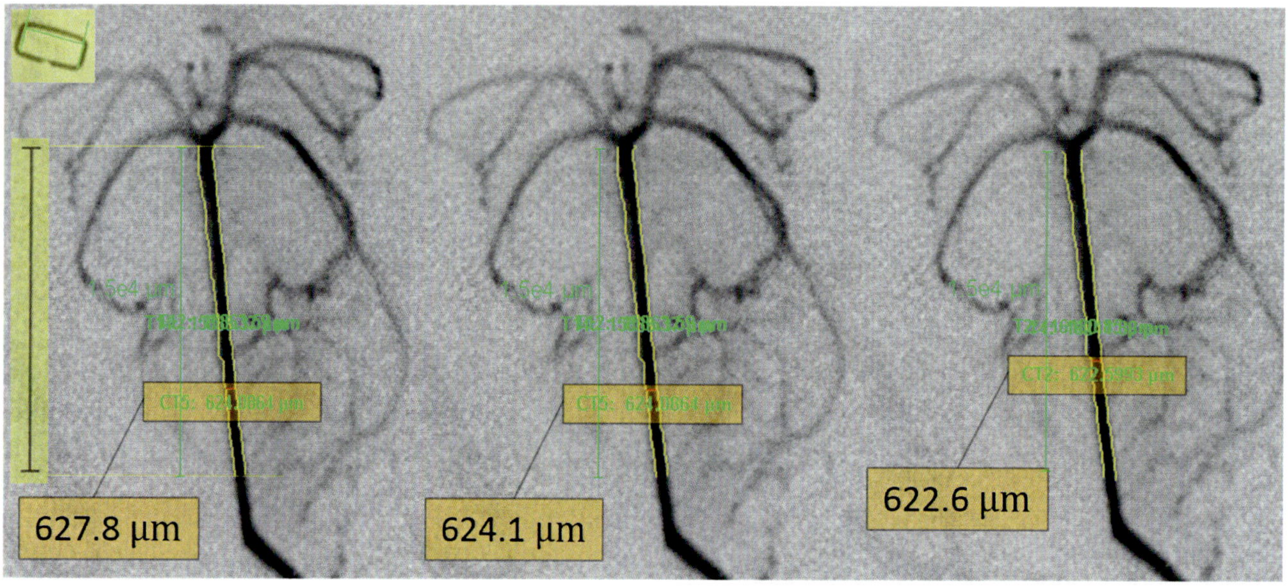

Fig. 3 Calibration and measurement of angiograms. Each angiogram is calibrated according to an external sizing device (skin stapler, *highlighted left upper corner*). The vessel diameter is measured along a predefined length (*highlighted scale on the left*) from the tip of the basilar artery using automatic measurement analysis software. The measurements are performed three times and the mean value is determined

Closed Cranium Condition and Cisterna Magna Puncture

To preserve the closed cranium condition, it is necessary to seal all burr holes with a thick plug of bone wax before SAH induction. After ICP reaches its nadir or intentional termination of the bleeding, the spinal access needle should be kept in place until ICP returns to a steady state close to baseline values. Incorrect positioning of the spinal access needle can result in significant morbidity and mortality. Therefore, one should be extremely careful with this step. After confirmation that the rabbit is fully anaesthetised, the needle can be slid down the down bony external protuberance until a gap is felt. Once having entered the cisterna magna, the needle should not be pushed any further unless spontaneous dripping of cerebrospinal fluid (head tilted down at 20° for at least 1 min) does not occur.

Outcome Measures

Neurological Grading

The four-point neurological grading system reported by Endo et al. [3] is a feasible tool often applied for evaluation of clinical signs after experimental SAH in rabbits. We graded neurological performance at 6, 12, 24, 48, and 72 h after SAH as follows. Grade 1, no neurological deficit; Grade 2, minimal or suspected neurological deficit; Grade 3, mild neurological deficit without abnormal movement; and Grade 4, severe neurological deficit with abnormal movement. Aggravation of neurological deficits was noted on days 1–3 after SAH induction. Previous studies confirmed that this grading system in rabbits correlates well with the onset of DCVS [4, 5]. More recently, other neurological scales developed to assess myelopathy in rabbits and SAH in dogs have been applied as clinical endpoints after single [8] and double [20] cisterna magna blood injection in rabbits.

SAH Bleeding Scale

An ultrasound flow probe mounted on the blood shunt allows quantitative assessment of haemorrhage volume. Although one needs to be aware of the rabbit's ability to rapidly clear subarachnoid blood, the severity of SAH based on the amount of blood can also be roughly estimated by grading the subarachnoid clots at the time of brain harvest [18, 20].

Applicability for Studying Early Brain Injury and Delayed Cerebral Vasospasm

The shunt model was originally developed to mimic pathophysiological mechanisms of acute SAH more closely in a closed cranium, thereby triggering moderate to severe degrees of DCVS [15]. Subsequent larger series using the model demonstrated an average of 30 % basilar artery narrowing on day 3 after SAH (unpublished data). These figures tempered the initial enthusiasm of >50 % of DCVS but are still at the upper end of what can be expected after single cisterna magna blood injection in rabbits [10, 12].

The blood shunt model has been shown to provoke acute hemodynamic disturbances and consistent early damage to the hippocampus, basal cortex, and cerebral vasculature 24 h after procedure [11]. Thus, the model seems to qualify for the study of the pathophysiology of EBI and their sequels after SAH. In light of the assumption that early damage to endothelial cells [1, 21] may trigger, aggravate, and maintain DCVS, the rabbit could play an increasingly important role in research of both the pre-vasospasm and DCVS phase after SAH, especially for the screening of potential preventive DCVS treatment modalities that act early in the pre-vasospasm phase.

Advantages and Limitations

Species-specific advantages of the rabbit model are the relatively low cost of the animal, the non-aggressive behaviour and therefore easy handling, and the fact that DCVS monitoring techniques including DSA [19], computed tomography angiography [7], and transcranial Doppler [17] are more readily applied than in smaller animals. A specific advantage of the shunt model is that the acute pathophysiological changes reflect those events seen during aneurysm rupture. Accordingly, SAH induction causes a rapid increase in ICP with a subsequent drop to almost zero in cerebral perfusion pressure (CPP), along with marked and equal reduction of regional cerebral blood flow in both cerebral hemispheres. The bleeding results in characteristic blood distribution with severe grades of SAH, with pronounced and consistent early ischemic brain and vessel damage on day 1. Furthermore, it provokes moderate to severe DCVS on day 3 after the onset of SAH. The shunt model allows for quantitative assessment of haemorrhage volume and corresponding time course. The model is reproducible, and "spontaneous" SAH induction is performed examiner-independently while simultaneously creating potential varying degrees of "controlled" SAH severity.

On the other hand, general disadvantages include possible sudden death during SAH because of respiratory arrest, and the overall rather limited availability of antibodies and transgenic animal models as compared with other species such as rats and mice. Moreover, the model presented represents a relatively recent technique that requires further evaluation to specify standard parameters and expected outcome. A pressurised saline-filled reservoir interposed in the shunt system would be needed to implement a saline control group. At the minimum, a sham-operation control group is needed to compensate for potential influence of anaesthetics (especially ketamine) on neuronal cells (neuroprotective and neurotoxic effects) and pathophysiology (changes in cerebral metabolic rate, CPP, ICP, systemic blood pressure). Finally, the exact time course of DCVS after blood shunt-induced SAH still needs to be established.

Conclusions

Our preliminary results using the blood shunt rabbit SAH model indicates its feasibility to study both early brain injury and DCVS after SAH. Notably, the technique needs further evaluation to specify standard parameters and expected outcome. Despite the straightforwardness of the model, successful implementation depends largely on technical details.

Acknowledgement This research was supported by the Department of Intensive Care Medicine, Bern University Hospital and University of Bern, Bern, Switzerland, the Department of Clinical Research, and the Research Fund from the Cantonal Hospital Aarau, Aarau, Switzerland.

Conflict of Interest Statement We declare that we have no conflict of interest.

References

1. Chen G, Wu J, Sun C, Qi M, Hang C, Gong Y, Han X, Shi J (2008) Potential role of JAK2 in cerebral vasospasm after experimental subarachnoid hemorrhage. Brain Res 1214:136–144
2. Egemen N, Sanlidilek U, Zorlutuna A, Baskaya M, Bilgic S, Caglar S, Unlu A (1992) Transclival approach to rabbit basilar artery for experimental induction of chronic vasospasm. Acta Neurochir (Wien) 115:123–126
3. Endo S, Branson PJ, Alksne JF (1988) Experimental model of symptomatic vasospasm in rabbits. Stroke 19:1420–1425
4. Hirashima Y, Endo S, Kato R, Takaku A (1996) Prevention of cerebrovasospasm following subarachnoid hemorrhage in rabbits by the platelet-activating factor antagonist, E5880. J Neurosurg 84:826–830
5. Jeon H, Ai J, Sabri M, Tariq A, Shang X, Chen G, Macdonald RL (2009) Neurological and neurobehavioral assessment of experimental subarachnoid hemorrhage. BMC Neurosci 10:103
6. Kikkawa Y, Kameda K, Hirano M, Sasaki T, Hirano K (2010) Impaired feedback regulation of the receptor activity and the myofilament Ca2+ sensitivity contributes to increased vascular reactiveness after subarachnoid hemorrhage. J Cereb Blood Flow Metab 30:1637–1650
7. Laslo AM, Eastwood JD, Chen FX, Lee TY (2006) Dynamic CT perfusion imaging in subarachnoid hemorrhage-related vasospasm. AJNR Am J Neuroradiol 27:624–631
8. Laslo AM, Eastwood JD, Pakkiri P, Chen F, Lee TY (2008) CT perfusion-derived mean transit time predicts early mortality and delayed vasospasm after experimental subarachnoid hemorrhage. AJNR Am J Neuroradiol 29:79–85
9. Logothetis J, Karacostas D, Karoutas G, Artemis N, Mansouri A, Milonas I (1983) A new model of subarachnoid hemorrhage in experimental animals with the purpose to examine cerebral vasospasm. Exp Neurol 81:257–278

10. Macdonald L, Weir B (2001) Cerebral vasospasm. Academic, San Diego
11. Marbacher S, Andereggen L, Neuschmelting V, Widmer HR, von Gunten M, Takala J, Jakob SM, Fandino J (2012) A new rabbit model for the study of early brain injury after subarachnoid hemorrhage. J Neurosci Methods 208:138–145
12. Marbacher S, Fandino J, Kitchen ND (2010) Standard intracranial in vivo animal models of delayed cerebral vasospasm. Br J Neurosurg 24:415–434
13. Marbacher S, Milavec H, Neuschmelting V, Andereggen L, Erhardt S, Fandino J (2011) Outer skull landmark-based coordinates for measurement of cerebral blood flow and intracranial pressure in rabbits. J Neurosci Methods 201:322–326
14. Marbacher S, Neuschmelting V, Graupner T, Jakob SM, Fandino J (2008) Prevention of delayed cerebral vasospasm by continuous intrathecal infusion of glyceroltrinitrate and nimodipine in the rabbit model in vivo. Intensive Care Med 34:932–938
15. Marbacher S, Sherif C, Neuschmelting V, Schlappi JA, Takala J, Jakob SM, Fandino J (2010) Extra-intracranial blood shunt mimicking aneurysm rupture: intracranial- pressure-controlled rabbit subarachnoid hemorrhage model. J Neurosci Methods 191:227–233
16. Nakajima M, Date I, Takahashi K, Ninomiya Y, Asari S, Ohmoto T (2001) Effects of aging on cerebral vasospasm after subarachnoid hemorrhage in rabbits. Stroke 32:620–628
17. Shao Z, Li J, Zhao Z, Gao C, Sun Z, Liu X (2010) Effects of tetramethylpyrazine on nitric oxide/cGMP signaling after cerebral vasospasm in rabbits. Brain Res 1361:67–75
18. Sugawara T, Ayer R, Jadhav V, Zhang JH (2008) A new grading system evaluating bleeding scale in filament perforation subarachnoid hemorrhage rat model. J Neurosci Methods 167:327–334
19. Zhang ZW, Yanamoto H, Nagata I, Miyamoto S, Nakajo Y, Xue JH, Iihara K, Kikuchi H (2010) Platelet-derived growth factor-induced severe and chronic vasoconstriction of cerebral arteries: proposed growth factor explanation of cerebral vasospasm. Neurosurgery 66:728–735; discussion 735
20. Zhou ML, Shi JX, Zhu JQ, Hang CH, Mao L, Chen KF, Yin HX (2007) Comparison between one- and two-hemorrhage models of cerebral vasospasm in rabbits. J Neurosci Methods 159:318–324
21. Zubkov AY, Aoki K, Parent AD, Zhang JH (2002) Preliminary study of the effects of caspase inhibitors on vasospasm in dog penetrating arteries. Life Sci 70:3007–3018

Blood Clot Placement Model of Subarachnoid Hemorrhage in Non-human Primates

Ali Reza Fathi, Kamran D. Bakhtian, Serge Marbacher, Javier Fandino, and Ryszard M. Pluta

Abstract Despite ongoing extensive and promising research to prevent and treat cerebrovascular vasospasm and delayed ischemic neurological deficits (DIND) after aneurysmal subarachnoid hemorrhage (aSAH), clinical outcomes remain unsatisfying. Neuroprotective strategies developed in basic science research laboratories need to be translated from bench-to-bedside using appropriate animal models. While a primate model is widely accepted as the best animal model mimicking development of delayed cerebral vasospasm after aSAH, its worldwide usage has dramatically decreased because of ethical and financial limitations. However, the use of primate models of subarachnoid hemorrhage (SAH) remains a recommended bridge for translation of early preclinical studies in rodents to human clinical trials. This paper discusses the technical aspects as well as advantages and disadvantages of a blood clot placement model of subarachnoid hemorrhage in non-human primates.

Keywords Subarachnoid hemorrhage • Animal model Primates • Blood clot placement

A.R. Fathi, MD (✉) • S. Marbacher, MD, MSc • J. Fandino, MD
Department of Neurosurgery, Kantonsspital Aarau,
Aarau, Switzerland
e-mail: ali-reza.fathi@ksa.ch; serge.marbacher@ksa.ch; javier.fandino@ksa.ch

K.D. Bakhtian, MS • R.M. Pluta, MD, PhD
Surgical Neurology Branch,
National Institute of Neurological Disorders and Stroke,
National Institutes of Health,
Bethesda, MD, USA

Introduction

Delayed ischemic neurological deficits (DIND) and ischemic brain injury following aneurysmal subarachnoid hemorrhage (aSAH) remain the most challenging and frustrating conditions for physicians dealing with patients after the rupture of an intracranial aneurysm [1]. Ongoing research is still of utmost importance because no effective treatment has been developed thus far. The traditional research roadmap to develop new treatment strategies or diagnostic paradigms usually is initiated by results of studies involving in vitro/ex vivo molecular mechanisms and cell-based targets. Then, the first-line in vivo experiments are performed in rodent models. For decades, non-human primate models served as a bridge for the translational clinical applications of innovative scientific findings. Primates have contributed to numerous major steps in medicine beginning from the early 1900s when typing of blood and use of plasma components were initiated. Numerous pharmacological agents and immunology treatments, including therapies for brain disorders, have become gold standards after successful confirmation of their usefulness in primate models. However, recent financial and well-founded ethical issues have raised concerns about the justification of primate experiments, subsequently leading to increasing levels of restriction for the use of these models.

The primate clot-placement model has served as the best available model for research of delayed events after subarachnoid hemorrhage (SAH) in the past decades [2–5]. Despite all of the concerns, it still remains crucial for the development of successful treatments for DIND and vasospasm following aSAH. This paper summarizes the key procedural steps of this model.

J. Fandino et al. (eds.), *Neurovascular Events After Subarachnoid Hemorrhage*, Acta Neurochirurgica Supplement, Vol. 120,
DOI 10.1007/978-3-319-04981-6_59, © Springer International Publishing Switzerland 2015

Animals

Cynomolgus monkeys (Macaca fascicularis) each weighing between 3.5 and 8 kg are used in this model. These animals have a gyrencephalic brain with similar cortical and subcortical anatomy to humans. They also have been used in permanent and transient middle cerebral artery (MCA) occlusion models [6, 7]. Their vascular anatomy very much resembles that of the human aside from a single pericallosal artery and more efficient collateralization than human neurovasculature. The primates rarely develop stroke or neurological deficits in the case of accidental ICA occlusion on one side. However, among the macaques, the neurovascular anatomy of the M. fascicularis has less collateralization than M. mulatta and might be more appropriate in stroke models where ischemic lesions are required [6]. The study goals and outcome parameters must be carefully taken into account when choosing the appropriate primate species. The clear advantage of using a non-human primate is their ability to deliver neurobehavioral information, including a greater series of tasks and neurological assessments for grade of consciousness, motor control, memory, and learning that mimics human testing.

Anesthesia

General anesthesia is induced by the injection of ketamine (10 mg/kg) and xylazine (1 mg/kg) followed by tracheal intubation. Anesthesia is maintained by inhaled isoflurane (0.5–1.0 %). Blood pressure, heart rate, rectal body temperature, and end-tidal CO_2 can be continuously monitored during anesthesia and for the duration of the experiment. Sodium thiopental (25 mg/kg) and cefazolin (500 mg) are injected at the beginning of cranial surgery.

Craniotomy and Clot Placement

This surgical technique has been slightly modified as described elsewhere [1, 3]. All procedures are performed under general anesthesia and aseptic conditions with the skin of the surgical field shaved. The animals are placed in a supine position with the head extended backwards and held in a slightly lateral position with tapes on a foam head holder. After shaving and the standard antiseptic preparation, the skin is incised in a semicircular fashion and the temporal muscle is dissected from the fronto-temporal bone using monopolar cautery. The fronto-temporal craniectomy is performed using high-speed cutting and diamond drills. After opening the dura mater, the Sylvian fissure is opened under the surgical microscope and the arachnoid is dissected from the proximal 14 mm of the right MCA, distal internal carotid artery, and proximal anterior cerebral artery. Autologous blood is collected from the left femoral artery and allowed to clot for approximately 15 min. Five milliliters of clot is placed around the exposed arteries. The dura is closed in a watertight fashion and the wound is closed. Animals are returned to their cages for monitoring of clinical parameters and neurological deficits. For sham controls, the same procedure is performed without placement of the blood clot. Because the pressure of the blood clot itself may cause some cortical damage or arterial irritation, the placement of fibrin glue or an artificial collagen clot without blood cell components might alternatively be considered.

Cerebrospinal Fluid (CSF) Collection

CSF can be collected from the cisterna magna via suboccipital puncture or more preferably from the lumbar spine. Macaques have 12 thoracic vertebrae and 7 lumbar vertebrae with the spinal cord usually ending at the T12 level. Animals are placed in a side position with the hips flexed. After shaving and skin disinfection, an 18- to 22-gauge needle (4–5 cm) with a short bevel is inserted between the spinous processes at a level lower than L2. The same needle can be used for cisterna magna puncture. The external protuberance and C1 process are palpated under aseptic conditions and the head is flexed without obstruction of the airways. The needle is inserted through the atlanto-occipital membrane until sudden loss of resistance and CSF flow occurs. Because of the risk of iatrogenic SAH, the suboccipital puncture could influence results in SAH models and should be carefully considered.

Outcome Measures

Arteriography

For digital subtraction arteriography (DSA), the right femoral artery is exposed and a 3-Fr catheter including guide wire (F3 polyethylene, Cook Group Co.) is introduced into the right carotid artery under fluoroscopic guidance. Next, 1–1.5 mL of contrast agent (Isovue-300, Bracco Diagnostics, Inc.) is injected, and arteriograms are acquired at a rate of eight images per second. For measurement calibration for image analysis, a ruler with a millimeter scale is placed at a standardized position underneath the head of the primate. Three blinded examiners should be available to measure the area of the proximal 14 mm of the right MCA using digital image analysis software (e.g., NIH Image J) three times each, and the mean value can be used for statistical analysis. The percent reduction in the ratio of the area measured on the serial arteriograms is then compared with the ratio computed from the baseline arteriogram, defining the degree of vasospasm by the equation: diameter = area/length.

Other imaging modalities such as computed tomography (CT), magnetic resonance imaging (MRI), and positron emission tomography (PET) can be performed under general anesthesia; although they are of great value at different time points after clot placement, they are not discussed in this paper.

Measurement of invasive and noninvasive physiological parameters during the experimental setup is simplified in large animal models compared with rodent models; nearly all methods used in the clinical setup to monitor humans after SAH can also be applied in primates. Standard parameters include heart rate, blood pressure, respiratory rate, temperature, etc. In addition, arterial and/or venous blood can be collected for blood/plasma parameters.

Invasive as well as noninvasive cerebral blood flow (CBF) analysis is crucial for early and delayed changes after SAH. Examples include intracranial pressure (ICP) monitoring, transcranial Doppler (TCD) and electroencephalogram (EEG) studies.

Neurological, neuropsychological, and neurobehavioral assessments are also critical and can be applied to primate studies in a standardized manner [8]. However, compared with the human grading scales for neurological and neurobehavioral assessment, there is a lack of standardized outcome scales for non-human primates. Neurological assessment includes vigilance, alertness of the animal, focal motor deficits, and repetition of previously trained tasks [9].

Discussion

To date, a sufficient level of evidence has not been achieved to establish a standardized primate model of aSAH that closely mimics the human condition. Moreover, none of the existing models have been able to predict the results of a human trial to the extent of achieving milestone improvements in patient outcome after aSAH. As an example, very promising neuroprotective substances, although effective in rodent models of stroke, were ultimately ineffective in humans [10]. However, primate studies may allow researchers to simulate the human condition more closely in the preclinical setting compared with other animal models [11].

On the other hand, many successful treatments in primates failed in human trials (i.e., Clazosentan). Therefore, anatomic and physiological similarities between the primate and human brain still need to be elucidated and more focused. This is supported by the fact that recent genomic mapping of various primate species reveals far more genetic variability than has been assumed [12]. Rapid proliferation and expansion of available genomic data must undoubtedly be taken into account for future SAH research in non-human primates. Still, alternatives should be discussed and weighed before using primate models.

Another limitation of the clot placement model is the lack of acute ICP increase, which is thought to be a central pathomechanism at the onset of aSAH.

As in the use of any other animal model for preclinical studies in stroke research, maximum consideration is essential to eliminating and minimizing pain, emotional distress, and anxiety, as well as in reducing unnecessary neurological deficits in primates [13]. At the same time, strict institutional regulations are necessary to avoid any disease transmission and pathogen contamination of the animals and human research members alike. As an example, one of the most feared conditions is hepatitis B virus infection [14].

Conclusion

Because of the tremendous financial, ethical, and resource requirements involved with primate experiments, highly elaborate research protocols must be established to minimize the total number of animals. For example, using the same animal for multiple studies under very strict ethical regulations is possible but this approach remains underused. This may be accomplished by starting with nonhazardous behavioral studies or animals that have previously been used in placebo groups for noninvasive pharmacological studies. Powerful statistical concepts and calculations should also use modern and alternative statistical methods such as Bayesian theory and statistics [15].

Conflict of Interest Statement We declare that we have no conflict of interest.

References

1. Weir B, Grace M, Hansen J, Rothberg C (1978) Time course of vasospasm in man. J Neurosurg 48(2):173–178
2. Megyesi JF, Vollrath B, Cook DA, Findlay JM (2000) In vivo animal models of cerebral vasospasm: a review. Neurosurgery 46(2):448–460; discussion 60–61
3. Espinosa F, Weir B, Overton T, Castor W, Grace M, Boisvert D (1984) A randomized placebo-controlled double-blind trial of nimodipine after SAH in monkeys. Part 1: clinical and radiological findings. J Neurosurg 60(6):1167–1175
4. Pluta RM, Dejam A, Grimes G, Gladwin MT, Oldfield EH (2005) Nitrite infusions to prevent delayed cerebral vasospasm in a primate model of subarachnoid hemorrhage. JAMA 293(12): 1477–1484

5. Fathi AR, Pluta RM, Bakhtian KD, Qi M, Lonser RR (2011) Reversal of cerebral vasospasm via intravenous sodium nitrite after subarachnoid hemorrhage in primates. J Neurosurg 115(6):1213–1220. doi:10.3171/2011.7.JNS11390, Epub 2011 Sep 2
6. West GA, Golshani KJ, Doyle KP, Lessov NS, Hobbs TR, Kohama SG et al (2009) A new model of cortical stroke in the rhesus macaque. J Cereb Blood Flow Metab 29(6):1175–1186
7. Qureshi AI, Suri MF, Ali Z, Ringer AJ, Boulos AS, Nakada MT et al (2005) Intraarterial reteplase and intravenous abciximab for treatment of acute ischemic stroke. A preliminary feasibility and safety study in a non-human primate model. Neuroradiology 47(11):845–854
8. Mack WJ, King RG, Hoh DJ, Coon AL, Ducruet AF, Huang J et al (2003) An improved functional neurological examination for use in nonhuman primate studies of focal reperfused cerebral ischemia. Neurol Res 25(3):280–284
9. Pluta RM, Skopets B, Kralik JD (2013) Relevance of animal models of subarachnoid hemorrhage for examining neurobehavioral changes. Acta Neurochir Suppl 115:225–232
10. O'Collins VE, Macleod MR, Donnan GA, Horky LL, van der Worp BH, Howells DW (2006) 1,026 experimental treatments in acute stroke. Ann Neurol 59(3):467–477
11. Cook DJ, Tymianski M (2012) Nonhuman primate models of stroke for translational neuroprotection research. Neurotherapeutics 9(2):371–379
12. Vallender EJ, Miller GM (2013) Nonhuman primate models in the genomic era: a paradigm shift. ILAR J 54(2):154–165
13. Rossi J (2009) Nonhuman primate research: the wrong way to understand needs and necessity. Am J Bioeth 9(5):21–23
14. Sa-Nguanmoo P, Rianthavorn P, Amornsawadwattana S, Poovorawan Y (2009) Hepatitis B virus infection in non-human primates. Acta Virol 53(2):73–82
15. Estey E (2009) Do commonly used clinical trial designs reflect clinical reality? Haematologica 94(10):1435–1439

Canine Double Hemorrhage Model of Experimental Subarachnoid Hemorrhage

Kentaro Mori, Kazuya Fujii, Satosi Tomura, Hideaki Ueno, Kojiro Wada, Naoki Otani, Hideo Osada, and Arata Tomiyama

Abstract Several animal subarachnoid hemorrhage (SAH) models have been proposed for the investigation of cerebral vasospasm. We describe the experimental procedures of a canine double-SAH model and also examine the model based on the canine physiological parameters and occurrence of angiographic delayed cerebral vasospasm using magnetic resonance (MR) imaging and digital subtraction angiography. Autologous blood was injected twice on days 1 and 3 in 36 beagles. All animals showed delayed angiographic vasospasm in the vertebrobasilar arteries on day 7. The degree of vasospasm was 29–42 % of the arterial caliber. MR imaging did not show any ischemic change. This animal model can produce definite delayed vasospasm without detectable cerebral infarction on MR imaging. The canine SAH model is suitable for the quantitative and chronological study of delayed angiographic vasospasm, but not for investigating early brain injury and delayed cerebral ischemia.

Keywords Subarachnoid hemorrhage • Cerebral vasospasm • Canine double-hemorrhage model

Introduction

Delayed ischemic neurological deficits caused by cerebral vasospasm are still a major cause of death and morbidity after subarachnoid hemorrhage (SAH). The pathogenesis of cerebral vasospasm is not completely understood and no definite treatment has been established. Therefore, appropriate animal models of SAH are required to investigate the pathogenesis and to develop new treatments. Various types of experimental SAH models using the mouse, rat, rabbit, cat, dog, and monkey have been advocated. We previously used a canine double-hemorrhage model of experimental SAH to develop the new treatment modality of vasospasm [4, 5]. In this study, we primarily describe how to perform the canine double-hemorrhage model to obtain stable angiographic vasospasm. We also discuss the merits and demerits of this canine model for the study of vasospasm.

Materials and Methods

Canine SAH Model and Experimental Protocols

All animal experiments were performed in accordance with the Institutional Guidelines and the Roles of Animal Experimentation, and the Guide for the Care and Use of Laboratory Animals of Juntendo University, Shizuoka Hospital. Thirty-six female beagle dogs weighing 9–11 kg were used. Cerebral vasospasm was induced by experimental SAH using the two-hemorrhage canine model [6].

The dogs were anesthetized using an intravenous bolus injection of 20 mg/kg of pentobarbital on day 1. The anesthesia was maintained by continuous intravenous infusion of 1 ml/kg/h propofol. Muscular relaxation was achieved by intravenous injection of 1 ml of vecuronium bromide, which was repeated every 30 min until the end of the procedure. The dogs were intubated using a 6-F tracheal cannula and respiration was controlled with a magnetic resonance (MR)-compatible mobile respirator (ParaPAC® Ventilator, Smiths Medical). A 4-F double-lumen sheath catheter was placed in the femoral artery for cerebral angiography, blood pressure monitoring, and arterial gas sampling. Partial pressure of

K. Mori, MD, PhD (✉) • K. Fujii • S. Tomura • H. Ueno
K. Wada • N. Otani • H. Osada • A. Tomiyama
Department of Neurosurgery, National Defense Medical College, 3-2 Namiki, Tokorozawa, Saitama 359-8513, Japan
e-mail: kmori@ndmc.ac.jp

DOI 10.1007/978-3-319-04981-6_60,

CO_2 was maintained between 35 and 45 mmHg. T2-weighted and diffusion-weighted MR imaging were performed using a 1.5-T Gyroscan (Philips). MR perfusion images were also obtained in several animals. At 1.5 h after the induction of anesthesia, the left vertebral artery was cannulated with a 4-F catheter under fluoroscopic control, and digital subtraction angiography was performed after injection of 3 ml of iopamidol (Bayer) using an automatic injector (2 ml/s). The diameters of the basilar artery (BA), vertebral artery (VA), and superior cerebellar artery (SCA) were quantitatively measured. After the control baseline images of the VA and BA were obtained, the cisterna magna was punctured using a 20-gauge needle, 0.3 ml/kg cerebrospinal fluid was drained by gravity flow, and 0.5 ml/kg autologous arterial blood was injected into the cerebellomedullary cistern (first SAH). During the cisterna magna puncture, the dog's neck was flexed to widen the cranio-cervical junction. After the blood injection, the dog's head was tilted downward at 30° for 15 min to permit pooling and clotting of the blood around the BA. The animals were then allowed to recover from the anesthesia. The second SAH was performed on day 3 using similar procedures as on Day 1.

The dogs were anesthetized and a tracheal cannula was intubated on day 7, as on day 1. A 4-F double-lumen sheath was also placed in the femoral artery. MR imaging was performed to assess any pathological changes, including ischemic change on T2-weighted and diffusion-weighted MR imaging. The Evans index was also calculated from the MR images on days 1 and 7. At 1.5 h after the induction of anesthesia, left vertebral angiography was performed to assess the morphological changes of the VA and BA after experimental SAH. Immediately after the angiography, the cisterna magna was punctured with a 20-gauge needle, 0.3 ml/kg of cerebrospinal fluid was collected, and 0.5 ml/kg of various concentrations (0–15 mmol/l) of magnesium sulfate ($MgSO_4$) solution in Ringer's solution was injected into the cerebellomedullary cistern. The dog's head was tilted downward at 30° for 15 min. At 1–1.5 h after $MgSO_4$ injection, left vertebral angiography was repeated to assess the changes after the intracisternal injection of $MgSO_4$ solution. The dogs were then killed by intravenous injection of overdoses of pentobarbital, and their brains were removed and immersed in 10 % formalin. The fixed brain containing the BA was sliced coronally and then stained with hematoxylin and eosin for histological examination of the spastic BA.

Statistical Analysis

The data are presented as means ± standard deviations. Statistical significance of differences was analyzed using the paired *t*-test with SPSS statistical software for Windows (version 7.5.1 J, SPSS Japan Inc.) Probability values <0.01 were considered statistically significant.

Table 1 Summary of physiological parameters, MR imaging findings, and diameters of the cerebral arteries before (Day 1) and after SAH (Day 7)

	Day 1 (pre-SAH)	Day 7 (post-SAH)	*P* value
Physiological parameters			
Body weight (kg)	10.3 ± 0.6	9.5 ± 0.6	<0.01
Mean blood pressure (mmHg)	123 ± 18	101 ± 13	<0.01
Heart rate (beats/min)	133 ± 30	92 ± 26	<0.01
Body temperature (°C)	38.3 ± 0.5	38.3 ± 0.4	NS
Hemoglobin (g/dl)	12.7 ± 1.1	11.4 ± 1.1	< 0.01
Hematocrit (%)	38 ± 3	34 ± 3	< 0.01
pH	7.36 ± 0.03	7.37 ± 0.02	NS
$PaCO_2$ (mmHg)	40 ± 3	40 ± 3	NS
PaO_2 (mmHg)	395 ± 34	422 ± 33	NS
MR imaging findings			
Cerebral infarct	none	none	
Evans index (%)	20.1 ± 1.4	22.8 ± 2.7	<0.01
Diameter (mm) and [% decrease]			
BA	1.04 ± 0.15	0.60 ± 0.14 [42 ± 12]	<0.01
VA	0.97 ± 0.19	0.69 ± 0.18 [29 ± 16]	<0.01
SCA	0.82 ± 0.16	0.49 ± 0.12 [39 ± 19]	<0.01

Data are presented as means ± standard deviations
NS not significant

Results

Table 1 list the mean physiological parameters, MR imaging findings, and diameters of the cerebral arteries on day 1 and day 7 before $MgSO_4$ intracisternal injection. The dogs showed appetite loss and their body weights had significantly decreased. The mean blood pressure, hemoglobin concentration, and hematocrit percentage on day 7 were significantly decreased. Blood gas levels had not changed. All dogs had hydrocephalus on day 7 (Fig. 1 upper), and the mean Evans index had significantly increased from 20.1 ± 1.4 % on day 1 to 22.8 ± 2.7 % on day 7. The MR perfusion images obtained on day 7 showed decreased cerebral blood flow (Fig.1 lower, data not shown). MR imaging showed no other changes including cerebral infarction caused by vasospasm. All dogs had angiographic vasospasm in the VA and BA (Fig. 2b). All cerebral arteries showed significant decreases in diameter after SAH on day 7. The percentage decreases were 42 ± 12,

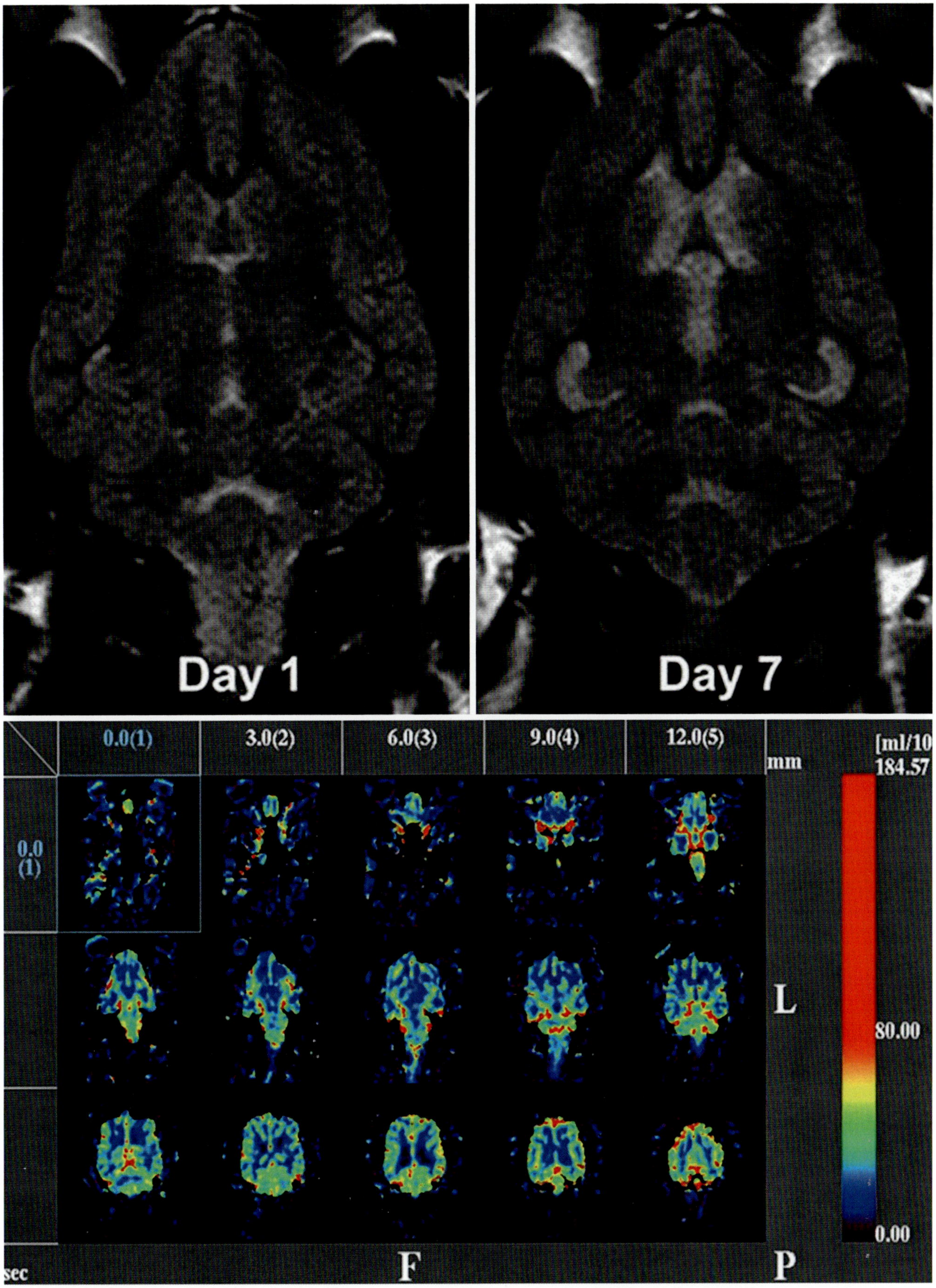

Fig. 1 MR images and MR perfusion images of a canine model of SAH. *Upper*: T2-weighted MR images obtained on day 1 (pre-SAH) and day 7 (post-SAH) showing the development of hydrocephalus. *Lower*: MR perfusion images on day 7 showing decreased cerebral blood flow

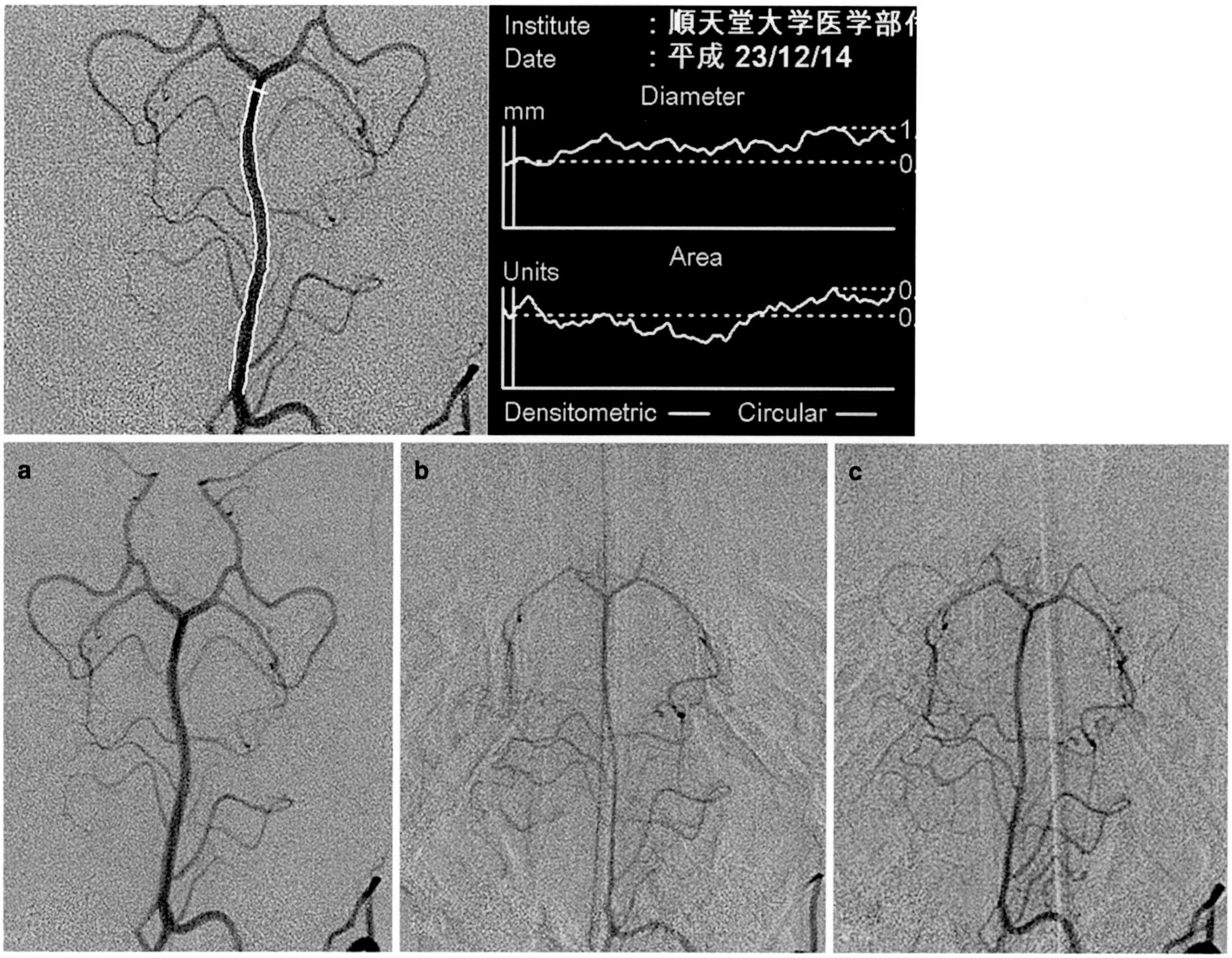

Fig. 2 Representative angiograms obtained on day 1 (**a**) and before (**b**) and after (**c**) infusion of intracisternal $MgSO_4$ solution on day 7 in a canine model of SAH. Note the severe angiographic delayed vasospasm and the reversal effect of $MgSO_4$ treatment on the spastic arteries

29 ± 16, and 39 ± 19 % in the BA, VA, and SCA, respectively. Intracisternal injection of $MgSO_4$ solution of more than 5 mmol/l dilated the spastic arteries (Fig. 2c, data not shown). Postmortem examination showed the SAH clot was located mainly in the prepontine cistern around the VA and BA (Fig. 3a). Histological examination of the BA showed prominent folding and corrugation of the intima and internal elastic lamina. The adventitia showed edematous changes with infiltration of inflammatory cells (Fig. 3b).

Discussion

The canine SAH model was originally established using a single injection of blood into the cisterna magna. The single injection model shows biphasic vasoconstriction at 30 min and on the second day after injection but does not cause enough delayed vasospasm [2]. Because the canine double-injection model provides adequate delayed angiographic vasospasm [6], the double-injection method has become the standard method. In the present study, we showed that the canine double-SAH model can produce 100 % angiographic delayed vasospasm with 29–42 % constriction. The dog is large enough to measure the arterial diameter quantitatively using digital subtraction angiography, as in the clinical setting, and this model can provide the temporal profile of arterial diameter change after the treatment in the same animal using serial angiography [4, 5]. The histological findings of the canine spastic artery are similar to those in humans. However, this model does not show any ischemic change on MR imaging, which implies that the canine SAH model is not suitable for the study of delayed cerebral infarction.

Delayed cerebral vasospasm is not the only cause of delayed ischemic neurological deficits after SAH. Future treatments for delayed cerebral ischemia after SAH should aim to not only ameliorate vasospasm but also prevent underlying possible causes such as early brain injury caused by initial cerebral

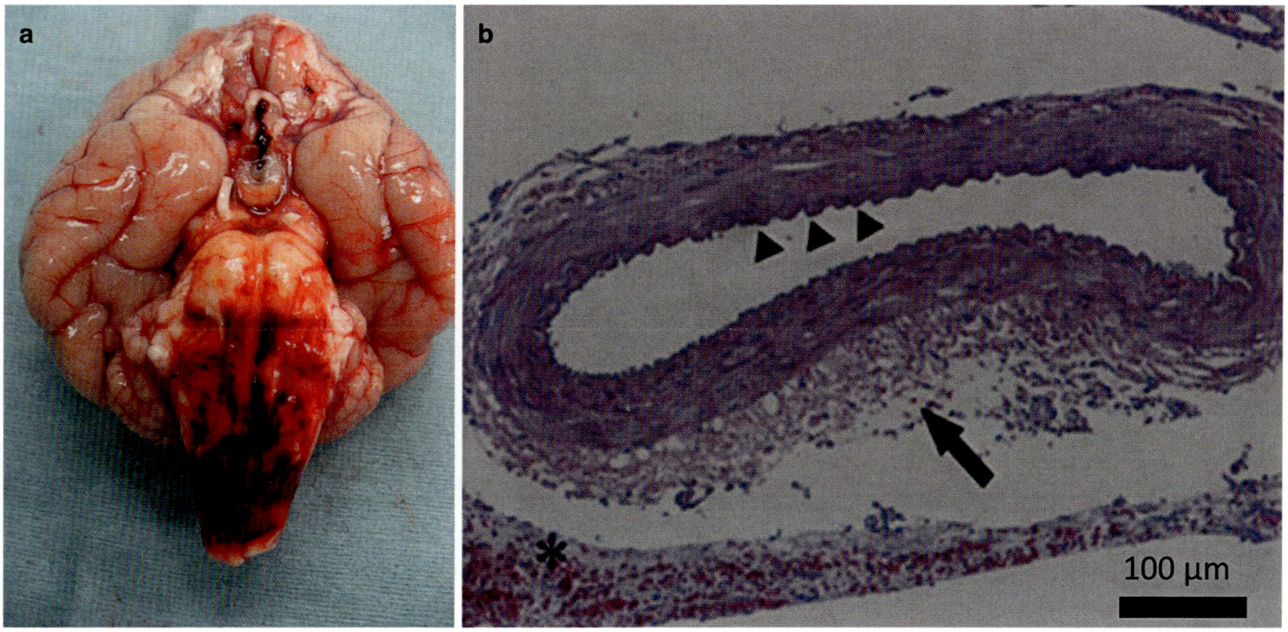

Fig. 3 Postmortem findings of brain (**a**) and photomicrograph (**b**) of a transverse section of the spastic BA in a canine model of SAH. The SAH clot is mainly located in the prepontine cistern (*asterisk*). The intima and internal elastic lamina show folding and corrugation (*arrow head*). The adventitia shows edematous change with infiltration of inflammatory cells (*arrow*)

global ischemic insult, cortical spreading ischemia, changes in nitric oxide production, and others [1]. The endovascular perforation rat model produces a rapid increase in intracranial pressure associated with decreased cerebral perfusion pressure similar to human SAH caused by ruptured cerebral aneurysm. Therefore, the endovascular perforation model is more suitable for the study of acute SAH sequelae such as early brain injury than cisterna magna injection models [3].

Conclusion

Canine double-SAH model can produce definite delayed angiographic vasospasm without detectable cerebral infarction on MR imaging. This model is suitable for the quantitative and chronological study of delayed angiographic vasospasm, but not for investigating delayed cerebral ischemia.

Conflict of Interest Statement The authors have no personal financial or institutional interest in any of the drugs, materials, or devices described in this article.

References

1. Fujii M, Yan J, Rolland WB, Soejima Y, Caner B, Zhang JH (2013) Early brain injury, an evolving frontier in subarachnoid hemorrhage research. Transl Stroke Res 4:432–446
2. Kuwayama A, Zervas NT, Belson R, Shintani A, Pickren K (1972) A model for experimental cerebral arterial spasm. Stroke 3:49–56
3. Mori K, Miyazaki M, Hara Y, Aiko Y, Yamamoto T, Nakao Y (2009) Novel vasodilatory effect of intracisternal injection of magnesium sulfate solution on spastic cerebral arteries in the canine two-hemorrhage model of subarachnoid hemorrhage. J Neurosurg 110:73–78
4. Mori K, Yamamoto T, Miyazaki M, Hara Y, Aiko Y, Koike N, Sakamoto S, Nakao Y, Esaki T (2011) Optimal cerebrospinal fluid magnesium ion concentration for vasodilatory effect and duration after intracisternal injection of magnesium sulfate solution in a canine subarachnoid hemorrhage model. J Neurosurg 114:1168–1175
5. Lee JY, Sagher O, Keep R, Hua Y, Xi G (2009) Comparison of experimental rat models of early brain injury after subarachnoid hemorrhage. Neurosurgery 65:331–343
6. Varsos VG, Liszcrak TM, Han DH, Kistler JP, Vielma J, Black PM, Heros RC, Zervas NT (1983) Delayed cerebral vasospasm is not reversible by aminophylline, nifedipine, or papaverine in a 'two-hemorrhage' canine model. J Neurosurg 58:11–17

Author Index

J. Fandino et al. (eds.), *Neurovascular Events After Subarachnoid Hemorrhage*, Acta Neurochirurgica Supplement, Vol. 120,
DOI 10.1007/978-3-319-04981-6, © Springer International Publishing Switzerland 2015

C

D

N

O

P

Q

R

S

T

U

V

Subject Index

D

T